Resistance to Targeted Anti-Cancer Therapeutics

Series Editor

Benjamin Bonavida, Los Angeles, CA, USA

More information about this series at http://www.springer.com/series/11727

Q. Ping Dou
Editor

Resistance to Proteasome Inhibitors in Cancer

Molecular Mechanisms and Strategies to Overcome Resistance

Springer

Editor
Q. Ping Dou
Wayne State University
Detroit, MI, USA

ISSN 2196-5501 ISSN 2196-551X (electronic)
ISBN 978-3-319-06751-3 ISBN 978-3-319-06752-0 (eBook)
DOI 10.1007/978-3-319-06752-0
Springer Cham Heidelberg New York Dordrecht London

Library of Congress Control Number: 2014947541

Printed on acid-free paper

Springer is part of Springer Science+Business Media (www.springer.com)

This book is dedicated to my loving family—my wife, Anna; my daughter, Eva; and my son, Dan.

Preface

A balance of protein synthesis and degradation is tightly regulated in our bodies in order to keep us healthy. Most intracellular proteins are degraded via the ubiquitin-proteasome pathway (UPP), and dysfunction of the UPP has been linked to the occurrence of many human diseases, including cancers. The clinical introduction of the first US Food and Drug Administration (FDA)-approved proteasome inhibitor bortezomib for the treatment of multiple myeloma (MM) and mantle cell lymphoma is an example of using the UPP as an anticancer target which has been met with success. Now, bortezomib-based therapies have become a staple for the MM treatment, contributing to a two- to threefold increase in the survival rate of the MM patients.

However, not all patients respond to bortezomib treatment and relapse occurs in many patients who initially responded. Also, bortezomib-based therapies had minimal effects in treating most of hematologic malignancies and almost all of the solid tumors. Furthermore, some neurotoxicities (such as peripheral neuropathy) were found to be associated with bortezomib treatment. Therefore, bortezomib resistance (both intrinsic and acquired) is a critical barrier to progress in bortezomib therapy for MM and other cancers.

This book, *Resistance to Proteasome Inhibitors in Cancer: Molecular mechanisms and strategies to overcome resistance*, focuses on the mechanisms of action and resistance of the proteasome inhibitor bortezomib in human cancers (including MM, mantle cell lymphoma, acute leukemia, and various solid tumors) and on cutting-edge strategies to overcome bortezomib clinical resistance. The second-generation 20S proteasome inhibitors carfilzomib, ixazomib, delanzomib, oprozomib, and marizomib, with different pharmacological properties and broader anticancer activities, have shown great promise in this respect; carfilzomib, the second FDA-approved proteasome inhibitor drug, induces responses in a minority of MM patients relapsed from or refractory to bortezomib. The potential reversal strategies for bortezomib resistance also include developing novel combinational therapies and identifying new targets in the UPP, such as ubiquitin E3 ligases, deubiquitinases, 26S proteasomal ATPases, histone deacetylases, oxidative stress and proteotoxic stress pathways, and pharmacogenomic signature profiling in resistant cancer cells. While bortezomib resistance could be reversed by several aforementioned strategies in several preclinical models, the confirmation under clinical settings is needed. There are high hopes in the field that the discovery of the mechanisms of proteasome inhibitor resistance will help illuminate the future of cancer treatment.

Due to the timely nature and keen interest in the subject matter of this book, it is my wish that this book will serve as an important resource for physicians, clinician scientists, translational researchers, basic researchers, graduate and medical students, patients, consumers, and pharmaceutical companies.

I would like to thank the authors, who are among the top leaders in their areas of research, for their exceptional contributions. This volume represents one in a new book series entitled *Resistance of Targeted Anti-Cancer Therapeutics* of which Professor Benjamin Bonavida of the University of California, Los Angeles, serves as the Series Editor (published by Springer Publishing Company). I wish to thank Professor Bonavida for his encouragement. I am also indebted to Ms. Fiona Sarne, the Editor of Cancer Research for Springer Science+Business Media, for her great effort and assistance.

Detroit, MI, USA Q. Ping Dou, Ph.D.

Contents

About the Editor

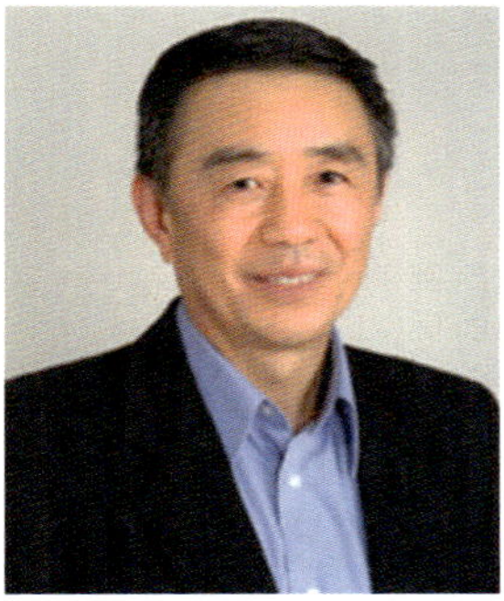

Dr. Q. Ping Dou obtained his B.S. degree in chemistry from Shandong University, People's Republic of China in 1981, Ph.D. degree in chemistry from Rutgers University in 1988, and postdoctoral training at the Dana-Farber Cancer Institute and Harvard Medical School from 1988 to 1993. He is currently a Professor of Oncology, Pharmacology, and Pathology at Barbara Ann Karmanos Cancer Institute, Wayne State University School of Medicine. Dr. Dou's research interests include targeted therapies, drug discovery, and chemoprevention. His laboratory is one of the first to provide preclinical evidence for the proteasome as a potential anticancer target. Dr. Dou's laboratory has also shown that certain tea polyphenols, curcumin, medicinal compounds, and metal complexes potently and specifically inhibit the tumor proteasome activity in vitro and in vivo. Dr. Dou is currently collaborating with physician scientists to translate some of the preclinical findings to clinical trials.

Chapter 1
Proteasome Inhibitors and Lessons Learned from Their Mechanisms of Action and Resistance in Human Cancer

Sara M. Schmitt, Rahul R. Deshmukh, and Q. Ping Dou

Abstract Selective protein degradation by the ubiquitin–proteasome pathway (UPP) is critical to cellular homeostasis, and dysregulation of the UPP has been associated with human diseases including cancer. Proteasome inhibition as a strategy for cancer treatment was validated by the US Food and Drug Administration approval of the proteasome inhibitor bortezomib for the treatment of multiple myeloma in 2003. After 10 years of success, bortezomib and its combinational therapies have become a staple for treating relapsed/refractory multiple myeloma. Unfortunately, bortezomib has several limitations, including, most notably, the emergence of resistance. To overcome bortezomib resistance, several approaches have been taken, including the development of novel second-generation proteasome inhibitors, application of rationalized bortezomib-based combinational therapies, and targeting sites outside the proteasomal core as well as factors involved in resistance mechanisms. Further understanding the mechanisms of resistance to proteasome inhibitors in human cancers will significantly improve current proteasome inhibitor therapies and patient care.

S.M. Schmitt
Barbara Ann Karmanos Cancer Institute and Department of Oncology, Wayne State University School of Medicine, 4100 John R St. HWCRC 516, Detroit, MI 48201, USA
e-mail: schmitts@karmanos.org

R.R. Deshmukh
Barbara Ann Karmanos Cancer Institute and Department of Pathology, Wayne State University School of Medicine, 4100 John R St. HWCRC 516, Detroit, MI 48201, USA
e-mail: deshmukr@karmanos.org

Q.P. Dou (✉)
Barbara Ann Karmanos Cancer Institute and Department of Oncology, Wayne State University School of Medicine, 4100 John R St. HWCRC 516, Detroit, MI 48201, USA

Barbara Ann Karmanos Cancer Institute and Department of Pathology, Wayne State University School of Medicine, 4100 John R St. HWCRC 516, Detroit, MI 48201, USA

Barbara Ann Karmanos Cancer Institute and Department of Pharmacology, Wayne State University School of Medicine, 4100 John R St. HWCRC 516, Detroit, MI 48201, USA
e-mail: doup@karmanos.org

Q.P. Dou (ed.), *Resistance to Proteasome Inhibitors in Cancer*, Resistance to Targeted Anti-Cancer Therapeutics, DOI 10.1007/978-3-319-06752-0_1

Keywords Ubiquitin–proteasome pathway • Cancer • Bortezomib • Carfilzomib • Resistance • Metals • Natural compounds

Abbreviations

BMSC	Bone marrow stromal cell
CQ	Clioquinol
CT	Chymotrypsin
DSF	Disulfiram
DUB	Deubiquitinating enzyme
(-)-EGCG	(-)-Epigallocatechin-3-gallate
ER	Endoplasmic reticulum
FDA	Food and Drug Administration
HDAC	Histone deacetylase
HSP	Heat shock protein
IGF-1	Insulin-like growth factor 1
IL-6	Interleukin-6
IPSI	Immunoproteasome-specific inhibitor
MAPK	Mitogen-activated protein kinase
MHC	Major histocompatibility complex
NSCLC	Non-small cell lung cancer
PBMC	Peripheral blood mononuclear cell
PGPH	Peptidyl-glutamyl peptide-hydrolyzing
RIP-1	Regulatory particle inhibitor peptoid-1
ROS	Reactive oxygen species
SAR	Structure–activity relationship
TNF-α	Tumor necrosis factor-α
UIM	Ubiquitin-interacting motif
UPP	Ubiquitin–proteasome pathway

1.1 Introduction

The ubiquitin–proteasome pathway (UPP) has gained considerable attention as a potential target for cancer therapeutics, owing to its extreme importance to normal cellular function and dysregulation in malignant cells. In fact, critical proteasomal target proteins are involved in processes important for carcinogenesis, including cell cycle progression, proliferation, and differentiation. The past decade has witnessed the emergence of proteasome inhibition as an effective therapeutic strategy for treating multiple myeloma. Bortezomib was the first proteasome inhibitor approved by the US Food and Drug Administration (FDA) in 2003, and the use of bortezomib and bortezomib-based combinational therapies has become a staple for the treatment of relapsed/refractory multiple myeloma. Unfortunately, further success of bortezomib has been hampered by tumor resistance (both intrinsic and acquired), severe toxicities, and low efficacy in solid tumors. To overcome these limitations, especially resistance, scientists have investigated the molecular mechanisms involved and developed novel strategies to improve proteasome inhibitor-based therapies and patient care. By improving chemical and biochemical properties, binding affinity and reversibility, potency and selectivity, several second-generation proteasome inhibitors have been developed, among them carfilzomib, which is more specific and less toxic than bortezomib, and has become the second FDA-approved proteasome inhibitor for multiple myeloma treatment. Other cutting-edge strategies to overcome bortezomib resistance include selectively targeting immunoproteasomes or sites outside the catalytic core (such as 19S deubiquitinases or ubiquitin E3 ligases) and developing novel combinational therapies. Definitively elucidating the mechanisms responsible for proteasome inhibitor resistance is key in designing new compounds to fully overcome this resistance.

1.2 Ubiquitin–Proteasome Pathway

The UPP is the major pathway responsible for regulating protein turnover in cells. The UPP is so critical to normal cellular function that its discoverers, Aaron Ciechanover and Avram Hershko, were awarded the 2004 Nobel Prize in Chemistry [1, 2]. Proteins degraded by the UPP are involved in many biological processes, including development, differentiation, proliferation, signal transduction, and apoptosis [3]. In addition to its critical role in protein homeostasis, the proteasome also functions in several non-proteolytic processes, such as transcription initiation and elongation [4], regulation of gene expression [5], and transcription-coupled nucleotide excision repair [6].

Protein degradation is carried out via two distinct steps: (1) conjugation of multiple ubiquitin molecules to the protein substrate and (2) degradation of the ubiquitin-tagged substrate by the 26S proteasome (Fig. 1.1) [7]. The 26S proteasome is a large (2.5 MDa), multi-subunit complex that is localized both in the cytosol and nucleus of cells [8–10]. The 26S proteasome is made up of the catalytic 20S core and one or two 19S regulatory caps (Fig. 1.2) [11, 12]. The 20S core is comprised of 28 subunits that form a barrel-like structure of four alternately stacked rings: two α-rings surrounding two β-rings, each with seven subunits [13–15]. The role of the α-subunits is to allow only unfolded proteins to enter the 20S core, while the β-subunits are responsible for the proteolytic activities of the proteasome, which are dependent on an amino-terminal nucleophilic Thr1 residue [15]: caspase or peptidyl-glutamyl peptide-hydrolyzing (PGPH)-like activity, carried out by β1, trypsin-like by β2 and chymotrypsin (CT)-like by β5 (Fig. 1.2) [15–17]. The 19S regulatory caps (700 kDa) can be divided into a base and a lid (Fig. 1.2); the base is responsible for the recognition and unfolding of ubiquitinated protein substrates, as well as

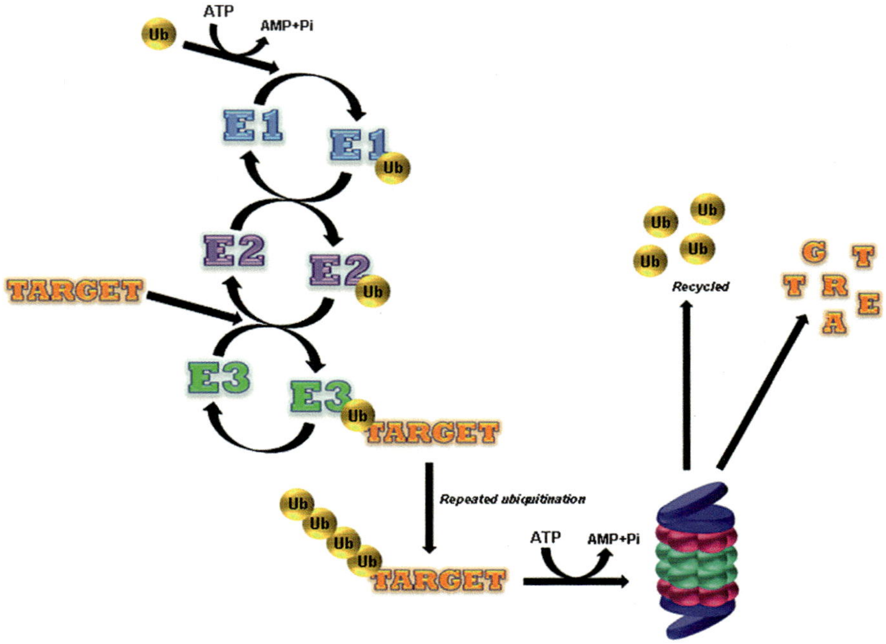

Fig. 1.1 The ubiquitin–proteasome pathway. There are two steps in the UPP: ubiquitination and target degradation. The ubiquitination step is carried out by three distinct types of enzymes, E1 (ubiquitin activating), E2s (ubiquitin conjugating), and E3s (ubiquitin ligating). First, ubiquitin is activated by E1, the activated ubiquitin is transferred to an E2 for conjugation, and finally, an E3 ubiquitin-ligating enzyme aids in the transfer of active ubiquitin to lysine residues within the target protein. The target protein is then recognized, deubiquitinated, and translocated to the 26S proteasome by components of the 19S regulatory cap, followed by degradation into small peptide fragments, and the ubiquitin molecules are recycled

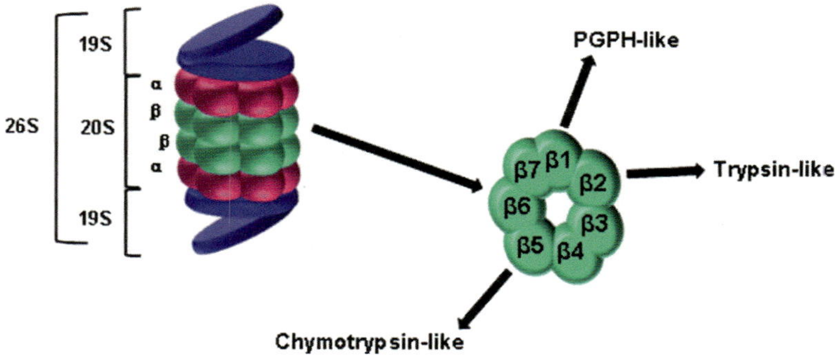

Fig. 1.2 Proteasome structure. The 26S constitutive proteasome is comprised of a 20S catalytic core and one or two 19S regulatory caps. The 20S core contains four stacked rings—two α-rings surrounding two β-rings, each consisting of seven subunits. The catalytic activity is carried out by three β-subunits: β1, β2, and β5 responsible for caspase or peptidyl-glutamyl peptide-hydrolyzing (PGPH)-like, trypsin-like, and chymotrypsin (CT)-like, respectively

opening the 20S pore and transport of protein substrates into the core, while the major responsibility of the lid component is deubiquitination of substrates before degradation. The base contains six ATPase subunits, Rpt1–6, which form a hexameric ring [18–20], as well as two non-ATPase subunits Rpn-1 and Rpn-2 [21, 22], and the lid consists of at least six non-ATPases, including Rpn-10/S5a and Rpn-13/Adrm1, which contain ubiquitin-interacting motifs (UIMs) [23]. Rpn-10/S5a has two UIMs that preferentially binds poly-ubiquitinated substrates [24], and Rpn-13/Adrm1 binds to the non-ATPase Rpn-2 to recruit deubiquitinating enzymes (DUBs) to the proteasome [25–27]. Deubiquitination is very highly regulated and is important for recycling ubiquitin molecules and controlling the rate of ubiquitin-dependent proteasomal degradation [27].

The ubiquitination step of the UPP is carried out by three distinct types of enzymes, E1 (ubiquitin activating), E2s (ubiquitin conjugating), and E3s (ubiquitin ligating). The first step in the pathway is ATP-dependent E1-mediated activation of ubiquitin, a small 76-amino-acid protein that is expressed ubiquitously and serves as a tag for protein substrates destined for various fates, including membrane trafficking, protein kinase activation, DNA repair and chromatin remodeling, as well as degradation by the UPP (Fig. 1.1) [28]. Activated ubiquitin is then transferred from E1 to an E2 enzyme, a group of enzymes responsible for ubiquitin conjugation, and then to an E3 ubiquitin-ligating enzyme, which aids in the transfer of active ubiquitin to lysine residues within the target protein (Fig. 1.1) [29, 30]. Following the conjugation of a sufficiently sized ubiquitin chain, which is four in most cases, except in rare cases such as mODC and HIF-1α, which require no ubiquitination for proteasomal degradation [31–33], the protein substrate is recognized, deubiquitinated, and translocated to the 26S proteasome by components of the 19S regulatory cap [34, 35]. Finally, the substrate is degraded into small peptide fragments and the ubiquitin molecules are recycled (Fig. 1.1) [36]. This process is tightly controlled and extremely crucial in the regulation of many cellular processes, including those involved in tumorigenesis [37], which makes it a promising target for anticancer therapeutic agents.

Because the UPP plays such a crucial role in normal cellular function, it is no surprise that it has also been implicated in the development, growth, and survival of various malignancies [38]. Thus, targeting factors involved in the synthesis and degradation of proteins, including the UPP, has been explored as a potential anticancer strategy [39]. Several studies have reported increased proteasome activity in various cancers, including colon, prostate, and leukemia [40–42], indicating that cancer cells may be more dependent on the UPP than normal cells and that targeting this pathway in the treatment of human cancer is a promising strategy. Specifically, inhibition of chymotrypsin (CT)-like activity has been associated with cell cycle arrest and apoptosis [43, 44], indicating that proteasome inhibition may effectively cause selective cell death in cancer cells, as well as sensitizing them to chemotherapeutics [45], with little toxicity in normal cells. Importantly, the use of proteasome inhibitors was validated by the US Food and Drug Administration (FDA) approval of bortezomib for the treatment of relapsed and refractory multiple myeloma and mantle cell lymphoma.

1.3 Proteasome Inhibitors

1.3.1 Early Inhibitors

Prior to the development and approval of bortezomib, numerous preclinical studies were carried out to validate the UPP as a valid druggable target. The most widely investigated early inhibitors include the peptide aldehydes, which are analogs of proteasome substrates that inhibit the CT-like activity of the proteasome and include MG-132 (Cbz-leu-leu-leucinal), MG-115 (Cbz-leu-leu-norvalinal), and ALLN (acetyl-leu-leu-norleucinal) [46, 47]. Importantly, in-depth studies using these complexes aided in elucidating the active site for compounds in this class, X-ray diffraction revealed that ALLN forms a hemiacetal complex with the N-terminal threonine hydroxyl groups of the catalytic β-subunits [14, 48]. Another peptide aldehyde inhibitor, PSI (Cbz-ile-glu(O-t-Bu)-alaleucinal), has been shown to suppress 26S proteasome-mediated proteolysis without affecting isopeptidase or ATPase activities [49]. These inhibitors are extremely potent (MG-132 K_i = low nanomolar in purified proteasome; IC_{50} = low micromolar in cultured cells) and their inhibitory activities are reversible by their removal from the system [46, 47]. Interestingly, because peptide aldehydes are also able to inhibit calpains and some lysosomal cysteine proteases, certain degradative processes that were originally believed to be carried out by calpains were shown to actually be proteasomal processes.

Vinyl sulfone peptides have also been reported to be potent inhibitors of the proteasome in cell models [50]. These peptides exert their proteasome-inhibitory activity through covalent binding to the hydroxyl groups of the active site threonine within the β-subunits, and their use in human lymphoma cells resulted in proteasome inhibition followed by the appearance of distinct cell variants expressing a compensatory proteolytic system, which has not been clearly identified [51].

Other early inhibitors of the proteasome include lactacystin and its derivative *clasto*-lactacystin β-lactone, the active form to which it is converted in aqueous solution [52]. These are naturally occurring products that differ structurally from the peptide aldehydes and are much more specific. Lactacystin was first isolated from actinomycetes because of its ability to promote neurite outgrowth and block cell division in cultured neurons [53]. These compounds have a mode of action similar to that of the vinyl sulfones [54, 55].

Other naturally occurring metabolites that have been used in the preclinical setting as inhibitors of the proteasome include TMC-95A and argyrin A. TMC-95A is a cyclic tripeptide that was isolated from *Apiospora montagnei*. TMC-95A specifically binds via hydrogen bonds to all three catalytic β-subunits and causes inhibition in the low nanomolar range [56, 57]. The tumor growth suppression caused by argyrin A, a cyclic octapeptide derived from *Archangium gephyra*, has been attributed to the inhibition of proteasomal degradation of $p27^{kip1}$ CDK inhibitor [58, 59]. Following the identification of these inhibitors, many other compounds were identified and designed to specifically target the tumor proteasome, ultimately resulting in the USFDA approval of bortezomib in 2003.

1.3.2 *Bortezomib, the First Clinically Approved Proteasome Inhibitor in Preclinical Studies*

Bortezomib (Velcade®) is a dipeptide boronic acid derivative that was first synthesized in 1995 by Myogenics Company and contains pyrazinoic acid, phenylalanine, and leucine in its structure. Bortezomib showed considerable apoptosis-inducing activity in a variety of tumor cell lines and animal models [60–62], and in 2003, seven years after its initial synthesis, bortezomib was approved by the USFDA for the treatment of relapsed multiple myeloma, and in 2006, it was approved for the treatment of mantle cell lymphoma. Bortezomib is able to enter nearly all tissues except brain and adipose, and is able to distribute to the plasma within 10 min of IV injection [63–66]. Furthermore, bortezomib is metabolized through intracellular cytochrome p450-mediated oxidative deboronation [67] and its half-life is more than 40 h [65].

Bortezomib is a reversible inhibitor of the 26S proteasome, with proteasome activity generally recovering within 72 h of administration [68]. Binding of the boronic acid group in bortezomib to the threonine hydroxyl group in the active site of the β5 subunit results in proteasome inhibition and, ultimately, cell death [69]. Bortezomib has been successful in hematological malignancies, but less than encouraging results have been observed in solid tumors [70, 71], limiting its use in the clinic.

Several preclinical studies demonstrated the potency of bortezomib against human tumor cells in vitro and in in vivo xenograft animal models. A standard NCI-60 screen revealed that bortezomib could potently inhibit cell proliferation [60] and induce apoptosis in many malignant cell lines, including multiple myeloma, prostate, pancreatic, renal and squamous cell carcinomas [72–77]. Importantly, the antitumor activity of bortezomib was observed in both chemoresistant and chemosensitive myeloma cells, and the sensitivity of resistant cells to chemotherapy was increased significantly when combined with a sublethal dose of bortezomib with no effect on normal hematopoietic cells [78, 79]. Additionally, in an in vitro study of four ovarian and three prostate cancer cell lines, bortezomib had comparable effects on cells derived from solid tumors and hematological malignancies [61]. Bortezomib was also able to potently inhibit the growth of multiple myeloma xenografts in mice [80].

Multiple targets of bortezomib have been identified in malignant cells, including the NF-κB signaling pathway. NF-κB is a p50/p65 heterodimer that usually exists in an inactive form in the cytoplasm bound to its inhibitory protein, IκB, and upon degradation of IκB, the NF-κB complex is activated and can translocate into the nucleus where it stimulates transcription of various genes including cytokines (IL-6, TNF-α), survival factors (IAPs, Bcl-X_L), and insulin-like growth factor 1 (IGF-1), ultimately resulting in proliferation, resistance to apoptosis, and drug resistance in cancer cells [81]. Bortezomib is able to prevent degradation of IκB, blocking activation of NF-κB and suppressing expression of related cytokines and survival factors in drug-resistant multiple myeloma cells expressing increased NF-κB activity [78, 82]. In contrast, other studies have shown that the NF-κB pathway may not be important in bortezomib-mediated tumor cell death. Specifically, in a study of mice bearing human multiple myeloma cells, treatment with bortezomib was associated with NF-κB activation, rather than inhibition [83].

Another possible target of bortezomib is NOXA (Latin for damage) [84], a pro-apoptotic member of the Bcl-2 family [85] that is involved in p53-mediated apoptosis, gene expression of which is associated with direct activation of its promoter by p53 [85]. Thus, upregulation of p53 and subsequent *Noxa* gene expression may be one mechanism of chemo- or radiotherapy-induced apoptosis. Studies have shown that NOXA upregulation induces apoptosis through interaction with, and inhibition of anti-apoptotic Bcl-xL and Bcl-2 proteins, or through stimulation of other pro-apoptotic factors [86, 87]. Importantly, bortezomib treatment in myeloma and melanoma cell lines resulted in p53-independent induction of NOXA and blockade of NOXA with an antisense oligonucleotide caused only 30 % to 50 % reduction in bortezomib-induced apoptosis [84]. Bortezomib induces NOXA in various p53-defective tumor cell lines [88], and clinical studies indicate that bortezomib suppresses tumor growth in a p53-independent manner [11, 89]. Importantly, NOXA induction by bortezomib is selective to cancer cells over normal cells, with levels unaffected in normal melanocytes [84, 90, 91].

Still other mechanisms of bortezomib-mediated apoptosis include inhibition of angiogenesis in human myeloma, pancreatic and squamous cell cancer xenografts [77, 92]; induction of endoplasmic reticulum (ER) stress and generation of reactive oxygen species (ROS) [93, 94]; induction of extrinsic and intrinsic apoptotic pathways via activation of caspase-8 and caspase-9 [95, 96]; activation of the p38 mitogen-activated protein kinase (MAPK) pathway [97]; and disruption of the interaction between tumor cells and dendritic cells [98]. Multiple targets generally play important roles in bortezomib-mediated apoptosis in some cancer cells, while different targets may be critical in other cells.

1.3.3 Bortezomib in Clinical Trials

1.3.3.1 Phase I/II Trials

The promising preclinical data involving bortezomib resulted in a series of clinical trials that ultimately led to the USFDA approval of bortezomib as a treatment for multiple myeloma. One phase I trial of 27 patients with relapsed multiple myeloma investigated bortezomib as a single agent, and found that bortezomib induced a dose-dependent inhibition of 20S proteasome activity [99], confirming preclinical findings that bortezomib could inhibit proteasome activity in a dose- and time-dependent manner. Two other phase I studies evaluated bortezomib in combination with doxorubicin. In the first, 42 patients with advanced hematologic malignancies were enrolled to obtain preliminary response data and to determine the maximum tolerated dose (1.30 mg/m^2) and dose-limiting toxicities (fatigue, thrombocytopenia, lymphopenia, nausea, constipation, peripheral neuropathy, and anemia) [100]. The other enrolled 22 patients with multiple myeloma, with eight patients achieving complete response (36 %) or near-complete response, and another eight partial responses (36 %) [100].

Additional phase I trials have investigated the effects of bortezomib either alone or in combination in solid tumors. Single-agent bortezomib showed antitumor activity in patients with advanced androgen-independent prostate cancer [101], but no significant responses were observed in patients with advanced metastatic breast cancer or neuroendocrine tumors [102, 103]. In combination with carboplatin, an overall response rate of 47 % was observed in recurrent ovarian or primary peritoneal cancer patients, but in combination with either docetaxel [104] or prednisone [105], hormone refractory and castrate-resistant metastatic prostate cancer patients achieved no significant responses. Therefore, while bortezomib has shown promise in hematological malignancies, it has proven quite ineffective against solid tumors.

The general success of phase I trials led to several phase II trials. In the SUMMIT (Study of Uncontrolled Multiple Myeloma Managed with Proteasome Inhibition Therapy) trial, 202 patients with relapsed or refractory myeloma with prior treatment were treated with 1.3 mg/m^2 bortezomib on days 1, 4, 8, and 11 of a 3-week cycle for as many as eight cycles, and an overall response rate of 35 % was observed [106]. In the CREST (Clinical Response and Efficacy Study of Bortezomib in the Treatment of Relapsing Multiple Myeloma) trial, 67 patients with relapsed/refractory multiple myeloma were randomly divided to receive either 1.0 or 1.3 mg/m^2 of bortezomib. The study ultimately showed that bortezomib was effective in relapsed multiple myeloma patients at a lower dose of 1.0 mg/m^2 [107].

Two other phase II trials examined bortezomib in combination with other agents. One study reported a 95 % response rate in relapsed multiple myeloma patients treated with a combination of bortezomib, dexamethasone, and doxorubicin [108]. Another study in patients with symptomatic multiple myeloma with no prior treatment compared single-agent bortezomib to bortezomib in combination with dexamethasone. Of the 32 patients, 22 were treated with the combination, and an increased response was seen in 15 of 22 patients (68 %) [45].

Additionally, the effects of bortezomib against mantle cell lymphoma and non-Hodgkin's lymphoma have also been investigated in clinical trials. A trial of patients with indolent non-Hodgkin's lymphoma and mantle cell lymphoma showed a 58 % overall response rate as a result of bortezomib treatment [109]. Another study conducted in patients with pretreated and untreated mantle cell lymphoma revealed response rates of 46.2 % and 46.7 %, respectively, following treatment with 1.3 mg/m^2 bortezomib, suggesting that bortezomib is an effective treatment for mantle cell lymphoma [110]. Finally, no significant response or survival advantage was observed in another phase II study evaluating the use of bortezomib and pemetrexed alone or in combination in advanced NSCLC with prior treatment, but bortezomib was better tolerated when given in combination with pemetrexed [111]. More clinical trials are being conducted to further explore the use of bortezomib in NSCLC. Unfortunately, phase II trials investigating the efficacy of bortezomib in solid tumors have yielded disappointing results.

1.3.3.2 Phase III Clinical Trials

Based on phase II trial results, a large international phase III trial in relapsed multiple myeloma patients with 1–3 prior therapies compared the effects of bortezomib to high-dose dexamethasone [75]. Patients ($n=669$) received either 1.3 mg/m^2 bortezomib (twice weekly for 2 weeks followed by a 1-week rest, intravenously) or high-dose dexamethasone (40 mg orally). Patients receiving bortezomib had a combined complete and partial response rate of 38 % compared to 18 % for the dexamethasone-treated patients, with median times to progression of 6.22 months in the bortezomib group versus 3.29 months in the dexamethasone group. Among patients taking bortezomib, the median time to progression was 6.22 months and 1-year survival rate was 80 %, while that for patients taking dexamethasone was 3.29 months and 66 % [75], demonstrating the advantage of bortezomib over dexamethasone in terms of response rate, time to progression, and survival.

Another study included 638 relapsed/refractory multiple myeloma patients who received 1.3 mg/m^2 bortezomib and achieved an overall response rate of 67 % [112]. After completion of at least two cycles for progressive and four cycles for stable disease, 20 mg/day dexamethasone was added on the day of and after each bortezomib dose. Of the patients receiving dexamethasone, enhanced response was observed in 34 %, suggesting that bortezomib, alone or in combination with dexamethasone, is both safe and effective for the treatment of relapsed/refractory multiple myeloma in patients with prior treatment [112]. The APEX (Assessment of Proteasome Inhibition for Extending Remissions) trial assessed the impact of dose modification on the severity and reversibility of peripheral neuropathy associated with bortezomib treatment in patients with relapsed multiple myeloma [113]. Peripheral neuropathy could be improved by dose modification without adverse effects on the outcome in 37 % of patients (124/331) following several cycles of bortezomib treatment [113], indicating that bortezomib-induced peripheral neuropathy is not only manageable, but also reversible in most relapsed myeloma patients.

The efficacy of bortezomib in combination with conventional chemotherapeutics was conducted at 151 centers in 22 countries. Patients with untreated multiple myeloma ($n=682$) were randomized to receive either a combination of bortezomib plus melphalan–prednisone or melphalan–prednisone alone [114]. Results revealed that bortezomib plus melphalan–prednisone may be a valuable frontline treatment option for myeloma patients [114]. Most recently, in the VISTA trial, bortezomib plus melphalan and prednisone was compared to melphalan and prednisone alone in multiple myeloma patients with no previous treatment. A prolonged follow-up (median = 36.7 months) indicated that bortezomib-based drugs as first-line treatments afford greater survival advantage than treatment with conventional drugs followed by salvage with bortezomib-based treatments [115]. Additionally, initial treatment with bortezomib, compared to initial treatment with traditional chemotherapeutics, resulted in less resistance to later therapies [115]. Overall, preclinical and clinical data evaluating the efficacy and safety of bortezomib have shown that the use of proteasome inhibitors as anticancer agents is a promising strategy that should be further investigated.

However, while bortezomib is successful in the clinic, toxicities and resistance have been reported, suggesting that further development of drugs like bortezomib is necessary. In fact, some second-generation proteasome inhibitors [116, 117] with different properties have been developed, with one, carfilzomib, being FDA approved. Additionally, inhibitors that specifically target the immunoproteasome (immunoproteasome-specific inhibitors, IPSIs) [117], as well as natural compounds that are able to inhibit the proteasome, may be sufficiently potent with significantly less adverse effects than currently approved drugs [118]. The use of these novel inhibitors may aid in overcoming bortezomib resistance or sensitizing resistant cells to bortezomib treatment, which could potentially result in increased clinical success.

1.3.4 *The Second Clinically Approved Proteasome Inhibitor, Carfilzomib*

Following the clinical success of bortezomib, the second-in-class proteasome inhibitor carfilzomib (Kyprolis®) was granted accelerated approval by the USFDA in July 2012 for the treatment of patients with MM progressing on or after treatment with bortezomib and an immunomodulatory agent. Carfilzomib is a peptide epoxyketone related to epoxomicin [119] that irreversibly inhibits the CT-like activity of the proteasome with high selectivity [120]. Preclinical studies revealed that carfilzomib inhibits CT-like activity in both the constitutive proteasome and the inducible immunoproteasome with IC_{50} values of 6 and 33 nM, respectively [121]. Carfilzomib was also extremely effective at suppressing tumor growth in cultured cell and tumor xenograft models, with prolonged proteasome inhibition for longer than one week in mice [121]. Importantly, carfilzomib was active against bortezomib-resistant cultured myeloma and patient plasma cells [119].

1.3.4.1 Phase I/II Trials

The data observed in cultured cell and xenograft models led to a series of clinical trials investigating the properties and efficacy of carfilzomib. In one phase I study, carfilzomib was administered on consecutive days twice weekly in patients with relapsed and refractory multiple myeloma or lymphoma. One hour following IV administration of 27 mg/m^2 carfilzomib, CT-like activity in whole blood and peripheral blood mononuclear cells (PBMCs) was inhibited by approximately 85 % and 90 % on average, respectively, and this inhibition was sustained throughout the trial [122]. Another small phase I dose-escalation study evaluated the safety and efficacy of carfilzomib in relapsed or refractory myeloma and lymphoma, with patients ($n = 29$) receiving carfilzomib for five consecutive days within 14-day cycles [123]. One unconfirmed complete response, one partial response, and two minimal responses were observed with observable antitumor activity at or above 11 mg/m^2 and a maximum tolerated dose of 15 mg/m^2. Grade 1–2 toxicities included nausea, diarrhea, and fatigue in more than one-third of patients. At the highest dose administered (20 mg/m^2), grade 3 febrile neutropenia and grade 4 thrombocytopenia were reported, and no grade 3 or 4 peripheral neuropathies were reported [123]. An additional phase I/II study investigated the tolerability, efficacy, and pharmacokinetic and pharmacodynamic profiles of carfilzomib in advanced solid tumors [124]. Carfilzomib was administered IV twice weekly on consecutive days within 28-day cycles. A small group of patients ($n=14$) received carfilzomib during the phase I dose escalation, and the single dose-limiting toxicity was determined to be grade 3 fatigue at the highest administered dose (36 mg/m^2). The maximum planned dose was determined based on the phase I cohort, and 65 additional patients then received carfilzomib at the maximum planned dose in a phase II study. The most common side effects were fatigue, nausea, anorexia, and dyspnea. No hepatotoxicity or ≥grade 2 peripheral neuropathy was reported. The half-life was determined to be <1 h, and one hour post treatment on day one of cycle two, proteasome CT-like activity in whole blood and PBMCs was inhibited by ≥80 %. Importantly, partial responses were reported in two patients (14 %) in the phase I study, with 21.5 % stable disease after four cycles in evaluable patients ($n=51$) in the phase II cohort [124].

Another phase I/II trial included patients with newly diagnosed multiple myeloma ($n=53$) and evaluated the efficacy and tolerability of the CRd combination treatment (carfilzomib + lenalidomide + dexamethasone) [125]. Carfilzomib was administered at 20, 27, or 36 mg/m^2 twice weekly on consecutive days, lenalidomide was given at a dose of 25 mg/day daily for the first 21 days, and weekly dexamethasone was given at 40 mg during cycles 1–4 and 20 mg during any additional cycles. The maximum planned dose (carfilzomib 36 mg/m^2) was expanded in the phase II study. Toxicities (grade 3–4) included anemia, thrombocytopenia, and neutropenia, hypophosphatemia, and hyperglycemia; no grade 3–4 peripheral neuropathy was observed and dose modification was not required in a majority of patients. A near-complete response was reported in 62 %, and complete response occurred in 42 % of patients ($n=53$) after an average of 12 cycles. After a median follow-up of 13 months, the 24-month progression-free survival estimate was 92 % [125]. Thus, the combination of carfilzomib, lenalidomide, and dexamethasone is highly effective and well tolerated in treatment-naïve multiple myeloma patients.

Finally, a single-arm multicenter phase II was completed in relapsed/refractory multiple myeloma patients ($n=46$) with at least two prior therapies [126]. Patients were given 20 mg/m^2 carfilzomib IV on consecutive days twice weekly every 28 days for up to 12 cycles. The overall response and clinical benefit response rates were 16.7 % and 23.8 %, respectively, in the 42 evaluable patients, with seven partial responses. Median durations of response were 7.2 months and 13.8 months, respectively. Anemia, fatigue, and thrombocytopenia were the most common treatment-related adverse effects, and events of neuropathy were rare [126]. The promising results of this pilot study resulted in an amendment to test a higher dose in additional patients (PX-171-003-A1). During the PX-171-003-A1 study [127], patients ($n=266$) received single-agent carfilzomib 20 mg/m^2 IV twice weekly for 3 of 4 weeks in cycle one, followed by 27 mg/m^2 for the remaining cycles (maximum = 12). The overall response rate (at least partial response) was 23.7 % with median duration of response of 7.8 months and median overall survival of 15.6 months. Manageable toxicities included anemia, nausea, fatigue, and thrombocytopenia, with grade 1–2 peripheral neuropathy in 12.4 % of evaluable patients [127]. Patients in this study had an average of five prior treatments, but the responses observed in this trial were quite durable and indicated that carfilzomib may be clinically beneficial in patients who fail on other chemotherapeutics, and based on this study, carfilzomib was approved by the FDA in July 2012 for relapsed and refractory multiple myeloma and mantle cell lymphoma.

1.3.4.2 Phase III Trials

Based on the promising phase I/II results, a randomized phase III study, FOCUS (Carfilzomib for Advanced Refractory Multiple Myeloma European Study), is being conducted to compare overall survival following single-agent carfilzomib treatment with best supportive care treatments in relapsed and refractory multiple myeloma patients who have received at least three previous treatments [128]. Enrolled patients ($n \approx 300$) have responded to at least one prior therapy and are refractory to their most recent therapy. Patients were randomized to receive either IV carfilzomib, 20 mg/m^2 on days 1–2 of cycle one, escalating to 27 mg/m^2 on days 8, 9, 15, and 16 for the remaining cycles (up to 16), or an active BSC regimen consisting of corticosteroid treatment of prednisolone 30 mg, dexamethasone 6 mg, or equivalent every other day with optional oral cyclophosphamide 50 mg once daily. Treatment will continue until disease progression or unacceptable adverse events occur. The primary endpoint will be overall survival with secondary endpoints of progression-free survival, overall response rate, and safety [128]. Enrollment has been completed and the study has begun with anticipated completion in 2015 [NCT01302392; Onyx Therapeutics, Inc.].

Another randomized phase III, open-label, multicenter study is comparing CRd (carfilzomib + lenalidomide + dexamethasone) and Rd (lenalidomide + dexamethasone) regimens in patients with relapsed multiple myeloma [NCT01080391; Onyx Therapeutics, Inc.]. Approximately 750 patients have been randomized to receive either Rd (40 mg oral dexamethasone on days 1, 8, 15, and 22 + 25 mg oral lenalidomide on days 1–21 in 28-day cycles) or CRd (20 mg/m^2 or 27 mg/m^2 IV carfilzomib + 40 mg oral dexamethasone on days 1, 8, 15, and 22 + 25 mg oral lenalidomide on days 1–21 in 28-day cycles; carfilzomib will be discontinued after completion of 18 cycles). Progression-free survival is the primary endpoint of this study, and overall survival, overall response rate, response duration, disease control, safety, time to progression, and quality of life are secondary endpoints. Severity and incidence of adverse effects will also be compared between the two treatment regimens. This study is expected to be completed in early 2014 [NCT01080391; Onyx Therapeutics, Inc.].

1.4 Resistance to Proteasome Inhibitors

Unfortunately, although clinical success has been achieved with proteasome inhibitors, resistance has emerged as a limiting factor in their continued clinical use. Resistance to proteasome inhibitors, as well as other drugs, can be either inherent or acquired. Inherent resistance is resistance which exists within cells without any exposure to a drug. This type of resistance is fairly uncommon in cancer, but has been reported in regard to antibiotics. Acquired resistance occurs following exposure to a drug, generally by genetic mutations and overexpression of target proteins. The exact mechanisms by which cells become resistant to proteasome inhibitors have yet to be fully elucidated, but several studies have explored potential mechanisms (Fig. 1.3).

1.4.1 Inherent Resistance

In a study of relapsed/refractory acute leukemia patients who had progressed on prior treatments, bortezomib treatment resulted in minimal responses [129], suggesting the potential for inherent resistance to proteasome inhibitors due to prior treatments. The ECOG E2A02 trial conducted with newly diagnosed high-risk

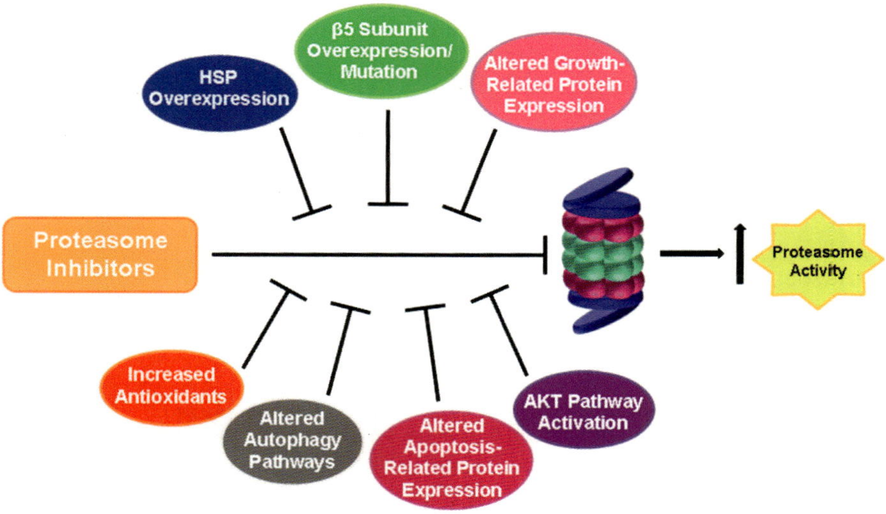

Fig. 1.3 Potential mechanisms of proteasome inhibitor resistance. Several factors have been implicated in resistance to proteasome inhibitors. These include overexpression or mutation of β5 subunits, overexpression of heat shock proteins (HSPs), AKT pathway activation, altered expression of apoptosis- and growth-related proteins, altered autophagy pathways, and increased antioxidants

multiple myeloma patients showed no clinical response following single-agent bortezomib treatment [130]. Bortezomib also failed to show clinical benefit in several other hematological and solid tumors [129]. The lack of benefit from bortezomib as an initial treatment suggests that some tumors may simply be inherently resistant to treatment with proteasome inhibitors.

1.4.2 Acquired Resistance

While little is known about inherent resistance to proteasome inhibitors like bortezomib, a number of cell-based studies have elucidated putative mechanisms of acquired resistance either at the proteasome level or its downstream effectors. These include overexpression or mutation of the proteasomal β5 subunit, upregulation of heat shock proteins (HSPs), altered expression of apoptosis-related proteins, AKT pathway activation, overexpression of other growth-related proteins, altered autophagy pathways, and increased antioxidant levels (Fig. 1.3).

1.4.2.1 β5 Subunit Overexpression/Mutation

When human monocytic/macrophage THP1 cells were treated with increasing concentrations of bortezomib, up to 60-fold overexpression of proteasomal β5 subunit (PSMB5) protein was observed. Additionally, the overexpressed β5 contained an alanine–threonine mutation at position 49 in the highly conserved bortezomib-binding pocket [131]. Together the overexpression and mutation resulted in resistance to bortezomib as well as cross-resistance to β5-targeted cytotoxic peptides 4A6, MG132, MG262, and ALLN [131]. Interestingly, there were no marked changes in the baseline CT-like activity, and when the *PSMB5* gene was silenced by siRNA, its sensitivity to bortezomib was restored [131]. A different set of mutations in the *PSMB5* protein at positions 49 and 50, including Ala49Val, Ala49Thr, and Ala50Val, as well as the Ala49Thr mutation, were reported in T lymphoblastic lymphoma/leukemia cells developed from the Jurkat cell line when treated with increasing concentrations of bortezomib [132]. Similarly, human leukemia K562 cells have been shown to be more resistant to bortezomib compared to other leukemia and myeloma cell lines due to inherent overexpression of proteasomal β5. However, there is no direct evidence that these phenomena, i.e., mutations or β5 overexpression, are responsible for bortezomib resistance in vivo [133]. In fact, a multiple myeloma patient who rapidly developed resistance to bortezomib (evident by sudden and accelerated disease progression and death) had no mutations in the *PSMB5* coding region, indicating that there may not be a correlation between bortezomib resistance and β5 mutation [134]. Further in-depth, large-scale studies are warranted to determine the role of β5 mutations and overexpression in in vivo resistance to proteasome inhibitors.

1.4.2.2 Upregulation of HSPs

The heat shock proteins are important in mediating resistance to apoptosis [135, 136], and many HSPs, especially HSP-72, are upregulated following proteasome inhibition. Several studies have reported dramatic HSP-72 upregulation resulting from treatment with a variety of proteasome inhibitors, including tripeptidyl aldehyde proteasome inhibitors, lactacystin and MG-132 [137–139]. Some studies demonstrated that proteasome inhibitor-mediated upregulation of HSP-72 was pro-apoptotic [138, 139], while others showed that MG-132 treatment caused an increase in HSP-72 expression and suppressed JNK activation, preventing JNK-mediated apoptosis by subsequent heat stress [139]. HSP-72 upregulation as a mechanism of proteasome inhibitor resistance was validated by a report showing that blocking HSP-72 by the introduction of an antisense oligonucleotide potentiated the apoptosis-inducing ability of MG-132 [140]. More recently, HSP-72 knockdown via siRNA was also shown to potentiate MG-132-induced cell death in prostate cancer cells [141].

Other HSP family members may also be involved in acquired resistance to proteasome inhibitors. Gene profiling of myeloma cells following bortezomib treatment revealed that several other HSPs are also induced by proteasome inhibition, including HSP-27, HSP-70, and HSP-90 [95, 142, 143]. One group demonstrated that bortezomib promotes increased phosphorylation of HSP-27 through activation of p38 and used p38 inhibitors and antisense-mediated downregulation of HSP-27 to reverse proteasome inhibitor resistance [142, 144]. HSP-70 has also been implicated in bortezomib resistance [143], and the flavonoid quercetin has been shown to inhibit HSP-70 mRNA and protein expression [145], suggesting that knockdown or inhibition of HSP-70 may also reverse acquired bortezomib resistance. Importantly, HSP-70 expression is high in pancreatic cancer cells, and inhibition of HSP-70 via quercetin treatment and siRNA knockdown both induced apoptosis in vitro [146].

Finally, HSP-90, which mediates the correct folding of various signal transduction intermediates, has also been implicated in proteasome inhibitor resistance [95]. In fact, synergistic cell death was observed in breast cancer cells treated with the combination of bortezomib and an HSP-90 inhibitor [147]. Additionally, in several preclinical multiple myeloma cell models, the combination resulted in increased apoptosis [147–149], but in pancreatic cancer the cell death resulting from combination treatment appears to be necrotic rather than apoptotic [150], indicating that the combination of HSP-90 antagonists with proteasome inhibitors must be further evaluated to more clearly understand their interactions with one another.

1.4.2.3 Altered Expression of Apoptosis-Related Proteins

As discussed previously, the Bcl-2 family members Bim [151] and Noxa [88] have been implicated in proteasome inhibitor-induced cell death in some cell types. While mutations causing inactivation of these proteins are rare in tumors [152, 153], cells may acquire resistance to proteasome inhibitors via epigenetic mechanisms. In fact, miR-17-92 and NFB2/p52 have recently been reported to repress Bim expression [154, 155], and Bmi-1-dependent methylation has been linked to Noxa expression [156]. The effects of Noxa and Bim could also be abrogated by overexpression of anti-apoptotic Bcl-2 proteins [157]. Small molecule inhibitors targeting Bcl-2, Bcl-xL (ABT-737), and MCL-1 (obatoclax) have been shown to significantly enhance bortezomib-induced cell death in various human cancer cell lines [158–160].

Other proteins that contribute to cell death, like p27, have also been reported to increase following proteasome inhibition [59, 161], and although inactivation of p27 through mutations is uncommon, its expression is often decreased due to increased Skp2 activity and proteasome-mediated degradation [162]. Methylation of p27 gene promoter occurs in almost 10 % of cancers [163], and proteasome inhibitor-resistant tumors may display increased methylation patterns that could contribute to the resistant phenotype. Additionally, p27 can be phosphorylated by AKT [164], which causes changes in its subcellular localization [164, 165], also potentially contributing to acquired proteasome inhibitor resistance.

1.4.2.4 Akt Pathway Activation

The pro-survival PI3K/Akt pathway is constitutively active in many cancers, and several pathways have been implicated in Akt activation, including amplification of PI3K [166] or Akt [167], growth factor receptor signaling [168], PTEN deletion [169], or mutation of Ras family members [170]. Akt activation, both constitutive and induced, can impair the activity of bortezomib [95, 171, 172]. Bortezomib can also directly activate Akt in some cell lines [173], and Akt inhibitors (both direct and indirect), including the PKC antagonist enzastaurin [174], PI3K inhibitors like perifosine, and the Raf inhibitor sorafenib [172] have been shown to enhance bortezomib-induced apoptosis. Additionally, Akt activation is regulated by receptor tyrosine kinase growth factor receptors like EGFR, and Akt activation can be reversed with selective RTK inhibitors in these cells [175], leading to increased bortezomib sensitivity [176, 177].

1.4.2.5 Overexpression of Other Growth-Related Proteins

Resistance to bortezomib has also been attributed to the overexpression of some proteins that are involved in cell growth, including interleukin-6 (IL-6) and insulin-like growth factor 1 (IGF-1), which are thought to confer resistance via activation of NF-κB through the PI3K/Akt and Raf/MEKKl pathways [178, 179]. IL-6 has been shown to play an important role in regulating drug sensitivity in multiple myeloma cells through inhibition of miRNA expression in bone marrow stromal cells (BMSCs) [180, 181]. In addition, IGF-1 receptor levels have also been shown to be high in multiple myeloma, and this overexpression, as well as increased IGF-1 levels, are associated with disease progression and poor patient prognosis [182, 183].

Increased IGF-1 signaling has been directly implicated in the resistance phenotype of bortezomib-resistant multiple myeloma cells with no β5 mutations. The role of IGF-1 signaling was further validated by gene expression profiling which showed that genes activated by IGF-1 were constitutively expressed in these bortezomib-resistant multiple myeloma cells. Importantly, blocking PI3K and mTOR downstream of IGF-1 partially overcame the bortezomib resistance. Direct inhibition of IGF-1R (insulin-like growth factor 1 receptor) was also able to sensitize cultured cells, in vivo models, and patient samples to bortezomib treatment [184], suggesting that combining bortezomib with IGF-1R inhibitors may be a promising strategy to prevent or overcome proteasome inhibitor resistance.

The receptor tyrosine kinase c-Met is also overexpressed in human myeloma cell lines and has been shown to promote drug resistance. One study showed that knockdown of c-Met in U266 human multiple myeloma cells enhanced their sensitivity to bortezomib via inhibition of the Akt/mTOR pathway [185]. Increased Akt/mTOR phosphorylation was also reported in bortezomib-resistant mantle cell lymphoma cells, and dual inhibition of PI3K and mTOR overcame acquired bortezomib resistance by suppressing the activated Akt/mTOR pathway [186]. Microarray analysis has also identified Rad (Ras associated with diabetes) as a potential factor in proteasome inhibitor resistance. Rad levels were increased in bortezomib-resistant Jurkat-R cells compared to parental controls, and knockdown resulted in induction of the mitochondrial apoptotic pathway via Noxa/Bcl-2, thus overcoming bortezomib resistance in these cells [187].

1.4.2.6 Altered Autophagy Pathways

Proteasome inhibitors are known to activate autophagy, but the exact role of autophagy in cancer cell death is a controversial one [188]. Studies have reported that inhibition of autophagy can both inhibit [189] and promote [190] proteasome inhibitor-mediated cell death depending on cell type. This may be due to the variable effects of these autophagy inhibitors, whereby they block macroautophagy but are unable to inhibit chaperone-mediated autophagy, which may play a critical role in clearing protein aggregates in some cells. These protein aggregates may be transferred to the lysosome via aggresomes during chaperone-mediated autophagy. HDAC6 is necessary for aggresome formation following proteasome inhibition, and HDAC inhibition has been shown to enhance proteasome inhibitor-induced cell death in proteasome inhibitor-sensitive cells and to reverse resistance in resistant cells [191, 192]. The combination of HDAC inhibition with proteasome inhibition has been extensively studied, and results suggest that this is the most promising combination. In fact, one phase I clinical trial investigating the combination of bortezomib and the pan-HDAC inhibitor SAHA was completed in patients with relapsed/refractory multiple myeloma [193], and another was completed in patients with solid tumors [NCT00310024; National Cancer Institute]. A phase II trial also investigated the combination in patients with progressive, recurrent glioblastoma [NCT00641706; National Cancer Institute], and results are forthcoming.

1.4.2.7 Increased Antioxidants

The production of ROS appears to play a role in cell death induced by some proteasome inhibitors, which suggests that antioxidant protection mechanisms may also contribute to proteasome inhibitor resistance. Sensitivity of multiple myeloma cells has been shown to increase following depletion of intracellular reduced glutathione by buthionine sulfoximine treatment [194]. Glutathione may promote resistance by acting as a cofactor for GSH-dependent enzymes; protein disulfide isomerase, glutathione peroxidase, and vitamin C, for example, inhibit toxicity induced by proteasome inhibitors, among other factors [195–199]. Thus, antioxidant levels may impact proteasome inhibitor sensitivity, so regulating these levels may be a strategy to overcome resistance.

1.5 Measures to Overcome Proteasome Inhibitor Resistance

1.5.1 Design of Novel Proteasome Inhibitors

Determination of exact molecular mechanisms of proteasome inhibitor resistance would help in the design of effective therapeutic strategies to overcome proteasome inhibitor resistance. Resistance at the proteasome level could be addressed by designing better, more potent inhibitors than bortezomib and carfilzomib. A new generation of irreversible proteasome inhibitors might be helpful in partially overcoming bortezomib resistance due to β5 overexpression. Targeting sites different than those targeted by bortezomib could also be explored for the design and development of next-generation proteasome inhibitors. Unfortunately, however, these next-generation inhibitors may not be effective in overcoming resistance due to downstream factors [133].

Bortezomib is administered intravenously and modification of its pharmacokinetic parameters affecting stability, metabolism, and tissue bioavailability may be a useful strategy for overcoming resistance [133]. Some orally bioavailable reversible second-generation inhibitors, like MLN9708 and CEP 18770, that can be hydrolyzed to an active form have been developed, and encouraging results in cultured cells and animal models have advanced these compounds to phase I clinical trials [200–202]. However, their similarities to bortezomib in terms of mode of action might hinder their ability to overcome bortezomib/carfilzomib resistance, but they may offer advantages in terms of pharmacokinetics and patient compliance due to their oral route of administration, dosing flexibility and convenience [133].

Structure–activity relationship (SAR) studies were conducted to develop orally bioavailable carfilzomib-like agents, and led to the discovery and development of ONX0912, a truncated carfilzomib analog with comparable potency, selectivity, and anticancer activities to its parent compound in vitro and in vivo in animal models [203, 204]. Carfilzomib and ONX0912 can be degraded by proteases and peptidases in the plasma due to their peptide-like structures, which decreases their half-life and efficacy [133]. Therefore, nonpeptidic, irreversible proteasome

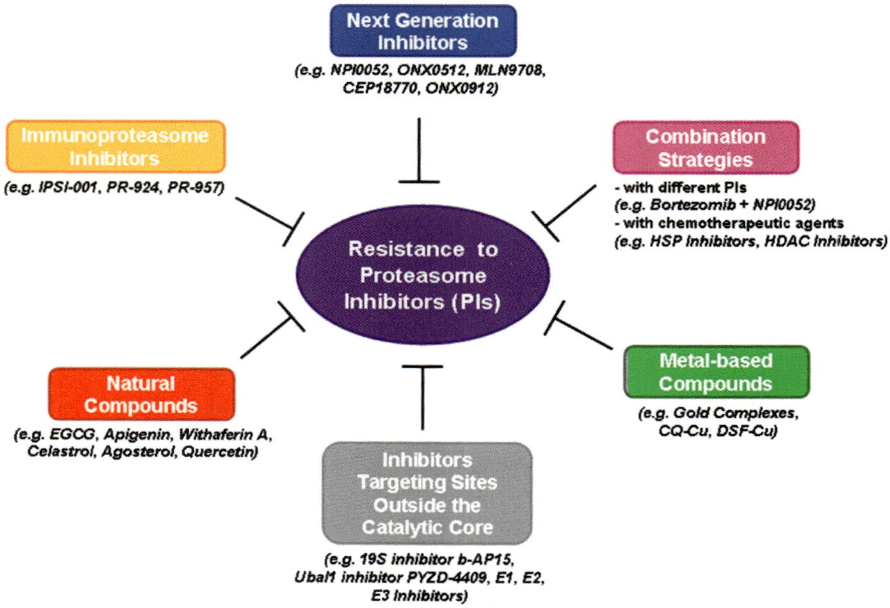

Fig. 1.4 Potential strategies to overcome proteasome inhibitor resistance. Many strategies have been suggested for overcoming proteasome inhibitor resistance. These include designing novel proteasome inhibitors, targeting sites outside the catalytic center (such as the 19S regulatory cap, E1, E2s, or E3s), targeting the immunoproteasome, combination strategies (like proteasome inhibitors + HSP or HDAC inhibitors), and using metal-based or natural compounds as inhibitors

inhibitors like NPI0052 (salinosporamide/marizomib) with better bioavailability have been developed [205]. NPI0052 is a β-lactone-γ-lactam isolated from the marine bacterium *Salinispora tropica* that shows potent irreversible inhibition of all three proteolytic activities of the proteasome through the formation of very stable acyl-ester bonds. Due to its anticancer activities in cell culture and animal models, NPI0052 has advanced into clinical trials for hematological and solid tumor malignancies (Fig. 1.4) [116, 206]. Larger in vitro studies should be conducted to further enhance the understanding of mechanisms associated with resistance to proteasome inhibitors. These studies could lead to the development of personalized therapeutic approaches by identifying subgroups of patients who are more likely to respond well or fail to respond to particular proteasome inhibitors.

1.5.2 Combination Strategies

In addition to designing new compounds to target the proteasome, combining current proteasome inhibitors with distinct modes of action could be an effective strategy to overcome resistance to particular proteasome inhibitors. For instance, NPI0052 in combination with bortezomib has been shown to induce synergistic cytotoxicity in vitro in cultured multiple myeloma cells as well as in multiple myeloma cells isolated from patients, and in multiple myeloma mouse models (Fig. 1.4) [207]. Alternatively, proteasome inhibitors could be combined with other chemotherapeutic agents targeting factors downstream of the proteasome to enhance efficacy. In fact, lenalidomide and NPI0052 in combination display synergistic anti-multiple myeloma activities in cultured and patient multiple myeloma cells, as well as in tumor xenografts in mice [208].

Because HSP overexpression has been suggested as a potential mechanism by which cells become resistant to proteasome inhibitors, combining HSP inhibitors with proteasome inhibitors may sensitize resistant cells to proteasome inhibition (Fig. 1.4). In fact, the combination of the HSP-90 inhibitor tanespimycin (17-allylamino-17-demethoxy-geldanamycin [17-AAG]; geldanamycin analog) with bortezomib resulted in bortezomib-mediated cell death and tumor regression in multiple myeloma cell and xenograft models, respectively [148]. A phase I trial combining these drugs has also been completed in relapsed/refractory multiple myeloma patients, some of whom had progressed to bortezomib resistance [209]. An overall response rate of 27 % was achieved, suggesting that this combination is effective at reversing bortezomib resistance in multiple myeloma.

As discussed previously, some HDACs have also been implicated in proteasome inhibitor resistance, indicating that combining HDAC inhibitors with proteasome inhibitors may be a promising strategy to overcome proteasome inhibitor resistance (Fig. 1.4). Several preclinical studies have reported synergism between these types of drugs. For example, knockdown of HDAC1 enhanced bortezomib-mediated apoptosis, while overexpression of HDAC1 resulted in bortezomib resistance in multiple myeloma cells and treatment with the HDAC inhibitor romidepsin restored bortezomib sensitivity in HDAC1 overexpressing cells and tumor xenografts [210]. Additionally, the combination of bortezomib and tubacin (HDAC6-specific inhibitor) inhibited proliferation in cultured multiple myeloma cells [211]. Selective inhibition of HDAC6 by ACY-1215, both alone and in combination with bortezomib, has also been shown to suppress multiple myeloma cell growth in a xenograft mouse model, again suggesting a synergistic relationship [212]. Finally, the combination of bortezomib and the HDAC inhibitor SAHA (vorinostat) has also been evaluated in a phase I clinical trial in patients with advanced multiple myeloma, the results of which reported an overall response rate of 30 % in bortezomib-resistant patients [193]. Another phase I trial investigating the efficacy of SAHA in combination with bortezomib resulted in one partial remission and one minimal response among three bortezomib-resistant patients [213]. Another trial in multiple myeloma patients combined the natural HDAC inhibitor romidepsin with bortezomib, and 60 % partial and 8 % complete responses were achieved [214]. The Vantage 095 phase IIb trial reported an overall response rate of 18 % with a median duration of response of 6.3 months in patients with bortezomib-refractory relapsed multiple myeloma [215]. A randomized, double-blind phase III trial, Vantage 088, compared SAHA or placebo in combination with bortezomib in 637 myeloma patients and reported an overall response rate of 54 % in the group treated with the SAHA–bortezomib combination, compared with 41 % in the placebo group [216]. Thus, HDAC inhibition may also be a promising strategy for overcoming proteasome inhibitor resistance in refractory cancers.

1.5.3 Immunoproteasome-Specific Inhibitors

The immunoproteasome is an inducible proteasome variant primarily expressed in lymphocytes and monocytes, as well as in cells exposed to inflammatory cytokines such as interferon-γ (IFN-γ) and tumor necrosis factor-α (TNF-α). The immunoproteasome is involved in the production of peptides for major histocompatibility complex-1 (MHC-1). During assembly of the immunoproteasome, the constitutive β1, β2, and β5 subunits are replaced by β1i (PSMB9/LMP2), β2i (PSMB10/LMP-10/MECL1), and β5i (PSMB8/LMP7), respectively. These are associated with the 11S peptidase regulator and the remaining subunits of the constitutive proteasome, which leads to alterations in substrate specificity [217, 218]. Although there may be some functional redundancy between the two proteasome isoforms [219–221], CT-like (β5i) and trypsin-like (β2i) proteolytic activities are upregulated, and PGPH-like activity (β1i) is decreased in the immuno-20S compared to the constitutive 20S [222]. Many conventional proteasome inhibitors (e.g., bortezomib, carfilzomib, NPI0052) designed to target the constitutive proteasome are also able to inhibit the immunoproteasome and thus offer broader activity at the cost of specificity, which may contribute to adverse effects [223].

Therefore, specifically targeting the immunoproteasome in hematological malignancies might be a novel approach toward increasing effectiveness and reducing negative off-target effects (Fig. 1.4) [223, 224], which ultimately led to the development of IPSIs. One such agent, IPSI-001, has shown selectivity for the immunoproteasome over the constitutive proteasome in binding assays and has been shown to induce apoptosis in a dose-dependent manner in patient derived cells of hematologic malignancies. IPSI-001 was also able to overcome resistance to conventional chemotherapeutic agents like doxorubicin, melphalan and, most importantly, bortezomib in vitro [224]. Other agents like the β5i selective tripeptide epoxyketone-based immunoproteasome inhibitors PR-924 [225] and PR-957 [226] have also shown promising results in preclinical cell culture and animal studies. Synthetic analogs of the epoxyketone dihydroeponemycin were also developed as molecular probes to study the effects of β1i (LMP2) inhibition. The combination of β1i inhibitors with the β5i inhibitor lactacystin resulted in enhanced inhibition of total CT-like activity compared to each agent alone. These inhibitors have also shown growth inhibitory effects in PC-3 prostate cancer cells overexpressing β1i [227]. Taken together, these results indicate that targeting the immunoproteasome may be an effective strategy for overcoming resistance to conventional proteasome inhibitors.

1.5.4 Targeting Sites Other than the Catalytic Center

1.5.4.1 E1, E2s, and E3s

Targeting other factors in the UPP may also prove effective in overcoming resistance associated with inhibitors of the 20S catalytic core (Fig. 1.4). Although inhibiting the ubiquitin E1 enzyme was initially disregarded due to potential lethality, the identification of two natural E1 inhibitors, panepophenanthrin and himeic acid, has suggested that this may indeed be a viable strategy. Both inhibitors specifically inhibit the formation of E1 ubiquitin thioester intermediates [228, 229]. Additionally, PYR-41, a synthetic pyrazone derivative, with E1 inhibitory activity that prevents protein degradation and cytokine-mediated activation of NF-κB has also been developed [230]. Another compound, PYZD-4409 induced cell death in malignant cells as well as in a leukemia mouse model, potentially by a mechanism similar to ER stress induced by proteasome inhibitors [231]. Similarly, cell-based screening identified NSC624206 as an E1 inhibitor, though more studies are necessary to determine its molecular effects [232]. Following the observation that functional knockdown of the E2 Ubc13 results in increased p53 activity [233], inhibition of the E2 enzymes has also been explored. In fact, leucettamol A, a natural compound, has been reported to inhibit the interaction between the E2 Ubc13 and the inactive conjugating enzyme variant Uev1A, which is required for efficient poly-ubiquitin chain formation [234].

Perhaps one of the most widely researched strategies for targeting factors upstream of the proteasomal catalytic core is inhibition of ubiquitin E3 ligases (Fig. 1.4), likely due to their role in identifying target proteins for ubiquitination. E3 ligases are divided into one of three classes, RING, HECT, and U-box, based on domain structure and mechanisms of target recognition. The p53-specific RING-type E3 MDM2/HDM2 is a popular target for inhibition, due to its high frequency of overexpression in human cancers [235]. Indeed, nutlin-3, a MDM2 small molecule inhibitor, has been shown to suppress tumor progression in mouse xenograft models [236], suggesting that MDM2 is a promising target. Additionally, in bortezomib-sensitive multiple myeloma and epithelial carcinoma cells, nutlin-3 in combination with bortezomib resulted in additive and synergistic cytotoxic effects, respectively [237]. Some natural products, including chlorofusin and (-)-hexylitaconic acid, that inhibit the interaction between MDM2 and p53 have also been identified [238–241]. Interestingly, disulfiram and its derivatives have also been investigated for their ability to inhibit zinc finger- and RING-finger-containing ubiquitin E3 ligases [242]. Thus, inhibition of upstream UPP factors should be further investigated as this may be a viable strategy for overcoming resistance to 20S inhibitors.

1.5.4.2 19S Regulatory Subunit

Inhibition of proteasomal regulators may also be effective in overcoming resistance to conventional proteasome inhibitors, as this inhibition should only hinder some proteasomal functions (Fig. 1.4). Indeed, screening of a library of purine analog-capped peptoids identified RIP-1 (regulatory particle inhibitor peptoid-1) as an inhibitor of protein unfolding through targeting of the ATPase Rpt4 [243, 244]. Reports have indicated that ubistatin A is capable of blocking recruitment of ubiquitinated proteins to the 26S proteasome by binding ubiquitin chains, ultimately suppressing proteasome-mediated proteolysis [245], indicating that ubiquitin chain receptors may also be good drug targets. Inhibition of deubiquitinase activity of the regulatory particle could be another useful strategy, and b-AP15, a small molecular weight compound that inhibits deubiquitinating enzymes like USP14 and UCHL5, but not POH1, has shown anticancer activity in solid tumor models [246]. Thus, it is clear that factors regulating the 20S catalytic core are good drug targets, and further investigation into this strategy as a way to overcome inhibitors of the 20S core would be very worthwhile.

1.6 Nontraditional Options Targeting the 20S Core

1.6.1 Metals in Cancer Development and Therapy

Just as proteasome activity levels have been shown to be altered in cancer, so have levels of various metals like copper [247–252] and zinc [253–256], a discovery which has led to extensive research regarding the roles of these metals in the development of human cancers as well as their potential as anticancer therapeutics.

The discovery that some metal-based compounds, like cisplatin, possess potent anticancer properties, coupled with the importance of copper and zinc to essential biological processes like tumorigenesis, has led to the investigation into copper and zinc as metal centers in anticancer drugs. Since its discovery over four decades ago, cisplatin has cured over 90 % of testicular cancer cases, and it has also played a critical role in the treatment of various other cancers, including lymphoma, melanoma, bladder, cervical, and ovarian [257]. Unfortunately, although cisplatin use has proven effective, it has also been associated with toxicity and resistance, which has limited its use [258, 259] and prompted the search for less toxic metal-based drugs, including second-generation platinum drugs, as well as complexes containing metals like cobalt, copper, gallium, gold, tin, and zinc, among others.

1.6.2 Metal-Based Complexes as Proteasome Inhibitors

1.6.2.1 Gold-Containing Complexes

Because of the successful use of gold compounds in other diseases [260, 261], gold compounds have also been investigated for their potential anticancer activity (Fig. 1.4). Gold (I) complexes, including auranofin analogs, exhibited potent cytotoxic activity against B16 melanoma and P388 leukemia cells [262], but phosphine-gold(I) thiosugars were the most potent, and while active against leukemia in vivo, these analogs were completely inactive in solid tumor models [263]. Gold(III) complexes have also been investigated, in spite of initial trepidation due to their high redox activity and poor stability. Au(III) is expected to be reduced to Au(I) and metallic Au in the reducing tumor microenvironment, potentially making Au(III) complexes less effective [264]. Various Au(III) compounds with ligand platforms containing nitrogen atoms as donor groups [265], exhibiting a superior chemotherapeutic index, increased cytotoxicity, and fewer toxic side effects than cisplatin [264], were investigated for their antitumor abilities. One example is Au (DMDT) Br_2, which significantly inhibited CT-like activity in purified 20S proteasome ($IC_{50}=7.4$ μM) and 26S proteasome in intact MDA-MB-231 breast cancer cells (10–20 μM) and breast tumor xenografts [266]. Another gold(III) compound, AUL12, was also shown to exhibit potent proteasome-inhibitory and cell death-inducing activities in MDA-MB-231 breast cancer cells ($IC_{50}=4.5$ μM, 70 % inhibition). Interestingly, treatment with this Au(III) compound was associated with redox processes, indicating that induction of oxidative stress may be partially responsible for the cytotoxicity of gold(III) compounds [267].

1.6.2.2 Metal Chelators as Proteasome Inhibitors

The success of metal-containing drugs, along with the functional importance of metals like copper and zinc to normal cellular function, has resulted in studies exploring chelation of these essential metals with chelators like dithiocarbamate and hydroxyquinolone compounds, several of which have been previously approved for the treatment of myriad diseases, such as AIDS, alcoholism, and bacterial and fungal infections [268–270].

Dithiocarbamates

Dithiocarbamate compounds, including disulfiram, are known to form metal complexes, a property that has been applied as a potential strategy to target the UPP in cancer. Disulfiram (tetraethylthiuram disulfide, DSF) is an irreversible aldehyde dehydrogenase inhibitor that is one of two drugs approved by the USFDA for the treatment of alcoholism [271–273]. When complexed with copper, disulfiram can potently inhibit both purified 20S ($IC_{50}=7.5$ μM) and intact 26S proteasome in MDA-MB-231 breast cancer cell lysates (20 μM; >95 % inhibition), as well as inducing apoptosis in the cultured cells [274]. DSF alone, however, had no effect, which is unsurprising, since cultured cells do not express high levels of copper. Significant inhibition (74 %) of tumor growth was also observed in female athymic nude mice bearing MDA-MB-231 tumor xenografts, associated with an 87 % decrease in CT-like activity [274]. Together, the results indicate that the increased copper levels observed in human tumors may be exploited as an anticancer mechanism (Fig. 1.4).

The results of these and other preclinical studies of DSF have also led to a number of clinical trials investigating the use of DSF in humans. One phase I/II clinical trial evaluated the efficacy of DSF in stage IV metastatic melanoma patients [NCT00256230; UC-Irvine] and another examined the effects of DSF on PSA levels in recurrent prostate cancer patients [NCT01118741; Johns Hopkins University]. Two other trials investigated the effects of DSF in combination treatments. The first evaluated the toxicity profile and safety of coadministration of DSF and copper gluconate in refractory malignancies with liver metastases

[NCT00742911; Huntsman Cancer Institute], and the other determined the effects of addition of DSF to current chemotherapeutic treatments in patients with non-small cell lung cancer [NCT00312819; Hadassah Medical Organization]. All of these trials have been completed, but results are as yet unavailable.

Hydroxyquinolones

Hydroxyquinolones are another class of metal-chelating compounds that have been investigated for their anticancer properties. One example is clioquinol (5-chloro-7-iodo-8-hydroxyuinoline, CQ), a lipophilic compound that can form stable complexes with copper (II) [275]. CQ has been shown to reduce and prevent the formation of amyloid plaques in Alzheimer's disease transgenic mice [276], a discovery that led to two clinical trials that validated the efficacy of CQ in Alzheimer's disease with no visible toxicity [277, 278]. Consequently, CQ is currently used for the treatment of Alzheimer's and Huntington's diseases [279, 280]. A CQ–Cu complex (1:1 molar ratio) inhibited both purified 20S ($IC_{50}=2.5$ μM) and intact proteasome (20 μM) in LNCaP and C4-2B prostate cancer cells (82 % and 83 %, respectively). Additionally, mice bearing C4-2B xenografts treated with CQ exhibited significant tumor growth inhibition (66 %), as well as inhibition of angiogenesis and the proteasome and induction of apoptosis [281]. These data clearly indicate that compounds like DSF and CQ require copper to be transported into cancer cells in order to exert their proteasome-inhibitory and apoptosis-inducing abilities [282], but that when copper is present, they are quite potent proteasome inhibitors that are minimally toxic toward normal cells (Fig. 1.4) and therefore, they may be exploited as potential novel strategies for overcoming resistance to traditional proteasome inhibitors like bortezomib.

1.6.3 Natural Compounds as Proteasome Inhibitors

While much emphasis has been placed on the development of synthetic proteasome inhibitors to overcome resistance to proteasome inhibitors, the use of natural compounds and their analogs or derivatives might be a better strategy as many phytochemicals and marine products have shown proteasome-inhibitory and subsequent anticancer activities (Fig. 1.4) [283]. Some examples of natural products investigated for their potential as proteasome inhibitors include Withaferin A, celastrol, agosterols, green tea polyphenols, and apigenin. Withaferins are isolated from the medicinal plant "Indian winter cherry" or "Indian ginseng" (*Withania somnifera*), and have been widely used in traditional Indian "Ayurveda" medicine. Specifically, Withaferin A has been reported to possess anticancer abilities, which may be partly attributed to inhibition of CT-like activity [284]. Celastrol, a triterpene isolated from the Chinese "Thunder of God Vine" (*Tripterygium wilfordii*) has also shown proteasome-inhibitory activity leading to the accumulation of ubiquitinated proteins and proteasomal target proteins in both androgen receptor positive and negative prostate cancer cell lines [285]. Agosterols, isolated from the marine sponge *Acanthodendrilla* sp., have shown inhibition of CT-like activity in rat proteasome in the low micromolar range and also induced cytotoxicity in HeLa cervical cancer cells [286]. The proteasome-inhibitory, apoptosis-inducing activities of green tea polyphenols and apigenin have been more extensively studied, with both advancing to clinical trials.

1.6.3.1 Green Tea Polyphenols

Tea, derived from the *Camellia sinensis* plant, is the most popular beverage in the world after water. Tea comes in many varieties, including green, black, and oolong, all of which contain many beneficial compounds. The most potent of these are polyphenols, which are characterized by the presence of more than one phenol group per molecule and are believed to provide the coloring in many plants [287].

The most active polyphenol in tea is (-)-epigallocatechin-3-gallate, or (-)-EGCG, which has been shown to possess anticancer activity in several cancer types, including bladder, breast, and B-cell malignancies (Fig. 1.4) [288–290]. The proteasome-inhibitory activity of (-)-EGCG has been explored in vitro and in vivo. (-)-EGCG inhibited CT-like activity in both purified 20S (IC_{50}=86–194 nM) and intact 26S (from Jurkat leukemia, LNCaP and PC-3 prostate cancer, and MCF-7 breast cancer cell extracts) proteasome, and increased ubiquitinated proteins, p27, and IκB-α were also observed [291]. Unfortunately, however, a recent study using experimental multiple myeloma models has revealed a direct interaction between (-)-EGCG and bortezomib that inhibits the efficacy of bortezomib [292], but whether green tea consumption affects the efficacy of bortezomib therapy in multiple myeloma patients needs to be confirmed.

The interesting preclinical data, coupled with the popularity of tea, have led to clinical trials using (-)-EGCG and other green tea polyphenols. One phase I trial evaluated the optimal dose and tolerability of (-)-EGCG in previously untreated, asymptomatic chronic lymphocytic leukemia patients, and results indicated that (-)-EGCG is tolerable and does result in some clinical benefit [293]. Another phase I study investigated the effects of (-)-EGCG supplementation on serum levels of prostate cancer biomarkers [294], with all prostate cancer-associated biomarkers, including hepatocyte growth factor (HGF), vascular endothelial growth factor (VEGF), insulin-like growth factor (IGF)-1, IGF-binding protein-3 (IGFBP-3), and prostate-specific antigen (PSA) decreasing significantly after treatment with no elevation of liver function enzymes. Therefore, even short-term (-)-EGCG treatment may be clinically beneficial to prostate cancer patients [294].

In addition, a number of phase I and II trials examining the effects of (-)-EGCG treatment in various types of cancer, including nonmetastatic bladder, breast, cervical, colorectal, prostate, non-small cell lung, and uterine carcinomas as well as multiple myeloma, are currently recruiting patients or are ongoing. Other studies are investigating the potential preventive effects of (-)-EGCG in patients at risk for cervical, esophageal, and lung cancers. Finally, still others are evaluating (-)-EGCG in combination with the EGFR inhibitor erlotinib in non-small cell lung cancer and premalignant lesions of the head and neck. The preclinical and clinical data, as well as the numerous recruiting/ongoing clinical trials, clearly support the use of (-)-EGCG as a chemopreventive or therapeutic agent, and its potential use following progression to resistance to other proteasome inhibitors should be explored.

1.6.3.2 Apigenin

Apigenin (5,7,4-trihydroxyflavone) has also been shown to possess antioxidant, antimutagenic, and chemopreventive properties (Fig. 1.4). Apigenin is a dietary flavonoid found in various natural products including celery seed, chamomile flowers, grapes, and parsley [295–298], and although the mechanism is not fully understood, chemoprevention by apigenin has been reported in several cancers including cervical [299], lung [300], prostate [301], and skin [302].

Studies have shown that the carbonyl carbon in the C4 position of apigenin binds to the β5 subunit in a suitable orientation for nucleophilic attack by the N-terminal Thr1 [303]. Apigenin potently inhibits CT-like activity of purified 20S (IC_{50} = 1.8–2.3 μM) and intact proteasome in Jurkat leukemia cell lysates (1–10 μM), with little to no toxicity in immortalized, non-transformed natural killer cells [303]. Proteasome inhibition-associated accumulation of ubiquitinated proteins and apoptosis-associated morphological changes, activation of caspase-3/-7, and cleavage of PARP were also observed, and similar proteasome inhibition and apoptosis induction were observed in breast cancer MBA-MD-231 cells and tumors, with no significant changes in body weight following apigenin treatment, indicating low toxicity in vivo [304]. The promising preclinical data have led to examination of the efficacy of apigenin in human patients. In one prospective study in patients with resected colon cancer or who had undergone polypectomy, one group received a flavonoid mixture and the other served as a matched control. The results suggested that dietary consumption of flavonoids like apigenin may reduce the risk of colorectal cancer [305]. This preventive effect has not been fully validated, however, and further studies are necessary to determine if apigenin could be used to overcome resistance to other proteasome inhibitors.

1.7 Conclusion

The clinical approval of the proteasome inhibitors bortezomib and carfilzomib was validation of the importance of the UPP as a critical anticancer therapeutic target. Unfortunately, intrinsic and acquired resistance in tumor cells is associated with the use of clinical proteasome inhibitors, so it is important to find novel strategies to overcome this resistance. Resistance may be due to a variety of factors including overexpression or mutation of the β5 subunit, overexpression of HSPs, altered expression of apoptosis- and growth-related proteins, Akt pathway activation, altered autophagy, and increased antioxidant levels. Toward the goal of overcoming this resistance, novel small molecules have been tested for their ability to selectively target and inhibit components of the UPP other than the catalytic 20S core. These novel targets include the 19S regulatory cap(s), deubiquitinating enzymes, and the enzymes involved in the ubiquitination cascade (E1, E2s, and E3s). Inhibitors containing metal centers and those derived from natural products may also be viable options for overcoming resistance associated with clinical proteasome inhibitors. Finally, targeting the specialized immunoproteasome also has potential as a valuable new strategy that may be more specific and could overcome resistance to constitutive 20S proteasome inhibitors. Therefore, the UPP is a promising target for cancer therapy, but further studies are necessary to develop inhibitors that can avoid the resistance associated with clinical proteasome inhibitors.

Acknowledgements This work was partially supported by NIH 1R01CA20009, 3R01CA120009-04S1, 5R01CA127258-05 and NCI R21CA184788 (to Dr. Dou), and NIH Center grant P30 CA022453 (to Karmanos Cancer Institute).

References

1. Ciehanover A, Hod Y, Hershko A (1978) A heat-stable polypeptide component of an ATP-dependent proteolytic system from reticulocytes. Biochem Biophys Res Commun 81: 1100–1105
2. Hershko A, Ciechanover A, Heller H, Haas AL, Rose IA (1980) Proposed role of ATP in protein breakdown: conjugation of protein with multiple chains of the polypeptide of ATP-dependent proteolysis. Proc Natl Acad Sci U S A 77:1783–1786
3. Nalepa G, Rolfe M, Harper JW (2006) Drug discovery in the ubiquitin-proteasome system. Nat Rev Drug Discov 5:596–613
4. Baker SP, Grant PA (2005) The proteasome: not just degrading anymore. Cell 123:361–363
5. Collins GA, Tansey WP (2006) The proteasome: a utility tool for transcription? Curr Opin Genet Dev 16:197–202
6. Krogan NJ, Lam MH, Fillingham J, Keogh MC, Gebbia M, Li J, Datta N, Cagney G, Buratowski S, Emili A, Greenblatt JF (2004) Proteasome involvement in the repair of DNA double-strand breaks. Mol Cell 16:1027–1034
7. Ciechanover A (1998) The ubiquitin-proteasome pathway: on protein death and cell life. EMBO J 17:7151–7160
8. Rivett AJ (1998) Intracellular distribution of proteasomes. Curr Opin Immunol 10:110–114
9. Hirsch C, Ploegh HL (2000) Intracellular targeting of the proteasome. Trends Cell Biol 10:268–272
10. Wojcik C, DeMartino GN (2003) Intracellular localization of proteasomes. Int J Biochem Cell Biol 35:579–589
11. Adams J (2004) The proteasome: a suitable antineoplastic target. Nat Rev Cancer 4:349–360
12. Peters JM, Cejka Z, Harris JR, Kleinschmidt JA, Baumeister W (1993) Structural features of the 26 S proteasome complex. J Mol Biol 234:932–937
13. Baumeister W, Walz J, Zuhl F, Seemuller E (1998) The proteasome: paradigm of a self-compartmentalizing protease. Cell 92:367–380
14. Groll M, Ditzel L, Lowe J, Stock D, Bochtler M, Bartunik HD, Huber R (1997) Structure of 20S proteasome from yeast at 2.4 A resolution. Nature 386:463–471

15. Groll M, Heinemeyer W, Jager S, Ullrich T, Bochtler M, Wolf DH, Huber R (1999) The catalytic sites of 20S proteasomes and their role in subunit maturation: a mutational and crystallographic study. Proc Natl Acad Sci U S A 96:10976–10983
16. DeMartino GN, Slaughter CA (1999) The proteasome, a novel protease regulated by multiple mechanisms. J Biol Chem 274:22123–22126
17. Goldberg AL, Cascio P, Saric T, Rock KL (2002) The importance of the proteasome and subsequent proteolytic steps in the generation of antigenic peptides. Mol Immunol 39: 147–164
18. Nickell S, Beck F, Scheres SH, Korinek A, Forster F, Lasker K, Mihalache O, Sun N, Nagy I, Sali A, Plitzko JM, Carazo JM, Mann M, Baumeister W (2009) Insights into the molecular architecture of the 26S proteasome. Proc Natl Acad Sci U S A 106:11943–11947
19. da Fonseca PC, Morris EP (2008) Structure of the human 26S proteasome: subunit radial displacements open the gate into the proteolytic core. J Biol Chem 283:23305–23314
20. Hartmann-Petersen R, Tanaka K, Hendil KB (2001) Quaternary structure of the ATPase complex of human 26S proteasomes determined by chemical cross-linking. Arch Biochem Biophys 386:89–94
21. Fu H, Doelling JH, Rubin DM, Vierstra RD (1999) Structural and functional analysis of the six regulatory particle triple-A ATPase subunits from the Arabidopsis 26S proteasome. Plant J 18:529–539
22. Rubin DM, Glickman MH, Larsen CN, Dhruvakumar S, Finley D (1998) Active site mutants in the six regulatory particle ATPases reveal multiple roles for ATP in the proteasome. EMBO J 17:4909–4919
23. Finley D (2009) Recognition and processing of ubiquitin-protein conjugates by the proteasome. Annu Rev Biochem 78:477–513
24. Deveraux Q, Ustrell V, Pickart C, Rechsteiner M (1994) A 26S protease subunit that binds ubiquitin conjugates. J Biol Chem 269:7059–7061
25. Hamazaki J, Iemura S, Natsume T, Yashiroda H, Tanaka K, Murata S (2006) A novel proteasome interacting protein recruits the deubiquitinating enzyme UCH37 to 26S proteasomes. EMBO J 25:4524–4536
26. Qiu XB, Ouyang SY, Li CJ, Miao S, Wang L, Goldberg AL (2006) hRpn13/ADRM1/GP110 is a novel proteasome subunit that binds the deubiquitinating enzyme, UCH37. EMBO J 25:5742–5753
27. Yao T, Song L, Xu W, DeMartino GN, Florens L, Swanson SK, Washburn MP, Conaway RC, Conaway JW, Cohen RE (2006) Proteasome recruitment and activation of the Uch37 deubiquitinating enzyme by Adrm1. Nat Cell Biol 8:994–1002
28. Chen ZJ, Sun LJ (2009) Nonproteolytic functions of ubiquitin in cell signaling. Mol Cell 33:275–286
29. Adams J (2003) The proteasome: structure, function, and role in the cell. Cancer Treat Rev 29(suppl 1):3–9
30. Ciechanover A, Orian A, Schwartz AL (2000) Ubiquitin-mediated proteolysis: biological regulation via destruction. Bioessays 22:442–451
31. Jariel-Encontre I, Bossis G, Piechaczyk M (2008) Ubiquitin-independent degradation of proteins by the proteasome. Biochim Biophys Acta 1786:153–177
32. Hoyt MA, Zhang M, Coffino P (2003) Ubiquitin-independent mechanisms of mouse ornithine decarboxylase degradation are conserved between mammalian and fungal cells. J Biol Chem 278:12135–12143
33. Hoyt MA, Coffino P (2004) Ubiquitin-free routes into the proteasome. Cell Mol Life Sci 61:1596–1600
34. Coux O, Tanaka K, Goldberg AL (1996) Structure and functions of the 20S and 26S proteasomes. Annu Rev Biochem 65:801–847
35. Nandi D, Tahiliani P, Kumar A, Chandu D (2006) The ubiquitin-proteasome system. J Biosci 31:137–155
36. Ciechanover A (2006) The ubiquitin proteolytic system: from a vague idea, through basic mechanisms, and onto human diseases and drug targeting. Neurology 66:S7–S19

37. Adams J (2004) The development of proteasome inhibitors as anticancer drugs. Cancer Cell 5:417–421
38. Smith L, Lind MJ, Drew PJ, Cawkwell L (2007) The putative roles of the ubiquitin/proteasome pathway in resistance to anticancer therapy. Eur J Cancer 43:2330–2338
39. Dou QP, Li B (1999) Proteasome inhibitors as potential novel anticancer agents. Drug Resist Updat 2:215–223
40. Loda M, Cukor B, Tam SW, Lavin P, Fiorentino M, Draetta GF, Jessup JM, Pagano M (1997) Increased proteasome-dependent degradation of the cyclin-dependent kinase inhibitor p27 in aggressive colorectal carcinomas. Nat Med 3:231–234
41. Li B, Dou QP (2000) Bax degradation by the ubiquitin/proteasome-dependent pathway: involvement in tumor survival and progression. Proc Natl Acad Sci U S A 97:3850–3855
42. Kumatori A, Tanaka K, Inamura N, Sone S, Ogura T, Matsumoto T, Tachikawa T, Shin S, Ichihara A (1990) Abnormally high expression of proteasomes in human leukemic cells. Proc Natl Acad Sci U S A 87:7071–7075
43. An B, Goldfarb RH, Siman R, Dou QP (1998) Novel dipeptidyl proteasome inhibitors overcome Bcl-2 protective function and selectively accumulate the cyclin-dependent kinase inhibitor p27 and induce apoptosis in transformed, but not normal, human fibroblasts. Cell Death Differ 5:1062–1075
44. Lopes UG, Erhardt P, Yao R, Cooper GM (1997) p53-dependent induction of apoptosis by proteasome inhibitors. J Biol Chem 272:12893–12896
45. Orlowski RZ, Kuhn DJ (2008) Proteasome inhibitors in cancer therapy: lessons from the first decade. Clin Cancer Res 14:1649–1657
46. Rock KL, Gramm C, Rothstein L, Clark K, Stein R, Dick L, Hwang D, Goldberg AL (1994) Inhibitors of the proteasome block the degradation of most cell proteins and the generation of peptides presented on MHC class I molecules. Cell 78:761–771
47. Lee DH, Goldberg AL (1996) Selective inhibitors of the proteasome-dependent and vacuolar pathways of protein degradation in Saccharomyces cerevisiae. J Biol Chem 271: 27280–27284
48. Lowe J, Stock D, Jap B, Zwickl P, Baumeister W, Huber R (1995) Crystal structure of the 20S proteasome from the archaeon T. acidophilum at 3.4 A resolution. Science 268:533–539
49. Figueiredo-Pereira ME, Berg KA, Wilk S (1994) A new inhibitor of the chymotrypsin-like activity of the multicatalytic proteinase complex (20S proteasome) induces accumulation of ubiquitin-protein conjugates in a neuronal cell. J Neurochem 63:1578–1581
50. Bogyo M, McMaster JS, Gaczynska M, Tortorella D, Goldberg AL, Ploegh H (1997) Covalent modification of the active site threonine of proteasomal beta subunits and the Escherichia coli homolog HslV by a new class of inhibitors. Proc Natl Acad Sci U S A 94:6629–6634
51. Glas R, Bogyo M, McMaster JS, Gaczynska M, Ploegh HL (1998) A proteolytic system that compensates for loss of proteasome function. Nature 392:618–622
52. Dick LR, Cruikshank AA, Grenier L, Melandri FD, Nunes SL, Stein RL (1996) Mechanistic studies on the inactivation of the proteasome by lactacystin: a central role for clasto-lactacystin beta-lactone. J Biol Chem 271:7273–7276
53. Omura S, Matsuzaki K, Fujimoto T, Kosuge K, Furuya T, Fujita S, Nakagawa A (1991) Structure of lactacystin, a new microbial metabolite which induces differentiation of neuroblastoma cells. J Antibiot 44:117–118
54. Fenteany G, Standaert RF, Lane WS, Choi S, Corey EJ, Schreiber SL (1995) Inhibition of proteasome activities and subunit-specific amino-terminal threonine modification by lactacystin. Science 268:726–731
55. Craiu A, Gaczynska M, Akopian T, Gramm CF, Fenteany G, Goldberg AL, Rock KL (1997) Lactacystin and clasto-lactacystin beta-lactone modify multiple proteasome beta-subunits and inhibit intracellular protein degradation and major histocompatibility complex class I antigen presentation. J Biol Chem 272:13437–13445
56. Koguchi Y, Kohno J, Nishio M, Takahashi K, Okuda T, Ohnuki T, Komatsubara S (2000) TMC-95A, B, C, and D, novel proteasome inhibitors produced by Apiospora montagnei Sacc. TC 1093. Taxonomy, production, isolation, and biological activities. J Antibiot 53:105–109

57. Groll M, Koguchi Y, Huber R, Kohno J (2001) Crystal structure of the 20 S proteasome: TMC-95A complex: a non-covalent proteasome inhibitor. J Mol Biol 311:543–548
58. Sasse F, Steinmetz H, Schupp T, Petersen F, Memmert K, Hofmann H, Heusser C, Brinkmann V, von Matt P, Hofle G, Reichenbach H (2002) Argyrins, immunosuppressive cyclic peptides from myxobacteria. I. Production, isolation, physico-chemical and biological properties. J Antibiot 55:543–551
59. Nickeleit I, Zender S, Sasse F, Geffers R, Brandes G, Sorensen I, Steinmetz H, Kubicka S, Carlomagno T, Menche D, Gutgemann I, Buer J, Gossler A, Manns MP, Kalesse M, Frank R, Malek NP (2008) Argyrin a reveals a critical role for the tumor suppressor protein p27(kip1) in mediating antitumor activities in response to proteasome inhibition. Cancer Cell 14:23–35
60. Adams J, Palombella VJ, Sausville EA, Johnson J, Destree A, Lazarus DD, Maas J, Pien CS, Prakash S, Elliott PJ (1999) Proteasome inhibitors: a novel class of potent and effective antitumor agents. Cancer Res 59:2615–2622
61. Frankel A, Man S, Elliott P, Adams J, Kerbel RS (2000) Lack of multicellular drug resistance observed in human ovarian and prostate carcinoma treated with the proteasome inhibitor PS-341. Clin Cancer Res 6:3719–3728
62. Hideshima T, Richardson P, Chauhan D, Palombella VJ, Elliott PJ, Adams J, Anderson KC (2001) The proteasome inhibitor PS-341 inhibits growth, induces apoptosis, and overcomes drug resistance in human multiple myeloma cells. Cancer Res 61:3071–3076
63. Ryan DP, O'Neil BH, Supko JG, Rocha Lima CM, Dees EC, Appleman LJ, Clark J, Fidias P, Orlowski RZ, Kashala O, Eder JP, Cusack JC Jr (2006) A phase I study of bortezomib plus irinotecan in patients with advanced solid tumors. Cancer 107:2688–2697
64. Ryan DP, Appleman LJ, Lynch T, Supko JG, Fidias P, Clark JW, Fishman M, Zhu AX, Enzinger PC, Kashala O, Cusack J Jr, Eder JP (2006) Phase I clinical trial of bortezomib in combination with gemcitabine in patients with advanced solid tumors. Cancer 107:2482–2489
65. Nix D, Milton M, Pligavko C, et al (2003) Pharmacokinetics of the proteasome inhibitor bortezomib (Velcade) in male cynomolgus monkeys (abstract C245). AACR-NCI-EORTC molecular targets and cancer therapeutics discovery, biology, and clinical applications meeting
66. Nix D, Press R, Wehrman T, et al (2003) Tissue distribution and mass balance of bortezomib (Velcade) in non-human primates (abstract M1336). AAPS annual meeting and exposition
67. Kane RC, Bross PF, Farrell AT, Pazdur R (2003) Velcade: U.S. FDA approval for the treatment of multiple myeloma progressing on prior therapy. Oncologist 8:508–513
68. Schwartz R, Davidson T (2004) Pharmacology, pharmacokinetics, and practical applications of bortezomib. Oncology 18:14–21
69. Crawford LJ, Walker B, Ovaa H, Chauhan D, Anderson KC, Morris TC, Irvine AE (2006) Comparative selectivity and specificity of the proteasome inhibitors BzLLLCOCHO, PS-341, and MG-132. Cancer Res 66:6379–6386
70. Engel RH, Brown JA, Von Roenn JH, O'Regan RM, Bergan R, Badve S, Rademaker A, Gradishar WJ (2007) A phase II study of single agent bortezomib in patients with metastatic breast cancer: a single institution experience. Cancer Invest 25:733–737
71. Yang CH, Gonzalez-Angulo AM, Reuben JM, Booser DJ, Pusztai L, Krishnamurthy S, Esseltine D, Stec J, Broglio KR, Islam R, Hortobagyi GN, Cristofanilli M (2006) Bortezomib (VELCADE) in metastatic breast cancer: pharmacodynamics, biological effects, and prediction of clinical benefits. Ann Oncol 17:813–817
72. Adams J (2002) Preclinical and clinical evaluation of proteasome inhibitor PS-341 for the treatment of cancer. Curr Opin Chem Biol 6:493–500
73. Jagannath S, Durie BG, Wolf J, Camacho E, Irwin D, Lutzky J, McKinley M, Gabayan E, Mazumder A, Schenkein D, Crowley J (2005) Bortezomib therapy alone and in combination with dexamethasone for previously untreated symptomatic multiple myeloma. Br J Haematol 129:776–783
74. Kondagunta GV, Drucker B, Schwartz L, Bacik J, Marion S, Russo P, Mazumdar M, Motzer RJ (2004) Phase II trial of bortezomib for patients with advanced renal cell carcinoma. J Clin Oncol 22:3720–3725

75. Richardson PG, Sonneveld P, Schuster MW, Irwin D, Stadtmauer EA, Facon T, Harousseau JL, Ben-Yehuda D, Lonial S, Goldschmidt H, Reece D, San-Miguel JF, Blade J, Boccadoro M, Cavenagh J, Dalton WS, Boral AL, Esseltine DL, Porter JB, Schenkein D, Anderson KC, Assessment of Proteasome Inhibition for Extending Remissions I (2005) Bortezomib or high-dose dexamethasone for relapsed multiple myeloma. N Engl J Med 352:2487–2498
76. Shah SA, Potter MW, McDade TP, Ricciardi R, Perugini RA, Elliott PJ, Adams J, Callery MP (2001) 26S proteasome inhibition induces apoptosis and limits growth of human pancreatic cancer. J Cell Biochem 82:110–122
77. Sunwoo JB, Chen Z, Dong G, Yeh N, Crowl Bancroft C, Sausville E, Adams J, Elliott P, Van Waes C (2001) Novel proteasome inhibitor PS-341 inhibits activation of nuclear factor-kappa B, cell survival, tumor growth, and angiogenesis in squamous cell carcinoma. Clin Cancer Res 7:1419–1428
78. Ma MH, Yang HH, Parker K, Manyak S, Friedman JM, Altamirano C, Wu ZQ, Borad MJ, Frantzen M, Roussos E, Neeser J, Mikail A, Adams J, Sjak-Shie N, Vescio RA, Berenson JR (2003) The proteasome inhibitor PS-341 markedly enhances sensitivity of multiple myeloma tumor cells to chemotherapeutic agents. Clin Cancer Res 9:1136–1144
79. Berenson JR, Ma HM, Vescio R (2001) The role of nuclear factor-kappaB in the biology and treatment of multiple myeloma. Semin Oncol 28:626–633
80. LeBlanc R, Catley LP, Hideshima T, Lentzsch S, Mitsiades CS, Mitsiades N, Neuberg D, Goloubeva O, Pien CS, Adams J, Gupta D, Richardson PG, Munshi NC, Anderson KC (2002) Proteasome inhibitor PS-341 inhibits human myeloma cell growth in vivo and prolongs survival in a murine model. Cancer Res 62:4996–5000
81. Chauhan D, Anderson KC (2003) Mechanisms of cell death and survival in multiple myeloma (MM): therapeutic implications. Apoptosis 8:337–343
82. Feinman R, Koury J, Thames M, Barlogie B, Epstein J, Siegel DS (1999) Role of NF-kappaB in the rescue of multiple myeloma cells from glucocorticoid-induced apoptosis by bcl-2. Blood 93:3044–3052
83. Hideshima T, Ikeda H, Chauhan D, Okawa Y, Raje N, Podar K, Mitsiades C, Munshi NC, Richardson PG, Carrasco RD, Anderson KC (2009) Bortezomib induces canonical nuclear factor-kappaB activation in multiple myeloma cells. Blood 114:1046–1052
84. Qin JZ, Ziffra J, Stennett L, Bodner B, Bonish BK, Chaturvedi V, Bennett F, Pollock PM, Trent JM, Hendrix MJ, Rizzo P, Miele L, Nickoloff BJ (2005) Proteasome inhibitors trigger NOXA-mediated apoptosis in melanoma and myeloma cells. Cancer Res 65:6282–6293
85. Oda E, Ohki R, Murasawa H, Nemoto J, Shibue T, Yamashita T, Tokino T, Taniguchi T, Tanaka N (2000) Noxa, a BH3-only member of the Bcl-2 family and candidate mediator of p53-induced apoptosis. Science 288:1053–1058
86. Adams JM, Cory S (1998) The Bcl-2 protein family: arbiters of cell survival. Science 281:1322–1326
87. Gross A, McDonnell JM, Korsmeyer SJ (1999) BCL-2 family members and the mitochondria in apoptosis. Genes Dev 13:1899–1911
88. Nikiforov MA, Riblett M, Tang WH, Gratchouck V, Zhuang D, Fernandez Y, Verhaegen M, Varambally S, Chinnaiyan AM, Jakubowiak AJ, Soengas MS (2007) Tumor cell-selective regulation of NOXA by c-MYC in response to proteasome inhibition. Proc Natl Acad Sci U S A 104:19488–19493
89. Caravita T, de Fabritiis P, Palumbo A, Amadori S, Boccadoro M (2006) Bortezomib: efficacy comparisons in solid tumors and hematologic malignancies. Nat Clin Pract Oncol 3:374–387
90. Qin JZ, Xin H, Sitailo LA, Denning MF, Nickoloff BJ (2006) Enhanced killing of melanoma cells by simultaneously targeting Mcl-1 and NOXA. Cancer Res 66:9636–9645
91. Fernandez Y, Verhaegen M, Miller TP, Rush JL, Steiner P, Opipari AW Jr, Lowe SW, Soengas MS (2005) Differential regulation of noxa in normal melanocytes and melanoma cells by proteasome inhibition: therapeutic implications. Cancer Res 65:6294–6304
92. Nawrocki ST, Bruns CJ, Harbison MT, Bold RJ, Gotsch BS, Abbruzzese JL, Elliott P, Adams J, McConkey DJ (2002) Effects of the proteasome inhibitor PS-341 on apoptosis and angiogenesis in orthotopic human pancreatic tumor xenografts. Mol Cancer Ther 1:1243–1253

93. Fribley A, Wang CY (2006) Proteasome inhibitor induces apoptosis through induction of endoplasmic reticulum stress. Cancer Biol Ther 5:745–748
94. Fribley A, Zeng Q, Wang CY (2004) Proteasome inhibitor PS-341 induces apoptosis through induction of endoplasmic reticulum stress-reactive oxygen species in head and neck squamous cell carcinoma cells. Mol Cell Biol 24:9695–9704
95. Mitsiades N, Mitsiades CS, Poulaki V, Chauhan D, Fanourakis G, Gu X, Bailey C, Joseph M, Libermann TA, Treon SP, Munshi NC, Richardson PG, Hideshima T, Anderson KC (2002) Molecular sequelae of proteasome inhibition in human multiple myeloma cells. Proc Natl Acad Sci U S A 99:14374–14379
96. Strauss SJ, Higginbottom K, Juliger S, Maharaj L, Allen P, Schenkein D, Lister TA, Joel SP (2007) The proteasome inhibitor bortezomib acts independently of p53 and induces cell death via apoptosis and mitotic catastrophe in B-cell lymphoma cell lines. Cancer Res 67:2783–2790
97. Lioni M, Noma K, Snyder A, Klein-Szanto A, Diehl JA, Rustgi AK, Herlyn M, Smalley KS (2008) Bortezomib induces apoptosis in esophageal squamous cell carcinoma cells through activation of the p38 mitogen-activated protein kinase pathway. Mol Cancer Ther 7:2866–2875
98. Kukreja A, Hutchinson A, Mazumder A, Vesole D, Angitapalli R, Jagannath S, O'Connor OA, Dhodapkar MV (2007) Bortezomib disrupts tumour-dendritic cell interactions in myeloma and lymphoma: therapeutic implications. Br J Haematol 136:106–110
99. Orlowski RZ, Stinchcombe TE, Mitchell BS, Shea TC, Baldwin AS, Stahl S, Adams J, Esseltine DL, Elliott PJ, Pien CS, Guerciolini R, Anderson JK, Depcik-Smith ND, Bhagat R, Lehman MJ, Novick SC, O'Connor OA, Soignet SL (2002) Phase I trial of the proteasome inhibitor PS-341 in patients with refractory hematologic malignancies. J Clin Oncol 20:4420–4427
100. Orlowski RZ, Voorhees PM, Garcia RA, Hall MD, Kudrik FJ, Allred T, Johri AR, Jones PE, Ivanova A, Van Deventer HW, Gabriel DA, Shea TC, Mitchell BS, Adams J, Esseltine DL, Trehu EG, Green M, Lehman MJ, Natoli S, Collins JM, Lindley CM, Dees EC (2005) Phase 1 trial of the proteasome inhibitor bortezomib and pegylated liposomal doxorubicin in patients with advanced hematologic malignancies. Blood 105:3058–3065
101. Papandreou CN, Daliani DD, Nix D, Yang H, Madden T, Wang X, Pien CS, Millikan RE, Tu SM, Pagliaro L, Kim J, Adams J, Elliott P, Esseltine D, Petrusich A, Dieringer P, Perez C, Logothetis CJ (2004) Phase I trial of the proteasome inhibitor bortezomib in patients with advanced solid tumors with observations in androgen-independent prostate cancer. J Clin Oncol 22:2108–2121
102. Dou QP, Goldfarb RH (2002) Bortezomib (millennium pharmaceuticals). IDrugs 5:828–834
103. Kong X, Alvarez-Castelao B, Lin Z, Castano JG, Caro J (2007) Constitutive/hypoxic degradation of HIF-alpha proteins by the proteasome is independent of von Hippel Lindau protein ubiquitylation and the transactivation activity of the protein. J Biol Chem 282:15498–15505
104. Dreicer R, Petrylak D, Agus D, Webb I, Roth B (2007) Phase I/II study of bortezomib plus docetaxel in patients with advanced androgen-independent prostate cancer. Clin Cancer Res 13:1208–1215
105. Hainsworth JD, Meluch AA, Spigel DR, Barton J Jr, Simons L, Meng C, Gould B, Greco FA (2007) Weekly docetaxel and bortezomib as first-line treatment for patients with hormone-refractory prostate cancer: a Minnie Pearl Cancer Research Network phase II trial. Clin Genitourin Cancer 5:278–283
106. Richardson PG, Barlogie B, Berenson J, Singhal S, Jagannath S, Irwin D, Rajkumar SV, Srkalovic G, Alsina M, Alexanian R, Siegel D, Orlowski RZ, Kuter D, Limentani SA, Lee S, Hideshima T, Esseltine DL, Kauffman M, Adams J, Schenkein DP, Anderson KC (2003) A phase 2 study of bortezomib in relapsed, refractory myeloma. N Engl J Med 348:2609–2617
107. Jagannath S, Barlogie B, Berenson J, Siegel D, Irwin D, Richardson PG, Niesvizky R, Alexanian R, Limentani SA, Alsina M, Adams J, Kauffman M, Esseltine DL, Schenkein DP, Anderson KC (2004) A phase 2 study of two doses of bortezomib in relapsed or refractory myeloma. Br J Haematol 127:165–172
108. Oakervee HE, Popat R, Curry N, Smith P, Morris C, Drake M, Agrawal S, Stec J, Schenkein D, Esseltine DL, Cavenagh JD (2005) PAD combination therapy (PS-341/bortezomib, doxorubicin and dexamethasone) for previously untreated patients with multiple myeloma. Br J Haematol 129:755–762

109. O'Connor OA, Wright J, Moskowitz C, Muzzy J, MacGregor-Cortelli B, Stubblefield M, Straus D, Portlock C, Hamlin P, Choi E, Dumetrescu O, Esseltine D, Trehu E, Adams J, Schenkein D, Zelenetz AD (2005) Phase II clinical experience with the novel proteasome inhibitor bortezomib in patients with indolent non-Hodgkin's lymphoma and mantle cell lymphoma. J Clin Oncol 23:676–684
110. Belch A, Kouroukis CT, Crump M, Sehn L, Gascoyne RD, Klasa R, Powers J, Wright J, Eisenhauer EA (2007) A phase II study of bortezomib in mantle cell lymphoma: the National Cancer Institute of Canada Clinical Trials Group trial IND.150. Ann Oncol 18:116–121
111. Scagliotti GV, Germonpre P, Bosquee L, Vansteenkiste J, Gervais R, Planchard D, Reck M, De Marinis F, Lee JS, Park K, Biesma B, Gans S, Ramlau R, Szczesna A, Makhson A, Manikhas G, Morgan B, Zhu Y, Chan KC, von Pawel J (2010) A randomized phase II study of bortezomib and pemetrexed, in combination or alone, in patients with previously treated advanced non-small-cell lung cancer. Lung Cancer 68:420–426
112. Mikhael JR, Belch AR, Prince HM, Lucio MN, Maiolino A, Corso A, Petrucci MT, Musto P, Komarnicki M, Stewart AK (2009) High response rate to bortezomib with or without dexamethasone in patients with relapsed or refractory multiple myeloma: results of a global phase 3b expanded access program. Br J Haematol 144:169–175
113. Richardson PG, Sonneveld P, Schuster MW, Stadtmauer EA, Facon T, Harousseau JL, Ben-Yehuda D, Lonial S, Goldschmidt H, Reece D, Blade J, Boccadoro M, Cavenagh JD, Boral AL, Esseltine DL, Wen PY, Amato AA, Anderson KC, San Miguel J (2009) Reversibility of symptomatic peripheral neuropathy with bortezomib in the phase III APEX trial in relapsed multiple myeloma: impact of a dose-modification guideline. Br J Haematol 144:895–903
114. San Miguel JF, Schlag R, Khuageva NK, Dimopoulos MA, Shpilberg O, Kropff M, Spicka I, Petrucci MT, Palumbo A, Samoilova OS, Dmoszynska A, Abdulkadyrov KM, Schots R, Jiang B, Mateos MV, Anderson KC, Esseltine DL, Liu K, Cakana A, van de Velde H, Richardson PG, Investigators VT (2008) Bortezomib plus melphalan and prednisone for initial treatment of multiple myeloma. N Engl J Med 359:906–917
115. Mateos MV, Richardson PG, Schlag R, Khuageva NK, Dimopoulos MA, Shpilberg O, Kropff M, Spicka I, Petrucci MT, Palumbo A, Samoilova OS, Dmoszynska A, Abdulkadyrov KM, Schots R, Jiang B, Esseltine DL, Liu K, Cakana A, van de Velde H, San Miguel JF (2010) Bortezomib plus melphalan and prednisone compared with melphalan and prednisone in previously untreated multiple myeloma: updated follow-up and impact of subsequent therapy in the phase III VISTA trial. J Clin Oncol 28:2259–2266
116. Potts BC, Albitar MX, Anderson KC, Baritaki S, Berkers C, Bonavida B, Chandra J, Chauhan D, Cusack JC Jr, Fenical W, Ghobrial IM, Groll M, Jensen PR, Lam KS, Lloyd GK, McBride W, McConkey DJ, Miller CP, Neuteboom ST, Oki Y, Ovaa H, Pajonk F, Richardson PG, Roccaro AM, Sloss CM, Spear MA, Valashi E, Younes A, Palladino MA (2011) Marizomib, a proteasome inhibitor for all seasons: preclinical profile and a framework for clinical trials. Curr Cancer Drug Targets 11:254–284
117. Kuhn DJ, Orlowski RZ, Bjorklund CC (2011) Second generation proteasome inhibitors: carfilzomib and immunoproteasome-specific inhibitors (IPSIs). Curr Cancer Drug Targets 11:285–295
118. Chen D, Frezza M, Schmitt S, Kanwar J, Dou QP (2011) Bortezomib as the first proteasome inhibitor anticancer drug: current status and future perspectives. Curr Cancer Drug Targets 11:239–253
119. Kuhn DJ, Chen Q, Voorhees PM, Strader JS, Shenk KD, Sun CM, Demo SD, Bennett MK, van Leeuwen FW, Chanan-Khan AA, Orlowski RZ (2007) Potent activity of carfilzomib, a novel, irreversible inhibitor of the ubiquitin-proteasome pathway, against preclinical models of multiple myeloma. Blood 110:3281–3290
120. Parlati F, Lee SJ, Aujay M, Suzuki E, Levitsky K, Lorens JB, Micklem DR, Ruurs P, Sylvain C, Lu Y, Shenk KD, Bennett MK (2009) Carfilzomib can induce tumor cell death through selective inhibition of the chymotrypsin-like activity of the proteasome. Blood 114:3439–3447
121. Demo SD, Kirk CJ, Aujay MA, Buchholz TJ, Dajee M, Ho MN, Jiang J, Laidig GJ, Lewis ER, Parlati F, Shenk KD, Smyth MS, Sun CM, Vallone MK, Woo TM, Molineaux CJ, Bennett MK (2007) Antitumor activity of PR-171, a novel irreversible inhibitor of the proteasome. Cancer Res 67:6383–6391

122. Alsina M, Trudel S, Furman RR, Rosen PJ, O'Connor OA, Comenzo RL, Wong A, Kunkel LA, Molineaux CJ, Goy A (2012) A phase I single-agent study of twice-weekly consecutive-day dosing of the proteasome inhibitor carfilzomib in patients with relapsed or refractory multiple myeloma or lymphoma. Clin Cancer Res 18:4830–4840
123. O'Connor OA, Stewart AK, Vallone M, Molineaux CJ, Kunkel LA, Gerecitano JF, Orlowski RZ (2009) A phase 1 dose escalation study of the safety and pharmacokinetics of the novel proteasome inhibitor carfilzomib (PR-171) in patients with hematologic malignancies. Clin Cancer Res 15:7085–7091
124. Papadopoulos KP, Burris HA III, Gordon M, Lee P, Sausville EA, Rosen PJ, Patnaik A, Cutler RE Jr, Wang Z, Lee S, Jones SF, Infante JR (2013) A phase I/II study of carfilzomib 2-10-min infusion in patients with advanced solid tumors. Cancer Chemother Pharmacol 72:861–868
125. Jakubowiak AJ, Dytfeld D, Griffith KA, Lebovic D, Vesole DH, Jagannath S, Al-Zoubi A, Anderson T, Nordgren B, Detweiler-Short K, Stockerl-Goldstein K, Ahmed A, Jobkar T, Durecki DE, McDonnell K, Mietzel M, Couriel D, Kaminski M, Vij R (2012) A phase 1/2 study of carfilzomib in combination with lenalidomide and low-dose dexamethasone as a frontline treatment for multiple myeloma. Blood 120:1801–1809
126. Jagannath S, Vij R, Stewart AK, Trudel S, Jakubowiak AJ, Reiman T, Somlo G, Bahlis N, Lonial S, Kunkel LA, Wong A, Orlowski RZ, Siegel DS (2012) An open-label single-arm pilot phase II study (PX-171-003-A0) of low-dose, single-agent carfilzomib in patients with relapsed and refractory multiple myeloma. Clin Lymphoma Myeloma Leuk 12:310–318
127. Siegel DS, Martin T, Wang M, Vij R, Jakubowiak AJ, Lonial S, Trudel S, Kukreti V, Bahlis N, Alsina M, Chanan-Khan A, Buadi F, Reu FJ, Somlo G, Zonder J, Song K, Stewart AK, Stadtmauer E, Kunkel L, Wear S, Wong AF, Orlowski RZ, Jagannath S (2012) A phase 2 study of single-agent carfilzomib (PX-171-003-A1) in patients with relapsed and refractory multiple myeloma. Blood 120:2817–2825
128. Hajek R, Bryce R, Ro S, Klencke B, Ludwig H (2012) Design and rationale of FOCUS (PX-171-011): a randomized, open-label, phase 3 study of carfilzomib versus best supportive care regimen in patients with relapsed and refractory multiple myeloma (R/R MM). BMC Cancer 12:415
129. Cortes J, Thomas D, Koller C, Giles F, Estey E, Faderl S, Garcia-Manero G, McConkey D, Ruiz SL, Guerciolini R, Wright J, Kantarjian H (2004) Phase I study of bortezomib in refractory or relapsed acute leukemias. Clin Cancer Res 10:3371–3376
130. Dispenzieri A, Jacobus S, Vesole DH, Callandar N, Fonseca R, Greipp PR (2010) Primary therapy with single agent bortezomib as induction, maintenance and re-induction in patients with high-risk myeloma: results of the ECOG E2A02 trial. Leukemia 24:1406–1411
131. Oerlemans R, Franke NE, Assaraf YG, Cloos J, van Zantwijk I, Berkers CR, Scheffer GL, Debipersad K, Vojtekova K, Lemos C, van der Heijden JW, Ylstra B, Peters GJ, Kaspers GL, Dijkmans BA, Scheper RJ, Jansen G (2008) Molecular basis of bortezomib resistance: proteasome subunit beta5 (PSMB5) gene mutation and overexpression of PSMB5 protein. Blood 112:2489–2499
132. Lu S, Yang J, Chen Z, Gong S, Zhou H, Xu X, Wang J (2009) Different mutants of PSMB5 confer varying bortezomib resistance in T lymphoblastic lymphoma/leukemia cells derived from the Jurkat cell line. Exp Hematol 37:831–837
133. Ruschak AM, Slassi M, Kay LE, Schimmer AD (2011) Novel proteasome inhibitors to overcome bortezomib resistance. J Natl Cancer Inst 103:1007–1017
134. Politou M, Karadimitris A, Terpos E, Kotsianidis I, Apperley JF, Rahemtulla A (2006) No evidence of mutations of the PSMB5 (beta-5 subunit of proteasome) in a case of myeloma with clinical resistance to Bortezomib. Leuk Res 30:240–241
135. Takayama S, Reed JC, Homma S (2003) Heat-shock proteins as regulators of apoptosis. Oncogene 22:9041–9047
136. Beere HM (2004) "The stress of dying": the role of heat shock proteins in the regulation of apoptosis. J Cell Sci 117:2641–2651

137. Zhou M, Wu X, Ginsberg HN (1996) Evidence that a rapidly turning over protein, normally degraded by proteasomes, regulates hsp72 gene transcription in HepG2 cells. J Biol Chem 271:24769–24775
138. Bush KT, Goldberg AL, Nigam SK (1997) Proteasome inhibition leads to a heat-shock response, induction of endoplasmic reticulum chaperones, and thermotolerance. J Biol Chem 272:9086–9092
139. Meriin AB, Gabai VL, Yaglom J, Shifrin VI, Sherman MY (1998) Proteasome inhibitors activate stress kinases and induce Hsp72. Diverse effects on apoptosis. J Biol Chem 273:6373–6379
140. Robertson JD, Datta K, Biswal SS, Kehrer JP (1999) Heat-shock protein 70 antisense oligomers enhance proteasome inhibitor-induced apoptosis. Biochem J 344(Pt 2):477–485
141. Gabai VL, Budagova KR, Sherman MY (2005) Increased expression of the major heat shock protein Hsp72 in human prostate carcinoma cells is dispensable for their viability but confers resistance to a variety of anticancer agents. Oncogene 24:3328–3338
142. Chauhan D, Li G, Shringarpure R, Podar K, Ohtake Y, Hideshima T, Anderson KC (2003) Blockade of Hsp27 overcomes Bortezomib/proteasome inhibitor PS-341 resistance in lymphoma cells. Cancer Res 63:6174–6177
143. Shringarpure R, Catley L, Bhole D, Burger R, Podar K, Tai YT, Kessler B, Galardy P, Ploegh H, Tassone P, Hideshima T, Mitsiades C, Munshi NC, Chauhan D, Anderson KC (2006) Gene expression analysis of B-lymphoma cells resistant and sensitive to bortezomib. Br J Haematol 134:145–156
144. Hideshima T, Podar K, Chauhan D, Ishitsuka K, Mitsiades C, Tai YT, Hamasaki M, Raje N, Hideshima H, Schreiner G, Nguyen AN, Navas T, Munshi NC, Richardson PG, Higgins LS, Anderson KC (2004) p38 MAPK inhibition enhances PS-341 (bortezomib)-induced cytotoxicity against multiple myeloma cells. Oncogene 23:8766–8776
145. Hosokawa N, Hirayoshi K, Nakai A, Hosokawa Y, Marui N, Yoshida M, Sakai T, Nishino H, Aoike A, Kawai K et al (1990) Flavonoids inhibit the expression of heat shock proteins. Cell Struct Funct 15:393–401
146. Aghdassi A, Phillips P, Dudeja V, Dhaulakhandi D, Sharif R, Dawra R, Lerch MM, Saluja A (2007) Heat shock protein 70 increases tumorigenicity and inhibits apoptosis in pancreatic adenocarcinoma. Cancer Res 67:616–625
147. Mimnaugh EG, Xu W, Vos M, Yuan X, Isaacs JS, Bisht KS, Gius D, Neckers L (2004) Simultaneous inhibition of hsp 90 and the proteasome promotes protein ubiquitination, causes endoplasmic reticulum-derived cytosolic vacuolization, and enhances antitumor activity. Mol Cancer Ther 3:551–566
148. Mitsiades CS, Mitsiades NS, McMullan CJ, Poulaki V, Kung AL, Davies FE, Morgan G, Akiyama M, Shringarpure R, Munshi NC, Richardson PG, Hideshima T, Chauhan D, Gu X, Bailey C, Joseph M, Libermann TA, Rosen NS, Anderson KC (2006) Antimyeloma activity of heat shock protein-90 inhibition. Blood 107:1092–1100
149. Davenport EL, Moore HE, Dunlop AS, Sharp SY, Workman P, Morgan GJ, Davies FE (2007) Heat shock protein inhibition is associated with activation of the unfolded protein response pathway in myeloma plasma cells. Blood 110:2641–2649
150. Nawrocki ST, Carew JS, Dunner K Jr, Boise LH, Chiao PJ, Huang P, Abbruzzese JL, McConkey DJ (2005) Bortezomib inhibits PKR-like endoplasmic reticulum (ER) kinase and induces apoptosis via ER stress in human pancreatic cancer cells. Cancer Res 65:11510–11519
151. Tan TT, Degenhardt K, Nelson DA, Beaudoin B, Nieves-Neira W, Bouillet P, Villunger A, Adams JM, White E (2005) Key roles of BIM-driven apoptosis in epithelial tumors and rational chemotherapy. Cancer Cell 7:227–238
152. Mestre-Escorihuela C, Rubio-Moscardo F, Richter JA, Siebert R, Climent J, Fresquet V, Beltran E, Agirre X, Marugan I, Marin M, Rosenwald A, Sugimoto KJ, Wheat LM, Karran EL, Garcia JF, Sanchez L, Prosper F, Staudt LM, Pinkel D, Dyer MJ, Martinez-Climent JA (2007) Homozygous deletions localize novel tumor suppressor genes in B-cell lymphomas. Blood 109:271–280

153. Lee SH, Soung YH, Lee JW, Kim HS, Lee JH, Kim HS, Lee JH, Park JY, Cho YG, Kim CJ, Kim SY, Park WS, Kim SH, Lee JY, Yoo NJ (2003) Mutational analysis of Noxa gene in human cancers. Acta Pathol Microbiol Immunol Scand 111:599–604
154. Xiao C, Srinivasan L, Calado DP, Patterson HC, Zhang B, Wang J, Henderson JM, Kutok JL, Rajewsky K (2008) Lymphoproliferative disease and autoimmunity in mice with increased miR-17-92 expression in lymphocytes. Nat Immunol 9:405–414
155. Wang Z, Zhang B, Yang L, Ding J, Ding HF (2008) Constitutive production of NF-kappaB2 p52 is not tumorigenic but predisposes mice to inflammatory autoimmune disease by repressing Bim expression. J Biol Chem 283:10698–10706
156. Yamashita M, Kuwahara M, Suzuki A, Hirahara K, Shinnaksu R, Hosokawa H, Hasegawa A, Motohashi S, Iwama A, Nakayama T (2008) Bmi1 regulates memory CD4 T cell survival via repression of the Noxa gene. J Exp Med 205:1109–1120
157. Letai A, Bassik MC, Walensky LD, Sorcinelli MD, Weiler S, Korsmeyer SJ (2002) Distinct BH3 domains either sensitize or activate mitochondrial apoptosis, serving as prototype cancer therapeutics. Cancer Cell 2:183–192
158. Chauhan D, Velankar M, Brahmandam M, Hideshima T, Podar K, Richardson P, Schlossman R, Ghobrial I, Raje N, Munshi N, Anderson KC (2007) A novel Bcl-2/Bcl-X(L)/Bcl-w inhibitor ABT-737 as therapy in multiple myeloma. Oncogene 26:2374–2380
159. Nguyen M, Marcellus RC, Roulston A, Watson M, Serfass L, Murthy Madiraju SR, Goulet D, Viallet J, Belec L, Billot X, Acoca S, Purisima E, Wiegmans A, Cluse L, Johnstone RW, Beauparlant P, Shore GC (2007) Small molecule obatoclax (GX15-070) antagonizes MCL-1 and overcomes MCL-1-mediated resistance to apoptosis. Proc Natl Acad Sci U S A 104: 19512–19517
160. Paoluzzi L, Gonen M, Bhagat G, Furman RR, Gardner JR, Scotto L, Gueorguiev VD, Heaney ML, Manova K, O'Connor OA (2008) The BH3-only mimetic ABT-737 synergizes the antineoplastic activity of proteasome inhibitors in lymphoid malignancies. Blood 112:2906–2916
161. Williams SA, McConkey DJ (2003) The proteasome inhibitor bortezomib stabilizes a novel active form of p53 in human LNCaP-Pro5 prostate cancer cells. Cancer Res 63:7338–7344
162. Yang G, Ayala G, De Marzo A, Tian W, Frolov A, Wheeler TM, Thompson TC, Harper JW (2002) Elevated Skp2 protein expression in human prostate cancer: association with loss of the cyclin-dependent kinase inhibitor p27 and PTEN and with reduced recurrence-free survival. Clin Cancer Res 8:3419–3426
163. Worm J, Bartkova J, Kirkin AF, Straten P, Zeuthen J, Bartek J, Guldberg P (2000) Aberrant p27Kip1 promoter methylation in malignant melanoma. Oncogene 19:5111–5115
164. Shin I, Yakes FM, Rojo F, Shin NY, Bakin AV, Baselga J, Arteaga CL (2002) PKB/Akt mediates cell-cycle progression by phosphorylation of p27(Kip1) at threonine 157 and modulation of its cellular localization. Nat Med 8:1145–1152
165. Ogino S, Kawasaki T, Ogawa A, Kirkner GJ, Loda M, Fuchs CS (2007) Cytoplasmic localization of p27 (cyclin-dependent kinase inhibitor 1B/KIP1) in colorectal cancer: inverse correlations with nuclear p27 loss, microsatellite instability, and CpG island methylator phenotype. Hum Pathol 38:585–592
166. Ma YY, Wei SJ, Lin YC, Lung JC, Chang TC, Whang-Peng J, Liu JM, Yang DM, Yang WK, Shen CY (2000) PIK3CA as an oncogene in cervical cancer. Oncogene 19:2739–2744
167. Osaki M, Oshimura M, Ito H (2004) PI3K-Akt pathway: its functions and alterations in human cancer. Apoptosis 9:667–676
168. Thompson JE, Thompson CB (2004) Putting the rap on Akt. J Clin Oncol 22:4217–4226
169. Cantley LC, Neel BG (1999) New insights into tumor suppression: PTEN suppresses tumor formation by restraining the phosphoinositide 3-kinase/AKT pathway. Proc Natl Acad Sci U S A 96:4240–4245
170. Guerrero S, Casanova I, Farre L, Mazo A, Capella G, Mangues R (2000) K-ras codon 12 mutation induces higher level of resistance to apoptosis and predisposition to anchorage-independent growth than codon 13 mutation or proto-oncogene overexpression. Cancer Res 60:6750–6756

171. Shi Y, Yan H, Frost P, Gera J, Lichtenstein A (2005) Mammalian target of rapamycin inhibitors activate the AKT kinase in multiple myeloma cells by up-regulating the insulin-like growth factor receptor/insulin receptor substrate-1/phosphatidylinositol 3-kinase cascade. Mol Cancer Ther 4:1533–1540
172. Yu C, Friday BB, Lai JP, Yang L, Sarkaria J, Kay NE, Carter CA, Roberts LR, Kaufmann SH, Adjei AA (2006) Cytotoxic synergy between the multikinase inhibitor sorafenib and the proteasome inhibitor bortezomib in vitro: induction of apoptosis through Akt and c-Jun NH2-terminal kinase pathways. Mol Cancer Ther 5:2378–2387
173. Shi YY, Small GW, Orlowski RZ (2006) Proteasome inhibitors induce a p38 mitogen-activated protein kinase (MAPK)-dependent anti-apoptotic program involving MAPK phosphatase-1 and Akt in models of breast cancer. Breast Cancer Res Treat 100:33–47
174. Moreau AS, Jia X, Ngo HT, Leleu X, O'Sullivan G, Alsayed Y, Leontovich A, Podar K, Kutok J, Daley J, Lazo-Kallanian S, Hatjiharissi E, Raab MS, Xu L, Treon SP, Hideshima T, Anderson KC, Ghobrial IM (2007) Protein kinase C inhibitor enzastaurin induces in vitro and in vivo antitumor activity in Waldenstrom macroglobulinemia. Blood 109:4964–4972
175. Shrader M, Pino MS, Lashinger L, Bar-Eli M, Adam L, Dinney CP, McConkey DJ (2007) Gefitinib reverses TRAIL resistance in human bladder cancer cell lines via inhibition of AKT-mediated X-linked inhibitor of apoptosis protein expression. Cancer Res 67:1430–1435
176. Cascone T, Morelli MP, Morgillo F, Kim WY, Rodolico G, Pepe S, Tortora G, Berrino L, Lee HY, Heymach JV, Ciardiello F (2008) Synergistic anti-proliferative and pro-apoptotic activity of combined therapy with bortezomib, a proteasome inhibitor, with anti-epidermal growth factor receptor (EGFR) drugs in human cancer cells. J Cell Physiol 216:698–707
177. An J, Rettig MB (2007) Epidermal growth factor receptor inhibition sensitizes renal cell carcinoma cells to the cytotoxic effects of bortezomib. Mol Cancer Ther 6:61–69
178. Rajkumar SV, Richardson PG, Hideshima T, Anderson KC (2005) Proteasome inhibition as a novel therapeutic target in human cancer. J Clin Oncol 23:630–639
179. Siegel DS (2012) Relapsed/refractory multiple myeloma: defining refractory disease and identifying strategies to overcome resistance. Semin Hematol 49(Suppl 1):S3–S15
180. Wang X, Li C, Ju S, Wang Y, Wang H, Zhong R (2011) Myeloma cell adhesion to bone marrow stromal cells confers drug resistance by microRNA-21 up-regulation. Leuk Lymphoma 52:1991–1998
181. Zang MR, Li F, An G, Xie ZQ, Li CH, Yu Z, Xu Y, Qiu LG, Hao M (2012) Regulation of miRNA-15a/-16 expression on the drug resistance of myeloma cells. Zhonghua Yi Xue Za Zhi 92:1100–1103
182. Bataille R, Robillard N, Avet-Loiseau H, Harousseau JL, Moreau P (2005) CD221 (IGF-1R) is aberrantly expressed in multiple myeloma, in relation to disease severity. Haematologica 90:706–707
183. Chng WJ, Gualberto A, Fonseca R (2006) IGF-1R is overexpressed in poor-prognostic subtypes of multiple myeloma. Leukemia 20:174–176
184. Kuhn DJ, Berkova Z, Jones RJ, Woessner R, Bjorklund CC, Ma W, Davis RE, Lin P, Wang H, Madden TL, Wei C, Baladandayuthapani V, Wang M, Thomas SK, Shah JJ, Weber DM, Orlowski RZ (2012) Targeting the insulin-like growth factor-1 receptor to overcome bortezomib resistance in preclinical models of multiple myeloma. Blood 120:3260–3270
185. Que W, Chen J, Chuang M, Jiang D (2012) Knockdown of c-Met enhances sensitivity to bortezomib in human multiple myeloma U266 cells via inhibiting Akt/mTOR activity. Acta Pathol Microbiol Immunol Scand 120:195–203
186. Kim A, Park S, Lee JE, Jang WS, Lee SJ, Kang HJ, Lee SS (2012) The dual PI3K and mTOR inhibitor NVP-BEZ235 exhibits anti-proliferative activity and overcomes bortezomib resistance in mantle cell lymphoma cells. Leuk Res 36:912–920
187. Yeom SY, Lee SJ, Kim WS, Park C (2012) Rad knockdown induces mitochondrial apoptosis in bortezomib resistant leukemia and lymphoma cells. Leuk Res 36:1172–1178
188. Levine B, Yuan J (2005) Autophagy in cell death: an innocent convict? J Clin Invest 115: 2679–2688

189. Yang W, Monroe J, Zhang Y, George D, Bremer E, Li H (2006) Proteasome inhibition induces both pro- and anti-cell death pathways in prostate cancer cells. Cancer Lett 243:217–227
190. Ding WX, Ni HM, Gao W, Yoshimori T, Stolz DB, Ron D, Yin XM (2007) Linking of autophagy to ubiquitin-proteasome system is important for the regulation of endoplasmic reticulum stress and cell viability. Am J Pathol 171:513–524
191. Hideshima T, Bradner JE, Chauhan D, Anderson KC (2005) Intracellular protein degradation and its therapeutic implications. Clin Cancer Res 11:8530–8533
192. Nawrocki ST, Carew JS, Pino MS, Highshaw RA, Andtbacka RH, Dunner K Jr, Pal A, Bornmann WG, Chiao PJ, Huang P, Xiong H, Abbruzzese JL, McConkey DJ (2006) Aggresome disruption: a novel strategy to enhance bortezomib-induced apoptosis in pancreatic cancer cells. Cancer Res 66:3773–3781
193. Badros A, Burger AM, Philip S, Niesvizky R, Kolla SS, Goloubeva O, Harris C, Zwiebel J, Wright JJ, Espinoza-Delgado I, Baer MR, Holleran JL, Egorin MJ, Grant S (2009) Phase I study of vorinostat in combination with bortezomib for relapsed and refractory multiple myeloma. Clin Cancer Res 15:5250–5257
194. Nerini-Molteni S, Ferrarini M, Cozza S, Caligaris-Cappio F, Sitia R (2008) Redox homeostasis modulates the sensitivity of myeloma cells to bortezomib. Br J Haematol 141:494–503
195. Uehara T, Nakamura T, Yao D, Shi ZQ, Gu Z, Ma Y, Masliah E, Nomura Y, Lipton SA (2006) S-nitrosylated protein-disulphide isomerase links protein misfolding to neurodegeneration. Nature 441:513–517
196. Kalivendi SV, Cunningham S, Kotamraju S, Joseph J, Hillard CJ, Kalyanaraman B (2004) Alpha-synuclein up-regulation and aggregation during MPP+-induced apoptosis in neuroblastoma cells: intermediacy of transferrin receptor iron and hydrogen peroxide. J Biol Chem 279:15240–15247
197. Keller JN, Huang FF, Zhu H, Yu J, Ho YS, Kindy TS (2000) Oxidative stress-associated impairment of proteasome activity during ischemia-reperfusion injury. J Cereb Blood Flow Metab 20:1467–1473
198. Catley L, Anderson KC (2006) Velcade and vitamin C: too much of a good thing? Clin Cancer Res 12:3–4
199. Zou W, Yue P, Lin N, He M, Zhou Z, Lonial S, Khuri FR, Wang B, Sun SY (2006) Vitamin C inactivates the proteasome inhibitor PS-341 in human cancer cells. Clin Cancer Res 12:273–280
200. Kupperman E, Lee EC, Cao Y, Bannerman B, Fitzgerald M, Berger A, Yu J, Yang Y, Hales P, Bruzzese F, Liu J, Blank J, Garcia K, Tsu C, Dick L, Fleming P, Yu L, Manfredi M, Rolfe M, Bolen J (2010) Evaluation of the proteasome inhibitor MLN9708 in preclinical models of human cancer. Cancer Res 70:1970–1980
201. Lee EC, Fitzgerald M, Bannerman B, Donelan J, Bano K, Terkelsen J, Bradley DP, Subakan O, Silva MD, Liu R, Pickard M, Li Z, Tayber O, Li P, Hales P, Carsillo M, Neppalli VT, Berger AJ, Kupperman E, Manfredi M, Bolen JB, Van Ness B, Janz S (2011) Antitumor activity of the investigational proteasome inhibitor MLN9708 in mouse models of B-cell and plasma cell malignancies. Clin Cancer Res 17:7313–7323
202. Sanchez E, Li M, Steinberg JA, Wang C, Shen J, Bonavida B, Li ZW, Chen H, Berenson JR (2010) The proteasome inhibitor CEP-18770 enhances the anti-myeloma activity of bortezomib and melphalan. Br J Haematol 148:569–581
203. Zhou HJ, Aujay MA, Bennett MK, Dajee M, Demo SD, Fang Y, Ho MN, Jiang J, Kirk CJ, Laidig GJ, Lewis ER, Lu Y, Muchamuel T, Parlati F, Ring E, Shenk KD, Shields J, Shwonek PJ, Stanton T, Sun CM, Sylvain C, Woo TM, Yang J (2009) Design and synthesis of an orally bioavailable and selective peptide epoxyketone proteasome inhibitor (PR-047). J Med Chem 52:3028–3038
204. Lawasut P, Chauhan D, Laubach J, Hayes C, Fabre C, Maglio M, Mitsiades C, Hideshima T, Anderson KC, Richardson PG (2012) New proteasome inhibitors in myeloma. Curr Hematol Malig Rep 7:258–266
205. Chauhan D, Catley L, Li G, Podar K, Hideshima T, Velankar M, Mitsiades C, Mitsiades N, Yasui H, Letai A, Ovaa H, Berkers C, Nicholson B, Chao TH, Neuteboom ST, Richardson P,

Palladino MA, Anderson KC (2005) A novel orally active proteasome inhibitor induces apoptosis in multiple myeloma cells with mechanisms distinct from Bortezomib. Cancer Cell 8:407–419
206. Fenical W, Jensen PR, Palladino MA, Lam KS, Lloyd GK, Potts BC (2009) Discovery and development of the anticancer agent salinosporamide A (NPI-0052). Bioorg Med Chem 17:2175–2180
207. Chauhan D, Singh A, Brahmandam M, Podar K, Hideshima T, Richardson P, Munshi N, Palladino MA, Anderson KC (2008) Combination of proteasome inhibitors bortezomib and NPI-0052 trigger in vivo synergistic cytotoxicity in multiple myeloma. Blood 111: 1654–1664
208. Chauhan D, Singh AV, Ciccarelli B, Richardson PG, Palladino MA, Anderson KC (2010) Combination of novel proteasome inhibitor NPI-0052 and lenalidomide trigger in vitro and in vivo synergistic cytotoxicity in multiple myeloma. Blood 115:834–845
209. Richardson PG, Chanan-Khan AA, Lonial S, Krishnan AY, Carroll MP, Alsina M, Albitar M, Berman D, Messina M, Anderson KC (2011) Tanespimycin and bortezomib combination treatment in patients with relapsed or relapsed and refractory multiple myeloma: results of a phase 1/2 study. Br J Haematol 153:729–740
210. Kikuchi J, Wada T, Shimizu R, Izumi T, Akutsu M, Mitsunaga K, Noborio-Hatano K, Nobuyoshi M, Ozawa K, Kano Y, Furukawa Y (2010) Histone deacetylases are critical targets of bortezomib-induced cytotoxicity in multiple myeloma. Blood 116:406–417
211. Hideshima T, Bradner JE, Wong J, Chauhan D, Richardson P, Schreiber SL, Anderson KC (2005) Small-molecule inhibition of proteasome and aggresome function induces synergistic antitumor activity in multiple myeloma. Proc Natl Acad Sci U S A 102:8567–8572
212. Santo L, Hideshima T, Kung AL, Tseng J-C, Tamang D, Yang M, Jarpe M, van Duzer JH, Mazitschek R, Cirstea D, Eda H, Scullen TA, Rodig S, Canavese M, Bradner J, Anderson KC, Jones S, Raje NS (2011) Selective HDAC6 inhibition via ACY-1215, either alone or in combination with bortezomib, restores osteoblast function and suppresses osteoclast differentiation in multiple myeloma. ASH Annual Meeting Abstracts 118:2908
213. Weber DM, Jagannath S, Mazumder A, Sobecks R, Schiller GJ, Gavino M, Sumbler C, McFadden C, Chen C, Ricker JL, Rizvi S, Oerth C, Brownell P, Hussein MA (2007) Phase I trial of oral vorinostat (suberoylanilide hydroxamic acid, SAHA) in combination with bortezomib in patients with advanced multiple myeloma. ASH Annual Meeting Abstracts 110:1172
214. Harrison SJ, Quach H, Link E, Seymour JF, Ritchie DS, Ruell S, Dean J, Januszewicz H, Johnstone R, Neeson P, Dickinson M, Nichols J, Prince HM (2011) A high rate of durable responses with romidepsin, bortezomib, and dexamethasone in relapsed or refractory multiple myeloma. Blood 118:6274–6283
215. Siegel DS, Dimopoulos MA, Yoon S-S, Laubach JP, Kaufman JL, Goldschmidt H, Reece DE, Leleu X, Durrant S, Offner FC, Cavo M, Nagler A, Jagannath S, Graef T, Houp J, Sun L, Howe J, Wear SM, Anderson KC (2011) Vantage 095: vorinostat in combination with bortezomib in salvage multiple myeloma patients: final study results of a global phase 2b trial. ASH Annual Meeting Abstracts 118:480
216. Dimopoulos MA, Jagannath S, Yoon S-S, Siegel DS, Lonial S, Hajek R, Facon T, Rosinol L, Blacklock HA, Goldschmidt H, Hungria V, Spencer A, Palumbo A, Reece DE, Graef T, Houp J, Sun L, Eid JE, Anderson KC (2011) Vantage 088: vorinostat in combination with bortezomib in patients with relapsed/refractory multiple myeloma: results of a global, randomized phase 3 trial. ASH Annual Meeting Abstracts 118:811
217. Heink S, Ludwig D, Kloetzel PM, Kruger E (2005) IFN-gamma-induced immune adaptation of the proteasome system is an accelerated and transient response. Proc Natl Acad Sci U S A 102:9241–9246
218. Kloetzel PM (2004) The proteasome and MHC class I antigen processing. Biochim Biophys Acta 1695:225–233
219. Noda C, Tanahashi N, Shimbara N, Hendil KB, Tanaka K (2000) Tissue distribution of constitutive proteasomes, immunoproteasomes, and PA28 in rats. Biochem Biophys Res Commun 277:348–354

220. Strehl B, Seifert U, Kruger E, Heink S, Kuckelkorn U, Kloetzel PM (2005) Interferon-gamma, the functional plasticity of the ubiquitin-proteasome system, and MHC class I antigen processing. Immunol Rev 207:19–30
221. Rivett AJ, Hearn AR (2004) Proteasome function in antigen presentation: immunoproteasome complexes, Peptide production, and interactions with viral proteins. Curr Protein Pept Sci 5:153–161
222. Gaczynska M, Rock KL, Goldberg AL (1993) Gamma-interferon and expression of MHC genes regulate peptide hydrolysis by proteasomes. Nature 365:264–267
223. Kuhn DJ, Orlowski RZ (2012) The immunoproteasome as a target in hematologic malignancies. Semin Hematol 49:258–262
224. Kuhn DJ, Hunsucker SA, Chen Q, Voorhees PM, Orlowski M, Orlowski RZ (2009) Targeted inhibition of the immunoproteasome is a potent strategy against models of multiple myeloma that overcomes resistance to conventional drugs and nonspecific proteasome inhibitors. Blood 113:4667–4676
225. Singh AV, Bandi M, Aujay MA, Kirk CJ, Hark DE, Raje N, Chauhan D, Anderson KC (2011) PR-924, a selective inhibitor of the immunoproteasome subunit LMP-7, blocks multiple myeloma cell growth both in vitro and in vivo. Br J Haematol 152:155–163
226. Muchamuel T, Basler M, Aujay MA, Suzuki E, Kalim KW, Lauer C, Sylvain C, Ring ER, Shields J, Jiang J, Shwonek P, Parlati F, Demo SD, Bennett MK, Kirk CJ, Groettrup M (2009) A selective inhibitor of the immunoproteasome subunit LMP7 blocks cytokine production and attenuates progression of experimental arthritis. Nat Med 15:781–787
227. Ho YK, Bargagna-Mohan P, Wehenkel M, Mohan R, Kim KB (2007) LMP2-specific inhibitors: chemical genetic tools for proteasome biology. Chem Biol 14:419–430
228. Sekizawa R, Ikeno S, Nakamura H, Naganawa H, Matsui S, Iinuma H, Takeuchi T (2002) Panepophenanthrin, from a mushroom strain, a novel inhibitor of the ubiquitin-activating enzyme. J Nat Prod 65:1491–1493
229. Tsukamoto S, Hirota H, Imachi M, Fujimuro M, Onuki H, Ohta T, Yokosawa H (2005) Himeic acid A: a new ubiquitin-activating enzyme inhibitor isolated from a marine-derived fungus, Aspergillus sp. Bioorg Med Chem Lett 15:191–194
230. Yang Y, Kitagaki J, Dai RM, Tsai YC, Lorick KL, Ludwig RL, Pierre SA, Jensen JP, Davydov IV, Oberoi P, Li CC, Kenten JH, Beutler JA, Vousden KH, Weissman AM (2007) Inhibitors of ubiquitin-activating enzyme (E1), a new class of potential cancer therapeutics. Cancer Res 67:9472–9481
231. Xu GW, Ali M, Wood TE, Wong D, Maclean N, Wang X, Gronda M, Skrtic M, Li X, Hurren R, Mao X, Venkatesan M, Beheshti Zavareh R, Ketela T, Reed JC, Rose D, Moffat J, Batey RA, Dhe-Paganon S, Schimmer AD (2010) The ubiquitin-activating enzyme E1 as a therapeutic target for the treatment of leukemia and multiple myeloma. Blood 115:2251–2259
232. Ungermannova D, Parker SJ, Nasveschuk CG, Chapnick DA, Phillips AJ, Kuchta RD, Liu X (2012) Identification and mechanistic studies of a novel ubiquitin E1 inhibitor. J Biomol Screen 17:421–434
233. Laine A, Topisirovic I, Zhai D, Reed JC, Borden KL, Ronai Z (2006) Regulation of p53 localization and activity by Ubc13. Mol Cell Biol 26:8901–8913
234. Tsukamoto S, Takeuchi T, Rotinsulu H, Mangindaan RE, van Soest RW, Ukai K, Kobayashi H, Namikoshi M, Ohta T, Yokosawa H (2008) Leucettamol A: a new inhibitor of Ubc13-Uev1A interaction isolated from a marine sponge, Leucetta aff. microrhaphis. Bioorg Med Chem Lett 18:6319–6320
235. Vassilev LT (2007) MDM2 inhibitors for cancer therapy. Trends Mol Med 13:23–31
236. Vassilev LT, Vu BT, Graves B, Carvajal D, Podlaski F, Filipovic Z, Kong N, Kammlott U, Lukacs C, Klein C, Fotouhi N, Liu EA (2004) In vivo activation of the p53 pathway by small-molecule antagonists of MDM2. Science 303:844–848
237. Ooi MG, Hayden PJ, Kotoula V, McMillin DW, Charalambous E, Daskalaki E, Raje NS, Munshi NC, Chauhan D, Hideshima T, Buon L, Clynes M, O'Gorman P, Richardson PG, Mitsiades CS, Anderson KC, Mitsiades N (2009) Interactions of the Hdm2/p53 and proteasome pathways may enhance the antitumor activity of bortezomib. Clin Cancer Res 15: 7153–7160

238. Duncan SJ, Gruschow S, Williams DH, McNicholas C, Purewal R, Hajek M, Gerlitz M, Martin S, Wrigley SK, Moore M (2001) Isolation and structure elucidation of Chlorofusin, a novel p53-MDM2 antagonist from a Fusarium sp. J Am Chem Soc 123:554–560
239. Clark RC, Lee SY, Boger DL (2008) Total synthesis of chlorofusin, its seven chromophore diastereomers, and key partial structures. J Am Chem Soc 130:12355–12369
240. Tsukamoto S, Yoshida T, Hosono H, Ohta T, Yokosawa H (2006) Hexylitaconic acid: a new inhibitor of p53-HDM2 interaction isolated from a marine-derived fungus, Arthrinium sp. Bioorg Med Chem Lett 16:69–71
241. Nakahashi A, Miura N, Monde K, Tsukamoto S (2009) Stereochemical studies of hexylitaconic acid, an inhibitor of p53-HDM2 interaction. Bioorg Med Chem Lett 19:3027–3030
242. Kona FR, Buac D, Burger A (2011) Disulfiram, and disulfiram derivatives as novel potential anticancer drugs targeting the ubiquitin-proteasome system in both preclinical and clinical studies. Curr Cancer Drug Targets 11:338–346
243. Lim HS, Archer CT, Kodadek T (2007) Identification of a peptoid inhibitor of the proteasome 19S regulatory particle. J Am Chem Soc 129:7750–7751
244. Lim HS, Cai D, Archer CT, Kodadek T (2007) Periodate-triggered cross-linking reveals Sug2/Rpt4 as the molecular target of a peptoid inhibitor of the 19S proteasome regulatory particle. J Am Chem Soc 129:12936–12937
245. Verma R, Peters NR, D'Onofrio M, Tochtrop GP, Sakamoto KM, Varadan R, Zhang M, Coffino P, Fushman D, Deshaies RJ, King RW (2004) Ubistatins inhibit proteasome-dependent degradation by binding the ubiquitin chain. Science 306:117–120
246. D'Arcy P, Linder S (2012) Proteasome deubiquitinases as novel targets for cancer therapy. Int J Biochem Cell Biol 44:1729–1738
247. Kuo SM, Huang CT, Blum P, Chang C (2001) Quercetin cumulatively enhances copper induction of metallothionein in intestinal cells. Biol Trace Elem Res 84:1–10
248. Rizk SL, Sky-Peck HH (1984) Comparison between concentrations of trace elements in normal and neoplastic human breast tissue. Cancer Res 44:5390–5394
249. Turecky L, Kalina P, Uhlikova E, Namerova S, Krizko J (1984) Serum ceruloplasmin and copper levels in patients with primary brain tumors. Klin Wochenschr 62:187–189
250. Nayak SB, Bhat VR, Upadhyay D, Udupa SL (2003) Copper and ceruloplasmin status in serum of prostate and colon cancer patients. Indian J Physiol Pharmacol 47:108–110
251. Diez M, Arroyo M, Cerdan FJ, Munoz M, Martin MA, Balibrea JL (1989) Serum and tissue trace metal levels in lung cancer. Oncology 46:230–234
252. Habib FK, Dembinski TC, Stitch SR (1980) The zinc and copper content of blood leucocytes and plasma from patients with benign and malignant prostates. Clin Chim Acta 104: 329–335
253. Gupta SK, Singh SP, Shukla VK (2005) Copper, zinc, and Cu/Zn ratio in carcinoma of the gallbladder. J Surg Oncol 91:204–208
254. Chakravarty PK, Ghosh A, Chowdhury JR (1986) Zinc in human malignancies. Neoplasma 33:85–90
255. Margalioth EJ, Schenker JG, Chevion M (1983) Copper and zinc levels in normal and malignant tissues. Cancer 52:868–872
256. Schwartz AE, Leddicotte GW, Fink RW, Friedman EW (1974) Trace elements in noraml and malignant human breast tissue. Surgery 76:325–329
257. Wong E, Giandomenico CM (1999) Current status of platinum-based antitumor drugs. Chem Rev 99:2451–2466
258. Galanski M, Arion VB, Jakupec MA, Keppler BK (2003) Recent developments in the field of tumor-inhibiting metal complexes. Curr Pharm Des 9:2078–2089
259. Galanski M, Jakupec MA, Keppler BK (2005) Update of the preclinical situation of anticancer platinum complexes: novel design strategies and innovative analytical approaches. Curr Med Chem 12:2075–2094
260. Forestier J (1935) Rheumatoid arthritis and its treatment with gold salts. The results of six years' experience. J Lab Clin Med 20:827–840
261. Tiekink ER (2003) Phosphinegold(I) thiolates—pharmacological use and potential. Bioinorg Chem Appl 1(1):53–67

262. Mirabelli CK, Johnson RK, Hill DT, Faucette LF, Girard GR, Kuo GY, Sung CM, Crooke ST (1986) Correlation of the in vitro cytotoxic and in vivo antitumor activities of gold(I) coordination complexes. J Med Chem 29:218–223
263. Milacic V, Fregona D, Dou QP (2008) Gold complexes as prospective metal-based anticancer drugs. Histol Histopathol 23:101–108
264. Ronconi L, Giovagnini L, Marzano C, Bettio F, Graziani R, Pilloni G, Fregona D (2005) Gold dithiocarbamate derivatives as potential antineoplastic agents: design, spectroscopic properties, and in vitro antitumor activity. Inorg Chem 44:1867–1881
265. Messori L, Marcon G, Orioli P (2003) Gold(III) compounds as new family of anticancer drugs. Bioinorg Chem Appl 1:177–187
266. Milacic V, Chen D, Ronconi L, Landis-Piwowar KR, Fregona D, Dou QP (2006) A novel anticancer gold(III) dithiocarbamate compound inhibits the activity of a purified 20S proteasome and 26S proteasome in human breast cancer cell cultures and xenografts. Cancer Res 66:10478–10486
267. Zhang X, Frezza M, Milacic V, Ronconi L, Fan Y, Bi C, Fregona D, Dou QP (2010) Inhibition of tumor proteasome activity by gold-dithiocarbamato complexes via both redox-dependent and -independent processes. J Cell Biochem 109:162–172
268. Malaguarnera L, Pilastro MR, DiMarco R, Scifo C, Renis M, Mazzarino MC, Messina A (2003) Cell death in human acute myelogenous leukemic cells induced by pyrrolidinedithiocarbamate. Apoptosis 8:539–545
269. Reymond JC (1950) Fight against alcoholism; a new product: antabuse. J Prat Rev Gen Clin Ther 64:64–66
270. Schreck R, Meier B, Mannel DN, Droge W, Baeuerle PA (1992) Dithiocarbamates as potent inhibitors of nuclear factor kappa B activation in intact cells. J Exp Med 175:1181–1194
271. Johansson B (1992) A review of the pharmacokinetics and pharmacodynamics of disulfiram and its metabolites. Acta Psychiatr Scand Suppl 369:15–26
272. Vallari RC, Pietruszko R (1982) Human aldehyde dehydrogenase: mechanism of inhibition of disulfiram. Science 216:637–639
273. Meyer RE (1989) Prospects for a rational pharmacotherapy of alcoholism. J Clin Psychiatry 50:403–412
274. Chen D, Cui QC, Yang H, Dou QP (2006) Disulfiram, a clinically used anti-alcoholism drug and copper-binding agent, induces apoptotic cell death in breast cancer cultures and xenografts via inhibition of the proteasome activity. Cancer Res 66:10425–10433
275. Di Vaira M, Bazzicalupi C, Orioli P, Messori L, Bruni B, Zatta P (2004) Clioquinol, a drug for Alzheimer's disease specifically interfering with brain metal metabolism: structural characterization of its zinc(II) and copper(II) complexes. Inorg Chem 43:3795–3797
276. Cherny RA, Atwood CS, Xilinas ME, Gray DN, Jones WD, McLean CA, Barnham KJ, Volitakis I, Fraser FW, Kim Y, Huang X, Goldstein LE, Moir RD, Lim JT, Beyreuther K, Zheng H, Tanzi RE, Masters CL, Bush AI (2001) Treatment with a copper-zinc chelator markedly and rapidly inhibits beta-amyloid accumulation in Alzheimer's disease transgenic mice. Neuron 30:665–676
277. Regland B, Lehmann W, Abedini I, Blennow K, Jonsson M, Karlsson I, Sjogren M, Wallin A, Xilinas M, Gottfries CG (2001) Treatment of Alzheimer's disease with clioquinol. Dement Geriatr Cogn Disord 12:408–414
278. Ritchie CW, Bush AI, Mackinnon A, Macfarlane S, Mastwyk M, MacGregor L, Kiers L, Cherny R, Li QX, Tammer A, Carrington D, Mavros C, Volitakis I, Xilinas M, Ames D, Davis S, Beyreuther K, Tanzi RE, Masters CL (2003) Metal-protein attenuation with iodochlorhydroxyquin (clioquinol) targeting Abeta amyloid deposition and toxicity in Alzheimer disease: a pilot phase 2 clinical trial. Arch Neurol 60:1685–1691
279. Ritchie CW, Bush AI, Masters CL (2004) Metal-protein attenuating compounds and Alzheimer's disease. Expert Opin Investig Drugs 13:1585–1592
280. Nguyen T, Hamby A, Massa SM (2005) Clioquinol down-regulates mutant huntingtin expression in vitro and mitigates pathology in a Huntington's disease mouse model. Proc Natl Acad Sci U S A 102:11840–11845

281. Chen D, Cui QC, Yang H, Barrea RA, Sarkar FH, Sheng S, Yan B, Reddy GP, Dou QP (2007) Clioquinol, a therapeutic agent for Alzheimer's disease, has proteasome-inhibitory, androgen receptor-suppressing, apoptosis-inducing, and antitumor activities in human prostate cancer cells and xenografts. Cancer Res 67:1636–1644
282. Zhai S, Yang L, Cui QC, Sun Y, Dou QP, Yan B (2010) Tumor cellular proteasome inhibition and growth suppression by 8-hydroxyquinoline and clioquinol requires their capabilities to bind copper and transport copper into cells. J Biol Inorg Chem 15:259–269
283. Rentsch A, Landsberg D, Brodmann T, Bulow L, Girbig AK, Kalesse M (2013) Synthesis and pharmacology of proteasome inhibitors. Angew Chem Int Ed Engl 52:5450–5488
284. Yang H, Shi G, Dou QP (2007) The tumor proteasome is a primary target for the natural anticancer compound Withaferin A isolated from "Indian winter cherry". Mol Pharmacol 71:426–437
285. Yang H, Chen D, Cui QC, Yuan X, Dou QP (2006) Celastrol, a triterpene extracted from the Chinese "Thunder of God Vine," is a potent proteasome inhibitor and suppresses human prostate cancer growth in nude mice. Cancer Res 66:4758–4765
286. Tsukamoto S, Tatsuno M, van Soest RW, Yokosawa H, Ohta T (2003) New polyhydroxy sterols: proteasome inhibitors from a marine sponge Acanthodendrilla sp. J Nat Prod 66:1181–1185
287. Scalbert A, Williamson G (2000) Dietary intake and bioavailability of polyphenols. J Nutr 130:2073S–2085S
288. Shanafelt TD, Lee YK, Call TG, Nowakowski GS, Dingli D, Zent CS, Kay NE (2006) Clinical effects of oral green tea extracts in four patients with low grade B-cell malignancies. Leuk Res 30:707–712
289. Sartippour MR, Heber D, Ma J, Lu Q, Go VL, Nguyen M (2001) Green tea and its catechins inhibit breast cancer xenografts. Nutr Cancer 40:149–156
290. Kemberling JK, Hampton JA, Keck RW, Gomez MA, Selman SH (2003) Inhibition of bladder tumor growth by the green tea derivative epigallocatechin-3-gallate. J Urol 170:773–776
291. Nam S, Smith DM, Dou QP (2001) Ester bond-containing tea polyphenols potently inhibit proteasome activity in vitro and in vivo. J Biol Chem 276:13322–13330
292. Golden EB, Lam PY, Kardosh A, Gaffney KJ, Cadenas E, Louie SG, Petasis NA, Chen TC, Schonthal AH (2009) Green tea polyphenols block the anticancer effects of bortezomib and other boronic acid-based proteasome inhibitors. Blood 113:5927–5937
293. Shanafelt TD, Call TG, Zent CS, LaPlant B, Bowen DA, Roos M, Secreto CR, Ghosh AK, Kabat BF, Lee MJ, Yang CS, Jelinek DF, Erlichman C, Kay NE (2009) Phase I trial of daily oral Polyphenon E in patients with asymptomatic Rai stage 0 to II chronic lymphocytic leukemia. J Clin Oncol 27:3808–3814
294. McLarty J, Bigelow RL, Smith M, Elmajian D, Ankem M, Cardelli JA (2009) Tea polyphenols decrease serum levels of prostate-specific antigen, hepatocyte growth factor, and vascular endothelial growth factor in prostate cancer patients and inhibit production of hepatocyte growth factor and vascular endothelial growth factor in vitro. Cancer Prev Res (Phila) 2:673–682
295. Lepley DM, Li B, Birt DF, Pelling JC (1996) The chemopreventive flavonoid apigenin induces G2/M arrest in keratinocytes. Carcinogenesis 17:2367–2375
296. Janssen K, Mensink RP, Cox FJ, Harryvan JL, Hovenier R, Hollman PC, Katan MB (1998) Effects of the flavonoids quercetin and apigenin on hemostasis in healthy volunteers: results from an in vitro and a dietary supplement study. Am J Clin Nutr 67:255–262
297. Manach C, Scalbert A, Morand C, Remesy C, Jimenez L (2004) Polyphenols: food sources and bioavailability. Am J Clin Nutr 79:727–747
298. Kaiser CS, Rompp H, Schmidt PC (2004) Supercritical carbon dioxide extraction of chamomile flowers: extraction efficiency, stability, and in-line inclusion of chamomile-carbon dioxide extract in beta-cyclodextrin. Phytochem Anal 15:249–256
299. Zheng PW, Chiang LC, Lin CC (2005) Apigenin induced apoptosis through p53-dependent pathway in human cervical carcinoma cells. Life Sci 76:1367–1379
300. Liu LZ, Fang J, Zhou Q, Hu X, Shi X, Jiang BH (2005) Apigenin inhibits expression of vascular endothelial growth factor and angiogenesis in human lung cancer cells: implication of chemoprevention of lung cancer. Mol Pharmacol 68:635–643

301. Gupta S, Afaq F, Mukhtar H (2002) Involvement of nuclear factor-kappa B, Bax and Bcl-2 in induction of cell cycle arrest and apoptosis by apigenin in human prostate carcinoma cells. Oncogene 21:3727–3738
302. Birt DF, Mitchell D, Gold B, Pour P, Pinch HC (1997) Inhibition of ultraviolet light induced skin carcinogenesis in SKH-1 mice by apigenin, a plant flavonoid. Anticancer Res 17:85–91
303. Chen D, Daniel KG, Chen MS, Kuhn DJ, Landis-Piwowar KR, Dou QP (2005) Dietary flavonoids as proteasome inhibitors and apoptosis inducers in human leukemia cells. Biochem Pharmacol 69:1421–1432
304. Chen D, Landis-Piwowar KR, Chen MS, Dou QP (2007) Inhibition of proteasome activity by the dietary flavonoid apigenin is associated with growth inhibition in cultured breast cancer cells and xenografts. Breast Cancer Res 9:R80
305. Hoensch H, Groh B, Edler L, Kirch W (2008) Prospective cohort comparison of flavonoid treatment in patients with resected colorectal cancer to prevent recurrence. World J Gastroenterol 14:2187–2193

Chapter 2
Resistance to Proteasome Inhibitors in Multiple Myeloma

Francesca Cottini, Anna Guidetti, Claudia Paba Prada, Teru Hideshima, Michelle Maglio, Cindy Varga, Dharminder Chauhan, Jacob Laubach, Kenneth C. Anderson, and Paul G. Richardson

Abstract Multiple myeloma (MM) is a clonal proliferation of malignant plasma cells in the bone marrow associated with a spectrum of clinical symptoms including bone destruction, anemia, hypercalcemia, and renal failure. Although MM remains incurable, a dramatic paradigm shift in the treatment of MM has occurred over the past decade through the introduction of novel agents, including the development of small molecule inhibitors targeting the proteasome. Among the proteasome inhibitors (PIs), bortezomib (BTZ) and carfilzomib (CFZ) have been approved by the FDA for treatment of relapsed/refractory MM in 2003 and 2012, respectively. Recently, other PIs, such as ixazomib (MLN-9708), oprozomib (ONX0912), and marizomib (NPI-0052), have been under evaluation in preclinical and clinical studies. Indeed, it is now well known that malignant plasma cells are exquisitely sensitive to proteasome inhibitors due to protein overload and ER stress. Unfortunately, relapse of myeloma develops due to acquisition of resistance to proteasome inhibitors. Specifically, mutations in overexpression of proteins belonging to the proteasome complex, upregulation of transporter channels or cytochrome components, induction of alternative compensative mechanisms such as the aggresome pathway, and modulation of downstream pathways have been all reported as possible mechanisms of

Authors contributed equally.

F. Cottini, M.D. • C.P. Prada, M.D. • T. Hideshima, M.D. Ph.D. • M. Maglio • C. Varga, M.D.
D. Chauhan, J.D. Ph.D. • J. Laubach, M.D. • K.C. Anderson, M.D. • P.G. Richardson, M.D. (✉)
Jerome Lipper Multiple Myeloma Center, Division of Hematologic Malignancy,
Department of Medical Oncology, Dana-Farber Cancer Institute,
450 Brookline Avenue, Boston, MA, USA
e-mail: francesca_cottini@dfci.harvard.edu; claudiap_prada@dfci.harvard.edu; teru_hideshima@dfci.harvard.edu; michelle_maglio@dfci.harvard.edu; cindy_varga@dfci.harvard.edu; dharminder_chauhan@dfci.harvard.edu; jacobp_laubach@dfci.harvard.edu; kenneth_anderson@dfci.harvard.edu; paul_richardson@dfci.harvard.edu

A. Guidetti, M.D.
Università degli Studi di Milano, Milan, Italy
e-mail: anna.guidetti@istitutotumori.mi.it

Q.P. Dou (ed.), *Resistance to Proteasome Inhibitors in Cancer*, Resistance to Targeted Anti-Cancer Therapeutics, DOI 10.1007/978-3-319-06752-0_2

proteasome inhibitor resistance. In this chapter, we will first briefly describe the structure and function of the proteasome in normal and malignant plasma cells, and then define the major mechanisms of resistance to proteasome inhibition, and clinical approaches to overcoming these pathways in the context of both clinical application of PIs and rational combinations of them with other agents in the treatment of MM.

Keywords Proteasome inhibitor • Carfilzomib • Bortezomib • Drug resistance • Multiple myeloma

Abbreviations

BTZ	Bortezomib
CFZ	Carfilzomib
C-L	Caspase-like
CT-L	Chymotrypsin-like
CR	Complete response
HDAC	Histone deacetylase
HDACIs	HDAC inhibitors
Ig	Immunoglobulin
MM	Multiple myeloma
MTD	Maximum-tolerated dose
OS	Overall survival
PI	Proteasome inhibitor
T-L	Trypsin-like
TTP	Time to progression

2.1 Introduction

Multiple myeloma (MM) is characterized by clonal expansion of malignant plasma cells with several genomic alterations. Plasma cells differentiate from B cells, which have limited immunoglobulin (Ig) synthesis and secretory capacity. Conversely, plasma cells have increased endoplasmic reticulum (ER) content, components for protein synthesis and quality control, and secretory pathways to synthesize and secrete Ig. Malignant plasma cells secrete even higher quantities of Ig, and are hence particularly sensitive to the detrimental effects associated with accumulation of incompletely or improperly folded proteins in the ER, relying on proteasome complexes to avoid protein overload [1–4].

Proteasomes (proteasome 26S), their protein structures conserved in both prokaryotic and eukaryotic organisms, are composed of a 20S core which binds one or two 19S regulatory particles [5]. The 20S core is a barrel-like structure composed of stacked heptameric rings, each of which consists of seven related, yet distinct,

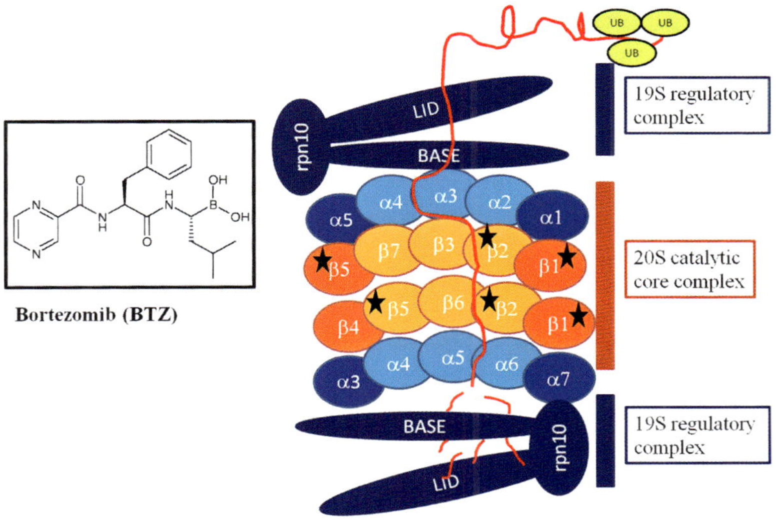

Fig. 2.1 Representative scheme of proteasome structure. 20S catalytic core and 19S regulatory complex are shown. Bortezomib (BTZ) and other proteasome inhibitors (PIs) bind to specific catalytic subunits

subunits (α1–α7 and β1–β7) organized in a fixed topological arrangement within each ring. Only a subset of β-subunits is catalytically active, and each of them preferentially cuts specific residues, such as basic, acidic, or hydrophobic amino acids. In particular, the chymotrypsin-like (CT-L), caspase-like (C-L), and trypsin-like (T-L) catalytic activities of the 20S proteasome are encoded by β5-, β1-, and β2-subunits, respectively. The 19S particles represent the lid or gate of the barrel and are important for substrate recognition, deubiquitination, unfolding, and translocation into the core particle. Indeed, protein degradation can occur only if the selected protein is recognized by the regulatory proteins, traverses the regulatory gate (19S structures, which bind to a ring and cause gate opening), and interacts with the catalytically active proteolytic enzymes of the core (Fig. 2.1). Additionally, in response to different biological stimuli such as interferon gamma and tumor necrosis factor-alpha, specific β-subunits can associate with a particular 11S regulatory particle, forming the so-called immunoproteasome (i20S). In the immunoproteasome, LMP7, LMP2, and MECL1, proteins represent the catalytically active subunits. 26S and i20S proteasomes are both present in MM cells: i20S is predominant in MM at diagnosis, while lower levels of i20S and increased levels of 26S proteasome are present in relapsed myelomas. Drugs targeting proteasomes are both reversible (BTZ, MLN9074, and CEP-18770) and irreversible competitive (CFZ, ONX 0912, and NPI-0052) inhibitors which differentially bind to proteasome catalytic subunits. Specifically, BTZ, MLN9074, and CEP-18770 are potent inhibitors of the C-L β5 subunits (PSMB5), NPI-0052 is a potent inhibitor of the T-L β1-subunits, whereas CFZ selectively inhibits both CT-L active sites and LMP7 subunits.

2.2 Preclinical Studies on Mechanisms of Resistance to BTZ

2.2.1 Genetic Abnormalities in Proteasome Subunits

PIs induce cytotoxicity in MM cells by multiple mechanisms including: induction of terminal ER stress and unfolded protein response (UPR), activation of c-Jun NH2 terminal kinase (JNK), inhibition of nuclear factor kappa B pathway, and induction of reactive oxygen species (ROS). One of the first mechanisms of proteasome resistance is the presence of mutations or altered and/or aberrant expression of proteasome subunits, which disrupt the ability of BTZ to bind and inhibit proteasomes. The first demonstration of this mechanism of BTZ resistance was in leukemia cells [6], and the results were later applied and confirmed in MM cells. Specifically, Oerlemans and colleagues generated BTZ-resistant human myelomonocytic THP1 cells by continuous culture with stepwise increasing concentrations (2.5–200 nM) of BTZ [6]. In this study, analysis of mRNA and protein expression of various proteasome subunits showed markedly increased (up to 60-fold) protein levels of β5-subunit (also known as PSMB5) and only modest (<2-fold) upregulation of β1- and β2-subunits. No increased mRNA was observed in PSMB5, indicating that posttranscriptional mechanisms were responsible for increased protein expression. Of note, upregulation of PSMB5 protein expression induced by BTZ treatment was reversible. Importantly, no additional alterations in expression of genes encoding ubiquitin-conjugating enzymes, ubiquitin-specific proteases, or ubiquitin C-terminal hydrolases were recognized.

In addition to PSMB5 overexpression, a point mutation in the β-subunit of BTZ-binding pocket (G322A mutant), introducing an Ala to Thr substitution at amino acid 49, was also reported [6]. This mutation has also been described in other cellular systems, such as BTZ-resistant Jurkat human lymphoblastic T cells by Lu and colleagues [7, 8]. Lu and colleagues also identified mutations in C323T (Ala49Val) alone or C326T in combination with G322A (Ala49Thr and Ala50Val) [8]. Ri and colleagues were the first to evaluate the mechanisms of BTZ resistance in myeloma by creating two BTZ-resistant cell lines (KMS-11 and OPM-2 cells). These BTZ-resistant cells were less prone to activate apoptotic pathways than the parental sensitive cells. Moreover, the BTZ-resistant cells have reduced amounts of polyubiquitinated proteins, thereby failing to trigger the UPR and induce CHOP and NOXA expression upon BTZ treatment [9]. These resistant-clones have a point mutation (G322A) in the PSMB5 gene as well. Balsas and colleagues generated another BTZ-resistant MM cell line (RPMI-8226/7B) [10]. Interestingly, these cells were morphologically larger than the parental cells, with about twofold DNA content per cell and overexpressed PSMB5 at both mRNA and protein levels; however, no mutation was recognized. Franke and colleagues also generated BTZ resistance in RPMI-8226 (MM) and CEM (acute lymphoblastic leukemia) cell lines. As expected, these cells show resistance to different types of PIs [11]. Consistent with previous studies, these cell lines upregulate PSMB5 gene together with other constitutive catalytic β-subunits, as well as the non-catalytic α7 subunit. Moreover, BTZ-resistant RPMI-8226 cells have a near-complete shift from the β5i

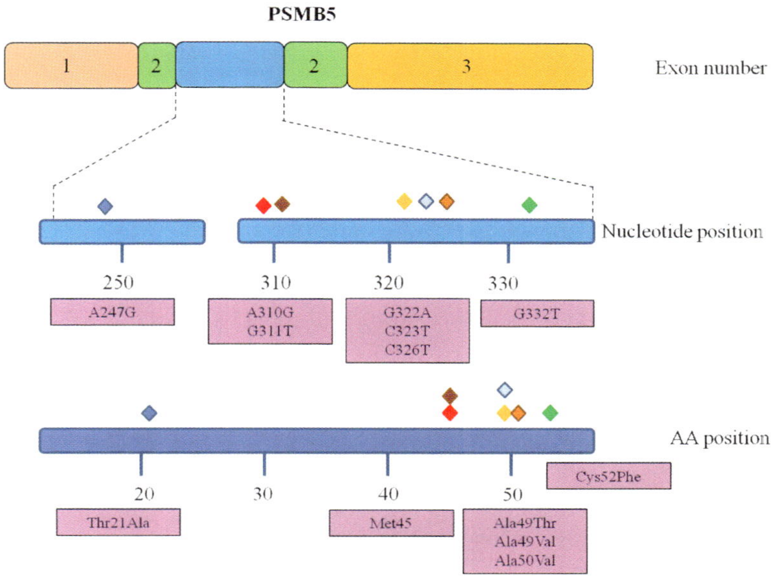

Fig. 2.2 Scheme of PSMB5 mutations identified in BTZ-resistant MM cell lines. Exons 1–3 create the S1-specific pocket of the β5-subunit and are the site of the most relevant mutations, which confer resistance to BTZ treatment. Both nucleotide- and amino acid-affected residues are shown

(immunoproteasome) subunit to the constitutive β5-subunit. To define the biologic relevance of PSMB5 mutations, they utilized a crystal structure and computer modeling system to characterize the physiological interactions between BTZ and the proteasome, showing that mutations involving PSMB5 create a functional protein. However, these mutations cluster together around the BTZ-binding pocket of proteasome, specifically around S1-specific pocket of the β5-subunit which recognizes the peptide bond of the substrate to be degraded [12, 13] (Fig. 2.2). In the S1 pocket, Ala49 and Ala50 residues are key positions for efficient binding of BTZ to the β5-subunit, and Ala49Val substitution in β5-subunit therefore hinders BTZ accessibility to the S1 pocket. They also identified additional mutations: G332T leading to Cys52Phe substitution, A247G to create Thr21Ala substitution, and G311T/A310G which changes Met45 residue. Thr21Ala substitution also decreases affinity of BTZ binding to the β5-subunit due to a loss of protein-ligand hydrogen bond. Met45 and Cys52 are not directly involved in BTZ-binding; however, Cys52Phe mutation leads to a slight repulsion of BTZ from the S1 pocket. Met45 also confers S1 pocket specificity and conformational change after BTZ binding [14]. Thus, all these mutations can alter the binding pocket's specificity and flexibility. Altogether, these studies in different cell types demonstrate two important findings that associate with PI resistance: first, the discovery of acquired mutations which decrease the affinity of the β5-binding pocket to proteasome inhibitors and second, compensatory upregulation of other proteasome subunits.

Although a number of in vitro studies of PI resistance have shown PSMB5 overexpression or mutations, no clinical data has identified these mechanisms in the subset of BTZ-resistant and/or refractory patients MM cells. Indeed, mutations in PBMS5 have not yet been identified by whole-genome sequencing of samples from patients with either newly diagnosed patients or relapsed MM [15]. Recently, another study tried to define more specifically the frequency and clinical relevance of PMSB5. In this study, DNA samples were isolated from MM patients ($n=16$) before and after BTZ treatment [16]. Ten patients were relatively resistant (minimal response, stable disease, or progressive disease) to BTZ monotherapy; six patients achieved PR and then subsequently relapsed. PSMB5 mutant variants were not detected in any case. Although the number of patients enrolled was small, these results suggest that clinical resistance to BTZ in patients with relapsed MM may not solely be due to PSMB5 mutations, which to date are shown only in cell lines.

Several single nucleotide polymorphisms (SNP) in the *PSMB5* gene have also been reported; however, they do not alter activity, but modulate transcription, of the proteasome [17]. Licther and colleagues identified three significant associations between SNP allelic frequencies (SNPs PSMB6 rs2304975, PSMB6 rs3169950, and PSMB9 rs241419) and overall survival (OS) or time to progression (TTP) of disease in patients treated with BTZ [16]. However, two of these variants were present only in 3–5 % patients, suggesting limited clinical relevance. In another small study, Shuqing and colleagues evaluated PSMB5 mRNA levels and DNA PSMB5 point mutations in MM cells from three patients whose MM was refractory to treatment with BADT regimen (BTZ, epirubicin, dexamethasone, and thalidomide) and normal bone marrow mononuclear cells from a healthy volunteer [18]. No mutations were present. Another single-case report from Politou and colleagues also failed to show PSMB5 mutations in one resistant patient [19].

The ubiquitin-proteasome pathway for protein degradation requires several enzymes, which could be altered and thereby mediate BTZ resistance. For example, upregulation of POMP (proteasome maturation protein) can promote BTZ resistance [20]. POMP plays a role in adding catalytically active β-subunits to the hemi-proteasome ring, which is initially composed of α-subunits. Li and colleagues identified higher mRNA level of POMP and nuclear factor erythroid-derived-2-like 2, its transcriptional regulator, in BTZ-resistant cells than in parental cells, thereby inducing higher chymotrypsin-like activity.

2.2.2 Alternative Pathways to Modulate Proteasome Activity

Another possible mechanism for acquired BTZ resistance is activation of alternative protein lysis/degradation systems, including the aggresome pathway, to degrade excessive or misfolded proteins [21]. Aggresomes or aggresomal particles form when nascent peptides do not fold correctly and create small protein aggregates in response to the presence of misfolded proteins. These structures are then transported towards the microtubule (MT) organizing center (MTOC), where they are sequestered into a bin-like structure called the aggresome. Acetylation of α-tubulin, which is reversed by histone deacetylase 6 (HDAC6), a class IIb HDAC, modulates the structure and function of MT, thereby playing a crucial role in autophagic (or lysosomal) lysis of protein aggregates [22]. Hideshima and colleagues showed that combination strategies directed against HDAC6 and proteasome activities, using tubacin and BTZ, respectively, significantly augment accumulation of polyubiquitinated proteins, followed by cell stress and cytotoxicity [23]. Catley et al. showed that BTZ strongly induces aggresome formation. A synergistic cytotoxic effect can be achieved when BTZ is combined with LBH589, a nonselective deacetylase inhibitor [24]. Interestingly, some cell lines were more responsive to LBH589 than BTZ or vice versa, suggesting that cell lines and perhaps patients can predominantly activate one of the two pathways.

Heat shock proteins (HSPs) are molecular chaperones presented which are rapidly upregulated when cells are exposed to a stress condition, such as treatments with chemotherapeutic agents. They play significant roles in accommodation of cells to stress conditions, including endoplasmic reticulum (ER) stress that is triggered by accumulation of unfolded proteins. Shringarpure and colleagues compared gene expression profiling in BTZ-resistant (SUDHL-4) and BTZ-sensitive (SUDHL-6) diffuse large B cell lymphoma cell lines, and identified overexpression of HSPs (i.e., Hsp27, Hsp70, Hsp90) in BTZ-resistant cells [25]. Subsequently, Chauhan and colleagues showed that silencing Hsp27 in BTZ-resistant SUDHL4 cells restores sensitivity to BTZ; conversely, overexpression of Hsp27 induces BTZ resistance in BTZ-sensitive SUDHL6 cells [26]. Although the mechanism of action of Hsp27 mediating BTZ resistance has not yet been fully delineated, one possible explanation is its antiapoptotic activity due to inhibition of mitochondrial apoptotic signaling. Specifically, Hsp27 can inhibit release of cytochrome-c/Smac by modulating the integrity of the actin network responsible for controlling translocation of proapoptotic factors from the actin cytoskeleton to mitochondria. Moreover, Hsp27 can also modulate autophagic cell death through ER stress [27]. Taken together, Hsp27 can modulate autophagy and ER stress triggered by BTZ [28], thereby, promoting survival in BTZ-treated cells. Most recently, it has been shown that nicotinamide phosphoribosyltransferase (Nampt) regulates NAD, and that its inhibition depletes intracellular NAD^+ level leading to autophagic cell death [29]. Moreover, higher Nampt mRNA levels are correlated with BTZ resistance in patient MM cells. Importantly, combining the NAD^+-depleting agent FK866 with BTZ induces synergistic MM cell death and overcomes BTZ resistance [30].

2.2.3 *Cell Dedifferentiation*

One of the major steps in plasma cell differentiation from B lymphocytes is linked to the activation of control mechanisms for protein folding which permit immunoglobulin synthesis and secretion. This response is mainly orchestrated by the activation of BLIMP1 transcription factor and the blockade of PAX5 (also known as

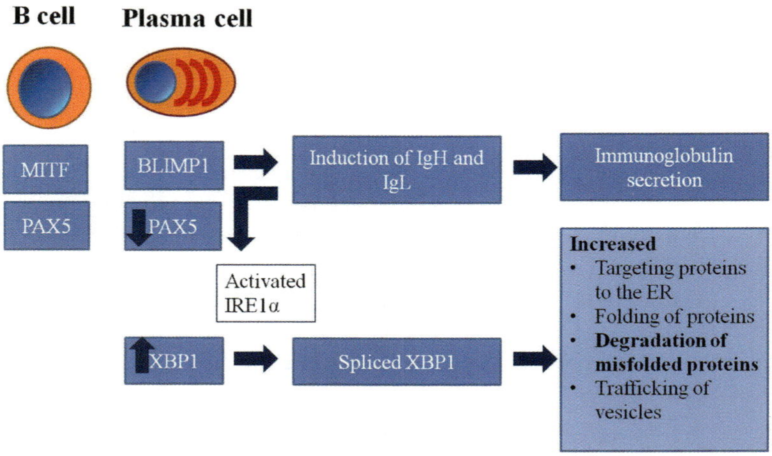

Fig. 2.3 Transition from B cell lymphocytes and plasma cells. MITF (microphthalmia-associated transcription factor) and PAX5 (paired box protein 5) transcription factors normally block plasma cell differentiation by repressing BLIMP1 (B lymphocyte-induced maturation protein 1). When PAX5 expression is downregulated, BLIMP1 represses B cell gene-expression programs and BLIMP1, XBP1 (X-box-binding protein 1), and IRF4 (interferon-regulatory factor 4) induce the expression of genes that are required for plasma cells. Specifically, there is an increase in immunoglobulin secretion and also in the control, folding, and degradation of misfolded proteins in plasma cells

BSAP, B cell-specific activator protein), thereby leading to X-box-binding protein (XBP1) transcription factor splicing and increased protein quality control (Fig. 2.3). Ling and colleagues observed that cell lines and primary MM cells which expressed low levels of XBP1 were more resistant to BTZ treatment, associated with lower levels of immunoglobulin secretion [31]. This effect was partially overcome by further inducing an UPR using alkylating agents or tunicamycin, a drug which creates ER stress by inhibiting the glycosylation of nascent proteins. Therefore, XBP1 levels can be used as a possible biomarker of response to BTZ treatment. In other study, Leung-Hagesteijn and colleagues hypothesized that BTZ resistance relies on the capabilities of MM cells to become less dependent to ER-stress control and dedifferentiate from plasma cells back to B lymphocytes [32]. In particular, they demonstrated that silencing Ire1or XBP1, but not Atf6 or Perk (other two ER stress sensor proteins), affects response to BTZ treatment. They confirmed that XBP1 levels correlate with clinical BTZ response: patients with progressive disease express lower levels of XBP1 target genes compared to patients with complete response. Moreover, they also suggested the importance of XBP1 mutations in BTZ resistance. Indeed, whole-genome sequencing has identified two mutations in samples from patients with relapsed MM. These mutations are considered to be inactivating mutations, which inhibit correct splicing and/or transcriptional activity of XBP1 [15]. Indeed, when plasmids containing mutant XBP1 were reintroduced into MM cells with silenced XBP1, these cells were not capable of overcoming the BTZ-resistant phenotypes. Even though the most intuitive role of Xpb1 in BTZ resistance was hyperactivation of PERK/ATF6 signaling as a compensatory mechanism, they observed that malignant plasma cells acquired a less-differentiated phenotype, characterized by decreased expression of CD138, CD38, and IL6R; upregulation of PAX5; and downregulation of heavy and light chains of Ig. These alterations lessen the high ER front loading of Ig, and so the attendant risk of harmful ER stress response. These data were shown in cell lines and confirmed in patients, since BTZ-sensitive tumors have a high proportion of mature plasma cells, while BTZ-resistant tumors contain subpopulations of plasma cell progenitor cells expressing low or absent levels of CD138, CD38, and XBP1. Moreover, when minimal residual disease was evaluated in bone marrow biopsies, patients in complete response (CR) still harbored a small subpopulation of less mature plasma cells, which might represent the principal source of relapse in responsive patients. Of note, they did not observe PSMB5 mutations or any correlation of PI resistance with expression levels of proteasome subunits. This is in contrast to in vitro models of PI resistance, where the majority of proteasome subunits including PSMB5 were upregulated. Therefore, they concluded that Ire1-XBP1 pathway is crucial to induce BTZ cytotoxicity. The Xbp-1 pathway can be shut down in malignant plasma cells without strongly affecting their survival, but reducing their dependency on protein control. A similar phenotypic change was also observed by Stessman et al. [33]. Comparing BTZ-sensitive and BTZ-resistant cells derived from tumors of the Bcl-XL/Myc mouse model of plasma cell malignancy, they identified a reduction of the levels of CD93 (a plasma cell maturation marker) and CD69 (a plasma cell activation marker) in cells with acquired PI resistance, as well as in subclones after 48 h BTZ treatment. They then evaluated CD93 mRNA expression in patient samples based on CD93 high or low expression and showed that CD93 levels correlate with better overall survival after BTZ treatment in the APEX trial. CD93, a marker of mature plasma cells in humans, also positively associates with BLIMP1 expression in MM patient samples. Thus, they proposed CD93 as a biomarker for BTZ sensitivity, together with XBP1. Hence, the loss of maturation markers is a strategy used by myeloma cells to escape BTZ-mediated apoptosis via reducing the UPR.

2.2.4 *Metabolism and Drug Efflux*

Another common mechanism involved in drug resistance consists in either upregulation of channel proteins/transporters which mediate expulsion of drug from the cells, or overexpression of catabolic proteins leading to rapid drug degradation. For example, overexpression of MDR-1 represents a critical mechanism of drug resistance in cancer. Rumpold and colleagues showed that both BTZ and MLN273 can be substrates of MDR-1, evidenced by sensitization of MDR-1-overexpressed K562/Dox cells to BTZ by knockdown of MDR-1 [34]. Other groups have also showed the association of activity of proteasome inhibitor with ATP-binding cassette transporter-mediated efflux expression [35]. Moreover, lymphoid CEM/VLB cells with Pgp-1 overexpression were more resistant than parental cells to carfilzomib (114-fold), ONX-0912 (23-fold), and ONX0914 (162-fold), as well as to BTZ; conversely, a Pgp transport inhibitor P121 (reversin 121) was able to restore proteasome activity. These results therefore confirm that expression of MDR-1 can also modulate sensitivity to BTZ treatment. In addition, differential expression of genes regulating multidrug resistance and drug metabolism in BTZ-sensitive versus BTZ-resistant DLBCL cell lines was also evaluated [25]. Specifically, two genes were overexpressed in BTZ-resistant SUDHL-4 cells: ATP-binding cassette (ABC) subfamily A member 1 (ABCA1) and cytochrome P450. However, their mechanism of actions and relevance in cellular entry or metabolism of BTZ have not yet been fully elucidated [25].

Another group identified a correlation between the active Notch pathway via Dll1/Notch2 receptors and BTZ resistance [36]. Indeed, Notch upregulates CYP1A1, a cytochrome P450 enzyme involved in drug metabolism; conversely, downregulation and inhibition of CYP1A1 restore sensitivity to BTZ treatment [36]. A gamma secretase inhibitor DAPT sensitizes the cells to BTZ treatment both in vitro and in vivo in murine human MM cell xenograft models.

2.2.5 Signaling Pathways Mediating MM Cell Survival and Drug Resistance

Constitutive activation or hyperactivation due to genetic abnormalities in signaling cascades, including NF-κB, β-catenin, IGFR, c-MET, MAF, and AKT, can also modulate sensitivity to BTZ (Fig. 2.4). Indeed, NF-κB is constitutively activated in primary patient MM cells and in MM cell lines, and its activity is further increased in response to soluble factors including IL-6, IGF-1, TNF-α, IL-1β, BAFF, SDF-1α, and APRIL in the bone marrow microenvironment. Although, the NF-κB pathway is involved in MM pathogenesis, its role in the context of sensitivity to BTZ is still controversial. Several molecules including IκB kinase (IKK) complex trigger phosphorylation of inhibitor protein IκBα, followed by its ubiquitination and subsequent degradation via the 26S proteasome. Degradation of IκBα allows the NF-κB complex to translocate to the nucleus. Importantly, IκBα can also be degraded in a proteasome-independent manner (PIR, proteasome inhibitor resistant), relying on calcium, calmodulin, and L-type calcium channels [37]. Interestingly, BTZ triggers NF-κB activation in MM cell lines and primary MM cells by proteasome-independent downregulation of IκBα associated with IKKβ activation, which enhances BTZ-induced cytotoxicity [38]. Two studies pointed out that primary tumor cells from MM and mantle cell lymphoma patients have relatively high constitutive NF-κB activation due to genetic abnormalities or microenvironment modulation, and that these cells are largely resistant to BTZ [39, 40]. Indeed, as also reported by Hideshima and colleagues, they observed that a significant fraction of patient MM cells treated with BTZ do not downregulate constitutive NF-κB activity, although BTZ effectively blocks proteasome activity. Even though the Markovina study suggests that BTZ resistance is mediated by NF-κB activation, data from our group showed that BTZ-treated MM cells with further induction of NF-κB activity nonetheless

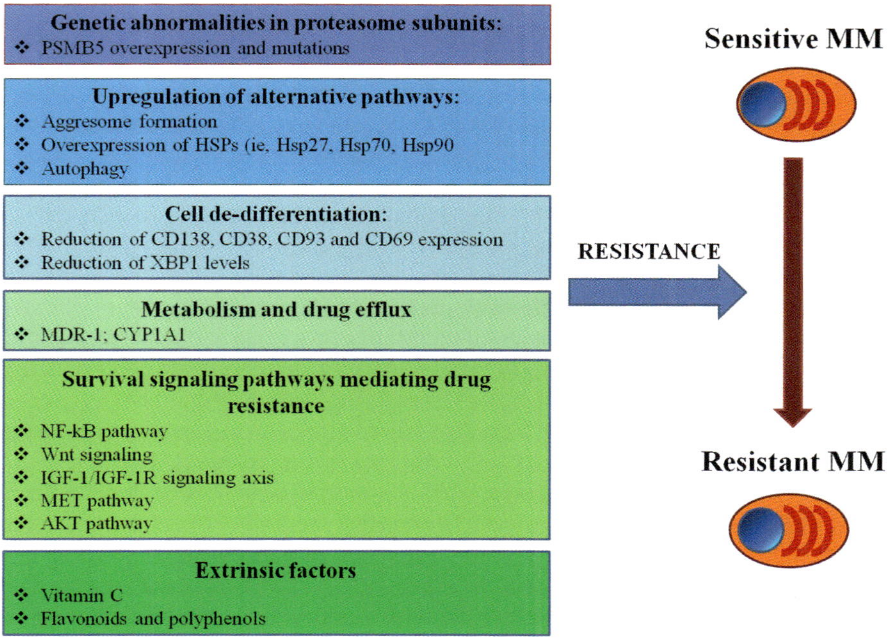

Fig. 2.4 Summary showing the state of the art in proteasome inhibitor resistance

remained responsive to BTZ treatment [38]. Hence, it remains controversial as to whether NF-κB activation represents a resistance mechanism or a compensatory strategy which only minimally affects cytotoxicity.

Myeloma cell lines with higher β-catenin levels are also resistant to BTZ treatment [41]. These cells have higher expression of TCF-4 transcription factor, which is a central player in Wnt signaling, regulating MM-relevant target genes including cyclin D1 and c-Myc, among others. IGF-1 pathway could also play a role on BTZ resistance. Kuhn and colleagues generated BTZ-resistant cells using RPMI8226, OPM-2, ANBL-6, and KAS-6/1 cell lines [42]. They showed that the IGF-1/IGF-1R signaling axis was the most deregulated in all BTZ-resistant cell lines, according to gene set enrichment analyses. Specifically, both the levels of soluble IGF-1 in cell culture supernatants, the levels of intracellular and membrane-bound IGF-1, as well as IGF-1R activity were increased in BTZ-resistant cells. Interestingly, AKT mRNA level was also higher in resistant than parental cells. Similar findings on the role of AKT in BTZ resistance was reported by Que and colleagues [43]. Moreover, they discovered that MET silencing was capable of increasing BTZ sensitivity, even though the mechanism was not defined. Indeed, c-MET has been implicated in proliferation, migration, and invasion of MM cells, and its overexpression correlates with short overall survival in MM patients. Additionally, the proto-oncogene MAF has also been associated with BTZ resistance, since both MM cell lines and patients with high MAF levels have lower response rates to BTZ treatment [44].

2.2.6 Extrinsic Factors

Drugs and vitamin supplements can potentially modulate BTZ metabolism and activity, hence reducing treatment responses. Specifically, vitamins having antioxidative effects, including vitamin C and E, are often taken by cancer patients. Previous reports show that BTZ induces production of ROS, which contributes to BTZ-induced cytotoxicity [45–48]. Interestingly, vitamin C (ascorbic acid) is capable of inhibiting BTZ-mediated cytotoxicity, while *N*-acetylcysteine and vitamin E are not [49]. Indeed given its chemical structure, a boronic acid class proteasome inhibitor BTZ can bind molecules with diol functional groups, including vitamin C. This binding causes the formation of an inactive form, thus reducing BTZ activity in MM cell lines [49]. Vitamin C effects on BTZ activity were also evaluated in vivo. Perrone and colleagues showed that plasma isolated from healthy volunteers taking increasing doses of vitamin C supplements, when added in cultured MM cells, can reduce BTZ cytotoxicity [50]. Moreover, when combination treatment of vitamin C with BTZ was evaluated in a murine xenograft model of human MM, antitumor activity of BTZ was significantly reduced [50]. Based on these results, vitamin C supplements should be avoided in patients who are receiving BTZ, or at least should be taken at low doses at least 12 h before BTZ treatment. A similar phenotype was observed in chronic lymphocytic leukemia cells treated with BTZ in the presence of quercetin or other dietary flavonoids (myricetin, kaempferol, and apigenin), which are commonly included in vegetables, fruits, and green tea. [51] Kim and colleagues screened a group of polyphenol compounds (catechin, epicatechin, gallic acid) which are present in cocoa, red wine, vegetables, and black/green tea, and showed that these agents block BTZ activity as well. Another group also showed inhibition of BTZ activity by green tea polyphenols [52]. Taken together, these results strongly recommend avoiding the intake of herbal supplements or foods containing polyphenols in large quantities during drug peaks or before clearance of BTZ.

2.2.7 Mechanisms to Sensitize Cells to BTZ Cytotoxicity

BTZ works predominantly by blocking degradation of excessive or misfolded proteins, leading to lethal ER stress. A similar phenotype can be observed by inhibition of deubiquitinating enzymes (DUBs) or ubiquitinating enzymes (E1, E2, and E3). DUBs are a family of proteins which are often dysregulated in cancers, promoting stabilization of oncogenic proteins. Specifically, ubiquitin-specific protease 7 (USP7) regulates important biological signaling pathways in tumorigenesis, including FOXO4 and PTEN [53] as well as HDM2 and HDMX, resulting in the destabilization of p53 and its transactivation activity [54]. Of note, USP7 is markedly elevated in MM cells, and its expression levels inversely correlate with overall survival in MM patients. A small molecule USP7 inhibitor P5091 triggers MM cell toxicity both in vitro and in vivo in a murine human MM cell xenograft model.

Importantly, P5091 induces cytotoxicity even in BTZ-resistant ANBL-6.BR cells. USP9X is another DUB highly expressed in MM, follicular lymphoma, and diffuse large B cell lymphoma cells, which regulates Mcl-1 stabilization. Mcl-1 is a well-known antiapoptotic protein, and small molecule inhibitors against Mcl-1, including WP1130 and PR-619, can enhance BTZ-induced cytotoxicity. E1/E2/E3 ubiquitin-modifying enzymes represent a diverse group of proteins with significant roles in ubiquitin conjugation [55]. The E1 ubiquitin-activating enzyme is generally not target-specific and therefore can broadly affect protein degradation, in a similar fashion to the proteasome. E3 ligases are more selective and identify recognition signals on target proteins; for example, HMDM2 is crucial to control p53 levels, and is often overexpressed or amplified in cancers, including myeloma. Nutlin-3a is a potent non-peptide HDM2 antagonist which blocks the interaction of p53 with HDM2 and stabilizes p53 and p21. In preclinical studies, Nutlin-3a induces additive cytotoxicity with BTZ [56]. Analogues of Nutlin-3a, such as R7112, RITA, or HLI98, are currently under evaluation in preclinical models and clinical trials in patients. Silencing of E1 enzyme also results in increased cell death in MM cells. Compounds such as PYR-41 and PYZD-4409 can behave as E1 inhibitors, reducing protein ubiquitylation and sumoylation, inducing signs of ER stress, and enhancing BTZ-mediated apoptosis [57]. Finally, cereblon (CRBN) is another protein which forms an E3 ligase complex with damaged DNA-binding protein 1 (DDB1) and Cul4A and is considered a target of thalidomide and lenalidomide, suggesting one possible explanation for the synergistic MM cytotoxicity observed when immunomodulatory drugs are combined with BTZ treatment.

Other strategies can also be applied to sensitize cells to BTZ. In particular, recent studies identified a relationship between drug activity and mitochondrial or iron homeostasis. Specifically, Song et al. evaluated the role of mitochondria in BTZ resistance. Specifically, they compared indices of mitochondrial function including oxygen consumption rates and ATP and Ca^{2+} concentrations, membrane potentials (Ψm), and depolarization of $\Delta\Psi$m, which trigger mitochondrial pore opening and apoptosis, in three MM cell lines, one with intrinsic resistance to BTZ treatment (KMS-20) and two which are sensitive (KMS-26 and KMS-28BM) to BTZ treatment [58]. They identified a higher stability of mitochondrial membrane potential ($\Delta\Psi$m) and a more modest increase in mitochondrial calcium response in BTZ-resistant cells (KMS-20) in comparison to sensitive cells. These studies, indicating that BTZ-resistant cells can better control the mitochondrial Ca^{2+} pool and hence minimize BTZ-induced Ca^{2+}, overload and related induction of apoptosis. Moreover, the levels of superoxide anion or ROS were lower in KMS-20 cells, suggesting that ROS induction can represent another modality through which BTZ triggers cell death. To explain this difference, several mitochondrial genes related to maintenance of $\Delta\Psi$m, elimination of ROS, and Ca^{2+} influx into mitochondria were evaluated. For example, SOD2 (an antioxidant protein that nullifies ROS toxicity) and pyruvate dehydrogenase (PDH)-E1α protein levels were decreased and MCU expression was increased in BTZ-sensitive cells, while CYPD, a regulator of mitochondrial permeability transition, was decreased in BTZ-resistant cells. The expression levels of the proteins mentioned above, apart from MCU (further induced by

BTZ), were not changed by BTZ, suggesting an intrinsic mechanism of resistance. Therefore, the resistance of KMS20 cells can be related to a reduced expression of CYPD, causing modifications in mitochondrial membrane potentials and a higher capacity of ROS elimination via SOD2, compared with sensitive cells. Indeed, SOD2 depletion induced cell death in KMS20 cells; and the combination of BTZ with 2-methoxyestradiol, a known SOD inhibitor, was capable of overcoming BTZ resistance in KMS-20 [59]. A similar phenotype was also observed when BTZ was combined with FCCP, which induces dissipation of $\Delta\Psi$m. Additionally, combining BTZ with PK-1195, an antagonist to mitochondrial peripheral benzodiazepine receptors which causes loss of $\Delta\Psi$m, generates superoxides and favors release of cytochrome-c and Smac, thereby prompting cytotoxicity even in resistant cells [60]. These data indicate that mitochondrial activity and differential expression of mitochondrial genes can be responsible for intrinsic resistance to BTZ, suggesting that some of these genes can be used to identify chemotherapeutic regimens capable of sensitizing BTZ activity.

Another mechanism to induce sensitivity to BTZ relies on the modulation of ROS by iron [61]. Indeed, the proteasome is crucial for iron homeostasis, since it mediates the degradation of iron regulatory proteins (IRP1 and IRP2) and ferritin [62–64]. Campanella and colleagues showed that BTZ abolishes the coordinated upregulation of FtH ferritin subunits and the reduction of transferrin receptor by decreasing its turnover. Interestingly, ferritin levels also positively correlated with BTZ resistance. Specifically, BTZ-resistant cells have higher levels of iron stored with ferritin to limit Fenton reaction and oxidative damage. Indeed, silencing of FtH increases sensitivity to BTZ, in comparison with control cells. Hence, interfering with iron homeostasis emerges as a potential novel synthetic lethality strategy to enhance proteasomal inhibitory effects specific for MM cells, since iron itself has no cytotoxic effects in the absence of BTZ. Approaches to overcome BTZ resistance by modulating iron in patients should focus mainly on finding strategies to selectively reduce ferritin levels in malignant plasma cells, or to specifically deliver iron supplements to cancer cells, using hepcidin antagonists or other inflammatory modulators, to relieve iron sequestration from macrophages.

2.3 Clinical Applications with a Focus on Proteasome Inhibitor-Based Combination Therapies

The introduction of proteasome inhibitors (PIs) and immunomodulatory drugs in clinical practice has revolutionized the treatment outcomes of patients with MM [65]. Bortezomib was the first proteasome inhibitor approved by the FDA for relapsed and refractory patients in 2003. Since then, this class of drug has emerged as a cornerstone of therapy for MM patients. Specifically, the use of bortezomib as part of induction, consolidation, and maintenance therapies after stem cell transplant, and then as part of salvage regimens for relapsed disease, has significantly improved the prognosis and overall survival of patients with MM.

Nevertheless, MM remains incurable, and the vast majority of patients ultimately die from their disease. In particular patients who are relapsed and/or refractory to bortezomib and immunomodulatory drugs (IMiDs) have a very poor prognosis with a median progression-free survival and overall survival of only 5 and 9 months, respectively [66].

Encouragingly, new PIs with activity to different catalytic sites within the proteasome have recently been introduced into the clinic in order to overcome resistance acquired during bortezomib and other treatments, and to so potentially improve outcome.

Carfilzomib is a selective proteasome inhibitor that has demonstrated potent anti-myeloma activity and a favorable tolerability profile with manageable toxicity as a single agent in heavily pretreated relapsed and refractory MM patients [67]. Carfilzomib has recently been approved by FDA for the treatment of MM patients who have received at least two prior lines of therapy, including bortezomib and an IMiD, and who have experienced disease progression during or within 60 days of completing their last therapy.

The family of second-generation PIs also includes marizomib (NPI-0052), oprozomib (ONX0912), and ixazomib citrate (MLN9708), each of which has demonstrated clinical activity in relapsed and refractory MM patients in phase I/II studies.

Thus, the availability of new drugs with greater efficacy than bortezomib may improve the outlook for MM patients, but nevertheless resistance to PIs remains a challenge that requires new strategies in order to obtain deeper and longer remissions in these patients, irrespective of the agents used, and typically requires a combinatorial approach, informed by preclinical studies.

The antitumor activity of PIs is a sum of various mechanisms including inhibition of the 26S subunit of the proteasome, induction of apoptosis and inhibition of NF-κB activity that result in disruption of cell-cycle progression and control, and inhibition of proliferation and angiogenesis. Caspase-mediated apoptosis is induced by bortezomib through three different pathways: the intrinsic mitochondrial apoptotic pathway involving caspase-9, the extrinsic death receptor pathway involving caspase-8, and the endoplasmic reticulum stress response pathway involving caspase-2, caspase-4, and caspase-12 [68]. Targeting different pathways using a combination of PIs with conventional therapies as well as new drugs may therefore result in synergistic activity, so overcoming resistance, as evidenced both preclinically and now clinically.

The hypothesis that a combination of drugs could overcome resistance of bortezomib was first tested in a study adding dexamethasone to bortezomib therapy in relapsed and refractory MM patients. In this study, the addition of dexamethasone to bortezomib resulted in clinical response in patients not responding to bortezomib alone [69]. With the aim of overcoming resistance, bortezomib has since been widely tested in combination with new and old drugs as summarized in Table 2.1, and as detailed below. Preliminary results of clinical trials of carfilzomib-based combination therapies have also been published, whereas studies investigating other new PIs are still ongoing, and only relatively limited preliminary results are therefore available.

Table 2.1 Studies of proteasome inhibitors in combination with conventional and novel drugs

Class of drugs	Combination regimen	Schedule	Study	*N*/*n*	ORR (≥PR)	ORR in PI rel/ref pts	Common toxicities of combination treatment
Alkylating	Bortezomib	Mel days: 1–4	Phase III	VMP: 344	VMP: 71 %	Na	G3 neuropathy 13 %
	Melphalan [71]	Bort days: 1, 4, 8, 11, 22, 25, 29, 32	VMP vs. MP	MP: 338	MP: 35 %		G3 neutropenia 30 %
		Prednisone	(VISTA Trial)				G3 thrombocytopenia 20 %
	Bortezomib	Bort days 1, 4, 8, 11	Phase II EVOLUTION trial	126/130 (evaluable)	VDC: 75 %		VCD
	Cyclophosphamide [76]	Cyclo days 1, 8 (15 VCD-mod)	VCD, VDR, VCD-mod, VCDR	140 patients enrolled	VDC-mod: 100 %		G3 neutropenia 30 %
		Dexa days 1, 8, 15 or			VDR: 85 %		G3 neuropathy 9 %
		Len 15 mg days 1–14 (VDR)			VDCR: 88 %		G3 thrombocytopenia 12 %
							VCD-mod
							G3 neutropenia 24 %
							G3 neuropathy 18 %
							G3 thrombocytopenia 10 %
Anthracycline	Bortezomib	PLD day 4	Phase III	PLD/Bor: 324	PLD/Bor: 44 %	Na	G≥3 neutropenia 29 %
	Pegylated Liposomal Doxorubicin (PLD) [94]	Bortezomib days: 1, 4, 8, 11	PLD/Bor vs. Bor	Bor: 322	Bor: 41 %		G≥3 thrombocytopenia 23 %
							G≥3 diarrhea 7 %
Immuno-modulatory drugs	Bortezomib	Len days 1–14	Phase I	38/36	61 %	50 %	G1–2 neuropathy 42 %
	Lenalidomide [95]	Bort days 1, 4, 8, 11					G3 neutropenia 63 %
		Dexa					G3 thrombocytopenia 45 %
	Carfilzomib	Len days 1–21	Phase II	52	76.90 %	69.20 %	G3 neutropenia 33 %
	Lenalidomide [77]	Carfilz days 1, 2, 8, 9, 15, 16					G3 thrombocytopenia 19 %
		Dexa					
	Carfilzomib	Pomalidomide days 1–14	Phase I	28/20	75 %	Na	G3 neutropenia 29 %
	Pomalidomide [79]	Bortezomib days 1, 4, 8, 11					G3 thrombocytopenia 19 %
		Dexa days 1, 2, 4, 5, 8, 9, 11, 12					
	Carfilzomib	Pomalidomide days 1–21	Phase I/II	72 (Phase I/II)	64 % (≥MR 81 %)	Na	G≥3 fatigue 48 %
	Pomalidomide [80]	Carfilzomib 1, 2, 8, 9, 15, 16					G≥3 neutropenia 20 %
		Dexa 1, 8, 15, 22					G≥3 thrombocytopenia 20 %
	Ixazomib citrate (MLN9708)	MLN9708 days 1, 4, 8, 11	Phase I/II	64/62	94 %		Any grade:
	Lenalidomide [78]	Len days 1–14					Neuropathy: 53 %
		Dexa days 1, 2, 4, 5, 8, 9, 11, 12					Rash: 50 %
							Thrombocytopenia 6 %
							Neutropenia 5 %

HDAC inhibitors	Bortezomib	Panobinostat 3 t/week	Phase II (PANORAMA 2)	55	34.50 %	25.90 %	G ≥ 3 thrombocytopenia 64 %
	Panobinostat [81]	Bortezomib days 1, 4, 8, 11					G ≥ 3 anemia 20 %
		Dexa					G ≥ 3 fatigue 20 %
	Bortezomib	Vorinostat days 1–14	Phase III	VB 317	VB 56.2 %	Na	G ≥ 3 thrombocytopenia 43 %
	Vorinostat [83]	Bortezomib days 1, 4, 8, 11	Vor/Bor vs. Pla/Bor (VANTAGE 088)	PlaB 320	PlaB 40.2 %	Na	G ≥ 3 neutropenia 24 %
							G ≥ 3 diarrhea 16 %
							G ≥ 3 fatigue 17 %
	Bortezomib	Romidepsin d 1, 8, 15, 22	Phase II	25	60 % (≥MR 72 %)	Na	G ≥ 3 thrombocytopenia 64 %
	Romidepsin [84]	Bortezomib d 1, 4, 8, 11					G ≥ 3 neutropenia 36 %
		Dexa days 1, 2, 4, 5, 8, 9, 11, 12					G ≥ 3 polyneuropathy 8 %
	Bortezomib	ACY1215 days 1–5, 8–12	Phase I/II	16	VGPR (1)	Na	G ≥ 3 thrombocytopenia n = 3
	ACY1215 [86]	Bortezomib days 1, 4, 8, 11			PR(2), MR (1)		G ≥ 3 anemia n = 1
AKT inhibitors	Bortezomib	Perifosine daily	Phase I/II	84	22 % (≥MR 41 %)	≥ MR 65 % in rel pts	G ≥ 3 thrombocytopenia 23 %
	Perifosine [90]	Bortezomib days 1, 4, 8, 11				≥MR 32 % in refr pts	G ≥ 3 neutropenia 15 %
							G ≥ 3 anemia 14 %
	Bortezomib	Perifosine daily	Phase III	PeriB 69	PeriB 20 %	Na	Na
	Perifosine [91]	Bortezomib days 1, 4, 8, 11	Per/Bor vs. Pla/bor	PlaB 66	PlaB 27 %	Na	
		Dexa					
Anti-CXCR4	Bortezomib	Plerixafor days 1, 2, 3, 6, 10, 13	Phase I/II	25/10	40 %	Na	G4 thrombocytopenia 20 %
	Plerixafor [88]	Bortezomib days 3, 6, 10, 13					G3 anemia 10 %
							G3 hyperglycemia 10 %
Antibodies	Bortezomib	Elotuzumab days 1, 11	Phase I	28	48 %	67 %	G ≥ 3 lymphopenia 25 %
	Elotuzumab [93]	Bortezomib days 1, 4, 8, 11					G ≥ 3 fatigue 14 %
Heat shock protein 90 inhibitors	Bortezomib	Tanespimycin days 1, 4, 8, 11	Phase I/II	72	15 % (≥MR 27 %)	22 %	G ≥ 3 thrombocytopenia 25%
	Tanespimycin [96]	Bortezomib days 1, 4, 8, 11					G ≥ 3 fatigue 7 %
							G ≥ 3 diarrhea 7 %

2.3.1 Proteasome Inhibitors and Conventional Drugs

2.3.1.1 Bortezomib and Melphalan

Melphalan and prednisone (MP) were the standard of care for patients ineligible for transplant for many years. The addition of bortezomib to this regimen was the first step done to improve the response rate of this combination. A study evaluating the combination of bortezomib (also known as Velcade) and MP (VMP) showed a very encouraging overall response rate of 89 % [70]. A subsequent randomized study (the so-called VISTA Trial) compared MP versus VMP in untreated patients and confirmed the superiority of the bortezomib-containing regimen in terms of both survival and response rate [71]. The major toxicities of VMP included neuropathy and gastrointestinal symptoms. A subsequent study investigating a new schedule of VMP with weekly bortezomib in association with melphalan and prednisone or in association with thalidomide and prednisone (VTP) followed. Both arms of the study were then subject to a second randomization to maintenance with VT versus VP. No major differences between the two arms were observed, except for a lower rate of neurotoxicity in the VP arm. [72] An Italian study investigating combination of VMP plus thalidomide (VMPT) followed by bortezomib and thalidomide (VT) maintenance compared with VMP alone showed an advantage in terms of progression-free survival, overall survival, and response rate for the VMPT-VT arm. With the addition of thalidomide, a higher incidence of neuropathies was observed. This study was also amended after inclusion of the first 139 patients, and the schedule was changed to a weekly administration of bortezomib with a remarkable improvement in the incidence of grade 3–4 neuropathy. In aggregate, synergistic activity of bortezomib and melphalan results in a higher response rate in comparison with single-agent bortezomib, and this combination continues to have a role in the treatment of newly diagnosed patients not eligible to stem cell transplant.

2.3.2 Proteasome Inhibitors and Immunomodulatory Drugs

2.3.2.1 Bortezomib and Lenalidomide

Lenalidomide is an IMiD that exerts its anti-myeloma activity through activation of the caspase-8-mediated apoptosis pathway and inhibition of NF-κB activity through a different mechanism than bortezomib. On this basis, the hypothesis of combining these two drugs to overcome resistance occurring with single bortezomib treatment was investigated. Synergistic activity of the combination of the two drugs was initially tested in relapsed and refractory MM, including patients who were refractory to bortezomib. [73] The MTD was lenalidomide 15 mg daily on days 1–14; bortezomib 1 mg/m^2 on days 1, 4, 8, and 11 of a 21-day cycle; and dexamethasone 40 or 20 mg on days 1–2, 4–5, 8–9, and 11–12. Promising activity and limited toxicity observed in this phase I and subsequent phase II studies prompted this combination to be treated in association with dexamethasone in newly diagnosed MM patients [74]. In this study, 66 patients were treated with lenalidomide, bortezomib, and dexamethasone (RVD) for at least eight cycles. Patients achieving at least a partial response (PR) after four cycles were allowed to proceed to transplant. The percentage of patients achieving PR or better was 100 %, with more than VGPR seen in 74 %, including nCR and CR in 52 %. Main side effects observed included predominantly grade 1–2 sensory neuropathy, rare motor neuropathy, and some neuropathic pain, with grade 3–4 neutropenia and thrombocytopenia observed in 5–10 % of patients, and an overall rate of thrombosis (including pulmonary embolism) of 6 %. Toxicities proved generally manageable, however, and the regimen was well tolerated overall with a low rate of discontinuation.

The very high response rate observed with the combination of lenalidomide and bortezomib led to the incorporation of this regimen in the posttransplant setting in patients with high-risk MM. New studies using this combination therapy as consolidation or as long-term maintenance after autologous stem cell transplant in order to obtain deeper and longer responses are underway. A recent published paper by Nooka AK et al. evaluated the impact of a consolidation/maintenance program with lenalidomide, bortezomib, and dexamethasone (RVD) after transplant in patients with high-risk MM and showed a benefit in terms of both progression-free survival and overall survival in this poor prognosis population [75].

2.3.2.2 Bortezomib and Dexamethasone in Combination with Cyclophosphamide and Lenalidomide

Bortezomib and dexamethasone in combination with cyclophosphamide (VCD) has shown significant efficacy in patients with MM. In the randomized, phase 2, EVOLUTION study, VCD was compared to bortezomib, lenalidomide, and dexamethasone (VDR) and to the quadruple regimen of cyclophosphamide combined with VDR (VDCR). One hundred and forty patients received eight 3-week cycles of induction therapy with standard bortezomib dose with dexamethasone 40 mg on days 1, 8, and 15, with either cyclophosphamide at 500 mg/m^2 on days 1, 8 and lenalidomide 25 mg from days 1 to 14 (VDCR) or cyclophosphamide 500 mg/m^2 on days 1, 8 (VCD) and lenalidomide 15 mg days 1–14 (VDR). All groups received maintenance therapy with weekly bortezomib. Following the interim analysis, the VCD arm was modified to add an additional dose of cyclophosphamide on day 15 (VDC-mod). Very good partial response (VGPR) or better was seen in 58 %, 51 %, 41 %, and 53 % of patients in the VDCR, VDR, VDC, and VDC-mod arms respectively with a 1-year progression-free survival of 86 %, 83 %, 93 %, and 100 %, respectively. No advantage was noted with VDCR over the 3-drug combinations. Although the numbers are relatively small, this trial suggests both VCD and VRD are excellent choices for newly diagnosed patients [76].

2.3.2.3 Carfilzomib and Lenalidomide

Carfilzomib is a second-generation selective proteasome inhibitor that irreversibly binds the chymotrypsin-like activity of the proteasome. Combination therapy with carfilzomib and lenalidomide in association with low dose of dexamethasone was initially tested in relapsed or progressive MM patients. The phase Ib escalation part of the study defined the maximum planned dose of carfilzomib at 20 mg/m^2 on days 1 and 2 and 27 mg/mq on days 8, 9, 15, 16 thereafter, lenalidomide 25 mg on days 1 to 21, and dexamethasone 40 mg weekly on a 28-day cycle. Results of the phase 2 dose expansion in 52 patients showed an overall response rate of 77 % and duration of response of 22.1 months. Among bortezomib-refractory patients, 69 % responded, and among lenalidomide refractory patients, 70 % responded. Grade 3–4 toxicities included lymphopenia (8 %), neutropenia (33 %), thrombocytopenia (19 %), and anemia (19.2 %) [77].

More information about efficacy of this very active drug combination is expected from results of a large phase III trial comparing the activity of carfilzomib plus lenalidomide and dexamethasone versus lenalidomide and dexamethasone alone in relapsed patients (the so-called ASPIRE Trial) which was recently completed, with data on outcome anticipated soon.

2.3.2.4 Ixazomib Citrate and Lenalidomide

Ixazomib citrate (MLN9708) is an oral proteasome inhibitor that rapidly hydrolyzes to the biologically active dipeptide boronic acid MLN2238. MLN2238 preferentially binds the β5-site of the 20S proteasome; at higher concentrations, it also inhibits the activity of the β1- and β2-sites. In preclinical studies, MLN2238 demonstrates a faster dissociation rate from the proteasome that may result in enhanced tumor penetration, and antitumor activity, and has more prolonged tissue penetration than bortezomib. Phase I studies of MLN9708 have shown promising activity and durable responses in heavily pretreated MM patients. Ixazomib citrate in combination with lenalidomide and dexamethasone has been investigated in a phase 1/2 study in newly diagnosed patients. Sixty four patients received MLN9708 3.0 or 3.7 mg on days 1, 4, 8, 11, lenalidomide 25 mg on days 1–14, and dexamethasone 20/10 mg (cycles 1–8/9–16; days 1, 2, 4, 5, 8, 9, 11, 12) for up to 16 on a 21-day cycle, followed by MLN9708 maintenance until progression. Transplant-eligible pts could undergo stem cell collection after four cycles of therapy. In 62 response-evaluable patients, 94 % achieved greater than a PR including 76 % VGPR. Most common grade 3 adverse events were rash (16 %), hyperglycemia (8 %), pneumonia (6 %), and PN (5 %), with the regimen otherwise generally well tolerated with manageable toxicity [78].

2.3.3 Proteasome Inhibitors and Pomalidomide

2.3.3.1 Bortezomib and Pomalidomide

Pomalidomide is a new generation immunomodulatory agent that exerts its anti-myeloma activity through different ways including modulation of cytokine production, immunomodulation, and interaction with the bone marrow microenvironment.

Pomalidomide has been demonstrated to be more effective and less toxic than lenalidomide. This new IMiD has been approved by the Food and Drug Administration (FDA) for patients with relapsed/refractory MM who have received more than two prior therapies, including lenalidomide and bortezomib, and have progressive disease on or within 60 days of completion of their last line of treatment. The marked anti-myeloma activity observed in clinical trials investigating the effect of the combination of pomalidomide with dexamethasone and the known synergism between immunomodulatory drugs and bortezomib suggested a potential activity of the combination with pomalidomide and bortezomib. Preliminary data of the phase I trial testing pomalidomide in combination with bortezomib and dexamethasone in myeloma patients refractory to lenalidomide and relapsed after bortezomib have been recently published. Twenty-two out of twenty-eight planned patients were evaluable for response. Patients received escalating doses of pomalidomide (1–4 mg, days 1–14), bortezomib (1 or 1.3 mg/mq, days 1, 4, 8, 11), and dexamethasone 20 mg on days 1–2, 4–8, 8–9, 10–11. Overall response rate was 75 % (15 of 20 evaluable patients) with 30 % of VGPR or better. Most common grade 3 and 4 toxicities were neutropenia (29 %) and thrombocytopenia (19 %). No grade 3–4 peripheral neuropathy was observed [79]. The combination of pomalidomide and bortezomib seems to have a strong anti-MM activity in patients already treated with bortezomib, thus suggesting that the addition of pomalidomide may have the ability to overcome resistance acquired during treatment with PIs, and phase III studies are now underway to validate this concept.

2.3.3.2 Carfilzomib and Pomalidomide

Carfilzomib has been evaluated with pomalidomide and dexamethasone in a phase I/II study in relapsed and refractory MM patients. Dosages of the combination included carfilzomib at 20/27 mg/m^2, pomalidomide 4 mg, and dexamethasone 40 mg. The effect of the addition of pomalidomide to carfilzomib was evaluated in 67 patients enrolled in the phase I and II of the study. Preliminary data showed an overall response rate (PR or better) in a population of heavily pretreated patients of 64 %, and 81 % of patients achieved minimal response or better. Responses were observed also among patients with intermediate and high-risk cytogenetics. Common >grade 3 side effects included fatigue, neutropenia, anemia, thrombocytopenia, and diarrhea [80].

2.3.4 Proteasome Inhibitors and Histone Deacetylase Inhibitors

Deacetylases are a family of enzymes that exerts their activity on histone proteins and on a large number of proteins involved in intracellular functions that are dysregulated in cancer: gene expression, DNA replication and repair, cell-cycle progression, and cytoskeletal reorganization. Histone deacetylases (HDAC) remove acetyl groups from protein and have been recognized as a target for the treatment of hematological malignancies. Although several HDAC inhibitors (HDACIs) have been investigated and are in clinical development, only two of them to date have been approved for treatment of hematological malignancies. Specifically, both vorinostat and romidepsin have been approved for treatment of T cell cutaneous lymphoma.

The first HDACI that demonstrated to have anti-myeloma activity was SAHA (vorinostat). Exposure of myeloma cells to SAHA resulted in antiproliferative and proapoptotic effect involving downregulation of transcripts for member of the insulin-like growth factor (IGF)/IGF1 receptor and IL-6 receptor signaling cascades, antiapoptotic molecules, oncogenic kinases, DNA synthesis/repair enzymes, and transcription factors. Preclinical studies of other HDACIs demonstrate that the anti-myeloma activity of this class of drugs is due to a various numbers of effect on myeloma cells and on their interactions with the microenvironment. HDACIs can induce direct cell-cycle arrest and apoptosis and also disrupt the signaling between MM cells and bone marrow stem cells. Vorinostat is able to induce expression of p21, leading to cell-cycle arrest and apoptosis. Romidepsin induces downregulation of antiapoptotic proteins BCL-2 and BCL-XL. Vorinostat suppresses the stimulation of IL-6 secretion in bone marrow stem cells by myeloma cells adhesion and also suppresses autocrine IGF production interrupting the IGF-I/IGF-IR/Akt signaling pathway. HDACIs are also involved in myeloma cell inhibition, and specifically the prevention of aggresome formation in MM cells treated with PIs. The aggresomes are an alternative way that the cell can use for catabolism of misfolded proteins when the production of misfolded protein exceeds the capacity of proteasomes, as detailed previously. Drugs like tubacin targeting HDAC6 or panHDAC inhibitors like panobinostat lead to increase ubiquitinated proteins through impairment of the transport of aggresome to lysosome [23].

Based on the important activities of HDACIs, the hypothesis of combining HDACI with bortezomib to induce synergistic activity and to overcome resistance has been investigated. As mentioned, the dual inhibition of the proteasome and aggresome pathways induces accumulation of ubiquitinated proteins, resulting in cell stress and apoptosis. In addition to this synergistic effect, the combination of the two classes of drugs also exerts an anti-myeloma activity through multiple other pathways including inhibition of NF-κB, suppression of production of IL-6 and IGF-1, and inhibition of angiogenesis resulting in growth inhibition, apoptosis, and reduction of survival of myeloma cell.

2.3.4.1 Bortezomib and Panobinostat

The efficacy of the combination of HDACI and bortezomib has been evaluated in various clinical trials in relapsed and refractory myeloma patients and subsequently in randomized trials. The combination of panobinostat with bortezomib in refractory and relapsed myeloma patients was comprehensively tested in the multicenter phase II PANORAMA-2 study. In this study, 55 patients with relapsed and refractory MM, all of whom were required to be refractory to bortezomib, received bortezomib with the usual biweekly schedule, panobinostat 20 mg three times per week, and dexamethasone. The overall response rate was 35 % and clinical benefit as reflected by minimal response or better was evident in 53 % of patients. Of note 40 out of the 55 patients enrolled in the study were progressing while on their last treatment with bortezomib and all of the patients being refractory to bortezomib at some point. [81] Common observed grade 3 and 4 adverse events included thrombocytopenia, fatigue, and diarrhea. Results of this study confirmed that the addition of panobinostat is able to overcome the resistance to proteasome inhibitor as demonstrated by the responses observed among patients progressing on bortezomib-based therapy. Additional information about this combination will be available from the recently completed phase III PANORAMA-1 study investigating the direct comparison between the combination of the proteasome inhibitor, dexamethasone, and panobinostat versus bortezomib, dexamethasone, and placebo in relapsed MM patients. Importantly, preliminary results of the PANORAMA-1 trial appear to strongly favor an advantage to adding panobinostat to bortezomib and dexamethasone [82].

2.3.4.2 Bortezomib and SAHA (Vorinostat)

The combination of bortezomib and vorinostat in relapsed and refractory myeloma patients was evaluated in the VANTAGE 095 study. In this study, the overall response rate was 42 %, with objective response also seen among patients refractory to bortezomib. Most common grade 3 and 4 toxicities were myelosuppression, fatigue, and diarrhea. Despite the encouraging results observed in this phase II study, the phase III VANTAGE 088 study investigating the efficacy of bortezomib plus vorinostat versus bortezomib and placebo failed to show a clinically significant difference in terms of PFS between the two groups [83]. Patients receiving the combination therapy with vorinostat and bortezomib had more objective responses, but this advantage did not result in a meaningfully longer PFS. Explanation for this unexpected result was probably related to higher toxicity observed in the vorinostat arm that required frequent dose reductions and/or treatment interruptions. In fact, in the vorinostat group the side effects were significantly higher than in the placebo group; specifically myelosuppression, fatigue, nausea, vomiting, and diarrhea were the most common drug-related toxicities. Although the evidence of synergism between HDACI and bortezomib in overcoming resistance to PIs has been demonstrated, it is also therefore clear that new less toxic HDACIs are needed in order to obtain a more efficacious combination therapy.

2.3.4.3 Bortezomib and Romidepsin

Romidepsin has been approved by the FDA in the United States for relapsed cutaneous T cell lymphoma. Preclinical studies have demonstrated its anti-MM activity through upregulation of p21, downregulation of antiapoptotic molecules, and induction of apoptosis. Single-agent romidepsin in MM patients showed modest activity, but the synergistic effects between HDACI and bortezomib observed in preclinical studies justified a clinical trial testing the combination. Twenty-five patients were enrolled in the combination study of romidepsin dose on day 1, 8, and 15 of a 28-day cycle and bortezomib on days 1, 4, 8, and 11 with dexamethasone. The MTD for romidepsin was fixed at 10 mg/mq. At least a minimal response was seen in 72 % of patients with a median time to progression of 7.2 months. Most common adverse events included grade 3 and 4 thrombocytopenia in 64 % of patients and grade 3 and 4 peripheral neuropathy in 8 % [84].

2.3.4.4 Bortezomib and ACY1215

In order to increase activity of the combination therapy with HDACI and PIs and to reduce the toxicity related to the association of the two drugs, new more specific HDACIs have been investigated both preclinically and in clinical trials. As mentioned above, HDAC6 plays a key role in the aggresome pathway and is involved in formation and transportation of aggresome to lysosomes, thus suggesting a potential strong synergism with inhibitors of the proteasome pathway. ACY-1215 is a first-in-class selective and potent oral HDAC6 inhibitor with an anti-myeloma activity demonstrated both in vitro and in vivo animal models [85]. It has been tested in phase I/II clinical trials in combination with bortezomib and also with lenalidomide. Preliminary data presented at the ASH Meeting in 2013 reported 4 responding patients among 16 patients receiving the combination of bortezomib at 1–1.3 mg/m^2 and ACY-1215 at different doses with very manageable and limited toxicity [86]. More information about the feasibility and the efficacy of this combination will be available over time, but these preliminary results appear very promising.

2.3.5 Proteasome Inhibitors and Plerixafor

Interactions of MM cells with extracellular matrix proteins and bone marrow cells play a key role for survival and proliferation of malignant cells. Chemokines regulate the adhesion of the myeloma cells to their microenvironment, and cells and cytokines of the bone marrow environment activate proliferative and antiapoptotic signals. In particular the chemokine stromal-derived factor-1 (SDF-1) and its receptor CXCR4 play a central role in trafficking of myeloma cells.

The hypothesis that inhibiting CXCR4 could increase the sensitivity of myeloma cells to anti-myeloma drugs by disrupting the interaction with bone marrow has been tested in preclinical studies. Azab et al. [87] have demonstrated that AMD3100 is able to disrupt the adhesion of myeloma cells and microenvironment and induce mobilization of cells leading to increase sensitivity to bortezomib. The use of anti-CXCR4 in combination with bortezomib has been investigated in a phase I/II in relapsed and refractory MM patients with the aim to evaluate the chemosensitization effect of AMD3100. Preliminary results of this study have been recently published. In the first part of the study, 25 relapsed/refractory MM patients were treated with AMD3100 and bortezomib in two different schedules of administration, and in the second part of the study, 11 patients received AMD3100 at the MTD dose (320 μg/ m^2) on days 1, 2, 3, 6, 10, and 13 and bortezomib 1.3 mg/m^2 on days 3, 6, 10, and 13 every 21 days. Ten patients were evaluable for response, and more than partial remission was observed in 40 % of patients. Grade 4 toxicities included lymphopenia (10 %) and thrombocytopenia (20 %); grade 3 toxicities included anemia (10 %), thrombocytopenia (10 %), lymphopenia (20 %), hyperglycemia (10 %), and hypophosphatemia (10 %) [88]. The preliminary results of this study are hopeful, with 40 % of patients achieved a clinical benefit from the combination therapy, including a subgroup of patients refractory to bortezomib.

2.3.6 Proteasome Inhibitors and Perifosine

Perifosine is a synthetic novel alkylphospholipid (ALP) that targets cell membrane and inhibits Akt activation. In myeloma cells, perifosine is able to inhibit Akt activation triggered by IL-6 and IGF-1. Moreover, perifosine exerts a potent cytotoxicity against myeloma cells adherent to bone marrow stromal cells and induces apoptosis by recruitment of death receptors such as tumor necrosis factor (TNF)-related apoptosis-inducing ligand (TRAIL)-R1/DR4 and TRAIL-R2/DR5. Myeloma cell apoptosis induced by bortezomib is associated with activation of Akt, and preclinical studies have demonstrated that perifosine enhances the cytotoxicity of bortezomib and dexamethasone [89].

Based on promising preclinical data, a phase I/II study was conducted in relapsed/ refractory MM population; patients preexposed to bortezomib were treated with perifosine and bortezomib + dexamethasone. The dose selected for the part II of the study was perifosine 50 mg every day and bortezomib 1.3 mg/mq on days 1, 4, 8, and 11 in a 21-day cycle; addition of 20 mg of dexamethasone was permitted if progression occurred in perifosine plus bortezomib alone.

The new combination was tested in 84 patients with relapsed or relapsed/refractory MM; all have been already treated with bortezomib and majority of them were refractory to bortezomib (73 %). A minimal response or better was observed in 41 % of patients, including an overall response rate of 65 % in bortezomib-relapsed patients and of 32 % in bortezomib-refractory patients. Observed toxicities were mild and manageable; grade 3 and 4 adverse events included thrombocytopenia (23 %), neutropenia (15 %), anemia (14 %), and pneumonia (12 %). Thirty-one percent of patients had polyneuropathy of any grade. No patients experienced polyneuropathy of grade 4 [90]. Based on the results of the phase II study, a placebo randomized controlled study was conducted in relapsed/refractory MM patients previously treated with bortezomib. The study enrolled 135 patients that were randomized to receive perifosine 50 mg every day; bortezomib 1.3 mg/m^2 on days 1, 4, 8, and 11; and dexamethasone 20 mg, or placebo, bortezomib, and dexamethasone.

The study was discontinued after the first planned interim analysis because although well tolerated, no major benefit was observed in overall response rate and progression-free survival by adding perifosine to bortezomib and dexamethasone, as well as the emergence of major resource constraints and slow enrollment prompting a recommendation for closure [91]. Despite disappointing results of the phase III study, inhibition of Akt pathway seems to be a promising target for the treatment of relapsed/refractory MM patients, and the development of new more potent inhibitors warrants additional studies.

2.3.7 Proteasome Inhibitors and Monoclonal Antibodies, Specifically Elotuzumab

Elotuzumab is a humanized immunoglobulin G1 mAb directed against the cell surface glycoprotein CS1, expressed on normal plasma cells and myeloma cells. Elotuzumab exerts its anti-myeloma activity by blocking the adhesion of myeloma cells to bone marrow stromal cells and activating the natural killer (NK) cell-mediated antibody-dependent cellular cytotoxicity (ADCC). Preclinical studies have demonstrated a synergism between elotuzumab and bortezomib. Bortezomib enhances ADCC-mediated myeloma cell death induced by elotuzumab via down-regulation of the cell surface expression of MHC class I, an inhibitor of NK activity. In vitro and in vivo studies have demonstrated that bortezomib enhanced the anti-myeloma activity of elotuzumab rendering myeloma cells more sensitive to NK cell-mediated lysis [92]. In a phase I clinical trial, 28 patients with relapsed/refractory myeloma patients were treated with escalation dosages of elotuzumab and bortezomib. The maximum-tolerated dose was not reached up to the maximum planned dose of elotuzumab of 20 mg/kg; the most frequent grade 3 and 4 adverse events were lymphopenia (25 %) and fatigue (14 %). The phase I study demonstrated clinical activity of the combination with favorable toxicity; a partial response or better was observed in 48 % of patients and a minimal response or better was observed in 63 % of patients, with the median time to progression being more than 9 months [93].

Phase III studies aimed to evaluate the anti-myeloma activity of the combination are ongoing and hopefully will confirm the synergism or at least additive effects between bortezomib and elotuzumab.

2.4 Conclusion

The introduction of PIs in the spectrum of chemotherapeutic agents used in MM patients has remarkably impacted on patient treatment and improved overall survival. BTZ as a first-in-class PI and subsequently other novel PIs (such as carfilzomib) are already and will remain a standard treatment for both newly diagnosed and relapsed/refractory MM patients, most often in combination regimens based upon results to date. Unfortunately, BTZ and other PI resistance can be acquired in patients and so reduce treatment efficacy. Several mechanisms have been proposed for resistance including mutations and overexpression of proteasome subunits, decommitment to less-differentiated B cell stages to reduce ER overload and stress, activation of compensatory pathways such as autophagy and aggresome formation; and increase support by survival pathways, including MAF, c-MET, IGFR-1, and AKT or bone marrow stromal cells (Fig. 2.4). Hence, strategies to overcome BTZ and other PI resistance consist of combining agents capable of blocking these compensatory mechanisms, such as AKT inhibitors or IGFR inhibitors, or compounds targeting aggresome formation (HDAC6 inhibitors) or autophagy (FK866). Several biomarkers have been proposed to predict BTZ activity, such as XBP1 levels and inactivating various mutations including CD93/CD69, CYPD or SOD2, NAMPT, USP7, and MAF, but none of them has yet been validated in the clinical setting.

More broadly, synergistic combinations with IMiDs, chemotherapeutics, glucocorticoids, and more recently MoAbs have already been broadly validated with multiple clinical studies confirming the benefit of these approaches, validating that PIs are a backbone in MM therapy [97, 98]. Strategies with PIs to further improve the therapeutic index remain an area of urgent unmet medical need and hold the real promise of further improving patient outcome in this otherwise incurable disease [99, 100].

References

1. Shapiro-Shelef M, Calame K (2005) Regulation of plasma-cell development. Nat Rev Immunol 5(3):230–242
2. Goldberg AL (2003) Protein degradation and protection against misfolded or damaged proteins. Nature 426(6968):895–899
3. Goldberg AL, Dice JF (1974) Intracellular protein degradation in mammalian and bacterial cells. Annu Rev Biochem 43:835–869
4. Goldberg AL, St John AC (1976) Intracellular protein degradation in mammalian and bacterial cells. Annu Rev Biochem 45:747–803
5. Voges D, Zwickl P, Baumeister W (1999) The 26S proteasome: a molecular machine designed for controlled proteolysis. Annu Rev Biochem 68:1015–1068
6. Oerlemans R, Franke NE, Assaraf YG, Cloos J, van Zantwijk I, Berkers CR, Scheffer GL, Debipersad K, Vojtekova K, Lemos C, van der Heijden JW, Ylstra B, Peters GJ, Kaspers GL, Dijkmans BA, Scheper RJ, Jansen G (2008) Molecular basis of bortezomib resistance: proteasome subunit beta5 (PSMB5) gene mutation and overexpression of PSMB5 protein. Blood 112(6):2489–2499
7. Lü S, Yang J, Song X, Gong S, Zhou H, Guo L, Song N, Bao X, Chen P, Wang J (2008) Point mutation of the proteasome beta5 subunit gene is an important mechanism of bortezomib resistance in bortezomib-selected variants of Jurkat T cell lymphoblastic lymphoma/leukemia line. J Pharmacol Exp Ther 326(2):423–431
8. Lü S, Chen Z, Yang J, Chen L, Gong S, Zhou H, Guo L, Wang J (2008) Overexpression of the PSMB5 gene contributes to bortezomib resistance in T-lymphoblastic lymphoma/leukemia cells derived from Jurkat line. Exp Hematol 36(10):1278–1284
9. Ri M, Iida S, Nakashima T, Miyazaki H, Mori F, Ito A, Inagaki A, Kusumoto S, Ishida T, Komatsu H, Shiotsu Y, Ueda R (2010) Bortezomib-resistant myeloma cell lines: a role for

mutated PSMB5 in preventing the accumulation of unfolded proteins and fatal ER stress. Leukemia 24(8):1506–1512
10. Balsas P, Galán-Malo P, Marzo I, Naval J (2012) Bortezomib resistance in a myeloma cell line is associated to PSMbeta5 overexpression and polyploidy. Leuk Res 36(2):212–218
11. Franke NE, Niewerth D, Assaraf YG, van Meerloo J, Vojtekova K, van Zantwijk CH, Zweegman S, Chan ET, Kirk CJ, Geerke DP, Schimmer AD, Kaspers GJ, Jansen G, Cloos J (2012) Impaired bortezomib binding to mutant beta5 subunit of the proteasome is the underlying basis for bortezomib resistance in leukemia cells. Leukemia 26(4):757–768
12. Groll M, Berkers CR, Ploegh HL, Ovaa H (2006) Crystal structure of the boronic acid-based proteasome inhibitor bortezomib in complex with the yeast 20S proteasome. Structure 14(3): 451–456
13. Borissenko L, Groll M (2007) 20S proteasome and its inhibitors: crystallographic knowledge for drug development. Chem Rev 107(3):687–717
14. Heinemeyer W, Fischer M, Krimmer T, Stachon U, Wolf DH (1997) The active sites of the eukaryotic 20 S proteasome and their involvement in subunit precursor processing. J Biol Chem 272(40):25200–25209
15. Chapman MA, Lawrence MS, Keats JJ, Cibulskis K, Sougnez C, Schinzel AC, Harview CL, Brunet JP, Ahmann GJ, Adli M, Anderson KC, Ardlie KG, Auclair D, Baker A, Bergsagel PL, Bernstein BE, Drier Y, Fonseca R, Gabriel SB, Hofmeister CC, Jagannath S, Jakubowiak AJ, Krishnan A, Levy J, Liefeld T, Lonial S, Mahan S, Mfuko B, Monti S, Perkins LM, Onofrio R, Pugh TJ, Rajkumar SV, Ramos AH, Siegel DS, Sivachenko A, Stewart AK, Trudel S, Vij R, Voet D, Winckler W, Zimmerman T, Carpten J, Trent J, Hahn WC, Garraway LA, Meyerson M, Lander ES, Getz G, Golub TR (2011) Initial genome sequencing and analysis of multiple myeloma. Nature 471(7339):467–472
16. Lichter DI, Danaee H, Pickard MD, Tayber O, Sintchak M, Shi H, Richardson PG, Cavenagh J, Bladé J, Façon T, Niesvizky R, Alsina M, Dalton W, Sonneveld P, Lonial S, van de Velde H, Ricci D, Esseltine DL, Trepicchio WL, Mulligan G, Anderson KC (2012) Sequence analysis of beta-subunit genes of the 20S proteasome in patients with relapsed multiple myeloma treated with bortezomib or dexamethasone. Blood 120(23):4513–4516
17. Wang L, Kumar S, Fridley BL, Kalari KR, Moon I, Pelleymounter LL, Hildebrandt MA, Batzler A, Eckloff BW, Wieben ED, Greipp PR (2008) Proteasome beta subunit pharmacogenomics: gene resequencing and functional genomics. Clin Cancer Res 14(11):3503–3513
18. Shuqing L, Jianmin Y, Chongmei H, Hui C, Wang J (2011) Upregulated expression of the PSMB5 gene may contribute to drug resistance in patient with multiple myeloma when treated with bortezomib-based regimen. Exp Hematol 39(12):1117–1118
19. Politou M, Karadimitris A, Terpos E, Kotsianidis I, Apperley JF, Rahemtulla A (2006) No evidence of mutations of the PSMB5 (beta-5 subunit of proteasome) in a case of myeloma with clinical resistance to Bortezomib. Leuk Res 30(2):240–241
20. Li B, Wang H, Orlowski RZ (2013) Proteasome maturation protein (pomp) is associated with proteasome inhibitor resistance in myeloma, and its suppression enhances the activity of bortezomib and carfilzomib. Annual Meeting of American Society of Hematology 2013. Blood 122:280
21. Johnston JA, Ward CL, Kopito RR (1998) Aggresomes: a cellular response to misfolded proteins. J Cell Biol 143(7):1883–1898
22. Kawaguchi Y, Kovacs JJ, McLaurin A, Vance JM, Ito A, Yao TP (2003) The deacetylase HDAC6 regulates aggresome formation and cell viability in response to misfolded protein stress. Cell 115(6):727–738
23. Hideshima T, Bradner JE, Wong J, Chauhan D, Richardson P, Schreiber SL, Anderson KC (2005) Small-molecule inhibition of proteasome and aggresome function induces synergistic antitumor activity in multiple myeloma. Proc Natl Acad Sci U S A 102(24):8567–8572
24. Catley L, Weisberg E, Kiziltepe T, Tai YT, Hideshima T, Neri P, Tassone P, Atadja P, Chauhan D, Munshi NC, Anderson KC (2006) Aggresome induction by proteasome inhibitor bortezomib and alpha-tubulin hyperacetylation by tubulin deacetylase (TDAC) inhibitor LBH589 are synergistic in myeloma cells. Blood 108(10):3441–3449
25. Shringarpure R, Catley L, Bhole D, Burger R, Podar K, Tai YT, Kessler B, Galardy P, Ploegh H, Tassone P, Hideshima T, Mitsiades C, Munshi NC, Chauhan D, Anderson KC (2006) Gene

expression analysis of B-lymphoma cells resistant and sensitive to bortezomib. Br J Haematol 134(2):145–156
26. Chauhan D, Li G, Shringarpure R, Podar K, Ohtake Y, Hideshima T, Anderson KC (2003) Blockade of Hsp27 overcomes Bortezomib/proteasome inhibitor PS-341 resistance in lymphoma cells. Cancer Res 63(19):6174–6177
27. Ito H, Iwamoto I, Inaguma Y, Takizawa T, Nagata K, Asano T, Kato K (2005) Endoplasmic reticulum stress induces the phosphorylation of small heat shock protein, Hsp27. J Cell Biochem 95(5):932–941
28. Kumano M, Furukawa J, Shiota M, Zardan A, Zhang F, Beraldi E, Wiedmann RM, Fazli L, Zoubeidi A, Gleave ME (2012) Cotargeting stress-activated Hsp27 and autophagy as a combinatorial strategy to amplify endoplasmic reticular stress in prostate cancer. Mol Cancer Ther 11(8):1661–1671
29. Cea M, Cagnetta A, Fulciniti M, Tai YT, Hideshima T, Chauhan D, Roccaro A, Sacco A, Calimeri T, Cottini F, Jakubikova J, Kong SY, Patrone F, Nencioni A, Gobbi M, Richardson P, Munshi N, Anderson KC (2012) Targeting NAD+ salvage pathway induces autophagy in multiple myeloma cells via mTORC1 and extracellular signal-regulated kinase (ERK1/2) inhibition. Blood 120(17):3519–3529
30. Cagnetta A, Cea M, Calimeri T, Acharya C, Fulciniti M, Tai YT, Hideshima T, Chauhan D, Zhong MY, Patrone F, Nencioni A, Gobbi M, Richardson P, Munshi N, Anderson KC (2013) Intracellular NAD(+) depletion enhances bortezomib-induced anti-myeloma activity. Blood 122(7):1243–1255
31. Ling SC, Lau EK, Al-Shabeeb A, Nikolic A, Catalano A, Iland H, Horvath N, Ho PJ, Harrison S, Fleming S, Joshua DE, Allen JD (2012) Response of myeloma to the proteasome inhibitor bortezomib is correlated with the unfolded protein response regulator XBP-1. Haematologica 97(1):64–72
32. Leung-Hagesteijn C, Erdmann N, Cheung G, Keats JJ, Stewart AK, Reece DE, Chung KC, Tiedemann RE (2013) Xbp1s-negative tumor B cells and pre-plasmablasts mediate therapeutic proteasome inhibitor resistance in multiple myeloma. Cancer Cell 24(3):289–304
33. Stessman HA, Mansoor A, Zhan F, Linden MA, Van Ness B, Baughn LB (2013) Bortezomib resistance can be reversed by induced expression of plasma cell maturation markers in a mouse in vitro model of multiple myeloma. PLoS One 8(10):e77608
34. Rumpold H, Salvador C, Wolf AM, Tilg H, Gastl G, Wolf D (2007) Knockdown of PgP resensitizes leukemic cells to proteasome inhibitors. Biochem Biophys Res Commun 361(2): 549–554
35. Verbrugge SE, Assaraf YG, Dijkmans BA, Scheffer GL, Al M, den Uyl D, Oerlemans R, Chan ET, Kirk CJ, Peters GJ, van der Heijden JW, de Gruijl TD, Scheper RJ, Jansen G (2012) Inactivating PSMB5 mutations and P-glycoprotein (multidrug resistance-associated protein/ATP-binding cassette B1) mediate resistance to proteasome inhibitors: ex vivo efficacy of (immuno)proteasome inhibitors in mononuclear blood cells from patients with rheumatoid arthritis. J Pharmacol Exp Ther 341(1):174–182
36. Xu D, Hu J, De Bruyne E, Menu E, Schots R, Vanderkerken K, Van Valckenborgh E (2012) Dll1/Notch activation contributes to bortezomib resistance by upregulating CYP1A1 in multiple myeloma. Biochem Biophys Res Commun 428(4):518–524
37. Shumway SD, Miyamoto S (2004) A mechanistic insight into a proteasome-independent constitutive inhibitor kappaBalpha (IkappaBalpha) degradation and nuclear factor kappaB (NF-kappaB) activation pathway in WEHI-231 B-cells. Biochem J 380(Pt 1):173–180
38. Hideshima T, Ikeda H, Chauhan D, Okawa Y, Raje N, Podar K, Mitsiades C, Munshi NC, Richardson PG, Carrasco RD, Anderson KC (2009) Bortezomib induces canonical nuclear factor-kappaB activation in multiple myeloma cells. Blood 114(5):1046–1052
39. Markovina S, Callander NS, O'Connor SL, Kim J, Werndli JE, Raschko M, Leith CP, Kahl BS, Kim K, Miyamoto S (2008) Bortezomib-resistant nuclear factor-kappaB activity in multiple myeloma cells. Mol Cancer Res 6(8):1356–1364
40. Yang DT, Young KH, Kahl BS, Markovina S, Miyamoto S (2008) Prevalence of bortezomib-resistant constitutive NF-kappaB activity in mantle cell lymphoma. Mol Cancer 7:40

41. Zhou L, Hou J, Fu W, Wang D, Yuan Z, Jiang H (2008) Arsenic trioxide and 2-methoxyestradiol reduce beta-catenin accumulation after proteasome inhibition and enhance the sensitivity of myeloma cells to Bortezomib. Leuk Res 32(11):1674–1683
42. Kuhn DJ, Berkova Z, Jones RJ, Woessner R, Bjorklund CC, Ma W, Davis RE, Lin P, Wang H, Madden TL, Wei C, Baladandayuthapani V, Wang M, Thomas SK, Shah JJ, Weber DM, Orlowski RZ (2012) Targeting the insulin-like growth factor-1 receptor to overcome bortezomib resistance in preclinical models of multiple myeloma. Blood 120(16):3260–3270
43. Que W, Chen J, Chuang M, Jiang D (2012) Knockdown of c-Met enhances sensitivity to bortezomib in human multiple myeloma U266 cells via inhibiting Akt/mTOR activity. APMIS 120(3):195–203
44. Ye S, Qiang W, Chen Y, Hu B, Zhang Q, Yaccoby S, van Rhee F, Barlogie B, Epstein J, Qiang YW (2013) MAF protein elicits innate resistance to bortezomib in multiple myeloma. Annual Meeting of American Society of Hematology 2013. Blood 122:281
45. Ling YH, Liebes L, Zou Y, Perez-Soler R (2003) Reactive oxygen species generation and mitochondrial dysfunction in the apoptotic response to Bortezomib, a novel proteasome inhibitor, in human H460 non-small cell lung cancer cells. J Biol Chem 278(36):33714–33723
46. Pei XY, Dai Y, Grant S (2003) The proteasome inhibitor bortezomib promotes mitochondrial injury and apoptosis induced by the small molecule Bcl-2 inhibitor HA14-1 in multiple myeloma cells. Leukemia 17(10):2036–2045
47. Pei XY, Dai Y, Grant S (2004) Synergistic induction of oxidative injury and apoptosis in human multiple myeloma cells by the proteasome inhibitor bortezomib and histone deacetylase inhibitors. Clin Cancer Res 10(11):3839–3852
48. Yu C, Rahmani M, Dent P, Grant S (2004) The hierarchical relationship between MAPK signaling and ROS generation in human leukemia cells undergoing apoptosis in response to the proteasome inhibitor Bortezomib. Exp Cell Res 295(2):555–566
49. Zou W, Yue P, Lin N, He M, Zhou Z, Lonial S, Khuri FR, Wang B, Sun SY (2006) Vitamin C inactivates the proteasome inhibitor PS-341 in human cancer cells. Clin Cancer Res 12(1): 273–280
50. Perrone G, Hideshima T, Ikeda H, Okawa Y, Calabrese E, Gorgun G, Santo L, Cirstea D, Raje N, Chauhan D, Baccarani M, Cavo M, Anderson KC (2009) Ascorbic acid inhibits antitumor activity of bortezomib in vivo. Leukemia 23(9):1679–1686
51. Liu FT, Agrawal SG, Movasaghi Z, Wyatt PB, Rehman IU, Gribben JG, Newland AC, Jia L (2008) Dietary flavonoids inhibit the anticancer effects of the proteasome inhibitor bortezomib. Blood 112(9):3835–3846
52. Golden EB, Lam PY, Kardosh A, Gaffney KJ, Cadenas E, Louie SG, Petasis NA, Chen TC, Schönthal AH (2009) Green tea polyphenols block the anticancer effects of bortezomib and other boronic acid-based proteasome inhibitors. Blood 113(23):5927–5937
53. Song MS, Salmena L, Carracedo A, Egia A, Lo-Coco F, Teruya-Feldstein J, Pandolfi PP (2008) The deubiquitinylation and localization of PTEN are regulated by a HAUSP-PML network. Nature 455(7214):813–817
54. Cummins JM, Rago C, Kohli M, Kinzler KW, Lengauer C, Vogelstein B (2004) Tumour suppression: disruption of HAUSP gene stabilizes p53. Nature 428(6982):1 p following 486
55. Hershko A, Heller H, Elias S, Ciechanover A (1983) Components of ubiquitin-protein ligase system. Resolution, affinity purification, and role in protein breakdown. J Biol Chem 258(13): 8206–8214
56. Ooi MG, Hayden PJ, Kotoula V, McMillin DW, Charalambous E, Daskalaki E, Raje NS, Munshi NC, Chauhan D, Hideshima T, Buon L, Clynes M, O'Gorman P, Richardson PG, Mitsiades CS, Anderson KC, Mitsiades N (2009) Interactions of the Hdm2/p53 and proteasome pathways may enhance the antitumor activity of bortezomib. Clin Cancer Res 15(23): 7153–7160
57. Xu GW, Ali M, Wood TE, Wong D, Maclean N, Wang X, Gronda M, Skrtic M, Li X, Hurren R, Mao X, Venkatesan M, Beheshti Zavareh R, Ketela T, Reed JC, Rose D, Moffat J, Batey RA, Dhe-Paganon S, Schimmer AD (2010) The ubiquitin-activating enzyme E1 as a therapeutic target for the treatment of leukemia and multiple myeloma. Blood 115(11):2251–2259

58. Song IS, Kim HK, Lee SR, Jeong SH, Kim N, Ko KS, Rhee BD, Han J (2013) Mitochondrial modulation decreases the bortezomib-resistance in multiple myeloma cells. Int J Cancer 133(6):1357–1367
59. Song IS, Jeong YJ, Jeong SH, Heo HJ, Kim HK, Lee SR, Ko TH, Youm JB, Kim N, Ko KS, Rhee BD, Han J (2013) Combination treatment with 2-methoxyestradiol overcomes bortezomib resistance of multiple myeloma cells. Exp Mol Med 45:e50
60. Chauhan D, Li G, Podar K, Hideshima T, Mitsiades C, Schlossman R, Munshi N, Richardson P, Cotter FE, Anderson KC (2004) Targeting mitochondria to overcome conventional and bortezomib/proteasome inhibitor PS-341 resistance in multiple myeloma (MM) cells. Blood 104(8):2458–2466
61. Campanella A, Santambrogio P, Fontana F, Frenquelli M, Cenci S, Marcatti M, Sitia R, Tonon G, Camaschella C (2013) Iron increases the susceptibility of multiple myeloma cells to bortezomib. Haematologica 98(6):971–979
62. De Domenico I, Vaughn MB, Li L, Bagley D, Musci G, Ward DM, Kaplan J (2006) Ferroportin-mediated mobilization of ferritin iron precedes ferritin degradation by the proteasome. EMBO J 25(22):5396–5404
63. Rouault TA (2006) The role of iron regulatory proteins in mammalian iron homeostasis and disease. Nat Chem Biol 2(8):406–414
64. Wang J, Fillebeen C, Chen G, Biederbick A, Lill R, Pantopoulos K (2007) Iron-dependent degradation of apo-IRP1 by the ubiquitin-proteasome pathway. Mol Cell Biol 27(7):2423–2430
65. Sonneveld P, Goldschmidt H, Rosinol L, Blade J, Lahuerta JJ, Cavo M, Tacchetti P, Zamagni E, Attal M, Lokhorst HM, Desai A, Cakana A, Liu K, van de Velde H, Esseltine DL, Moreau P (2013) Bortezomib-based versus nonbortezomib-based induction treatment before autologous stem-cell transplantation in patients with previously untreated multiple myeloma: a meta-analysis of phase III randomized, controlled trials. J Clin Oncol 31(26):3279–3287
66. Kumar SK, Lee JH, Lahuerta JJ, Morgan G, Richardson PG, Crowley J, Haessler J, Feather J, Hoering A, Moreau P, LeLeu X, Hulin C, Klein SK, Sonneveld P, Siegel D, Blade J, Goldschmidt H, Jagannath S, Miguel JS, Orlowski R, Palumbo A, Sezer O, Rajkumar SV, Durie BG (2012) Risk of progression and survival in multiple myeloma relapsing after therapy with IMiDs and bortezomib: a multicenter international myeloma working group study. Leukemia 26(1):149–157
67. Siegel DS, Martin T, Wang M, Vij R, Jakubowiak AJ, Lonial S, Trudel S, Kukreti V, Bahlis N, Alsina M, Chanan-Khan A, Buadi F, Reu FJ, Somlo G, Zonder J, Song K, Stewart AK, Stadtmauer E, Kunkel L, Wear S, Wong AF, Orlowski RZ, Jagannath S (2012) A phase 2 study of single-agent carfilzomib (PX-171-003-A1) in patients with relapsed and refractory multiple myeloma. Blood 120(14):2817–2825
68. Mitsiades N, Mitsiades CS, Poulaki V, Chauhan D, Fanourakis G, Gu X, Bailey C, Joseph M, Libermann TA, Treon SP, Munshi NC, Richardson PG, Hideshima T, Anderson KC (2002) Molecular sequelae of proteasome inhibition in human multiple myeloma cells. Proc Natl Acad Sci U S A 99(22):14374–14379
69. Richardson PG, Barlogie B, Berenson J, Singhal S, Jagannath S, Irwin D, Rajkumar SV, Srkalovic G, Alsina M, Alexanian R, Siegel D, Orlowski RZ, Kuter D, Limentani SA, Lee S, Hideshima T, Esseltine DL, Kauffman M, Adams J, Schenkein DP, Anderson KC (2003) A phase 2 study of bortezomib in relapsed, refractory myeloma. N Engl J Med 348(26): 2609–2617
70. Mateos MV, Hernández JM, Hernández MT, Gutiérrez NC, Palomera L, Fuertes M, Díaz-Mediavilla J, Lahuerta JJ, de la Rubia J, Terol MJ, Sureda A, Bargay J, Ribas P, de Arriba F, Alegre A, Oriol A, Carrera D, García-Laraña J, García-Sanz R, Bladé J, Prósper F, Mateo G, Esseltine DL, van de Velde H, San Miguel JF (2006) Bortezomib plus melphalan and prednisone in elderly untreated patients with multiple myeloma: results of a multicenter phase 1/2 study. Blood 108(7):2165–2172
71. San Miguel JF, Schlag R, Khuageva NK, Dimopoulos MA, Shpilberg O, Kropff M, Spicka I, Petrucci MT, Palumbo A, Samoilova OS, Dmoszynska A, Abdulkadyrov KM, Schots R,

Jiang B, Mateos MV, Anderson KC, Esseltine DL, Liu K, Cakana A, van de Velde H, Richardson PG (2008) Bortezomib plus melphalan and prednisone for initial treatment of multiple myeloma. N Engl J Med 359(9):906–917
72. Mateos MV, Oriol A, Martinez-Lopez J, Gutierrez N, Teruel AI, de Paz R, Garcia-Larana J, Bengoechea E, Martin A, Mediavilla JD, Palomera L, de Arriba F, Gonzalez Y, Hernandez JM, Sureda A, Bello JL, Bargay J, Penalver FJ, Ribera JM, Martin-Mateos ML, Garcia-Sanz R, Cibeira MT, Ramos ML, Vidriales MB, Paiva B, Montalban MA, Lahuerta JJ, Blade J, Miguel JF (2010) Bortezomib, melphalan, and prednisone versus bortezomib, thalidomide, and prednisone as induction therapy followed by maintenance treatment with bortezomib and thalidomide versus bortezomib and prednisone in elderly patients with untreated multiple myeloma: a randomised trial. Lancet Oncol 11(10):934–941
73. Richardson PG, Weller E, Jagannath S, Avigan DE, Alsina M, Schlossman RL, Mazumder A, Munshi NC, Ghobrial IM, Doss D, Warren DL, Lunde LE, McKenney M, Delaney C, Mitsiades CS, Hideshima T, Dalton W, Knight R, Esseltine DL, Anderson KC (2009) Multicenter, phase I, dose-escalation trial of lenalidomide plus bortezomib for relapsed and relapsed/refractory multiple myeloma. J Clin Oncol 27(34):5713–5719
74. Richardson PG, Weller E, Lonial S, Jakubowiak AJ, Jagannath S, Raje NS, Avigan DE, Xie W, Ghobrial IM, Schlossman RL, Mazumder A, Munshi NC, Vesole DH, Joyce R, Kaufman JL, Doss D, Warren DL, Lunde LE, Kaster S, Delaney C, Hideshima T, Mitsiades CS, Knight R, Esseltine DL, Anderson KC (2010) Lenalidomide, bortezomib, and dexamethasone combination therapy in patients with newly diagnosed multiple myeloma. Blood 116(5):679–686
75. Nooka AK, Kaufman JL, Muppidi S, Langston A, Heffner LT, Gleason C, Casbourne D, Saxe D, Boise LH, Lonial S (2014) Consolidation and maintenance therapy with lenalidomide, bortezomib and dexamethasone (RVD) in high-risk myeloma patients. Leukemia 28(3):690–693
76. Kumar S, Flinn I, Richardson PG, Hari P, Callander N, Noga SJ, Stewart AK, Turturro F, Rifkin R, Wolf J, Estevam J, Mulligan G, Shi H, Webb IJ, Rajkumar SV (2012) Randomized, multicenter, phase 2 study (EVOLUTION) of combinations of bortezomib, dexamethasone, cyclophosphamide, and lenalidomide in previously untreated multiple myeloma. Blood 119(19):4375–4382
77. Wang M, Martin T, Bensinger W, Alsina M, Siegel DS, Kavalerchik E, Huang M, Orlowski RZ, Niesvizky R (2013) Phase 2 dose-expansion study (PX-171-006) of carfilzomib, lenalidomide, and low-dose dexamethasone in relapsed or progressive multiple myeloma. Blood 122(18):3122–3128
78. Kumar SK, Roy V, Reeder C, LaPlant BR, Lacy MQ, Gertz MA, Laumann K, Thompson MA, Witzig TE, Buadi FK, Rivera CE, Mikhael JR, Bergsagel PL, Hwa L, Rajkumar V, Dispenzieri A (2013) Phase 2 trial of single agent MLN9708 in patients with relapsed multiple myeloma not refractory to bortezomib. Annual Meeting of American Society of Hematology 2013. Blood 122(21):1944
79. Richardson PG, Hofmeister CC, Siegel D, Lonial S, Laubach JP, Efebera YA, Vesole DH, Nooka AK, Rosenblatt J, Raje N, Zaki MH, Hua Y, Li Y, Shah S, Wang J, Anderson KC (2013) MM-005: a phase 1 trial of pomalidomide, bortezomib, and low-dose dexamethasone (PVD) in relapsed and/or refractory multiple myeloma (RRMM). Annual Meeting of American Society of Hematology 2013. Blood 122(21):1969a
80. Shah JJ, Stadtmauer EA, Abonour R, Cohen AD, Bensinger W, Gasparetto C, Kaufman JL, Lentzsch S, Vogl DT, Orlowski RL, Kim L, Bialas N, Smith DD, Durie BGM (2013) Phase I/II dose expansion of a multi-center trial of carfilzomib and pomalidomide with dexamethasone (Car-Pom-d) in patients with relapsed/refractory multiple myeloma. Annual Meeting of American Society of Hematology 2013. Blood 122(21):690a
81. Richardson PG, Schlossman RL, Alsina M, Weber DM, Coutre SE, Gasparetto C, Mukhopadhyay S, Ondovik MS, Khan M, Paley CS, Lonial S (2013) PANORAMA 2: panobinostat in combination with bortezomib and dexamethasone in patients with relapsed and bortezomib-refractory myeloma. Blood 122(14):2331–2337

82. Richardson PG, Schlossman RL, Alsina M, Weber DM, Coutre SE, Gasparetto C, Mukhopadhyay S, Ondovik MS, Khan M, Paley CS, Lonial S (2013) Time to event analyses in PANORAMA 2: a phase 2 study of panobinostat, bortezomib, and dexamethasone in patients with relapsed and bortezomib-refractory multiple myeloma. Annual Meeting of American Society of Hematology 2013. Blood 122(21):1970
83. Dimopoulos M, Siegel DS, Lonial S, Qi J, Hajek R, Facon T, Rosinol L, Williams C, Blacklock H, Goldschmidt H, Hungria V, Spencer A, Palumbo A, Graef T, Eid JE, Houp J, Sun L, Vuocolo S, Anderson KC (2013) Vorinostat or placebo in combination with bortezomib in patients with multiple myeloma (VANTAGE 088): a multicentre, randomised, double-blind study. Lancet Oncol 14(11):1129–1140
84. Harrison SJ, Quach H, Link E, Seymour JF, Ritchie DS, Ruell S, Dean J, Januszewicz H, Johnstone R, Neeson P, Dickinson M, Nichols J, Prince HM (2011) A high rate of durable responses with romidepsin, bortezomib, and dexamethasone in relapsed or refractory multiple myeloma. Blood 118(24):6274–6283
85. Santo L, Hideshima T, Kung AL, Tseng JC, Tamang D, Yang M, Jarpe M, van Duzer JH, Mazitschek R, Ogier WC, Cirstea D, Rodig S, Eda H, Scullen T, Canavese M, Bradner J, Anderson KC, Jones SS, Raje N (2012) Preclinical activity, pharmacodynamic, and pharmacokinetic properties of a selective HDAC6 inhibitor, ACY-1215, in combination with bortezomib in multiple myeloma. Blood 119(11):2579–2589
86. Raje N, Vogl DT, Hari PN, Jagannath S, Jones SS, Supko JG, Leone G, Wheeler C, Orlowski RZ, Richardson PG, Lonial S (2013) ACY-1215, a selective histone deacetylase (HDAC) 6 inhibitor: interim results of combination therapy with bortezomib in patients with multiple myeloma (MM). Annual Meeting of American Society of Hematology 2013. Blood 122(21):759a
87. Azab AK, Runnels JM, Pitsillides C, Moreau AS, Azab F, Leleu X, Jia X, Wright R, Ospina B, Carlson AL, Alt C, Burwick N, Roccaro AM, Ngo HT, Farag M, Melhem MR, Sacco A, Munshi NC, Hideshima T, Rollins BJ, Anderson KC, Kung AL, Lin CP, Ghobrial IM (2009) CXCR4 inhibitor AMD3100 disrupts the interaction of multiple myeloma cells with the bone marrow microenvironment and enhances their sensitivity to therapy. Blood 113(18):4341–4351
88. Ghobrial IM, Shain K, Hanlon C, Banwait R, Azab AK, Laubach JP, Armand P, Munshi NC, Schlossman RL, Chuma S, Boswell EN, Mostyn P, Houry L, Anderson KC, Richardson PG (2013) Phase I/II trial of plerixafor and bortezomib as a chemosensitization strategy in relapsed or relapsed/refractory multiple myeloma. Annual Meeting of American Society of Hematology 2013. Blood 122(21):1947a
89. Hideshima T, Catley L, Raje N, Chauhan D, Podar K, Mitsiades C, Tai YT, Vallet S, Kiziltepe T, Ocio E, Ikeda H, Okawa Y, Hideshima H, Munshi NC, Yasui H, Richardson PG, Anderson KC (2007) Inhibition of Akt induces significant downregulation of survivin and cytotoxicity in human multiple myeloma cells. Br J Haematol 138(6):783–791
90. Richardson PG, Wolf J, Jakubowiak A, Zonder J, Lonial S, Irwin D, Densmore J, Krishnan A, Raje N, Bar M, Martin T, Schlossman R, Ghobrial IM, Munshi N, Laubach J, Allerton J, Hideshima T, Colson K, Poradosu E, Gardner L, Sportelli P, Anderson KC (2011) Perifosine plus bortezomib and dexamethasone in patients with relapsed/refractory multiple myeloma previously treated with bortezomib: results of a multicenter phase I/II trial. J Clin Oncol 29(32):4243–4249
91. Richardson PG, Nagler A, Ben-Yehuda D, Badros A, Hari P, Hajek R, Spicka I, Kaya H, Le Blanc R, Yoon S, Kim K, Martinez-Lopez J, Mittelman M, Shpilberg O, Tothova E, Laubach JP, Ghobrial IM, Leiba M, Gatt ME, Sportelli P, Chen M, Anderson KC (2013) Randomized placebo-controlled phase III study of perifosine combined with bortezomib and dexamethasone in relapsed, refractory multiple myeloma patients previously treated with bortezomib Annual Meeting of American Society of Hematology 2013. Blood 122(21):3189
92. van Rhee F, Szmania SM, Dillon M, van Abbema AM, Li X, Stone MK, Garg TK, Shi J, Moreno-Bost AM, Yun R, Balasa B, Ganguly B, Chao D, Rice AG, Zhan F, Shaughnessy JD Jr, Barlogie B, Yaccoby S, Afar DE (2009) Combinatorial efficacy of anti-CS1 monoclonal antibody elotuzumab (HuLuc63) and bortezomib against multiple myeloma. Mol Cancer Ther 8(9):2616–2624

93. Jakubowiak AJ, Benson DM, Bensinger W, Siegel DS, Zimmerman TM, Mohrbacher A, Richardson PG, Afar DE, Singhal AK, Anderson KC (2012) Phase I trial of anti-CS1 monoclonal antibody elotuzumab in combination with bortezomib in the treatment of relapsed/refractory multiple myeloma. J Clin Oncol 30(16):1960–1965
94. Orlowski RZ, Nagler A, Sonneveld P, Blade J, Hajek R, Spencer A, San Miguel J, Robak T, Dmoszynska A, Horvath N, Spicka I, Sutherland HJ, Suvorov AN, Zhuang SH, Parekh T, Xiu L, Yuan Z, Rackoff W, Harousseau JL (2007) Randomized phase III study of pegylated liposomal doxorubicin plus bortezomib compared with bortezomib alone in relapsed or refractory multiple myeloma: combination therapy improves time to progression. J Clin Oncol 25(25):3892–3901
95. Richardson PG, Xie W, Mitsiades C, Chanan-Khan AA, Lonial S, Hassoun H, Avigan DE, Oaklander AL, Kuter DJ, Wen PY, Kesari S, Briemberg HR, Schlossman RL, Munshi NC, Heffner LT, Doss D, Esseltine DL, Weller E, Anderson KC, Amato AA (2009) Single-agent bortezomib in previously untreated multiple myeloma: efficacy, characterization of peripheral neuropathy, and molecular correlations with response and neuropathy. J Clin Oncol 27(21):3518–3525
96. Richardson PG, Chanan-Khan AA, Lonial S, Krishnan AY, Carroll MP, Alsina M, Albitar M, Berman D, Messina M, Anderson KC (2011) Tanespimycin and bortezomib combination treatment in patients with relapsed or relapsed and refractory multiple myeloma: results of a phase 1/2 study. Br J Haematol 153(6):729–740
97. Lonial S, Mitsiades CS, Richardson PG (2011) Treatment options for relapsed and refractory multiple myeloma. Clin Cancer Res 17(6):1264–1277
98. Laubach JP, Voorhees PM, Hassoun H, Jakubowiak A, Lonial S, Richardson PG (2014) Current strategies for treatment of relapsed/refractory multiple myeloma. Expert Rev Hematol 7(1):97–111
99. Ocio EM, Mitsiades CS, Orlowski RZ, Anderson KC (2014) Future agents and treatment directions in multiple myeloma. Expert Rev Hematol 7(1):127–141
100. Kyle RA, Rajkumar SV (2014) An overview of the progress in the treatment of multiple myeloma. Expert Rev Hematol 7(1):5–7

Chapter 3
Overcoming Bortezomib Resistance: A Review of the Second-Generation Proteasome Inhibitor Carfilzomib in the Treatment of Multiple Myeloma

Hans C. Lee and Robert Z. Orlowski

Abstract Proteasome inhibitors now form the backbone of many myeloma therapeutic regimens in either the upfront or relapsed settings, but both innate and acquired drug resistance have emerged as significant clinical challenges. The second-generation proteasome inhibitor carfilzomib recently received regulatory approval after showing promising activity in bortezomib-resistant preclinical models and human studies. Although similar to its predecessor in targeting the chymotrypsin-like activity of both the constitutive proteasome and the immunoproteasome, carfilzomib has distinct mechanistic and structural properties. These allow it to bind irreversibly and provide a more sustained target inhibition than bortezomib, which is characterized by slowly reversible binding kinetics, and may in part contribute to its ability to overcome proteasome inhibitor resistance. Numerous clinical studies with carfilzomib are now underway investigating its use in various clinical settings and in combination with other novel agents that will provide valuable insight on its optimal use. However, despite the important advance in myeloma therapeutics that carfilzomib represents, cross-resistance between proteasome inhibitors remains a significant problem. This highlights the need for a better understanding of proteasome inhibitor resistance biology to inform the design of next-generation proteasome inhibitors and the development of rational drug combinations to overcome such resistance.

H.C. Lee, M.D.
Division of Cancer Medicine, The University of Texas MD Anderson Cancer Center, Houston, TX, USA
e-mail: hclee@mdanderson.org

R.Z. Orlowski, M.D., Ph.D. (✉)
Department of Lymphoma/Myeloma, The University of Texas MD Anderson Cancer Center, Houston, TX, USA

Department of Experimental Therapeutics, The University of Texas MD Anderson Cancer Center, 1515 Holcombe Boulevard, Unit 429, Houston, TX 77030, USA
e-mail: rorlowsk@mdanderson.org

Q.P. Dou (ed.), *Resistance to Proteasome Inhibitors in Cancer*, Resistance to Targeted Anti-Cancer Therapeutics, DOI 10.1007/978-3-319-06752-0_3

Keywords Proteasome inhibitor • Carfilzomib • Bortezomib • Drug resistance • Multiple myeloma

Abbreviations

AE	Adverse event
ChT-L	Chymotrypsin-like activity
C-L	Caspase-like
DLTs	Dose-limiting toxicities
FDA	Food and Drug Administration
IMiD	Immunomodulatory drug
JNK	c-Jun NH2-terminal kinase
MM	Multiple myeloma
MRs	Minor responses
MTD	Maximum tolerated dose
nCR	Near-complete responses
NDA	New Drug Application
NF-κB	Nuclear factor kappa B
NHL	Non-Hodgkin lymphoma
ODAC	Oncologic Drugs Advisory Committee
ORR	Overall response rate
PFS	Progression-free survival
PR	Partial response
PSMB	Proteasome subunit β type
SD	Stable disease
T-L	Trypsin-like
TTP	Time to progression
uCR	Unconfirmed complete response
VGPRs	Very good partial responses
WM	Waldenström's macroglobulinemia

3.1 Introduction

The regulatory approval of the first-in-class proteasome inhibitor bortezomib has contributed to substantial improvements in outcomes in multiple myeloma (MM) patients over the last decade [1] and validated the ubiquitin-proteasome pathway as a viable target in MM and other hematologic malignancies [2, 3]. However, primary, or de novo, and secondary, or acquired, bortezomib resistance [4, 5], and its dose-limiting toxicities (DLTs) such as peripheral neuropathy and thrombocytopenia [6, 7], have driven the development of new classes of proteasome inhibitors aimed to overcome these limitations. Carfilzomib, a novel second-generation proteasome inhibitor, recently received accelerated United States Food and Drug Administration (FDA) approval in 2012 for use in patients who have been exposed to bortezomib and an immunomodulatory drug (IMiD) and whose disease was refractory to their last therapy. Like bortezomib, carfilzomib also inhibits the chymotrypsin-like activity (ChT-L) of the constitutive proteasome and immunoproteasome, although its irreversible binding to its target leads to prolonged proteasome inhibition compared to bortezomib. This may explain its ability to overcome bortezomib resistance in certain subsets of patients and provides a proof of concept that rationally designed, next-generation proteasome inhibitors based on insights in proteasome resistance mechanisms may be one strategy to overcome drug resistance. In this chapter, the preclinical and clinical development of carfilzomib and its current role in myeloma therapy will be reviewed.

3.2 Discovery and Chemistry

The epoxyketone class of proteasome inhibitors was first discovered in the early 1990s, when the α′,β′-epoxyketone-containing natural products eponemycin and epoxomicin were isolated from different Actinobacteria, and demonstrated potent in vitro and in vivo antitumor activity against B16 murine melanoma [8, 9]. However, their precise mechanism of action was unclear at the time, and subsequent studies by Meng et al. [10] showed that epoxomicin covalently bound to the catalytic subunits of the 20S proteasome. This produced a highly selective inhibition of the ChT-L activity of the β5 subunit at low nanomolar concentrations. There was less selectivity for the trypsin-like (T-L) activity of the β2 subunit, and the post-glutamyl peptide hydrolyzing, or caspase-like (C-L) activity of the β1 subunit, requiring 100-fold and 1,000-fold higher epoxomicin concentrations, respectively, for enzymatic inhibition. Importantly, it also did not display any inhibitory activity of non-proteasomal intracellular proteases, such as calpain, papain, chymotrypsin, trypsin, and cathepsin, as seen with the peptide aldehyde, peptide vinyl sulfone, and boronate classes of proteasome inhibitors [10]. Cocrystallization studies with epoxomicin and the *S. cerevisiae* 20S proteasome indeed confirmed epoxomicin's covalent interaction with the β5 proteasomal subunit, and the formation of an irreversible morpholino adduct between the epoxyketone pharmacophore and the N-terminal nucleophilic threonine residue on the *β*5 subunit active site. Because other non-proteasomal proteases do not contain an N-terminal nucleophilic residue required for epoxomicin binding, this also explained the unique specificity of epoxomicin for its target [11]. Shortly thereafter, the first synthesis of epoxomicin was reported [12], and additional α′, β′-epoxyketone peptides were synthesized and screened with varying lengths and amino acid combinations to identify analogues with greater potency and selectivity toward the β5 subunit ChT-L activity [13]. This ultimately yielded the compound YU-101, and with the addition of an N-terminal morpholine ring for greater solubility, carfilzomib was created under the development of Proteolix, Inc., which was later acquired by Onyx Pharmaceuticals (Fig. 3.1).

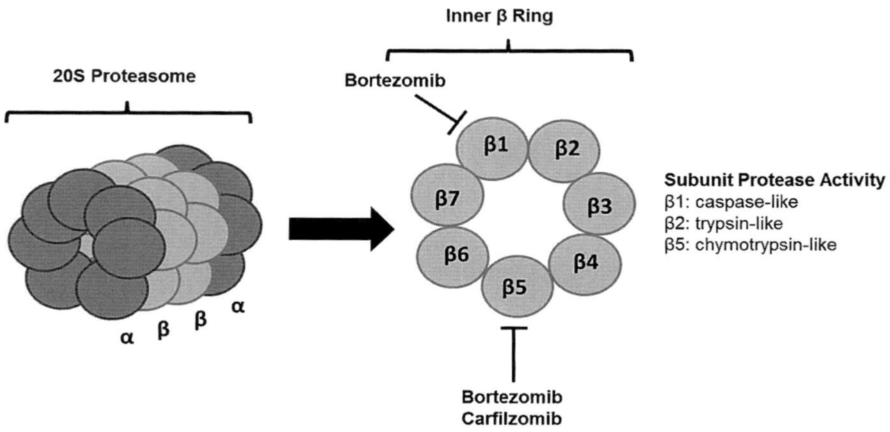

Fig. 3.1 Structure of 20S proteasome and sites of action of carfilzomib and bortezomib

3.3 Preclinical Activity

Early studies with carfilzomib in myeloma in vitro models demonstrated its potent and selective inhibition of the ChT-L activity of both the constitutive β5 proteasome subunit and the β5i (LMP-7) immunoproteasome subunit more commonly expressed in cells of hematopoietic origin [14, 15]. While near-complete inhibition of the ChT-L activity was achieved at doses of 10 nM, there was minimal effect on the β1 C-L activity, and the β2 T-L activity at drug concentrations up to 100 nM. Carfilzomib treatment also induced a dose- and time-dependent decrease in cell proliferation and a corresponding increase in apoptosis. This was also observed when cells were treated with a 1-h pulse of carfilzomib followed by recovery in drug-free media, to mimic the in vivo pharmacokinetics of proteasome inhibitor treatment and the rapid clearance of carfilzomib from the plasma. As with bortezomib, both the intrinsic and extrinsic apoptotic pathways were implicated as contributing to cell death, as there was an increase in caspase-8, caspase-9, and caspase-3 activity after a 1-h carfilzomib pulse. In addition, there was also increased c-Jun NH_2-terminal kinase (JNK) activation, a key player in stress-induced release of mitochondrial cytochrome *c*, and a well-described mechanism of proteasome-mediated apoptosis [16, 17]. Several other mechanisms of apoptosis common to proteasome inhibitors have also similarly been ascribed to carfilzomib. These include prevention of nuclear factor kappa B (NF-κB) activation through stabilization of its functional inhibitor, IκBα, stabilization of proapoptotic proteins such as p53, and induction of the unfolded protein response (UPR) due to excessive accumulation of polyubiquinated proteins [5, 10, 18–20].

In comparison to bortezomib, pulse doses of carfilzomib produced a statistically significant greater decrease in cell proliferation across a panel of MM cell lines. In addition, carfilzomib was more potent in inducing JNK phosphorylation and caspase-3, caspase-9, and caspase-8 activation [14]. The kinetics of proteasome recovery were also assessed, given the reversible nature of bortezomib-proteasome adducts compared to the irreversible inhibitor-enzyme complexes formed by carfilzomib. Interestingly, recovery of ChT-L activity was only modestly slower in lysates prepared from HT-29 adenocarcinoma and RPMI 8226 MM cells after pulse doses of bortezomib compared with carfilzomib [19]. In contrast, when proteasome recovery was tested in mice and rat tissue in vivo, there was a rapid recovery of ChT-L activity within 24 h with both bortezomib and carfilzomib. In anucleate whole red blood cells, where new proteasome synthesis cannot occur, complete recovery of proteasome activity after bortezomib pulse treatment eventually occurred after 72 h, which was attributable to the slow dissociation of bortezomib adducts with the β5 subunit. However, in the same model, there was still less than 50 % recovery of ChT-L activity after 7 days of the initial pulse dose of carfilzomib, consistent with its irreversible inhibition. In addition, whereas pulse treatments of carfilzomib demonstrated greater cytotoxicity than bortezomib, these differences were eliminated when drug exposure time was extended to 72 h [19]. Together, these observations suggested that, in tissue other than blood, transcriptional upregulation of proteasome subunit genes and synthesis of new proteasomes is the primary mechanism of proteasome recovery after treatment with proteasome inhibitors [21].

The potent antitumor activity of carfilzomib and its irreversible proteasome inhibition raised hope that it could potentially overcome innate and secondary resistance to bortezomib, an unfortunate and frequent observation seen in patients since the advent of its clinical use. Overexpression of proteasome subunit genes such as proteasome subunit β type 4 (*PSMB4*) and proteasome subunit β type 5 (*PSMB5*) has been identified as one possible mechanism of bortezomib resistance [22–24]. Therefore, while recovery of proteasome activity after bortezomib treatment would be aided by its slow dissociation from its binding target, irreversible proteasome inhibition with carfilzomib would force cells to assemble new proteasomes to recover their proteolytic activity resulting in more sustained drug activity. Consistent with this hypothesis, bortezomib-resistant ANBL-6, RPMI 8226, and OMP-2 MM cell lines generated in the laboratory did indeed demonstrate 2.0-, 1.5-, and 2.1-fold increased sensitivity, respectively, to carfilzomib compared with bortezomib. Enhanced cytotoxic effect was also observed with carfilzomib in two primary tumor samples of patients who had progressed on bortezomib therapy. However, some cross-resistance was observed, as bortezomib-resistant cell lines were notably less sensitive to carfilzomib compared with bortezomib-naïve cells [14].

Further evidence of carfilzomib's ability to overcome bortezomib resistance was demonstrated in HT-29 colorectal adenocarcinoma cells. Basal rates of proteasome subunit expression and activity level were increased 7–11-fold in the bortezomib-resistant cells compared to their parental clones. Faster proteasome recovery after brief bortezomib exposure was also observed in bortezomib-resistant cells relative to bortezomib-naïve cells. However, this effect was also retained in cells that were co-treated with cycloheximide, a protein translation inhibitor, suggesting that bortezomib resistance was not due to an increase in proteasome turnover and de novo proteasome synthesis. Instead, sequence analysis of the proteasomal subunits revealed a novel Cys63Phe mutation in the β5 subunit in the resistant cell lines, resulting in a conformational shift and altered binding kinetics with bortezomib. In contrast, brief exposure to carfilzomib in bortezomib-resistant cells resulted in prolonged proteasome inhibition and a tenfold lower IC_{50} compared with bortezomib. These results suggested that carfilzomib binding kinetics were unaffected by the Cys63Phe mutation, and hence, carfilzomib was able to overcome bortezomib resistance caused by mutations in the β5 subunit binding domain [25]. However, while such mutations in the β5 subunit have been described in acquired in vitro proteasome inhibitor resistance models [26, 23], they have not been detected yet to date in any primary samples from patients whose disease was bortezomib refractory, and hence, the true significance of these mutations is uncertain [27–29].

3.4 Pharmacodynamics and Pharmacokinetics

Pharmacodynamic studies in rats and monkeys demonstrated widespread distribution of radiolabeled carfilzomib and a corresponding dose-dependent reduction in ChT-L activity in all tissue except the brain 1 h after intravenous drug administration. The increased selectivity of carfilzomib for the ChT-L activity was also seen in vivo, as suggested by earlier in vitro studies [10]. Mice treated with intravenous carfilzomib and bortezomib with doses that induced >80 % inhibition of the ChT-L activity also showed significant inhibition (>60 %) of the β1 C-L activity in bortezomib-treated cells, but <25 % inhibition with carfilzomib. Neither drug displayed significant inhibition of the β2 T-L activity [19].

Like bortezomib [30, 31], carfilzomib was also rapidly cleared from the plasma after a single intravenous bolus administration of 2–8 mg/kg in rats, with a $T_{1/2}$ ranging from 5 to 20 min. Pretreatment with another irreversible proteasome inhibitor, ONX 0912, did not affect carfilzomib clearance, suggesting that carfilzomib clearance was not due to irreversible binding to the proteasome. Moreover, carfilzomib plasma clearance was faster at all dose levels than the reported hepatic blood flow for rats, suggesting that, unlike bortezomib, a substantial portion of carfilzomib clearance was mediated by extrahepatic metabolism. Indeed, major carfilzomib metabolites were recovered in both bile and urine and accounted for 26 % and 31 %, respectively, of the total carfilzomib dose at 24 h. These metabolites were primarily derived from peptidase cleavage or epoxide hydrolysis, and they lacked the epoxyketone pharmacophore, suggesting that they lacked any residual activity as proteasome inhibitors. Metabolites of carfilzomib were detected within 10 s of drug administration and peaked at 5 min, consistent with its rapid clearance from the plasma [32].

Pharmacokinetic data from a phase I/II study for patients with advanced solid tumors [33] who received intravenous carfilzomib at a dose of 20 mg/m^2 also revealed rapid plasma clearance and significant extrahepatic drug metabolism. In human liver microsomes, carfilzomib did exhibit an inhibitory effect on the cytochrome P450 CYP3A enzyme activity and midazolam metabolism, although there was no clinically relevant drug-drug interaction when tested in humans. This discrepancy may be explained by carfilzomib's short half-life, which would limit the actual exposure of cytochrome P450 enzymes to intact drug. In addition, carfilzomib was extensively plasma protein bound, further limiting hepatocyte exposure to free circulating drug [34].

While biweekly dosing on days 1 and 4 has been established as the standard for bortezomib, more intense and frequent carfilzomib dosing schedules were explored in animal models to maintain proteasome suppression between doses. Daily dosing up to 2 mg/kg for five consecutive days resulted in peak inhibition of the ChT-L activity of >80 % and was well tolerated in rodents. Antitumor activity and various dosing schedules of carfilzomib were also evaluated in HT-29 colorectal adenocarcinoma, RL B cell lymphoma, and HS-Sultan Burkitt's lymphoma murine xenograft models. Notably, efficacy was most pronounced when carfilzomib at 5 mg/kg was given on days 1 and 2 of each week compared with a biweekly, day 1 and 4 schedule, or a weekly, 10 mg/kg schedule. It was also more effective than bortezomib given at 1 mg/kg on days 1 and 4, considered the maximum tolerated dose (MTD) for mice. These results suggested that carfilzomib efficacy is schedule dependent and may be attributed to suppression of proteasome recovery between doses when the drug is given on consecutive days [19].

3.5 Clinical Studies

3.5.1 Phase I Monotherapy Studies in Hematologic Malignancies

Based on its encouraging in vitro and in vivo preclinical efficacy, the first-in-human PX-171-001 phase I clinical trial with carfilzomib was initiated in 2005 to evaluate the safety and tolerability of the drug [35]. Patients with relapsed and refractory MM, non-Hodgkin lymphoma (NHL), Hodgkin lymphoma (HL), or Waldenström's macroglobulinemia (WM) were enrolled in this study. Carfilzomib was administered on days 1–5 every 14 days starting at 1.2 mg/m^2 per day and progressively dose-escalated up to 20 mg/m^2. DLTs were only observed at the highest dosing level of 20 mg/m^2, with one patient experiencing grade 3 febrile neutropenia and one patient experiencing grade 4 thrombocytopenia. Hence, the preceding dose level of 15 mg/m^2 was deemed to be the MTD. Overall, carfilzomib was well tolerated, with the most common side effects being nausea and fatigue. Of 29 total patients enrolled in the study across all dose cohorts, 14 (48 %) patients experienced a grade 3/4 adverse event (AE), although only 4 (14 %) patients discontinued treatment due to an AE. Notably, there was no grade 3/4 peripheral neuropathy reported, despite having patients with preexisting neuropathy enrolled in the study. Among the patients who received at least six cycles of therapy, the most common reason for treatment discontinuation was the inability to maintain compliance with the intensive daily dosing schedule. There was one unconfirmed complete response (uCR) in a mantle cell lymphoma patient, one partial response (PR) in a bortezomib-refractory MM patient, and two minor responses in one MM patient and one WM patient. Nine patients had stable disease, and 15 patients ultimately had progression of disease while on study.

Table 3.1 Phase 1 trials reported to date with single-agent carfilzomib in MM

Study	Disease	Dosing regimen	*N*	MTD
PX-171-001	Hematologic malignancies	1.2–20 mg/m² D1–5 (14-day cycle)	29 Total	15 mg/m²
O'Connor et al. [35]			10 MM	
PX-171-002	Hematologic malignancies	Dose escalation: 1.2–27 mg/m² D1–2, 8–9, 15–16 (28-day cycle)	37 Total	Not reached
Alsina et al. [36]		Dose expansion: 20/27 mg/m² D1–2, 8–9, 15–16 (28-day cycle)	21 MM	
			11 Total	
			7 MM	
PX-171-007	R/R MM	20 mg/m² C1D1–2, then dose-escalated to 36–70 mg/m² D8–9, 15–16 (28-day cycle)[a]	20	56 mg/m²
Papadopoulos et al. [65]				

D day, *N* number, *C* cycle, *R/R* relapsed/refractory, *MM* multiple myeloma, *MTD* maximum tolerated dose

[a]30-min carfilzomib infusion

An alternative dosing schedule was explored in the PX-171-002 phase I study, in which carfilzomib was given on days 1, 2, 8, 9, 15, and 16 of an every 28-day cycle [36]. A total of 37 patients with relapsed and refractory MM, NHL, or HL were enrolled in the dose-escalation portion of the study, and 11 additional patients were enrolled in the dose-expansion arm, in which patients received carfilzomib, 20 mg/m², on days 1 and 2, followed by a dose-escalation to 27 mg/m² for subsequent doses. The most common carfilzomib-related grade 3/4 toxicities were anemia (36 %) and thrombocytopenia (27 %) in the dose-expansion cohort, and no grade 3/4 peripheral neuropathy was reported. Pharmacodynamic studies demonstrated >90 % inhibition of the ChT-L activity after day 2 with the 27 mg/m² dose, similar to what was seen after completion of five consecutive 15 mg/m² doses in the PX-171-001 study [35], and greater than the 65–70 % inhibition that was seen with biweekly bortezomib dosing in a previous study [37]. Of the 45 response-evaluable patients, 17 (38 %) had objective responses, and all but one had MM. Responses were generally seen at doses of 15 mg/m² or greater, at which inhibition of ChT-L activity exceeded 70 %. Overall tolerability was similar between the two dosing schedules in the PX-171-001 and PX-171-002 studies, although the less frequent twice-weekly regimen led to fewer treatment discontinuations and was therefore chosen as the preferred dosing schedule in subsequent trials (Table 3.1).

3.5.2 Phase II Monotherapy Studies in MM

The safety and tolerability of carfilzomib, and early evidence of its efficacy, prompted further investigation in phase II studies. The PX-171-003-A0 pilot phase II study began in 2007 and enrolled 46 patients with relapsed and refractory MM who had received at last two prior therapies, including bortezomib and an IMiD [38]. Patients received carfilzomib, 20 mg/m², on days 1, 2, 8, 9, 15, and 16 on a 28-day cycle for up to 12 cycles. Overall response rate (ORR, ≥PR) was 17 %, with 7 (17 %) PRs,

3 (7 %) minor responses (MRs), and 17 (40 %) patients with stable disease (SD) as defined by the International Myeloma Working Group Uniform Response criteria [39] with MR assessed by the European Group for Blood and Marrow Transplantation criteria [40]. Median duration of response was 7.2 months among PR patients, and median time to progression (TTP) for all patients was 3.5 months. As seen in the phase I trials, the most common grade 3/4 AEs were hematologic in nature, including anemia (37 %), thrombocytopenia (26 %), and lymphopenia (13 %). Grade 3/4 nonhematologic AEs were rare although, notably, 6 (13 %) patients did experience grade 3/4 renal failure, among which four of these events were thought to be unrelated to carfilzomib. Only 7 (15 %) patients experienced treatment-emergent peripheral neuropathy, despite 40 (87 %) patients having preexisting neuropathy at the time of study entry. Overall, carfilzomib was well tolerated, with disease progression being the most common reason for treatment discontinuation.

Shortly after the initiation of the PX-171-003-A0 study, accrual began for a significantly larger phase IIB expansion cohort (PX-171-003-A1) in 2008 [41]. A total of 266 patients with relapsed MM after at least two therapies, and with disease that was refractory to their most recent treatment, were enrolled in the study. Every patient had received prior IMiD therapy, and all but one patient had received prior bortezomib therapy. Patients initially received twice-weekly carfilzomib, 20 mg/m^2, and were dose-escalated to 27 mg/m^2 for all subsequent doses if cycle 1 was well tolerated. Among these patients, 73 % were refractory to bortezomib in any line of therapy, and 45 % were refractory to bortezomib during their most recent therapy. Of 257 response-evaluable patients, the ORR was 24 %, with 47 (18.3 %) PRs, 13 (5.1 %) very good partial responses (VGPRs), and 1 (0.4 %) CR. In 61 patients who achieved a PR or better, the median duration of response was 7.8 months. Median progression-free survival (PFS) was 3.7 months, and median overall survival (OS) was 15.6 months for the entire study population. While these results were certainly encouraging considering the heavily pretreated study cohort, evidence of proteasome inhibitor cross-resistance to carfilzomib was seen in a subset of patients, as response rates were notably lower in patients with ≥2 lines of bortezomib therapy (18.5 %) compared to those with <2 lines (29.5 %). Response rates were also lower in patients who were refractory to bortezomib in their last line of therapy (18.6 %) versus patients who did not receive bortezomib in their most recent therapy (28.3 %). Notably, the ORR was comparable in patients with high-risk (26 %) and standard-risk cytogenetic profiles (25 %), with a trend toward shorter duration of response in high-risk patients [42]. Overall, carfilzomib was well tolerated, with the most common grade 3/4 AEs being thrombocytopenia (29 %) and anemia (24 %).

Similar to the phase I results, only 33 (12 %) patients reported any degree of treatment-emergent peripheral neuropathy, with the majority of cases (91 %) being of grade 1/2 severity. This was a significant improvement from the 38 % rate of treatment-emergent peripheral neuropathy reported with subcutaneous bortezomib, and 53 % reported with intravenous bortezomib [43]. The basis for this difference in side effect profiles was further investigated in vitro on neuronal cell lines treated with either bortezomib or carfilzomib. Only bortezomib induced shortening of neurite length, despite equivalent inhibition of proteasome activity with both drugs [44]. Using an activity-based probe approach, bortezomib was found to inhibit multiple non-proteasomal serine proteases, such as cathepsin G, cathepsin A, chymase, dipeptidyl peptidase II, and HtrA2/Omi with similar potencies compared to its activity against the ChT-L activity of the proteasome. Bortezomib-induced inhibition of mitochondrial HtrA2/Omi was thought to be of particular consequence, given its known protective role against neurodegeneration, although additional confirmatory studies characterizing the precise mechanisms of bortezomib-induced neuropathy are still needed. Nevertheless, as suggested in earlier studies, these experiments highlighted the specificity of carfilzomib's epoxyketone pharmacophore due to its interaction with the N-terminal nucleophilic threonine residue found exclusively on the β5 proteasome subunit, in contrast with the more promiscuous boronate pharmacophore [11].

The positive results from the PX-171-003-A1 phase IIB expansion cohort prompted the filing of a New Drug Application (NDA) for carfilzomib in late 2011. Data from the trial and earlier phase I and preclinical studies were presented to the Oncologic Drugs Advisory Committee (ODAC) of the FDA in June 2012. Despite initial concerns for drug safety and efficacy outlined in the FDA briefing document [45], ODAC strongly voted in favor of recommending carfilzomib's regulatory approval. One month later, the FDA granted accelerated approval of carfilzomib 20 mg/m^2 for cycle 1 and 27 mg/m^2 for cycle 2 and thereafter in patients who had received at least two prior therapies, including bortezomib and an IMiD, and who had progressed during or within 60 days of their most recent therapy.

Following its initial NDA filing, additional single-agent carfilzomib phase II studies were reported looking at its efficacy in various patient populations. The PX-171-004 trial, a parallel study to the PX-171-003-A1 study, evaluated the efficacy of carfilzomib in a less heavily pretreated patient population including a large cohort of relapsed and refractory bortezomib-naïve MM patients [46]. Among 59 bortezomib-naïve patients who received twice-weekly carfilzomib at 20 mg/m^2, the ORR was 42 %, including 2 (3.4 %) CRs, 8 (13.6 %) VGPRs, and 15 (25.4 %) PRs. A second cohort of 70 bortezomib-naïve patients who were dose-escalated to twice-weekly carfilzomib at 27 mg/m^2 after cycle 1 had a higher ORR of 52 %, including 1 (1.5 %) CR, 18 (26.9 %) VGPRs, and 16 (23.9 %) PRs. Reponses were durable, with a median PFS of 54 % at 9 months follow-up between the two cohorts. While the high ORR in the dose-escalation cohort was very promising, the lower limit of its 95 % confidence interval did not exceed the 40 % chosen for the study based on historical response rates of single-agent bortezomib in a similar patient population [47, 48]. Given the limitations and pitfalls of inter-study comparisons, the results of the ongoing phase III ENDEAVOR (Randomized, Open-label, Phase III Study of Carfilzomib Plus Dexamethasone vs Bortezomib Plus Dexamethasone in Patients With Relapsed Multiple Myeloma) trial will provide important insight as to any added benefit of the use of carfilzomib in this setting.

The increase in the ORR from 42 to 52 % between the 20 and 27 mg/m^2 dosing groups, respectively, also raised the question of whether a greater dose-dependent proteasome inhibition is correlated with improved efficacy. Although phase I studies established the MTD of carfilzomib at 27 mg/m^2 given over a 2–10 min intravenous bolus, preclinical studies in rats suggested that higher doses could be administered at slower infusion rates with greater tolerability and equivalent levels of proteasome inhibition compared with bolus administration [32]. This was the rationale of the phase Ib/II PX-171-007 study, in which relapsed/refractory MM patients were given carfilzomib, 20 mg/m^2, on days 1 and 2 over 30 min and were then dose-escalated to levels up to 70 mg/m^2 in subsequent weeks. The MTD was determined to be 56 mg/m^2, and of 24 patients in the 20/56 mg/m^2 cohort, the ORR was 60 % with a median duration of response of 8.0 months at the interim analysis [49]. Pharmacodynamic studies demonstrated a >95 % inhibition of the ChT-L activity in peripheral blood mononuclear cells at the 56 mg/m^2 dose versus >80 % inhibition at 20 mg/m^2. The most common grade 3/4 AEs in the 20/56 mg/m^2 cohort were thrombocytopenia (38 %) and anemia (21 %), and only one case of peripheral neuropathy (grade 1) was reported. Based on these results, infusional carfilzomib at 20/56 mg/m^2 was chosen as the dose for the ongoing phase III ENDEAVOR trial in its direct head-to-head comparison with bortezomib in relapsed MM patients. This also provided the rationale of the recently activated SWOG S1304 randomized phase II study in its comparison of high-dose carfilzomib 20/56 mg/m^2 versus low-dose carfilzomib 20/27 mg/m^2 combined with dexamethasone in both arms.

Finally, the PX-171-005 phase II study evaluated the efficacy of carfilzomib in patients with varying degrees of renal insufficiency [50]. Patients were divided into four cohorts depending on their creatinine clearance (>80 ml/min, 50–80 ml/min, 30–49 ml/min, or <30 ml/min and on chronic hemodialysis) and were progressively dose-escalated from twice-weekly carfilzomib at 15 mg/m^2 for cycle 1, 20 mg/m^2 for cycle 2, and 27 mg/m^2 for cycle 3 and beyond. The ORR was 26 % for the entire study population with a median duration of response of 7.9 months. Importantly, there was no difference in carfilzomib clearance, degree of proteasome inhibition, or incidence of grade 3/4 AEs between the patient cohorts, thus confirming the safety and efficacy of carfilzomib in patients with renal impairment (Table 3.2).

Table 3.2 Phase 2 trials reported to date with single-agent carfilzomib in MM

Study	Disease	Dosing regimen (28-day cycle)	*N*	ORR, PR, VGPR, CR
PX-171-003-A0	R/R MM	20 mg/m^2 D1–2, 8–9, 15–16	46	16.7 %, 16.7 %, 0 %, 0 %
Jagannath et al. [38]				
PX-171-003-A1	R/R MM	20/27 mg/m^2 D1–2, 8–9, 15–16	266	23.5 %,18.3 %, 5.1 %, 0.4 %
Siegel et al. [41]				
PX-171-004	R/R MM, bortezomib naïve	Cohort 1: 20 mg/m^2 D1–2, 8–9, 15-16	59	42.4 % 25.4 %, 13.6 %, 3.4 %
Vij et al. [46]		Cohort 2: 20/27 mg/m^2 D1–2, 8–9, 15–16	70	52.2 %, 23.9 %, 26.9 %, 1.5 %
PX-171-005	R/R MM with renal impairment	15/20/27 mg/m^2 D1–2, 8–9, 15–16	50	25.5 %, 25.5 %
Badros et al. [50]				0 %, 0 %
PX-171-007	Newly diagnosed MM	20/56 mg/m^2 D1–2, 8–9, 15–16[a]	20	60 %, 35 %
Papadopoulos et al. [49]				20 %, 5 %[b]

D day, *N* number, *MM* multiple myeloma, *R/R* relapsed/refractory, *ORR* overall response rate, *PR* partial response, *VGPR* very good partial response, *CR* complete response
[a]30-min carfilzomib infusion
[b]Stringent CR

3.5.3 Carfilzomib Combination Studies

With the demonstration of the efficacy of single-agent carfilzomib in relapsed MM patients, many trials are now underway investigating its safety, tolerability, and efficacy in combination with other novel agents. In the phase Ib/II PX-171-006 trial, patients with relapsed and/or refractory MM were dose-escalated to the MTD of carfilzomib 20 mg/m^2 on days 1 and 2, and 27 mg/m^2 thereafter, along with lenalidomide at 25 mg on days 1–21, and low-dose dexamethasone at 40 mg once weekly on a 28-day cycle [51]. Of 52 patients who received the MTD, 42 (81 %) had received prior bortezomib therapy, of which 14 (27 %) had disease that was refractory to such treatment. The ORR was 77 % in the MTD study population, and 71 % in the subset of bortezomib-refractory patients, an improvement on the historical ORR of 60 % with lenalidomide and dexamethasone [52, 53], and 68 % with the combination of bortezomib, lenalidomide, and dexamethasone [54] in the relapsed setting. Overall, the combination was well tolerated, with one-third of study patients completing 12 or more cycles of therapy. The ongoing phase III ASPIRE (Carfilzomib, Lenalidomide, and Dexamethasone versus Lenalidomide and Dexamethasone for the treatment of Patients with Relapsed Multiple Myeloma) trial has finished accrual and is awaiting data maturation, and its results will provide additional insight as to the potential added benefit of carfilzomib use in this setting.

Several phase I and II trials looking at carfilzomib combinations in newly diagnosed MM patients have also been reported. An impressive 98 % ORR, including 81 % VGPR and 62 % near-complete responses (nCR), were recently reported in 53 patients enrolled in a phase I/II study who received carfilzomib in combination with lenalidomide and low-dose dexamethasone in the frontline setting [55]. While the ORR in a phase II study with bortezomib, lenalidomide, and dexamethasone in newly diagnosed patients was 100 %, the depth of response was slightly lower in the bortezomib combination, with 57 % of patients achieving ≥nCR, and 74 % of patients achieving ≥VGPR [56]. Again, given the limitations and pitfalls of inter-study comparisons, ongoing randomized studies such as the Eastern Cooperative Group E1A11 phase III trial comparing carfilzomib or bortezomib with lenalidomide and dexamethasone in newly diagnosed MM patients will be important in determining if these incremental improvements with carfilzomib hold true.

A number of other phase I/II studies with carfilzomib in combination with other novel agents are currently ongoing, with early interim results reporting favorable safety profiles and encouraging efficacy data. In the relapsed and refractory setting, these have included carfilzomib in combination with the novel kinesin spindle protein inhibitor ARRY-520 [57], histone deacetylase inhibitors such as panobinostat [58, 59], and the third-generation IMiD pomalidomide [60]. In newly diagnosed patients, carfilzomib is being tested in combination with thalidomide and dexamethasone [61]; thalidomide, cyclophosphamide, and dexamethasone [62]; or cyclophosphamide and dexamethasone [63]. Lastly, the safety and efficacy of carfilzomib is also being explored in the transplant-ineligible population in combination with melphalan and prednisone [64]. Final results from these studies and other ongoing trials are eagerly anticipated as rational drug combinations with carfilzomib continue to be developed in both the upfront and relapsed/refractory settings.

3.6 Conclusions

While the introduction of the first-in-class proteasome inhibitor bortezomib and the second-generation IMiD lenalidomide to the MM therapeutic armamentarium has led to substantial improvements in patient outcomes, eventual drug resistance to such novel agents remains an emerging problem of great significance and an area of intense research focus. The second-generation proteasome inhibitor carfilzomib has shown promise as having potent activity in bortezomib-resistant MM in both pre-clinical models and human clinical studies. This may be explained in part due to its distinct mechanistic and structural properties allowing for irreversible binding of the β5 proteasome subunit, leading to more sustained proteasome inhibition. Moreover, its greater selectivity for the ChT-L activity of the β5 subunit and lack of inhibition of non-proteasomal proteases may explain the significant decrease in treatment-emergent peripheral neuropathy seen with carfilzomib compared with bortezomib, although additional studies are needed to further characterize these differences in side effect profile between the two drugs.

Despite these advances, response rates to single-agent carfilzomib remain only 20 % in bortezomib-refractory patients. While upregulation of proteasomal subunit genes may explain carfilzomib's efficacy in certain subsets of bortezomib-refractory patients, cross-resistance through other mechanisms that have been implicated in models of primary or secondary proteasome inhibitor resistance is also likely involved as described in detail in Chap. 1. An improved understanding and validation of emerging mechanisms of resistance will be critical in the development of next-generation proteasome inhibitors and rational drug combinations to overcome resistance and to establish predictive biomarkers to help individualize therapy in patients with MM.

Acknowledgments R.Z.O. would like to acknowledge support from the National Cancer Institute in the form of The MD Anderson Cancer Center SPORE in Multiple Myeloma (P50 CA142509) and the Southwest Oncology Group (U10 CA032102). H.C.L. would like to acknowledge support from the Conquer Cancer Foundation (American Society of Clinical Oncology Young Investigator Award).

References

1. Kumar SK, Rajkumar SV, Dispenzieri A, Lacy MQ, Hayman SR, Buadi FK, Zeldenrust SR, Dingli D, Russell SJ, Lust JA, Greipp PR, Kyle RA, Gertz MA (2008) Improved survival in multiple myeloma and the impact of novel therapies. Blood 111(5):2516–2520
2. Richardson PG, Barlogie B, Berenson J, Singhal S, Jagannath S, Irwin D, Rajkumar SV, Srkalovic G, Alsina M, Alexanian R, Siegel D, Orlowski RZ, Kuter D, Limentani SA, Lee S, Hideshima T, Esseltine DL, Kauffman M, Adams J, Schenkein DP, Anderson KC (2003) A phase 2 study of bortezomib in relapsed, refractory myeloma. N Engl J Med 348(26): 2609–2617
3. Chen D, Frezza M, Schmitt S, Kanwar J, Dou QP (2011) Bortezomib as the first proteasome inhibitor anticancer drug: current status and future perspectives. Curr Cancer Drug Targets 11(3):239–253
4. Kale AJ, Moore BS (2012) Molecular mechanisms of acquired proteasome inhibitor resistance. J Med Chem 55(23):10317–10327

5. McConkey DJ, Zhu K (2008) Mechanisms of proteasome inhibitor action and resistance in cancer. Drug Resist Updat 11(4–5):164–179
6. Lonial S, Waller EK, Richardson PG, Jagannath S, Orlowski RZ, Giver CR, Jaye DL, Francis D, Giusti S, Torre C, Barlogie B, Berenson JR, Singhal S, Schenkein DP, Esseltine DL, Anderson J, Xiao H, Heffner LT, Anderson KC (2005) Risk factors and kinetics of thrombocytopenia associated with bortezomib for relapsed, refractory multiple myeloma. Blood 106(12):3777–3784
7. Argyriou AA, Iconomou G, Kalofonos HP (2008) Bortezomib-induced peripheral neuropathy in multiple myeloma: a comprehensive review of the literature. Blood 112(5):1593–1599
8. Hanada M, Sugawara K, Kaneta K, Toda S, Nishiyama Y, Tomita K, Yamamoto H, Konishi M, Oki T (1992) Epoxomicin, a new antitumor agent of microbial origin. J Antibiot (Tokyo) 45(11):1746–1752
9. Sugawara K, Hatori M, Nishiyama Y, Tomita K, Kamei H, Konishi M, Oki T (1990) Eponemycin, a new antibiotic active against B16 melanoma. I. Production, isolation, structure and biological activity. J Antibiot (Tokyo) 43(1):8–18
10. Meng L, Mohan R, Kwok BH, Elofsson M, Sin N, Crews CM (1999) Epoxomicin, a potent and selective proteasome inhibitor, exhibits in vivo antiinflammatory activity. Proc Natl Acad Sci U S A 96(18):10403–10408
11. Groll M, Kim K, Kairies N, Huber R, Crews C (2000) Crystal structure of epoxomicin: 20s proteasome reveals a molecular basis for selectivity of α′, β′-epoxyketone proteasome inhibitors. J Am Chem Soc 122(6):1237–1238
12. Sin N, Kim KB, Elofsson M, Meng L, Auth H, Kwok BH, Crews CM (1999) Total synthesis of the potent proteasome inhibitor epoxomicin: a useful tool for understanding proteasome biology. Bioorg Med Chem Lett 9(15):2283–2288
13. Elofsson M, Splittgerber U, Myung J, Mohan R, Crews CM (1999) Towards subunit-specific proteasome inhibitors: synthesis and evaluation of peptide alpha′, beta′-epoxyketones. Chem Biol 6(11):811–822
14. Kuhn DJ, Chen Q, Voorhees PM, Strader JS, Shenk KD, Sun CM, Demo SD, Bennett MK, van Leeuwen FW, Chanan-Khan AA, Orlowski RZ (2007) Potent activity of carfilzomib, a novel, irreversible inhibitor of the ubiquitin-proteasome pathway, against preclinical models of multiple myeloma. Blood 110(9):3281–3290
15. Parlati F, Lee SJ, Aujay M, Suzuki E, Levitsky K, Lorens JB, Micklem DR, Ruurs P, Sylvain C, Lu Y, Shenk KD, Bennett MK (2009) Carfilzomib can induce tumor cell death through selective inhibition of the chymotrypsin-like activity of the proteasome. Blood 114(16):3439–3447
16. Tsuruta F, Sunayama J, Mori Y, Hattori S, Shimizu S, Tsujimoto Y, Yoshioka K, Masuyama N, Gotoh Y (2004) JNK promotes Bax translocation to mitochondria through phosphorylation of 14-3-3 proteins. EMBO J 23(8):1889–1899
17. Yang Y, Ikezoe T, Saito T, Kobayashi M, Koeffler HP, Taguchi H (2004) Proteasome inhibitor PS-341 induces growth arrest and apoptosis of non-small cell lung cancer cells via the JNK/c-Jun/AP-1 signaling. Cancer Sci 95(2):176–180
18. Sacco A, Aujay M, Morgan B, Azab AK, Maiso P, Liu Y, Zhang Y, Azab F, Ngo HT, Issa GC, Quang P, Roccaro AM, Ghobrial IM (2011) Carfilzomib-dependent selective inhibition of the chymotrypsin-like activity of the proteasome leads to antitumor activity in Waldenstrom's Macroglobulinemia. Clin Cancer Res 17(7):1753–1764
19. Demo SD, Kirk CJ, Aujay MA, Buchholz TJ, Dajee M, Ho MN, Jiang J, Laidig GJ, Lewis ER, Parlati F, Shenk KD, Smyth MS, Sun CM, Vallone MK, Woo TM, Molineaux CJ, Bennett MK (2007) Antitumor activity of PR-171, a novel irreversible inhibitor of the proteasome. Cancer Res 67(13):6383–6391
20. Mitsiades N, Mitsiades CS, Poulaki V, Chauhan D, Fanourakis G, Gu X, Bailey C, Joseph M, Libermann TA, Treon SP, Munshi NC, Richardson PG, Hideshima T, Anderson KC (2002) Molecular sequelae of proteasome inhibition in human multiple myeloma cells. Proc Natl Acad Sci U S A 99(22):14374–14379

21. Meiners S, Heyken D, Weller A, Ludwig A, Stangl K, Kloetzel PM, Kruger E (2003) Inhibition of proteasome activity induces concerted expression of proteasome genes and de novo formation of Mammalian proteasomes. J Biol Chem 278(24):21517–21525
22. Shaughnessy JD Jr, Qu P, Usmani S, Heuck CJ, Zhang Q, Zhou Y, Tian E, Hanamura I, van Rhee F, Anaissie E, Epstein J, Nair B, Stephens O, Williams R, Waheed S, Alsayed Y, Crowley J, Barlogie B (2011) Pharmacogenomics of bortezomib test-dosing identifies hyperexpression of proteasome genes, especially PSMD4, as novel high-risk feature in myeloma treated with Total Therapy 3. Blood 118(13):3512–3524
23. Oerlemans R, Franke NE, Assaraf YG, Cloos J, van Zantwijk I, Berkers CR, Scheffer GL, Debipersad K, Vojtekova K, Lemos C, van der Heijden JW, Ylstra B, Peters GJ, Kaspers GL, Dijkmans BA, Scheper RJ, Jansen G (2008) Molecular basis of bortezomib resistance: proteasome subunit beta5 (PSMB5) gene mutation and overexpression of PSMB5 protein. Blood 112(6):2489–2499
24. Lu S, Chen Z, Yang J, Chen L, Gong S, Zhou H, Guo L, Wang J (2008) Overexpression of the PSMB5 gene contributes to bortezomib resistance in T-lymphoblastic lymphoma/leukemia cells derived from Jurkat line. Exp Hematol 36(10):1278–1284
25. Suzuki E, Demo S, Deu E, Keats J, Arastu-Kapur S, Bergsagel PL, Bennett MK, Kirk CJ (2011) Molecular mechanisms of bortezomib resistant adenocarcinoma cells. PLoS One 6(12):e27996
26. Franke NE, Niewerth D, Assaraf YG, van Meerloo J, Vojtekova K, van Zantwijk CH, Zweegman S, Chan ET, Kirk CJ, Geerke DP, Schimmer AD, Kaspers GJ, Jansen G, Cloos J (2012) Impaired bortezomib binding to mutant β5 subunit of the proteasome is the underlying basis for bortezomib resistance in leukemia cells. Leukemia 26(4):757–768
27. Politou M, Karadimitris A, Terpos E, Kotsianidis I, Apperley JF, Rahemtulla A (2006) No evidence of mutations of the PSMB5 (beta-5 subunit of proteasome) in a case of myeloma with clinical resistance to Bortezomib. Leuk Res 30(2):240–241
28. Lichter DI, Danaee H, Pickard MD, Tayber O, Sintchak M, Shi H, Richardson PG, Cavenagh J, Blade J, Facon T, Niesvizky R, Alsina M, Dalton W, Sonneveld P, Lonial S, van de Velde H, Ricci D, Esseltine DL, Trepicchio WL, Mulligan G, Anderson KC (2012) Sequence analysis of beta-subunit genes of the 20S proteasome in patients with relapsed multiple myeloma treated with bortezomib or dexamethasone. Blood 120(23):4513–4516
29. Wang L, Kumar S, Fridley BL, Kalari KR, Moon I, Pelleymounter LL, Hildebrandt MA, Batzler A, Eckloff BW, Wieben ED, Greipp PR (2008) Proteasome beta subunit pharmacogenomics: gene resequencing and functional genomics. Clin Cancer Res 14(11):3503–3513
30. Papandreou CN, Daliani DD, Nix D, Yang H, Madden T, Wang X, Pien CS, Millikan RE, Tu SM, Pagliaro L, Kim J, Adams J, Elliott P, Esseltine D, Petrusich A, Dieringer P, Perez C, Logothetis CJ (2004) Phase I trial of the proteasome inhibitor bortezomib in patients with advanced solid tumors with observations in androgen-independent prostate cancer. J Clin Oncol 22(11):2108–2121
31. Hemeryck A, Geerts R, Monbaliu J, Hassler S, Verhaeghe T, Diels L, Verluyten W, van Beijsterveldt L, Mamidi RN, Janssen C, De Coster R (2007) Tissue distribution and depletion kinetics of bortezomib and bortezomib-related radioactivity in male rats after single and repeated intravenous injection of 14 C-bortezomib. Cancer Chemother Pharmacol 60(6):777–787
32. Yang J, Wang Z, Fang Y, Jiang J, Zhao F, Wong H, Bennett MK, Molineaux CJ, Kirk CJ (2011) Pharmacokinetics, pharmacodynamics, metabolism, distribution, and excretion of carfilzomib in rats. Drug Metab Dispos 39(10):1873–1882
33. Rosen PJ, Gordon P, Lee E, Sausville K, Papadopoulous A, Wong M, Vallone L, Kunkel L, Infante J, Burris H (2012) Phase II results of study PX-171-007: a phase Ib/II study of carfilzomib (CFZ), a selective proteasome inhibitor, in patients with selected advanced metastatic solid tumors. J Clin Oncol 27(15S):(suppl; abstr 3515)
34. Wang Z, Yang J, Kirk C, Fang Y, Alsina M, Badros A, Papadopoulos K, Wong A, Woo T, Bomba D, Li J, Infante JR (2013) Clinical pharmacokinetics, metabolism, and drug-drug interaction of carfilzomib. Drug Metab Dispos 41(1):230–237

35. O'Connor OA, Stewart AK, Vallone M, Molineaux CJ, Kunkel LA, Gerecitano JF, Orlowski RZ (2009) A phase 1 dose escalation study of the safety and pharmacokinetics of the novel proteasome inhibitor carfilzomib (PR-171) in patients with hematologic malignancies. Clin Cancer Res 15(22):7085–7091
36. Alsina M, Trudel S, Furman RR, Rosen PJ, O'Connor OA, Comenzo RL, Wong A, Kunkel LA, Molineaux CJ, Goy A (2012) A phase I single-agent study of twice-weekly consecutive-day dosing of the proteasome inhibitor carfilzomib in patients with relapsed or refractory multiple myeloma or lymphoma. Clin Cancer Res 18(17):4830–4840
37. Orlowski RZ, Stinchcombe TE, Mitchell BS, Shea TC, Baldwin AS, Stahl S, Adams J, Esseltine DL, Elliott PJ, Pien CS, Guerciolini R, Anderson JK, Depcik-Smith ND, Bhagat R, Lehman MJ, Novick SC, O'Connor OA, Soignet SL (2002) Phase I trial of the proteasome inhibitor PS-341 in patients with refractory hematologic malignancies. J Clin Oncol 20(22):4420–4427
38. Jagannath S, Vij R, Stewart AK, Trudel S, Jakubowiak AJ, Reiman T, Somlo G, Bahlis N, Lonial S, Kunkel LA, Wong A, Orlowski RZ, Siegel DS (2012) An open-label single-arm pilot phase II study (PX-171-003-A0) of low-dose, single-agent carfilzomib in patients with relapsed and refractory multiple myeloma. Clin Lymphoma Myeloma Leuk 12(5):310–318
39. Durie BG, Harousseau JL, Miguel JS, Blade J, Barlogie B, Anderson K, Gertz M, Dimopoulos M, Westin J, Sonneveld P, Ludwig H, Gahrton G, Beksac M, Crowley J, Belch A, Boccadaro M, Cavo M, Turesson I, Joshua D, Vesole D, Kyle R, Alexanian R, Tricot G, Attal M, Merlini G, Powles R, Richardson P, Shimizu K, Tosi P, Morgan G, Rajkumar SV (2006) International uniform response criteria for multiple myeloma. Leukemia 20(9):1467–1473
40. Blade J, Samson D, Reece D, Apperley J, Bjorkstrand B, Gahrton G, Gertz M, Giralt S, Jagannath S, Vesole D (1998) Criteria for evaluating disease response and progression in patients with multiple myeloma treated by high-dose therapy and haemopoietic stem cell transplantation. Myeloma Subcommittee of the EBMT. European Group for Blood and Marrow Transplant. Br J Haematol 102(5):1115–1123
41. Siegel DS, Martin T, Wang M, Vij R, Jakubowiak AJ, Lonial S, Trudel S, Kukreti V, Bahlis N, Alsina M, Chanan-Khan A, Buadi F, Reu FJ, Somlo G, Zonder J, Song K, Stewart AK, Stadtmauer E, Kunkel L, Wear S, Wong AF, Orlowski RZ, Jagannath S (2012) A phase 2 study of single-agent carfilzomib (PX-171-003-A1) in patients with relapsed and refractory multiple myeloma. Blood 120(14):2817–2825
42. Jakubowiak AJ, Siegel DS, Martin T, Wang M, Vij R, Lonial S, Trudel S, Kukreti V, Bahlis N, Alsina M, Chanan-Khan A, Buadi F, Reu FJ, Somlo G, Zonder J, Song K, Stewart AK, Stadtmauer E, Harrison BL, Wong AF, Orlowski RZ, Jagannath S (2013) Treatment outcomes in patients with relapsed and refractory multiple myeloma and high-risk cytogenetics receiving single-agent carfilzomib in the PX-171-003-A1 study. Leukemia 27(12):2351–2356
43. Moreau P, Pylypenko H, Grosicki S, Karamanesht I, Leleu X, Grishunina M, Rekhtman G, Masliak Z, Robak T, Shubina A, Arnulf B, Kropff M, Cavet J, Esseltine DL, Feng H, Girgis S, van de Velde H, Deraedt W, Harousseau JL (2011) Subcutaneous versus intravenous administration of bortezomib in patients with relapsed multiple myeloma: a randomised, phase 3, non-inferiority study. Lancet Oncol 12(5):431–440. doi:10.1016/S1470-2045(11)70081-X
44. Arastu-Kapur S, Anderl JL, Kraus M, Parlati F, Shenk KD, Lee SJ, Muchamuel T, Bennett MK, Driessen C, Ball AJ, Kirk CJ (2011) Nonproteasomal targets of the proteasome inhibitors bortezomib and carfilzomib: a link to clinical adverse events. Clin Cancer Res 17(9): 2734–2743
45. New Drug Application (NDA) 202714, carfilzomib (Kyprolis): Food and Drug Administration briefing document, Oncologic Drugs Advisory Committee Meeting, June 20, 2012.
46. Vij R, Wang M, Kaufman JL, Lonial S, Jakubowiak AJ, Stewart AK, Kukreti V, Jagannath S, McDonagh KT, Alsina M, Bahlis NJ, Reu FJ, Gabrail NY, Belch A, Matous JV, Lee P, Rosen P, Sebag M, Vesole DH, Kunkel LA, Wear SM, Wong AF, Orlowski RZ, Siegel DS (2012) An open-label, single-arm, phase 2 (PX-171-004) study of single-agent carfilzomib in bortezomib-naive patients with relapsed and/or refractory multiple myeloma. Blood 119(24): 5661–5670

47. Richardson PG, Sonneveld P, Schuster MW, Irwin D, Stadtmauer EA, Facon T, Harousseau JL, Ben-Yehuda D, Lonial S, Goldschmidt H, Reece D, San-Miguel JF, Blade J, Boccadoro M, Cavenagh J, Dalton WS, Boral AL, Esseltine DL, Porter JB, Schenkein D, Anderson KC (2005) Bortezomib or high-dose dexamethasone for relapsed multiple myeloma. N Engl J Med 352(24):2487–2498
48. Orlowski RZ, Nagler A, Sonneveld P, Blade J, Hajek R, Spencer A, San Miguel J, Robak T, Dmoszynska A, Horvath N, Spicka I, Sutherland HJ, Suvorov AN, Zhuang SH, Parekh T, Xiu L, Yuan Z, Rackoff W, Harousseau JL (2007) Randomized phase III study of pegylated liposomal doxorubicin plus bortezomib compared with bortezomib alone in relapsed or refractory multiple myeloma: combination therapy improves time to progression. J Clin Oncol 25(25):3892–3901
49. Papadopoulos K, Lee P, Singhal S, Holahan J, Vesole D, Rosen S, Kunkel L, Zojwalla N, Hannah A, Siegel D (2011) A phase 1b/2 study of prolonged infusion carfilzomib in patients with relapsed and/or refractory (R/R) multiple myeloma: updated efficacy and tolerability from the completed 20/56mg/m^2 expansion cohort of PX-171-007. Blood 118(21):2930
50. Badros AZ, Vij R, Martin T, Zonder JA, Kunkel L, Wang Z, Lee S, Wong AF, Niesvizky R (2013) Carfilzomib in multiple myeloma patients with renal impairment: pharmacokinetics and safety. Leukemia 27(8):1707–1714
51. Wang M, Martin T, Bensinger W, Alsina M, Siegel D, Kavalerchik E, Niesvizky R (2013) Final results from the phase Ib/II study (PX-171-006) of carfilzomib, lenalidomide, and low-dose dexamethasone (CRd) in patients with relapsed or progressive multiple myeloma. J Clin Oncol 31:(suppl; abstr 8529)
52. Dimopoulos M, Spencer A, Attal M, Prince HM, Harousseau JL, Dmoszynska A, San Miguel J, Hellmann A, Facon T, Foa R, Corso A, Masliak Z, Olesnyckyj M, Yu Z, Patin J, Zeldis JB, Knight RD (2007) Lenalidomide plus dexamethasone for relapsed or refractory multiple myeloma. N Engl J Med 357(21):2123–2132
53. Weber DM, Chen C, Niesvizky R, Wang M, Belch A, Stadtmauer EA, Siegel D, Borrello I, Rajkumar SV, Chanan-Khan AA, Lonial S, Yu Z, Patin J, Olesnyckyj M, Zeldis JB, Knight RD (2007) Lenalidomide plus dexamethasone for relapsed multiple myeloma in North America. N Engl J Med 357(21):2133–2142
54. Anderson K, Jagannath S, Jakubowiak S, Lonial S, Raje N, Alsina M, Ghobrial I, Knight R, Esseltine D, Richardson P (2009) Lenalidomide, bortezomib, and dexamethasone in relapsed/ refractory multiple myeloma (MM): encouraging outcomes and tolerability in a phase II study J Clin Oncol 27 (15S):(suppl; abstr 8536)
55. Jakubowiak AJ, Dytfeld D, Griffith KA, Lebovic D, Vesole DH, Jagannath S, Al-Zoubi A, Anderson T, Nordgren B, Detweiler-Short K, Stockerl-Goldstein K, Ahmed A, Jobkar T, Durecki DE, McDonnell K, Mietzel M, Couriel D, Kaminski M, Vij R (2012) A phase 1/2 study of carfilzomib in combination with lenalidomide and low-dose dexamethasone as a frontline treatment for multiple myeloma. Blood 120(9):1801–1809
56. Richardson PG, Weller E, Lonial S, Jakubowiak AJ, Jagannath S, Raje NS, Avigan DE, Xie W, Ghobrial IM, Schlossman RL, Mazumder A, Munshi NC, Vesole DH, Joyce R, Kaufman JL, Doss D, Warren DL, Lunde LE, Kaster S, Delaney C, Hideshima T, Mitsiades CS, Knight R, Esseltine DL, Anderson KC (2010) Lenalidomide, bortezomib, and dexamethasone combination therapy in patients with newly diagnosed multiple myeloma. Blood 116(5):679–686
57. Shah JJ, Weber DM, Thomas SK, Alexanian R, Wang M, Qazilbash MH, Parmar S, Shah N, Bashir Q, Popat UR, Hilder B, Orlowski RZ (2012) Phase 1 study of the novel kinesin spindle protein inhibitor ARRY-520 + carfilzomib in patients with relapsed and/or refractory multiple myeloma. ASH Annual Meeting Abstracts 120(21):4082
58. Berdeja JG, Hart L, Lamar R, Murphy P, Morgan S, Flinn IW (2012) Phase I/II study of panobinostat and carfilzomib in patients (pts) with relapsed or refractory multiple myeloma (MM), interim phase I safety analysis. ASH Annual Meeting Abstracts 120(21):4048
59. Shah JJ, Thomas SK, Weber DM, Wang M, Alexanian R, Qazilbash MH, Bashir Q, Parmar S, Shah N, Popat UR, Orlowski RZ (2012) Phase 1/1b study of the efficacy and safety of the combination of panobinostat + carfilzomib in patients with relapsed and/or refractory multiple myeloma. ASH Annual Meeting Abstracts 120(21):4081

60. Shah JJ, Stadtmauer EA, Abonour R, Cohen AD, Bensinger WI, Gasparetto C, Kaufman JL, Lentzsch S, Vogl DT, Orlowski RZ, Kim EL, McKinley MB, Durie BGM (2012) A multi-center phase I/II trial of carfilzomib and pomalidomide with dexamethasone (Car-Pom-d) in patients with relapsed/refractory multiple myeloma. ASH Annual Meeting Abstracts 120(21):74
61. Sonneveld P, Hacker E, Zweegman S, Kersten MJ, Vellenga E, van Marwijk-Kooy M, de Weerdt O, Lonergan S, Palumbo A, Lokhorst HM (2011) Carfilzomib combined with thalidomide and dexamethasone (CARTHADEX) as induction treatment prior to high-dose melphalan (HDM) in newly diagnosed patients with multiple myeloma (MM). a trial of the European Myeloma Network EMN. ASH Annual Meeting Abstracts 118(21):633
62. Mikhael JR, Reeder CB, Libby EN III, Costa LJ, Bergsagel PL, Buadi F, Mayo A, Gano K, Wolf C, Dueck AC, Stewart AK (2012) Results from the phase II dose expansion of cyclophosphamide, carfilzomib, thalidomide and dexamethasone (CYCLONE) in patients with newly diagnosed multiple myeloma. ASH Annual Meeting Abstracts 120(21):445
63. Palumbo A, Bringhen S, Villani O, Siniscalchi A, Russo E, Uccello G, Cerrato C, Gilestro M, Rossi D, Boccadoro M (2012) Carfilzomib, cyclophosphamide and dexamethasone (CCd) for newly diagnosed multiple myeloma (MM) patients. ASH Annual Meeting Abstracts 120(21):730
64. Kolb B, Hulin C, Caillot D, Benboubker L, Tiab M, Blin M, Leleu X, Roussel M, Attal M, Facon T, Moreau P (2012) Phase I/II study of carfilzomib plus melphalan-prednisone (CMP) in elderly patients with de novo multiple myeloma. J Clin Oncol 30:(suppl; abstr 8009)
65. Papadopoulos K, Lee P, Singhal S, Holahan J, Tolcher A, Patnaik A, Vesole D, Rosen S, Rosen P, Bilotti E, Woo T, Lee S, Hannah A, Siegel D (2011) PX-171-007: a phase 1b study of evaluation the safety and efficacy of a 30-min IV infusion of carfilzomib in patients with relapsed and/or refractory (R/R) multiple myeloma (MM). Haematology 96(S2):374

Chapter 4
Proteasome Inhibitors in the Treatment of Multiple Myeloma and AL Amyloidosis

Jeffrey A. Zonder

Abstract Therapeutic advances in the last decade have led to improved outcomes for people diagnosed with multiple myeloma (MM) and primary systemic (AL) amyloidosis. Foremost among these advances is the incorporation of proteasome inhibitors (PIs) and immunomodulatory drugs (IMiDs) into treatment regimens. Induction regimens for MM which incorporate one or both of these drug classes are associated with response rates ranging from 80 to 100 % in various studies. Myeloma remains a generally incurable disease with most patients relapsing within 5 years of initial therapy. Specific "high-risk" cytogenetic abnormalities in the malignant clone predict particularly short disease control. Results of therapy for relapsed disease are typically inferior to initial treatment, both in terms of likelihood and duration of response. Thus, resistance to proteasome inhibitor-based therapies, both inherent and acquired, remains a problem in the therapy of clonal plasma cell disorders. This chapter will provide a general overview of the use of PIs in myeloma and AL amyloidosis, with particular emphasis on the limitations of such therapy.

Keywords Bortezomib • Carfilzomib • Ixazomib • Oprozomib • Marizomib • Multiple myeloma • Amyloidosis • Proteasome inhibitors

Abbreviations

AL	Amyloidosis
ASCT	Autologous stem cell transplant
BTZ	Bortezomib
CFZ	Carfilzomib
CR	Complete response
DEX	Dexamethasone
DLZ	Delanzomib, CEP-18770

J.A. Zonder, M.D. (✉)
Departments of Oncology and Medicine, Karmanos Cancer Institute, Wayne State University School of Medicine, Detroit, MI, USA
e-mail: zonderj@karmanos.org

Q.P. Dou (ed.), *Resistance to Proteasome Inhibitors in Cancer*, Resistance to Targeted Anti-Cancer Therapeutics, DOI 10.1007/978-3-319-06752-0_4

IMiDs	Immunomodulatory drugs
IV	Intravenously
IXZ	Ixazomib, MLN-9708
LEN	Lenalidomide
MEL	Melphalan
MM	Multiple myeloma
MRZ	Marizomib, NPI-0052, salinosporamide A
OPZ	Oprozomib, ONX-0912, PR-047
PAD	BTZ + doxorubicin + DEX
PIs	Proteasome inhibitors
PN	Peripheral neuropathy
PR	Partial response
SC	Subcutaneously
UPS	Ubiquitin-proteasome system
VAD	Vincristine-adriamycin [doxorubicin]-dexamethasone
VGPR	Very good partial response
VMP	BTZ + MEL + PRED
VRD	BTZ + LEN + DEX
VTD	BTZ + THAL + DEX

4.1 Introduction

Multiple myeloma (MM) is a malignant plasma cell disorder associated with renal insufficiency, anemia, and altered bone metabolism with destructive bone lesions and increased risk for pathologic fractures. Most patients with MM have a measurable monoclonal immunoglobulin and/or free light chain in the serum or urine. Primary systemic (AL) amyloidosis is a related clonal plasma cell disorder in which abnormally folded monoclonal light chains aggregate into extracellular fibrillar protein deposits, resulting in organ dysfunction. There is some overlap between these two conditions, with approximately 10–15 % (perhaps higher) of MM cases complicated by coexisting AL [1]. Therapy for MM has evolved significantly over the last two decades, notably with the widespread use of high-dose chemotherapy with autologous stem cell transplant (ASCT) and also the development of two important classes of drugs, proteasome inhibitors (PIs), and immunomodulatory drugs (IMiDs). Therapy for AL has largely paralleled that of MM, albeit with some lag, as the condition is significantly less common and survival is often shorter.

The ubiquitin-proteasome system (UPS) is primarily responsible for the degradation of the majority of intracellular proteins, thereby playing a key role in protein homeostasis. The proteasome itself is a multiunit protease complex with a cylindrical catalytic core comprised of subunits which possess varying proteolytic functions [2]. Three specific subunits—β1, β2, and β5, which possess caspase-like, trypsin-like, and chymotrypsin-like function, respectively—account for the bulk of the proteolytic function of the organelle. Proteasome inhibition leads to intracellular accumulation of ubiquitinated proteins, ultimately triggering cell death [3]. Malignant cells are particularly susceptible to the effects of targeted proteasomal inhibition, largely through the resultant effects on NF-κB signaling [4, 5].

Bortezomib (BTZ) was the first FDA-approved proteasome inhibitor. The drug is currently approved for treatment of MM and also mantle cell lymphoma. This dipeptide boronic acid derivative preferentially inhibits the β5 subunit, and to a lesser degree the β1 subunit, in a reversible fashion [6]. BTZ may be administered either intravenously (IV) or subcutaneously (SC). Carfilzomib (CFZ) is an intravenous second-generation irreversible epoxyketone PI with increased binding specificity for the β5 subunit [7]. The pharmacodynamic properties of BTZ and CFZ likely account for much of the observed differences in efficacy and toxicity, although "off-target" effects may also play a role [8]. In 2012, CFZ was approved in the United States as treatment for myeloma relapsing after prior BTZ and IMiD therapy. Newer PIs are currently in clinical development, including the oral agents ixazomib (IXZ) and oprozomib (OPZ). Currently none of these drugs are FDA-approved for treatment of AL, but as will be discussed below, BTZ has emerged as one of the most widely used agents.

Herein, the use of BTZ and CFZ, as well as newer PIs, as treatment for all stages of MM and AL will be discussed.

4.2 Frontline Therapy of Multiple Myeloma with Bortezomib-Containing Regimens

Up until the 1980s therapy for MM generally consisted of combinations of corticosteroids (e.g., prednisone or dexamethasone), alkylating agents (e.g., melphalan or cyclophosphamide), vinca alkaloids (e.g., vincristine), and/or anthracyclines (e.g., doxorubicin) administered in repeating cycles until disease progression [9]. Such regimens typically induced responses (usually partial) 55–70 % of the time. Responses generally lasted 1–2 years, after which time salvage options were limited. Thus, median survival after a diagnosis of MM was generally accepted to be 2–3 years at that time [10]. The advent and widespread adoption of high-dose melphalan (MEL) therapy with ASCT changed expectations somewhat for younger, fitter patients. Some patients who failed to respond to induction regimens of the era would respond to subsequent therapy with high-dose MEL/ASCT. This modality resulted in higher overall response rates, higher complete response rates, longer time until disease progression, and—in some studies—improved survival. A common strategy for transplant-eligible patients throughout the 1990s involved three or four 28-day cycles of induction therapy with a regimen like VAD (vincristine-adriamycin [doxorubicin]-dexamethasone) followed by high-dose MEL and then ASCT. Within a few years of the first report describing the use of thalidomide as treatment for MM [11], this IMiD became one of the most widely used frontline drugs [12]. It was in this setting that proteasome inhibitors began to be explored as initial therapy for MM.

There is relatively little published experience with single-agent BTZ as initial therapy of MM. In a phase II study involving 49 previously untreated, symptomatic MM patients treated with BTZ (with or without DEX) for a maximum of six 3-week cycles, 90 % of patients ultimately achieved at least a partial response to therapy [13, 14]. All patients were initially treated with BTZ monotherapy, with DEX only added after cycle 2 (if less than a partial response [PR]) or cycle 4 (if less than a complete response [CR]). DEX was eventually added in 36 of the patients, with subsequent improvement in response in 28 cases. More than half of the patients in this small study went on to receive MEL/ASCT, hampering assessment of response duration, but in the patients who did not get MEL/ASCT, the median time until subsequent therapy was approximately 22 months. In the IFM 2005-01 phase III trial, the overall response rate among 240 MM patients randomized to initial therapy comprised of four cycles of BTZ+DEX was 78.5 % [15]. Although this is slightly lower than the rate reported by Jagannath et al. [14], it was superior to VAD. Additionally, subsequent MEL/ASCT increased the overall response rate to just over 90 %, with 61 % of patients achieving at least a 90 % reduction in their myeloma m-protein. It should be noted that over half of the patients treated with BTZ+DEX induction on the IFM 2005-001 study developed treatment-emergent peripheral neuropathy (PN), including functionally significant in a third of cases. This high incidence was likely due in large part to the twice-weekly IV BTZ schedule. It has since been shown that weekly dosing and/or SC administration attenuates the risk of severe PN [16–19].

BTZ-containing combination regimens incorporating IMiDs and/or older anti-myeloma drugs have been studied extensively. The HOVON-65/GMMG-HD4 Trial [20] evaluated BTZ+doxorubicin+DEX [PAD] induction, and the IFM2007-02 [21], GIMEMA MM-BO2005 [22], and GEM05-MENOS65 [23] Trials evaluated BTZ+THAL+DEX (VTD) induction in patients eligible for MEL/ASCT. As demonstrated in Table 4.1, the overall response rates after induction with such regimens is in excess of 90 %. As was seen following BTZ+DEX induction, subsequent MEL/ASCT improved the quality of responses, with half or more of the patients achieving a CR. The median time to progression after BTZ-based induction and subsequent MEL/ASCT was just over 3 years in a meta-analysis of these studies, slightly superior to the pooled results observed in the non-BTZ-containing comparator arms [24]. In the United States, the most commonly used induction combination regimen for transplantable MM patients is BTZ+LEN+DEX (VRD), despite only phase II data being available thus far [25]. Overall response rates with the combination approach are 100 %, with a large percentage of patients achieving at least a 90 % reduction in the m-protein. As both BTZ and LEN are associated with peripheral neuropathy, it is not surprising that the incidence of PN reported for this combination is >50 % [25, 26]. MEL/ASCT is readily feasible following limited VRD induction [25]. Currently there are several ongoing phase III studies utilizing VRD (e.g., S-0777 comparing VRD to RD and the DFCI/IFM Trial utilizing VRD as induction followed by immediate or delayed MEL/ASCT). Another regimen that has become widely used based on the results of phase II data is CyBorD [27, 28], particularly in patients with impaired renal function.

Table 4.1 Key bortezomib trials in newly diagnosed myeloma patients

Patient population	Study	Regimen	*N*	Response rate (%)[a]	Response duration	Survival	Reference
Non-ASCT	VISTA	VMP	344	71 (CR 30)	24.0 months	56.4 months	[27]
		MP	338	35 (CR 4)	16.6 months	43.1 months	
Non-ASCT	GIMEMA-MM-03-05	VMPT-VT	254	89 (CR 38)	56 % 3 year PFS	89 % 3 years OS	[16]
		VMP	257	81 (CR 24)	41 % 3 years PFS	87 % 3 years OS	
Non-ASCT	GEM05MAS65	VMP	130	80 (≥nCR 32)	34 months	74 % 3 years OS	[29]
	Induction	VTP	130	81 (≥nCR 36)	25 months	65 % 3 years OS	
	Maintenance	VT	91	95 (≥nCR 56)	39 months	69 % 5 years OS	
		VP	87	97 (≥nCR 50)	32 months	60 % 5 years OS	
Non-ASCT	UPFRONT	VD-V	168	73 (≥nCR 30)	14.3 months	73.7 % 2 years OS	[30]
		VTD-V	167	80 (≥nCR 40)	14.9 months	73.6 % 2 years OS	
		VMP-V	167	69 (≥nCR 33)	17.3 months	77.6 % 2 years OS	
ASCT	HOVON65-GMMG-HD4	PAD-V maintenance	371	91 (≥nCR 49)	36 months	78 % 3 years OS	[20]
		VAD-T maintenance	373	83 (≥nCR 34)	27 months	70 % 3 years OS	
ASCT	IFM2005-01	VD-ASCT	240	90.9 (≥nCR 39.6)	36 months	81.4 % 3 years OS	[15]
		VAD-ASCT	242	91.3 (≥nCR 21.7)	20.7 months	77.4 % 3 years OS	
ASCT	GEM05-MEN0565	VTD-ASCT	130	85 (≥nCR 35)	NR	NR	[23]
		TD-ASCT	127	64 (≥nCR 14)			
		Chemo/Btz-ASCT	129	75 (≥nCR 21)			
ASCT	GIMEMA	VTD-ASCT	241	93 (≥nCR 73)	68 % 3 years PFS	86 % 3 years OS	[22]
		TD-ASCT	239	99 (≥nCR 61)	56 % 3 years PFS	84 % 3 years OS	
ASCT	IFM2007-02	VTD-ASCT	100	89 (CR 29)	26 months	NR ("No difference")	[21]
		VD-ASCT	99	86 (CR 31)	30 months		
Mixed	Phase II	RVD	66	100 (CR 29)	75 % 18 months PFS (97 % w ASCT)	NR	[25]
Mixed	Phase II	CyBorD	63	90 (≥nCR 41)	2.7 years	88 % 3 years OS	[27]

[a]Response rates in ASCT trials are the posttransplant results

BTZ-containing combination regimens have also been developed in older, non-transplantable MM patients. Studies in this patient population provide more insight regarding the emergence of resistance to BTZ-containing therapy without the confounding influence of subsequent high-dose therapy. The VISTA trial, in which nine 6-week cycles of BTZ+MEL+PRED (VMP) was compared to MP, established the former as a widely used standard in older patients, due to the higher overall response rate (71 % vs. 35 %), CR rate (30 % vs. 4 %), time to disease progression (19.9 months vs. 13.1 months), and overall survival [29]. As in other studies, PN was observed in the VMP arm. Herpes zoster reactivation ("shingles") was common in the VMP arm, as well, though the incidence was reduced with the addition of antiviral prophylaxis [29, 30]. Other trials have largely confirmed the clinical efficacy of VMP [16, 31, 32].

4.3 Bortezomib-Based Regimens for Previously Treated Multiple Myeloma

BTZ, with or without dexamethasone, is an FDA-approved therapy for patients with myeloma progressing after prior treatment. The CREST and SUMMIT trials were phase II studies in which a total of 256 patients with previously treated myeloma received intravenous BTZ on days 1, 4, 8, and 11 of repeating 21-day cycles [33, 34]. DEX could be added if necessary for suboptimal response to initial monotherapy. The response rates reported for CREST and SUMMIT were in the 30–40 % range with BTZ monotherapy; adding DEX increased the likelihood of response somewhat. The duration of responses was short, with a median of just over a year for patients in the SUMMIT trial. The APEX trial was a subsequent randomized trial comparing BTZ monotherapy to DEX alone as treatment for relapsed multiple myeloma [35]. The response rate among patients randomized to BTZ was 38 %, with responses lasting a median of 8 months. Response rate and duration were slightly improved in the subset of patients who had had only prior line of therapy before enrollment in the APEX trial. As none of the patients in APEX, SUMMIT, or CREST had had prior BTZ, one can conclude that relapsing myeloma has a higher degree of inherent PI resistance than does myeloma that has not been previously treated. This is not surprising, as resistance to other drug classes, including corticosteroids, alkylating agents, and IMiDs, also increases after prior therapy. Combination regimens may partially overcome drug resistance. Reported response rates to combinations like VRD [36], PAD [37], and CyBorD are generally higher than those reported for BTZ alone in patients with relapsed myeloma, though not as high the response rates observed for the same regimens when used as initial therapy.

Retreatment with BTZ after prior use of the drug has been studied. A fairly large prospective study evaluated the efficacy of BTZ (with DEX in most cases) in myeloma patients who had previously responded to BTZ-based therapy [38]. The response rate (40 %) and duration (6.5 months) are similar to that seen after treatment with other classes of drugs. This confirmed previously reported retrospective analyses of BTZ retreatment [39, 40]. One retrospective analysis reported patients who achieved a partial response or better with BTZ retreatment after having failed to do so during initial therapy, albeit in a small minority of such cases. This provides indirect clinical evidence supporting the concept that subclones with varying sensitivity to particular classes of drugs may emerge, regress, and reemerge at different time points in the course of the disease [41].

Preclinical studies exploring mechanisms of PI resistance and pharmacologic interventions designed to circumvent it have led to clinical trials combining other agents with BTZ. These have been variably successful. For example, preclinical work showed that aggresomal inhibition by histone deacetylase inhibitors enhanced myeloma cell line sensitivity to BTZ. Despite this, the VANTAGE 088 study, which compared BTZ + the histone deacetylase inhibitor vorinostat to BTZ alone as treatment for patients with myeloma progressing after one to three prior lines of therapy, showed essentially no clinically meaningful improvement in outcomes in the combination arm [42]. A phase II study of the more potent pan-deacetylase inhibitor panobinostat, on the other hand, reported an overall response rate of 35 % among a group of patients who were relapsed and refractory to prior BTZ therapy [43]. Little benefit was gained by adding the Akt inhibitor perifosine to BTZ, despite a strong preclinical rationale and promising phase II data [44]. These experiences suggest that development of resistance to proteasome inhibitors may derive from redundant intracellular alterations or transition to a proteasome-independent homeostasis.

4.4 Bortezomib Consolidation and Maintenance Therapy for Multiple Myeloma

BTZ has been studied as post-ASCT consolidation therapy. In a randomized trial involving 370 patients, 20 doses of BTZ given over 21 weeks (starting 3 months post-ASCT) improved progression-free survival and also increased the likelihood of achieving a very good partial response (VGPR) [45]. The GIMEMA Italian Myeloma Network conducted another phase 3 study in which two 35-day cycles of VTD was compared to TD as post-ASCT consolidation therapy. PFS was longer in the BTZ-containing arm, and also more patients in that arm had upgrading of their posttransplant response [46]. The potential importance of upgrading response, particularly to CR, is hinted at in another report in which the likelihood of both CR and molecular CR (often prolonged) improved after four cycles of post-ASCT consolidation [47]. Taken together, these reports suggest that a relatively brief period of post-ASCT BTZ-based therapy may be able to improve clinical outcomes.

There is also data supporting the use of prolonged BTZ-based therapy after non-ASCT induction therapy. Palumbo et al. compared VMP as given in the VISTA study to a four-drug combination (VMP + THAL) followed by BTZ + THAL maintenance and found that VMPT + VT therapy was associated with prolonged disease control compared to VMP [16]. Subsequent trials utilizing BTZ alone [20] or in combination with either THAL or PRED [48] have confirmed the feasibility and efficacy of this approach. Sonneveld et al. suggest that BTZ maintenance partially overcomes the adverse impact of certain high-risk cytogenetic features, namely del17p, though the noted median progression-free survival of only 22 months in this group remains short compared to published results for standard risk patients. Based largely on this, some experts have recommended that at least 1 year of BTZ-based maintenance therapy be considered for all patients with intermediate- or high-risk myeloma [49].

4.5 Carfilzomib (CFZ) as Treatment for Multiple Myeloma

CFZ is currently used as therapy for patients with myeloma progressing on or immediately after at least two prior lines of therapy that include an IMiD and BTZ. As might be predicted based on the previous discussion on BTZ, sensitivity to CFZ varies according to the amount of prior therapy and also prior sensitivity to BTZ-containing regimens. In BTZ-naïve patients, an overall response rate of 52 % was reported [50], essentially double the response rate seen in a study in which most patients were resistant to BTZ [51]. Responses to CFZ can be seen even in patients refractory to BTZ as the last prior therapy, suggesting that residual BTZ-resistant cells may still be sensitive to CFZ. The median duration of responses to CFZ is generally less than a year in patients with relapsed myeloma, but a minority of patients can enjoy extended disease control. CFZ-containing combinations are being developed as treatment for previously treated and newly diagnosed myeloma [52–56] (Table 4.2).

As stated above, the toxicity profile of CFZ differs somewhat from that of BTZ. Both drugs are associated with fatigue, myelosuppression (particularly thrombocytopenia), and gastrointestinal side effects. The incidence of treatment-emergent peripheral sensory neuropathy is significantly lower with CFZ compared to intravenous BTZ [57]. The frequency of treatment-emergent toxicity does not seem to worsen over time with prolonged CFZ therapy, but the twice-weekly schedule presents a formidable challenge in terms of developing the drug as prolonged (maintenance) therapy.

4.6 Ixazomib (MLN-9708/2238)

Ixazomib (MLN-9708; IXZ) is the first orally bioavailable reversible proteasome inhibitor to enter clinical investigation in MM patients. In preclinical studies, the anti-myeloma activity of the drug compared favorably to BTZ [58, 59]. Phase I and

Table 4.2 Carfilzomib combination trials in multiple myeloma patients

Patient population	Regimen	N	Response rate (%)	Response duration	Survival	Reference
Newly diagnosed	CRd	53	98 (≥nCR 62))	2 years PFS 92 %	NR	[53]
Newly diagnosed	CCyD	54	91 (CR 18)	1 year PFS 90 %	1 year OS 98 %	[56]
Relapsed	CRd	52	77	PFS 15.4 months	NR	[55]

II trials suggest that single-agent IXZ has clinical activity in heavily pretreated relapsed and/or refractory MM patients, with infrequent peripheral neuropathy. It is currently being tested in many clinical trials in a wide range of clinical indications, including previously untreated MM, relapsed MM, advanced stage solid tumors, lymphoblastic leukemia, non-Hodgkin's lymphoma, and AL amyloidosis. There is interest in developing the drug as maintenance therapy in MM.

4.7 Delanzomib (CEP-18770)

Delanzomib (DLZ) is another reversibly binding boronate-based, second-generation proteasome inhibitor with both oral and IV bioavailability. DLZ has been shown to have proteasome-inhibitory activity similar to that of BTZ in hematologic and solid tumor cell lines, as well as in primary cells from multiple myeloma patients. DLZ is currently in phase I/II clinical investigations for myeloma, lymphoma, and solid tumors still using intravenous administration [60]. The initial clinical report suggests a favorable safety profile with minimal neurotoxicity. Preclinical work evaluating the drug in combination with other anti-myeloma drugs has been reported [61].

4.8 Oprozomib (ONX-0912, PR-047)

OPZ is an orally bioavailable peptide epoxyketone-based, irreversible proteasome inhibitor that showed similar potency to CFZ in cytotoxicity assays [62]. Orally administered OPZ showed equivalent antitumor activity to intravenously administered CFZ in human tumor xenograft and mouse syngeneic models. Early studies were hampered by significant gastrointestinal toxicity, prompting the manufacturer to develop a modified formulation. The formulation currently being investigated in phase I and II trials for patients with hematological cancers (including multiple myeloma) or solid tumors appears more tolerable. The optimal dosing schedule of the drug is still being worked out. A phase I/II trial combining OPZ with lenalidomide and DEX in newly diagnosed MM patients is being planned.

4.9 Marizomib (NPI-0052, Salinosporamide A)

Marizomib (MRZ) is an irreversible proteasome inhibitor with a β-lactone backbone. Compared to other proteasome inhibitors, MRZ produces rapid, broad, and prolonged inhibition of all three 20S proteasome catalytic subunits [63]. MRZ is the only non-peptide-based inhibitor in clinical trials. It is administrated intravenously twice weekly and is being investigated for phase Ib for recurrent MM, solid tumors, lymphoma, and leukemia. MRZ exhibits an extremely short half-life (<5 min) wide tissue distribution [64]. Responses to MRZ were found in patients with BTZ-refractory MM. The safety profile of MRZ differs from BTZ, with no significant treatment-emergent peripheral neuropathy, myelosuppression, or thrombocytopenia reported. The dose limiting toxicities include transient hallucinations, cognitive changes, and loss of balance, perhaps reflecting CNS penetration.

4.10 Proteasome Inhibitor Therapy for AL Amyloidosis

Based on the efficacy of BTZ and other proteasome inhibitors vs. myeloma, this class of drugs has also been studied as therapy for another clonal plasma cell dyscrasia, AL amyloidosis. In the first reported use of BTZ for AL, 18 patients (seven previously treated) were treated with BTZ+DEX, resulting in a 94 % hematologic response rate—including CR in 44 % [65]. Improvement in organ function was observed in a minority of patients, in some cases quite quickly. This has been postulated to be due to rapid reduction in cytotoxic soluble light chains [66, 67] and mitigating effects of proteasome inhibition on the inflammatory cascade in affected organs, notably the kidney [68].

A larger subsequent analysis of 94 AL patients treated with BTZ at three major European amyloid centers described somewhat more modest results, with an overall hematologic response rate of 71 %, with 25 % of patients achieving CR [69]. Patients in this analysis were not treated in a uniform fashion: DEX use was variable, and the BTZ schedule ranged from once to twice each week. The twice-weekly schedule was associated with a somewhat faster time to response, a finding reconfirmed in another trial, the CAN2007 study [70, 71]. In this phase I/II trial, once- and twice-weekly BTZ dosing schedules were explored. Hematologic responses were seen in approximately two-thirds of patients regardless of schedule. Time to response was shorter for the patients getting twice-weekly dosing. Importantly, the majority of patients who had hematologic responses remained free from hematologic relapse 1 year after completion of therapy. Renal and cardiac improvement was observed in 29 % and 13 % of patients, respectively.

BTZ-containing combinations have been explored in AL amyloidosis. The "CyBorD" regimen, in which BTZ was co-administered with cyclophosphamide and dexamethasone on a weekly basis, induced responses in 16 of 17 patients (including hematologic CRs in 12 patients) [72]. Therapy was relatively brief, with patients receiving between two and six cycles of therapy. A few patients who started their treatment non-transplant eligible became eligible after responding to CyBorD. BTZ has also been added to standard MEL-DEX ("VMD" regimen) [73]. As seen with CyBorD, the overall hematologic response rate was quite high, with hematologic CRs and some organ function improvement noted. Currently, a multicenter study combining BTZ, DEX, and the IMiD pomalidomide as first-line therapy for AL is ongoing.

BTZ has been evaluated as part of ASCT conditioning and post-ASCT consolidation therapy in AL patients. Ten patients received four doses of BTZ along with standard high-dose melphalan conditioning. One patient was removed from protocol prior to receiving study therapy, but eight of the remaining nine treated patients did exhibit hematologic responses (including six CRs) [74]. Toxicity was manageable. In another study, of 40 patients with AL amyloidosis undergoing ASCT, more than half (23) failed to achieve a CR and were then treated with BTZ+DEX. Most of these patients had improved responses after that, including 40 % still in CR after 1 year of follow-up [75].

Clinical studies in AL amyloidosis utilizing other proteasome inhibitors—ixazomib and CFZ—are currently ongoing.

4.11 Conclusions

The advent of proteasome inhibitors and their incorporation into treatment regimens have dramatically improved clinical outcomes of patients with multiple myeloma and AL amyloidosis. Almost all patients with these conditions respond to initial therapy, sometimes for prolonged periods. Despite this, as described in this review, the effectiveness of this class of drugs is diminished when used in a second-line therapy or beyond. Resistance to PIs and strategies for overcoming it will be explored in other chapters of this book.

References

1. Bahlis NJ, Lazarus HM (2006) Multiple myeloma-associated AL amyloidosis: is a distinctive therapeutic approach warranted? Bone Marrow Transplant 38(1):7–15. doi:10.1038/sj.bmt.1705395
2. Groll M, Ditzel L, Lowe J, Stock D, Bochtler M, Bartunik HD, Huber R (1997) Structure of 20S proteasome from yeast at 2.4 A resolution. Nature 386(6624):463–471. doi:10.1038/386463a0
3. Adams J (2003) The proteasome: structure, function, and role in the cell. Cancer Treat Rev 29(Suppl 1):3–9
4. Dou QP, Li B (1999) Proteasome inhibitors as potential novel anticancer agents. Drug Resist Updat 2(4):215–223. doi:10.1054/drup.1999.0095
5. Yang H, Zonder JA, Dou QP (2009) Clinical development of novel proteasome inhibitors for cancer treatment. Expert Opin Investig Drugs 18(7):957–971. doi:10.1517/13543780903002074
6. Boccadoro M, Morgan G, Cavenagh J (2005) Preclinical evaluation of the proteasome inhibitor bortezomib in cancer therapy. Cancer Cell Int 5(1):18. doi:10.1186/1475-2867-5-18
7. Kuhn DJ, Chen Q, Voorhees PM, Strader JS, Shenk KD, Sun CM, Demo SD, Bennett MK, van Leeuwen FW, Chanan-Khan AA, Orlowski RZ (2007) Potent activity of carfilzomib, a novel, irreversible inhibitor of the ubiquitin-proteasome pathway, against preclinical models of multiple myeloma. Blood 110(9):3281–3290. doi:10.1182/blood-2007-01-065888
8. Kuhn DJ, Orlowski RZ, Bjorklund CC (2011) Second generation proteasome inhibitors: carfilzomib and immunoproteasome-specific inhibitors (IPSIs). Curr Cancer Drug Targets 11(3):285–295
9. Zonder JA (2007) Initial treatment approach to multiple myeloma. In: Bolwell B, Sekeres M, Kalacyio M (eds) Clinical Malignant Hematology. McGraw-Hill, New York, pp 873–888
10. Kumar SK, Rajkumar SV, Dispenzieri A, Lacy MQ, Hayman SR, Buadi FK, Zeldenrust SR, Dingli D, Russell SJ, Lust JA, Greipp PR, Kyle RA, Gertz MA (2008) Improved survival in multiple myeloma and the impact of novel therapies. Blood 111(5):2516–2520. doi:10.1182/blood-2007-10-116129

11. Singhal S, Mehta J, Desikan R, Ayers D, Roberson P, Eddlemon P, Munshi N, Anaissie E, Wilson C, Dhodapkar M, Zeddis J, Barlogie B (1999) Antitumor activity of thalidomide in refractory multiple myeloma. N Engl J Med 341(21):1565–1571. doi:10.1056/NEJM199911183412102
12. Rajkumar SV, Rosinol L, Hussein M, Catalano J, Jedrzejczak W, Lucy L, Olesnyckyj M, Yu Z, Knight R, Zeldis JB, Blade J (2008) Multicenter, randomized, double-blind, placebo-controlled study of thalidomide plus dexamethasone compared with dexamethasone as initial therapy for newly diagnosed multiple myeloma. J Clin Oncol 26(13):2171–2177. doi:10.1200/JCO.2007.14.1853
13. Jagannath S, Durie BG, Wolf J, Camacho E, Irwin D, Lutzky J, McKinley M, Gabayan E, Mazumder A, Schenkein D, Crowley J (2005) Bortezomib therapy alone and in combination with dexamethasone for previously untreated symptomatic multiple myeloma. Br J Haematol 129(6):776–783. doi:10.1111/j.1365-2141.2005.05540.x
14. Jagannath S, Durie BG, Wolf JL, Camacho ES, Irwin D, Lutzky J, McKinley M, Potts P, Gabayan AE, Mazumder A, Crowley J, Vescio R (2009) Extended follow-up of a phase 2 trial of bortezomib alone and in combination with dexamethasone for the frontline treatment of multiple myeloma. Br J Haematol 146(6):619–626. doi:10.1111/j.1365-2141.2009.07803.x
15. Harousseau JL, Attal M, Avet-Loiseau H, Marit G, Caillot D, Mohty M, Lenain P, Hulin C, Facon T, Casassus P, Michallet M, Maisonneuve H, Benboubker L, Maloisel F, Petillon MO, Webb I, Mathiot C, Moreau P (2010) Bortezomib plus dexamethasone is superior to vincristine plus doxorubicin plus dexamethasone as induction treatment prior to autologous stem-cell transplantation in newly diagnosed multiple myeloma: results of the IFM 2005-01 phase III trial. J Clin Oncol 28(30):4621–4629. doi:10.1200/JCO.2009.27.9158
16. Palumbo A, Bringhen S, Rossi D, Cavalli M, Larocca A, Ria R, Offidani M, Patriarca F, Nozzoli C, Guglielmelli T, Benevolo G, Callea V, Baldini L, Morabito F, Grasso M, Leonardi G, Rizzo M, Falcone AP, Gottardi D, Montefusco V, Musto P, Petrucci MT, Ciccone G, Boccadoro M (2010) Bortezomib-melphalan-prednisone-thalidomide followed by maintenance with bortezomib-thalidomide compared with bortezomib-melphalan-prednisone for initial treatment of multiple myeloma: a randomized controlled trial. J Clin Oncol 28(34):5101–5109. doi:10.1200/JCO.2010.29.8216
17. Wang Y, Ai L, Cui G, Gowrea B, Li M, Hu Y (2012) Once- versus twice-weekly bortezomib induction therapy with dexamethasone in newly diagnosed multiple myeloma. J Huazhong Univ Sci Technolog Medical Sci 32(4):495–500. doi:10.1007/s11596-012-0086-7
18. Bringhen S, Larocca A, Rossi D, Cavalli M, Genuardi M, Ria R, Gentili S, Patriarca F, Nozzoli C, Levi A, Guglielmelli T, Benevolo G, Callea V, Rizzo V, Cangialosi C, Musto P, De Rosa L, Liberati AM, Grasso M, Falcone AP, Evangelista A, Cavo M, Gaidano G, Boccadoro M, Palumbo A (2010) Efficacy and safety of once-weekly bortezomib in multiple myeloma patients. Blood 116(23):4745–4753. doi:10.1182/blood-2010-07-294983
19. Moreau P, Pylypenko H, Grosicki S, Karamanesht I, Leleu X, Grishunina M, Rekhtman G, Masliak Z, Robak T, Shubina A, Arnulf B, Kropff M, Cavet J, Esseltine DL, Feng H, Girgis S, van de Velde H, Deraedt W, Harousseau JL (2011) Subcutaneous versus intravenous administration of bortezomib in patients with relapsed multiple myeloma: a randomised, phase 3, non-inferiority study. Lancet Oncol 12(5):431–440. doi:10.1016/S1470-2045(11)70081-X
20. Sonneveld P, Schmidt-Wolf IG, van der Holt B, El Jarari L, Bertsch U, Salwender H, Zweegman S, Vellenga E, Broyl A, Blau IW, Weisel KC, Wittebol S, Bos GM, Stevens-Kroef M, Scheid C, Pfreundschuh M, Hose D, Jauch A, van der Velde H, Raymakers R, Schaafsma MR, Kersten MJ, van Marwijk-Kooy M, Duehrsen U, Lindemann W, Wijermans PW, Lokhorst HM, Goldschmidt HM (2012) Bortezomib induction and maintenance treatment in patients with newly diagnosed multiple myeloma: results of the randomized phase III HOVON-65/GMMG-HD4 trial. J Clin Oncol 30(24):2946–2955. doi:10.1200/JCO.2011.39.6820
21. Moreau P, Avet-Loiseau H, Facon T, Attal M, Tiab M, Hulin C, Doyen C, Garderet L, Randriamalala E, Araujo C, Lepeu G, Marit G, Caillot D, Escoffre M, Lioure B, Benboubker L, Pegourie B, Kolb B, Stoppa AM, Fuzibet JG, Decaux O, Dib M, Berthou C, Chaleteix C, Sebban C, Traulle C, Fontan J, Wetterwald M, Lenain P, Mathiot C, Harousseau JL (2011) Bortezomib plus dexamethasone versus reduced-dose bortezomib, thalidomide plus dexamethasone as induction treatment before autologous stem cell transplantation in newly diagnosed multiple myeloma. Blood 118(22):5752–5758. doi:10.1182/blood-2011-05-355081; quiz 5982

22. Cavo M, Tacchetti P, Patriarca F, Petrucci MT, Pantani L, Galli M, Di Raimondo F, Crippa C, Zamagni E, Palumbo A, Offidani M, Corradini P, Narni F, Spadano A, Pescosta N, Deliliers GL, Ledda A, Cellini C, Caravita T, Tosi P, Baccarani M, Network GIM (2010) Bortezomib with thalidomide plus dexamethasone compared with thalidomide plus dexamethasone as induction therapy before, and consolidation therapy after, double autologous stem-cell transplantation in newly diagnosed multiple myeloma: a randomised phase 3 study. Lancet 376(9758):2075–2085. doi:10.1016/S0140-6736(10)61424-9
23. Rosinol L, Oriol A, Teruel AI, Hernandez D, Lopez-Jimenez J, de la Rubia J, Granell M, Besalduch J, Palomera L, Gonzalez Y, Etxebeste MA, Diaz-Mediavilla J, Hernandez MT, de Arriba F, Gutierrez NC, Martin-Ramos ML, Cibeira MT, Mateos MV, Martinez J, Alegre A, Lahuerta JJ, San Miguel J, Blade J, Programa para el Estudio y la Terapeutica de las Hemopatias Malignas/ Grupo Espanol de Mieloma g (2012) Superiority of bortezomib, thalidomide, and dexamethasone (VTD) as induction pretransplantation therapy in multiple myeloma: a randomized phase 3 PETHEMA/GEM study. Blood 120(8):1589–1596. doi:10.1182/blood-2012-02-408922
24. Sonneveld P, Goldschmidt H, Rosinol L, Blade J, Lahuerta JJ, Cavo M, Tacchetti P, Zamagni E, Attal M, Lokhorst HM, Desai A, Cakana A, Liu K, van de Velde H, Esseltine DL, Moreau P (2013) Bortezomib-based versus nonbortezomib-based induction treatment before autologous stem-cell transplantation in patients with previously untreated multiple myeloma: a meta-analysis of phase III randomized, controlled trials. J Clin Oncol 31(26):3279–3287. doi:10.1200/JCO.2012.48.4626
25. Richardson PG, Weller E, Lonial S, Jakubowiak AJ, Jagannath S, Raje NS, Avigan DE, Xie W, Ghobrial IM, Schlossman RL, Mazumder A, Munshi NC, Vesole DH, Joyce R, Kaufman JL, Doss D, Warren DL, Lunde LE, Kaster S, Delaney C, Hideshima T, Mitsiades CS, Knight R, Esseltine DL, Anderson KC (2010) Lenalidomide, bortezomib, and dexamethasone combination therapy in patients with newly diagnosed multiple myeloma. Blood 116(5):679–686. doi:10.1182/blood-2010-02-268862
26. Voorhees PM, Laubach J, Anderson KC, Richardson PG (2013) Peripheral neuropathy in multiple myeloma patients receiving lenalidomide, bortezomib, and dexamethasone (RVD) therapy. Blood 121(5):858. doi:10.1182/blood-2012-11-465765
27. Reeder CB, Reece DE, Kukreti V, Chen C, Trudel S, Hentz J, Noble B, Pirooz NA, Spong JE, Piza JG, Zepeda VH, Mikhael JR, Leis JF, Bergsagel PL, Fonseca R, Stewart AK (2009) Cyclophosphamide, bortezomib and dexamethasone induction for newly diagnosed multiple myeloma: high response rates in a phase II clinical trial. Leukemia 23(7):1337–1341. doi:10.1038/leu.2009.26
28. Reeder CB, Reece DE, Kukreti V, Chen C, Trudel S, Laumann K, Hentz J, Pirooz NA, Piza JG, Tiedemann R, Mikhael JR, Bergsagel PL, Leis JF, Fonseca R, Stewart AK (2010) Once- versus twice-weekly bortezomib induction therapy with CyBorD in newly diagnosed multiple myeloma. Blood 115(16):3416–3417. doi:10.1182/blood-2010-02-271676
29. San Miguel JF, Schlag R, Khuageva NK, Dimopoulos MA, Shpilberg O, Kropff M, Spicka I, Petrucci MT, Palumbo A, Samoilova OS, Dmoszynska A, Abdulkadyrov KM, Schots R, Jiang B, Mateos MV, Anderson KC, Esseltine DL, Liu K, Cakana A, van de Velde H, Richardson PG, Investigators VT (2008) Bortezomib plus melphalan and prednisone for initial treatment of multiple myeloma. N Engl J Med 359(9):906–917. doi:10.1056/NEJMoa0801479
30. Vickrey E, Allen S, Mehta J, Singhal S (2009) Acyclovir to prevent reactivation of varicella zoster virus (herpes zoster) in multiple myeloma patients receiving bortezomib therapy. Cancer 115(1):229–232. doi:10.1002/cncr.24006
31. Mateos MV, Oriol A, Martinez-Lopez J, Gutierrez N, Teruel AI, de Paz R, Garcia-Larana J, Bengoechea E, Martin A, Mediavilla JD, Palomera L, de Arriba F, Gonzalez Y, Hernandez JM, Sureda A, Bello JL, Bargay J, Penalver FJ, Ribera JM, Martin-Mateos ML, Garcia-Sanz R, Cibeira MT, Ramos ML, Vidriales MB, Paiva B, Montalban MA, Lahuerta JJ, Blade J, Miguel JF (2010) Bortezomib, melphalan, and prednisone versus bortezomib, thalidomide, and prednisone as induction therapy followed by maintenance treatment with bortezomib and thalidomide versus bortezomib and prednisone in elderly patients with untreated multiple myeloma: a randomised trial. Lancet Oncol 11(10):934–941. doi:10.1016/S1470-2045(10)70187-X
32. Niesvizky RF, Flinn IW, Rifkin RM, Gabrail NY, Charu V, Clowney B, Essell J, Gaffar YA, Warr TA, Neuwirth R, Corzo D, Reeves JA (2013) Phase 3b UPFRONT study: safety and efficacy of

weekly bortezomib maintenance therapy after bortezomib-based induction regimens in elderly, newly diagnosed multiple myeloma patients. Blood 122(21):suppl. Abstract #619
33. Richardson PG, Barlogie B, Berenson J, Singhal S, Jagannath S, Irwin D, Rajkumar SV, Srkalovic G, Alsina M, Alexanian R, Siegel D, Orlowski RZ, Kuter D, Limentani SA, Lee S, Hideshima T, Esseltine DL, Kauffman M, Adams J, Schenkein DP, Anderson KC (2003) A phase 2 study of bortezomib in relapsed, refractory myeloma. N Engl J Med 348(26):2609–2617. doi:10.1056/NEJMoa030288
34. Jagannath S, Barlogie B, Berenson J, Siegel D, Irwin D, Richardson PG, Niesvizky R, Alexanian R, Limentani SA, Alsina M, Adams J, Kauffman M, Esseltine DL, Schenkein DP, Anderson KC (2004) A phase 2 study of two doses of bortezomib in relapsed or refractory myeloma. Br J Haematol 127(2):165–172. doi:10.1111/j.1365-2141.2004.05188.x
35. Richardson PG, Sonneveld P, Schuster MW, Irwin D, Stadtmauer EA, Facon T, Harousseau JL, Ben-Yehuda D, Lonial S, Goldschmidt H, Reece D, San-Miguel JF, Blade J, Boccadoro M, Cavenagh J, Dalton WS, Boral AL, Esseltine DL, Porter JB, Schenkein D, Anderson KC, Assessment of Proteasome Inhibition for Extending Remissions I (2005) Bortezomib or high-dose dexamethasone for relapsed multiple myeloma. N Engl J Med 352(24):2487–2498. doi:10.1056/NEJMoa043445
36. Richardson PG, Xie W, Jagannath S, Jakubowiak A, Lonial S, Raje NS, Alsina M, Ghobrial IM, Schlossman RL, Munshi NC, Mazumder A, Vesole DH, Kaufman JL, Colson K, McKenney M, Lunde LE, Feather J, Maglio ME, Warren D, Francis D, Hideshima T, Knight R, Esseltine DL, Mitsiades CS, Weller E, Anderson KC (2014) A phase II trial of lenalidomide, bortezomib and dexamethasone in patients with relapsed and relapsed/refractory myeloma. Blood 123(10):1461–1469. doi:10.1182/blood-2013-07-517276
37. Orlowski RZ, Nagler A, Sonneveld P, Blade J, Hajek R, Spencer A, San Miguel J, Robak T, Dmoszynska A, Horvath N, Spicka I, Sutherland HJ, Suvorov AN, Zhuang SH, Parekh T, Xiu L, Yuan Z, Rackoff W, Harousseau JL (2007) Randomized phase III study of pegylated liposomal doxorubicin plus bortezomib compared with bortezomib alone in relapsed or refractory multiple myeloma: combination therapy improves time to progression. J Clin Oncol 25(25):3892–3901. doi:10.1200/JCO.2006.10.5460
38. Petrucci MT, Giraldo P, Corradini P, Teixeira A, Dimopoulos MA, Blau IW, Drach J, Angermund R, Allietta N, Broer E, Mitchell V, Blade J (2013) A prospective, international phase 2 study of bortezomib retreatment in patients with relapsed multiple myeloma. Br J Haematol 160(5):649–659. doi:10.1111/bjh.12198
39. Wolf J, Richardson PG, Schuster M, LeBlanc A, Walters IB, Battleman DS (2008) Utility of bortezomib retreatment in relapsed or refractory multiple myeloma patients: a multicenter case series. Clin Adv Hematol Oncol 6(10):755–760
40. Conner TM, Doan QD, Walters IB, LeBlanc AL, Beveridge RA (2008) An observational, retrospective analysis of retreatment with bortezomib for multiple myeloma. Clin Lymphoma Myeloma 8(3):140–145. doi:10.3816/CLM.2008.n.016
41. Keats JJ, Chesi M, Egan JB, Garbitt VM, Palmer SE, Braggio E, Van Wier S, Blackburn PR, Baker AS, Dispenzieri A, Kumar S, Rajkumar SV, Carpten JD, Barrett M, Fonseca R, Stewart AK, Bergsagel PL (2012) Clonal competition with alternating dominance in multiple myeloma. Blood 120(5):1067–1076. doi:10.1182/blood-2012-01-405985
42. Dimopoulos M, Siegel DS, Lonial S, Qi J, Hajek R, Facon T, Rosinol L, Williams C, Blacklock H, Goldschmidt H, Hungria V, Spencer A, Palumbo A, Graef T, Eid JE, Houp J, Sun L, Vuocolo S, Anderson KC (2013) Vorinostat or placebo in combination with bortezomib in patients with multiple myeloma (VANTAGE 088): a multicentre, randomised, double-blind study. Lancet Oncol 14(11):1129–1140. doi:10.1016/S1470-2045(13)70398-X
43. Richardson PG, Schlossman RL, Alsina M, Weber DM, Coutre SE, Gasparetto C, Mukhopadhyay S, Ondovik MS, Khan M, Paley CS, Lonial S (2013) PANORAMA 2: panobinostat in combination with bortezomib and dexamethasone in patients with relapsed and bortezomib-refractory myeloma. Blood 122(14):2331–2337. doi:10.1182/blood-2013-01-481325
44. Richardson PG, Wolf J, Jakubowiak A, Zonder J, Lonial S, Irwin D, Densmore J, Krishnan A, Raje N, Bar M, Martin T, Schlossman R, Ghobrial IM, Munshi N, Laubach J, Allerton J,

Hideshima T, Colson K, Poradosu E, Gardner L, Sportelli P, Anderson KC (2011) Perifosine plus bortezomib and dexamethasone in patients with relapsed/refractory multiple myeloma previously treated with bortezomib: results of a multicenter phase I/II trial. J Clin Oncol 29(32):4243–4249. doi:10.1200/JCO.2010.33.9788

45. Mellqvist UH, Gimsing P, Hjertner O, Lenhoff S, Laane E, Remes K, Steingrimsdottir H, Abildgaard N, Ahlberg L, Blimark C, Dahl IM, Forsberg K, Gedde-Dahl T, Gregersen H, Gruber A, Guldbrandsen N, Haukas E, Carlson K, Kvam AK, Nahi H, Lindas R, Andersen NF, Turesson I, Waage A, Westin J, Nordic Myeloma Study G (2013) Bortezomib consolidation after autologous stem cell transplantation in multiple myeloma: a Nordic Myeloma Study Group randomized phase 3 trial. Blood 121(23):4647–4654. doi:10.1182/blood-2012-11-464503
46. Cavo M, Pantani L, Petrucci MT, Patriarca F, Zamagni E, Donnarumma D, Crippa C, Boccadoro M, Perrone G, Falcone A, Nozzoli C, Zambello R, Masini L, Furlan A, Brioli A, Derudas D, Ballanti S, Dessanti ML, De Stefano V, Carella AM, Marcatti M, Nozza A, Ferrara F, Callea V, Califano C, Pezzi A, Baraldi A, Grasso M, Musto P, Palumbo A, Network GIM (2012) Bortezomib-thalidomide-dexamethasone is superior to thalidomide-dexamethasone as consolidation therapy after autologous hematopoietic stem cell transplantation in patients with newly diagnosed multiple myeloma. Blood 120(1):9–19. doi:10.1182/blood-2012-02-408898
47. Ladetto M, Pagliano G, Ferrero S, Cavallo F, Drandi D, Santo L, Crippa C, De Rosa L, Pregno P, Grasso M, Liberati AM, Caravita T, Pisani F, Guglielmelli T, Callea V, Musto P, Cangialosi C, Passera R, Boccadoro M, Palumbo A (2010) Major tumor shrinking and persistent molecular remissions after consolidation with bortezomib, thalidomide, and dexamethasone in patients with autografted myeloma. J Clin Oncol 28(12):2077–2084. doi:10.1200/JCO.2009.23.7172
48. Mateos MV, Oriol A, Martinez-Lopez J, Gutierrez N, Teruel AI, Lopez de la Guia A, Lopez J, Bengoechea E, Perez M, Polo M, Palomera L, de Arriba F, Gonzalez Y, Hernandez JM, Granell M, Bello JL, Bargay J, Penalver FJ, Ribera JM, Martin-Mateos ML, Garcia-Sanz R, Lahuerta JJ, Blade J, San-Miguel JF (2012) Maintenance therapy with bortezomib plus thalidomide or bortezomib plus prednisone in elderly multiple myeloma patients included in the GEM2005MAS65 trial. Blood 120(13):2581–2588. doi:10.1182/blood-2012-05-427815
49. Mikhael JR, Dingli D, Roy V, Reeder CB, Buadi FK, Hayman SR, Dispenzieri A, Fonseca R, Sher T, Kyle RA, Lin Y, Russell SJ, Kumar S, Bergsagel PL, Zeldenrust SR, Leung N, Drake MT, Kapoor P, Ansell SM, Witzig TE, Lust JA, Dalton RJ, Gertz MA, Stewart AK, Rajkumar SV, Chanan-Khan A, Lacy MQ, Mayo C (2013) Management of newly diagnosed symptomatic multiple myeloma: updated Mayo Stratification of Myeloma and Risk-Adapted Therapy (mSMART) consensus guidelines 2013. Mayo Clin Proc 88(4):360–376. doi:10.1016/j.mayocp.2013.01.019
50. Vij R, Wang M, Kaufman JL, Lonial S, Jakubowiak AJ, Stewart AK, Kukreti V, Jagannath S, McDonagh KT, Alsina M, Bahlis NJ, Reu FJ, Gabrail NY, Belch A, Matous JV, Lee P, Rosen P, Sebag M, Vesole DH, Kunkel LA, Wear SM, Wong AF, Orlowski RZ, Siegel DS (2012) An open-label, single-arm, phase 2 (PX-171-004) study of single-agent carfilzomib in bortezomib-naive patients with relapsed and/or refractory multiple myeloma. Blood 119(24):5661–5670. doi:10.1182/blood-2012-03-414359
51. Siegel DS, Martin T, Wang M, Vij R, Jakubowiak AJ, Lonial S, Trudel S, Kukreti V, Bahlis N, Alsina M, Chanan-Khan A, Buadi F, Reu FJ, Somlo G, Zonder J, Song K, Stewart AK, Stadtmauer E, Kunkel L, Wear S, Wong AF, Orlowski RZ, Jagannath S (2012) A phase 2 study of single-agent carfilzomib (PX-171-003-A1) in patients with relapsed and refractory multiple myeloma. Blood 120(14):2817–2825. doi:10.1182/blood-2012-05-425934
52. Moreau P (2014) The emerging role of carfilzomib combination therapy in the management of multiple myeloma. Expert Rev Hematol 7(2):265–290. doi:10.1586/17474086.2014.873699
53. Jakubowiak AJ, Dytfeld D, Griffith KA, Lebovic D, Vesole DH, Jagannath S, Al-Zoubi A, Anderson T, Nordgren B, Detweiler-Short K, Stockerl-Goldstein K, Ahmed A, Jobkar T, Durecki DE, McDonnell K, Mietzel M, Couriel D, Kaminski M, Vij R (2012) A phase 1/2 study of carfilzomib in combination with lenalidomide and low-dose dexamethasone as a frontline treatment for multiple myeloma. Blood 120(9):1801–1809. doi:10.1182/blood-2012-04-422683

54. Niesvizky R, Martin TG 3rd, Bensinger WI, Alsina M, Siegel DS, Kunkel LA, Wong AF, Lee S, Orlowski RZ, Wang M (2013) Phase Ib dose-escalation study (PX-171-006) of carfilzomib, lenalidomide, and low-dose dexamethasone in relapsed or progressive multiple myeloma. Clin Cancer Res 19(8):2248–2256. doi:10.1158/1078-0432.CCR-12-3352
55. Wang M, Martin T, Bensinger W, Alsina M, Siegel DS, Kavalerchik E, Huang M, Orlowski RZ, Niesvizky R (2013) Phase 2 dose-expansion study (PX-171-006) of carfilzomib, lenalidomide, and low-dose dexamethasone in relapsed or progressive multiple myeloma. Blood 122(18):3122–3128. doi:10.1182/blood-2013-07-511170
56. Mikhael JR, Reeder CB, Libby EN, Costa LJ, Bergsagel L, Buadi F, Mayo A, Gano K, Wolf C, Dueck AC, Stewart AK (2013) A phase I/II Trial of cyclophosphamide, carfilzomib, thalidomide and dexamethasone (cyclone) in patients with newly diagnosed multiple myeloma: final results of MTD expansion cohort. Blood 122(21):suppl. Abstract #653
57. Siegel D, Martin T, Nooka A, Harvey RD, Vij R, Niesvizky R, Badros AZ, Jagannath S, McCulloch L, Rajangam K, Lonial S (2013) Integrated safety profile of single-agent carfilzomib: experience from 526 patients enrolled in 4 phase II clinical studies. Haematologica 98(11):1753–1761. doi:10.3324/haematol.2013.089334
58. Kupperman E, Lee EC, Cao Y, Bannerman B, Fitzgerald M, Berger A, Yu J, Yang Y, Hales P, Bruzzese F, Liu J, Blank J, Garcia K, Tsu C, Dick L, Fleming P, Yu L, Manfredi M, Rolfe M, Bolen J (2010) Evaluation of the proteasome inhibitor MLN9708 in preclinical models of human cancer. Cancer Res 70(5):1970–1980. doi:10.1158/0008-5472.CAN-09-2766
59. Chauhan D, Tian Z, Zhou B, Kuhn D, Orlowski R, Raje N, Richardson P, Anderson KC (2011) In vitro and in vivo selective antitumor activity of a novel orally bioavailable proteasome inhibitor MLN9708 against multiple myeloma cells. Clin Cancer Res 17(16):5311–5321. doi:10.1158/1078-0432.CCR-11-0476
60. Gallerani E, Zucchetti M, Brunelli D, Marangon E, Noberasco C, Hess D, Delmonte A, Martinelli G, Bohm S, Driessen C, De Braud F, Marsoni S, Cereda R, Sala F, D'Incalci M, Sessa C (2013) A first in human phase I study of the proteasome inhibitor CEP-18770 in patients with advanced solid tumours and multiple myeloma. Eur J Cancer 49(2):290–296. doi:10.1016/j.ejca.2012.09.009
61. Sanchez E, Li M, Li J, Wang C, Chen H, Jones-Bolin S, Hunter K, Ruggeri B, Berenson JR (2012) CEP-18770 (delanzomib) in combination with dexamethasone and lenalidomide inhibits the growth of multiple myeloma. Leuk Res 36(11):1422–1427. doi:10.1016/j.leukres.2012.07.018
62. Zang Y, Thomas SM, Chan ET, Kirk CJ, Freilino ML, DeLancey HM, Grandis JR, Li C, Johnson DE (2012) The next generation proteasome inhibitors carfilzomib and oprozomib activate prosurvival autophagy via induction of the unfolded protein response and ATF4. Autophagy 8(12):1873–1874. doi:10.4161/auto.22185
63. Potts BC, Albitar MX, Anderson KC, Baritaki S, Berkers C, Bonavida B, Chandra J, Chauhan D, Cusack JC Jr, Fenical W, Ghobrial IM, Groll M, Jensen PR, Lam KS, Lloyd GK, McBride W, McConkey DJ, Miller CP, Neuteboom ST, Oki Y, Ovaa H, Pajonk F, Richardson PG, Roccaro AM, Sloss CM, Spear MA, Valashi E, Younes A, Palladino MA (2011) Marizomib, a proteasome inhibitor for all seasons: preclinical profile and a framework for clinical trials. Curr Cancer Drug Targets 11(3):254–284
64. Singh AV, Palladino MA, Lloyd GK, Potts BC, Chauhan D, Anderson KC (2010) Pharmacodynamic and efficacy studies of the novel proteasome inhibitor NPI-0052 (marizomib) in a human plasmacytoma xenograft murine model. Br J Haematol 149(4):550–559. doi:10.1111/j.1365-2141.2010.08144.x
65. Kastritis E, Anagnostopoulos A, Roussou M, Toumanidis S, Pamboukas C, Migkou M, Tassidou A, Xilouri I, Delibasi S, Psimenou E, Mellou S, Terpos E, Nanas J, Dimopoulos MA (2007) Treatment of light chain (AL) amyloidosis with the combination of bortezomib and dexamethasone. Haematologica 92(10):1351–1358. doi:10.3324/haematol.11325
66. Merlini G, Palladini G (2013) Light chain amyloidosis: the heart of the problem. Haematologica 98(10):1492–1495. doi:10.3324/haematol.2013.094482

67. Liao R, Jain M, Teller P, Connors LH, Ngoy S, Skinner M, Falk RH, Apstein CS (2001) Infusion of light chains from patients with cardiac amyloidosis causes diastolic dysfunction in isolated mouse hearts. Circulation 104(14):1594–1597
68. Sitia R, Palladini G, Merlini G (2007) Bortezomib in the treatment of AL amyloidosis: targeted therapy? Haematologica 92(10):1302–1307. doi:10.3324/haematol.12136
69. Kastritis E, Wechalekar AD, Dimopoulos MA, Merlini G, Hawkins PN, Perfetti V, Gillmore JD, Palladini G (2010) Bortezomib with or without dexamethasone in primary systemic (light chain) amyloidosis. J Clin Oncol 28(6):1031–1037. doi:10.1200/JCO.2009.23.8220
70. Reece DE, Sanchorawala V, Hegenbart U, Merlini G, Palladini G, Fermand JP, Vescio RA, Liu X, Elsayed YA, Cakana A, Comenzo RL, Group VCS (2009) Weekly and twice-weekly bortezomib in patients with systemic AL amyloidosis: results of a phase 1 dose-escalation study. Blood 114(8):1489–1497. doi:10.1182/blood-2009-02-203398
71. Reece DE, Hegenbart U, Sanchorawala V, Merlini G, Palladini G, Blade J, Fermand JP, Hassoun H, Heffner L, Vescio RA, Liu K, Enny C, Esseltine DL, van de Velde H, Cakana A, Comenzo RL (2011) Efficacy and safety of once-weekly and twice-weekly bortezomib in patients with relapsed systemic AL amyloidosis: results of a phase 1/2 study. Blood 118(4):865–873. doi:10.1182/blood-2011-02-334227
72. Mikhael JR, Schuster SR, Jimenez-Zepeda VH, Bello N, Spong J, Reeder CB, Stewart AK, Bergsagel PL, Fonseca R (2012) Cyclophosphamide-bortezomib-dexamethasone (CyBorD) produces rapid and complete hematologic response in patients with AL amyloidosis. Blood 119(19):4391–4394. doi:10.1182/blood-2011-11-390930
73. Gasparetto CS, Sanchorawala V, Snyder R, Matous J, Terebelo HR, Janakiraman N, Mapara MY, Webb C, Abrams J, Zonder J (2010) Use of Melphalan, Dexamethasone, and Bortezomib in AL Amyloidois. J Clin Oncol 28(155):suppl. Abstract 8024
74. Sanchorawala V, Quillen K, Sloan JM, Andrea NT, Seldin DC (2011) Bortezomib and high-dose melphalan conditioning for stem cell transplantation for AL amyloidosis: a pilot study. Haematologica 96(12):1890–1892. doi:10.3324/haematol.2011.049858
75. Landau H, Hassoun H, Rosenzweig MA, Maurer M, Liu J, Flombaum C, Bello C, Hoover E, Riedel E, Giralt S, Comenzo RL (2013) Bortezomib and dexamethasone consolidation following risk-adapted melphalan and stem cell transplantation for patients with newly diagnosed light-chain amyloidosis. Leukemia 27(4):823–828. doi:10.1038/leu.2012.274

Chapter 5
Profiling Bortezomib Resistance in Multiple Myeloma: Implications in Personalized Pharmacotherapy

Amit Kumar Mitra, Holly Stessman, John Shaughnessy, and Brian Van Ness

Abstract Treatment regimens for MM patients have undergone considerable modifications from the 1960s in an attempt to achieve that elusive "complete cure." Proteasome inhibitors such as bortezomib (Bz) have recently become effective chemotherapeutic agents in the treatment of MM, used alone or in combination with other anticancer agents like alkylating agents, immunomodulators (IMiDs), topoisomerase inhibitors, corticosteroids, and histone deacetylase inhibitors (HDACis). However, wide interindividual variation in response to treatment with Bz is a major limitation in achieving consistent therapeutic effect in MM. In addition, patients who respond commonly develop resistance to proteasome inhibitors, with subsequent aggressive relapses. Drug resistance may be categorized into innate resistance with nonspecific resistance already present in Bz-refractory drug-naive patients who never respond to Bz treatment or emerging (acquired) resistance where a patient's tumor cells "acquire" the ability to resist therapy in the course of treatment leading to eventual Bz-resistant relapse. We discuss molecular profiling approaches to characterize bortezomib resistance, including analysis of genomic variations, gene expression patterns, epigenetic patterns, and protein patterns. We conclude that robust approaches using multiple data types are of primary importance in profiling drug resistance in MM. The ultimate purpose of such an effort will be to create a pharmacogenomic profiling-guided therapeutic response score that can be cross-validated using clinical trials on MM patients undergoing Bz-based therapy or any chemotherapy, so that it can be routinely applied in clinical settings to improve selective response to available drugs, predict effective combinations, and identify secondary therapies to circumvent the challenges in the relapsed patient.

A.K. Mitra • H. Stessman • B. Van Ness (✉)
Department of Genetics, Cell Biology and Development, University of Minnesota, Cancer Center, Minneapolis, MN 55455, USA
e-mail: vanne001@umn.edu

J. Shaughnessy
Signal Genetics and Myeloma Institute, University of Arkansas Medical Center, Little Rock, AK, USA

Q.P. Dou (ed.), *Resistance to Proteasome Inhibitors in Cancer*, Resistance to Targeted Anti-Cancer Therapeutics, DOI 10.1007/978-3-319-06752-0_5

Keywords Myeloma • Bortezomib • Drug resistance • Pharmacogenomics • Genomic profile

Abbreviations

alloSCT	Allogeneic stem cell transplantation
autoSCT	Autologous stem cell transplantation
BMSCs	Bone marrow stromal cells
Bz	Bortezomib/Velcade®
ChIP	Chromatin immunoprecipitation
CMAP	Connectivity map
COBRA	Combined bisulfite restriction analysis
CR	Complete response
CRD	Complete response duration
Cz	Carfilzomib/Kyprolis®
Dex	Dexamethasone
EMD	Extramedullary disease
ERK	Extracellular signal-regulated kinase
FDA	Food and Drug Administration
FGF	Fibroblast growth factor
GEP	Gene expression profiling
GSEA	Gene set enrichment analysis
HDACis	Histone deacetylase inhibitors
HPLC	High-performance liquid chromatography
IGF-1	Insulin-like growth factor 1
IL-6	Interleukin 6
IM	Intermediate metabolizers
IMiDs	Immunomodulatory drugs
JAK	Janus kinase
KMT	Lysine methyltransferases
LPS	Lipopolysaccharide
5-mC	5-Methylcytosine
MDR1	Multidrug resistance 1 or P-glycoprotein
MEK	RAS/RAF/MAPK kinase
MGUS	Monoclonal gammopathy of undetermined significance
MM	Multiple myeloma
MM-BMSCs	MM cells and bone marrow stromal cells
MR	Minimal response
MSDA	Multiple linear discriminant analysis
Ms-SNuPE	Methylation-sensitive single-nucleotide primer extension
NC	No change
NGS	Next-generation sequencing
OS	Overall survival

PD	Progressive disease
PI3K	Phosphatidylinositol-3 kinase
PLD	Pegylated liposomal doxorubicin
PM	Poor metabolizers
PN	Peripheral neuropathy
PR	Partial response
PSGL-1	P-selectin glycoprotein ligand-1
SDF-1α	SC-derived factor 1α
SMM	Smoldering multiple myeloma
SNPs	Single-nucleotide polymorphisms (or "snips")
STAT3	Signal transducers and activators of transcription 3
TNF	Tumor necrosis factor
TNT	Time-to-next treatment
TT3	Total therapy 3
UPR	Unfolded protein response
VEGF	Vascular endothelial growth factor
VRC2	Velcade resensitizing compound 2

5.1 Introduction

5.1.1 Multiple Myeloma (MM)

Multiple myeloma (MM) is an incurable age-dependent plasma cell neoplasm characterized by clonal expansion of malignant antibody producing post-germinal-center B-cell-derived plasma cells within the bone marrow with significant complexity and heterogeneity at the molecular level [1, 2]. It is the second most common hematopoietic malignancy in the United States after non-Hodgkin's lymphoma accounting for 1 % of all cancers and 10 % of all hematologic malignancies with around 20,000 new cases per year and an annual age-adjusted incidence of about 4 per 100,000 [3, 4]. The median age at diagnosis is around 62 years with 90 % and 98 % of patients being older than 50 years and 40 years, respectively [5]. The major clinical manifestations associated with MM include presence of monoclonal immunoglobulin in the serum and/or urine, osteocytic bone lesions, anemia, hypercalcemia, renal failure, increase risk of infections, and extramedullary disease (EMD) [4]. MM is considered a continuum disorder which is preceded by a precondition called monoclonal gammopathy of undetermined significance (MGUS) that progresses to the earliest stage of MM called smoldering multiple myeloma (SMM) [6, 7]. MGUS is characterized by low disease burden and an absence of organ involvement which means that many patients likely go undiagnosed until progression to MM. MGUS is present in 1 % of adults over the age of 25 years and progresses to MM at a rate of 0.5–3 % per year [8–10]. SMM is accompanied by increased serum paraprotein and/or increased clonal plasma cells in the bone marrow but not accompanied by organ dysfunction [7]. The rate of progression from

SMM to intramedullary MM is 10 % in the first 5 years following diagnosis [9]. Diagnosis of intramedullary MM is followed by EMD that finally culminates in plasma cell leukemia at end stages.

Despite recent improvements in treatment strategies, MM still remains mostly an incurable disease with median survival rate of around 7 years [1, 11].

5.1.2 Bortezomib (Bz)

Treatment regimens for MM patients have undergone considerable modifications since the 1960s in an attempt to achieve that elusive "complete cure." Although the standard of care for MM continues to include a cocktail of classical agents (corticosteroids, alkylating agents, anthracyclines, mitotic inhibitors), over the years, this cocktail regimen has incorporated additional treatment options including next-generation drugs (IMiDs and proteasome inhibitors) and autologous (autoSCT) or allogeneic stem cell transplantation (alloSCT) from a sibling or close relative and high-dose treatment (HDT) with stem cell support [12–20].

Proteasome inhibitors are effective chemotherapeutic agents in the treatment of MM, used alone or in combination with other anticancer agents like alkylating agents, topoisomerase inhibitors, corticosteroids, and histone deacetylase inhibitors (HDACis) [4, 21]. Bortezomib/Velcade® (Bz) was the first proteasome inhibitor to be approved by the US Food and Drug Administration (FDA) for clinical application in 2003 for the treatment of relapsed and refractory MM [4, 11, 22]. Recently, a second-generation proteasome inhibitor carfilzomib/Kyprolis® (Cz) that irreversibly inhibits the proteasome has been approved by the FDA for treating MM. Other examples of second-generation proteasome inhibitors include marizomib and MLN9708 (ixazomib) [11, 22–24]. Key to the newer proteasome inhibitors is the formulations that can be orally administered, rather than intravenous administration.

Bz is a peptidyl boronic acid that specifically inhibits the ATP-independent chymotrypsin-like activity of the of 26S proteasome through reversible binding to the PSMB5 subunit of the central 20S multi-catalytic protease core. Bz has been shown to interfere with tumor metastasis and angiogenesis by accelerating unfolded protein response (UPR) or the ubiquitin-dependent proteolysis of important regulatory proteins involved in key physiological and pathophysiological cellular processes in cancer cells, by interfering with the NF-κB-enabled regulation of cell adhesion-mediated drug resistance, by disrupting IL-6-induced signaling pathways, and by cleaving DNA repair enzymes [25–28]. It has been shown to be effective against MM in drug trials with mouse models [29] and relapsed and refractory MM patients [30]. Currently, Bz has proven very successful when used in drug cocktails for treating newly diagnosed MM. However, Bz resistance and potential side effects including peripheral neuropathy, thrombocytopenia, and shingles can negatively impact patient's quality of life and hinder the use of this drug in a large section of MM patients [31–34].

5.1.3 *Bortezomib Resistance*

Wide interindividual variation in response to treatment with Bz is a major limitation in achieving consistent therapeutic effect in MM [35–37]. Drug resistance may be categorized into innate resistance with nonspecific resistance already present in Bz-refractory drug-naive patients who never respond to Bz treatment or emerging (acquired) resistance where a patient's tumor cells "acquire" the ability to resist therapy in the course of treatment leading to eventual Bz-resistant relapse [38–40]. As will be discussed below, this becomes an important consideration in effective patient management.

5.1.3.1 Mechanisms of Bortezomib Resistance

Heterogeneity in Bz response is governed by the underlying molecular characteristics of the tumor and its microenvironment. Although the exact mechanisms of Bz resistance in the treatment of MM is not well understood, decades of research using multiple model systems have provided evidence to the potential mechanisms for the occurrence of innate or acquired resistance to Bz (Fig. 5.1). Among these, influence of cell–cell interactions with the bone marrow microenvironment on the Bz sensitivity of MM cells seems to be the most well-studied and widely accepted mechanism of Bz resistance [41–44]. Extracellular matrix proteins like fibronectin, collagen,

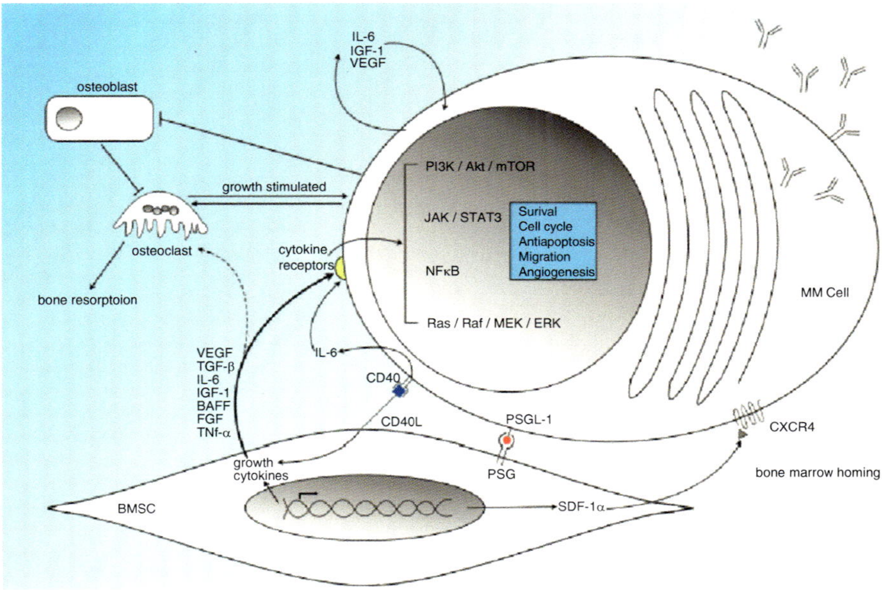

Fig. 5.1 Mechanisms of bortezomib resistance

laminin, and osteopontin and supporting cell types HSCs, progenitor and precursor cells, immune cells, erythroid cells, bone marrow stromal cells (BMSCs), endothelial cells, adipocytes, osteoclasts, and osteoblasts in the bone marrow compartment produce and secrete an incessant supply of growth cytokines like interleukin 6 (IL-6), insulin-like growth factor 1 (IGF-1), B cell-activating factor, fibroblast growth factor (FGF), SC-derived factor 1α (SDF-1α), tumor necrosis factor α (TNF-α), transformation growth factor β (TGF-β), and vascular endothelial growth factor (VEGF) [45] that support the survival of MM cells. Furthermore, physical interactions between MM and BMSCs through cell-surface molecules like CD40, CXCR4, and P-selectin glycoprotein ligand-1 (PSGL-1) escalate the secretion of these cytokines by BMSCs which subsequently stimulate the phosphatidylinositol-3 kinase (PI3K)/AKT, RAS/RAF/MAPK kinase (MEK)/extracellular signal-regulated kinase (ERK), and Janus kinase 2 (JAK)/signal transducers and activators of transcription 3 (STAT3) downstream survival by decreasing drug sensitivity, enhancing cell migration and antibody secretion, upregulating cell cycle regulatory proteins, and increasing telomerase activity [45–49]. Furthermore, interactions between MM cells and bone marrow stromal cells (MM-BMSCs) lead to the production of much higher levels of growth cytokines IL-6 and VEGF which alter drug sensitivity through enhanced survival of MM cells and may also control the expression of microRNA within MM cells [50–54]. Constitutively activating mutations within genes involved in growth cytokine signaling pathways (IL-6) and mutations resulting in the loss of adhesion proteins CD40 [55] and CXCR4 [56] result in the disruption of interaction between MMs and BMSCs which increases migratory capabilities of MM cells which can now survive away from the bone marrow compartment giving rise to EMD in end-stage patients with considerable Bz resistance [42].

Mutations at the drug active site within the protein PSMB5, a β subunit of the 20S catalytic core responsible for chymotrypsin-like proteasome activity, are considered to be the most common mechanism for acquired Bz resistance in in vitro model systems following dose escalation over time [57]. These mutations include Met56Ile, Cys63Phe, Ala49Thr, Met45Val and Cys52Phe, or Ala49Val changes within the PSMB5 binding pocket, an Arg24Cys change in the propeptide region that results in the increase of PSMB5 transcript and protein as well as proteasome chymotrypsin-like activity and in some cases increase in immunoproteasome activity [58–70]. Interestingly, however, none of the non-synonymous coding PSMB5 variants found in Bz-refractory MM patients were associated with survival or differences in proteasome activity. Moreover, none of the mutations identified in Bz-resistant cells in vitro were found in drug-naïve Bz-refractory MM patient samples [58, 71–73]. Additionally, reduction of Bz sensitivity has also been attributed to changes that increase cell viability like inhibition of the pro-apoptotic gene NOXA upregulation, loss of wild-type TP53 activity, and overexpression of anti-apoptotic genes like BCL-2, MCL-1, and BAG3 [74–82]. Furthermore, constitutive activation of the oncogene NOTCH, PI3K/AKT/mTOR, Hedgehog, NF-κB, MEK/ERK, and/or JAK/STAT3 signaling pathways has been observed in several model systems of MM cells to avoid Bz-induced cell death [83–92]. Other mechanisms of Bz resistance include overexpression of the receptor tyrosine kinase c-MET [93–95]; reduction of cellular oxidative stress through the increase of baseline expression of the stress response proteins HSPA2, GRP78/BiP, NRF2, HSP27, HSP70, and HSP90 [96–102]; and activation of autophagy as alternative pathways in Bz-resistant cells that may help shunt unfolded and/or misfolded proteins towards degradation [103–106]. Increased expression of drug efflux pumps like the P-glycoprotein/multidrug resistance 1 (MDR1) may also contribute towards reduction of Bz sensitivity by keeping intracellular levels of Bz low [60]. Furthermore, proteasome inhibition by Bz results in the formation of aggregates of misfolded ubiquitin-conjugated proteins (called aggresomes) which activate an alternative protein catabolism pathway through lysosome-mediated protein degradation in the autophagosomes that may lead to Bz resistance [107].

5.2 Profiling of Bortezomib Resistance

Multiple complex genetic and epigenetic alterations underline the basis of the wide interindividual variations in response to proteasome inhibitors. A number of efforts have been undertaken to profile resistance to the proteasome inhibitor Bz from genomic, transcriptome, and epigenetic standpoints, to generate signature profiles of Bz response/resistance that can be translated into predictive scores for clinical application (Table 5.1).

Table 5.1 Studies pertaining to profiling bortezomib resistance and discussed in this chapter

Study type	Major contribution	Reference
Gene expression profiling	Generated gene-based survival and response classifiers in humans	[108]
	Created GEP-derived 70-gene and 17-gene risk-stratification models	[109]
	Reconstructed and refined the 17-gene-based stratification model	[110]
	Used the GEP-derived 70-gene-based risk score in Bz-containing clinical trials	[111]
	Developed a post-Bz GEP80 using gene expression analysis before and after 48 h of Bz treatment	[112]
	Identified GEP signatures associated with Bz response using time-course-based analysis of kinetic gene expression profiles in mouse and human models	[113]
Epigenetic profiling	Global and gene-specific DNA methylation analysis following Bz treatment	[114]
SNP-based profiling	Association of candidate gene polymorphisms with Bz resistance	[36, 115–118]
	Association of candidate gene polymorphisms with peripheral neuropathy (PN) following Bz treatment	[119, 120]
RNAi-based screening	Large-scale RNAi screen to find genes that synergistically potentiate the growth inhibitory effects of Bz	[121]
Immunophenotyping	Loss of plasma cell maturation markers results in Bz resistance	[122, 123]

5.2.1 Gene Expression Profiling

Gene expression-based profiling or the measurement of relative expression of genes at a global scale to obtain a gene expression signature that distinguishes between cells or patients based on Bz response has so far been the most common method of choice to generate gene-based predictive signatures of Bz resistance and treatment outcome.

The first such effort aimed at the creation and subsequent validation of a genomic predictive signature of clinical response to Bz in MM patients dates back to 2007 [108]. In this study by Mulligan et al., a DNA microarray-based gene expression profiling (GEP) study was used to develop predictive signatures of survival and response to Bz in pretreatment samples from patients with relapsed myeloma enrolled in phase 2 (SUMMIT 025 [124] and CREST 024 [125]) and phase 3 (APEX 039 and 040) [30] multicenter international clinical trials of Bz in MM. Clinical response was categorized into complete response (CR), partial response (PR), minimal response (MR), no change (NC), or progressive disease (PD) based on the European Group for Bone Marrow Transplantation criteria [126], while overall survival (OS) was used as a measure for survival. A 100 probe set response classifier was developed from the 025 and 040 trials that were validated on data from the 039 trial. Genes most significantly associated with response included ribosomal (RPS7, RPS13), mitochondrial (COX7C, UQCRH), ER stress (SERP1), DNA repair (APEX1, REC14), and cancer-associated (NRAS, NPM1) genes, components of the PI3 kinase pathway (PIK3R1, DAPP1), and other signaling molecules (TYROBP, RRAGC, LYK5). As identified by gene set enrichment analysis (GSEA) [127], major pathways (gene sets) most relatively highly expressed in patients with higher response include adhesion, cytokines, NF-κB activity, and hypoxia gene sets, elevated protein synthesis, mitochondrial function and RNA transcription/splicing and the NF-κB targets IL8, IL15, CXCL5, CFLAR, ICAM, and NFKB2. Gene expression data from 025 to 040 trials were used then to develop a survival classifier that was validated on data from the 039 trial. When tested on independent data, the response and survival classifiers generated could successfully stratify the Bz-treated 039 patients into high-risk and low-risk groups and were significantly associated with clinical outcome of Bz treatment having very high overall accuracy. Although the survival classifier could also stratify patients in the dexamethasone (Dex)-treated arm of the 039 trial, the authors opined that there could still be Bz sensitivity in the prognostic significance of the probe sets since Bz was also eventually used in most of the patients in the Dex arm. Furthermore, the predictive gene signatures for survival showed great complementarity with clinical variables-based International Staging System [128] since it could further enable the risk stratification in patients demarcated as low and high risk. The probe sets included in the survival classifier did not overlap with those in the response classifier.

In another study, Shaughnessy et al. [109] performed GEP analysis on purified plasma cells obtained prior to initiation of therapy from 532 newly diagnosed patients with MM treated on two separate protocols (351 samples in training set/UARK 98-026 and 181 samples in the validation set/UARK03-033) to molecularly

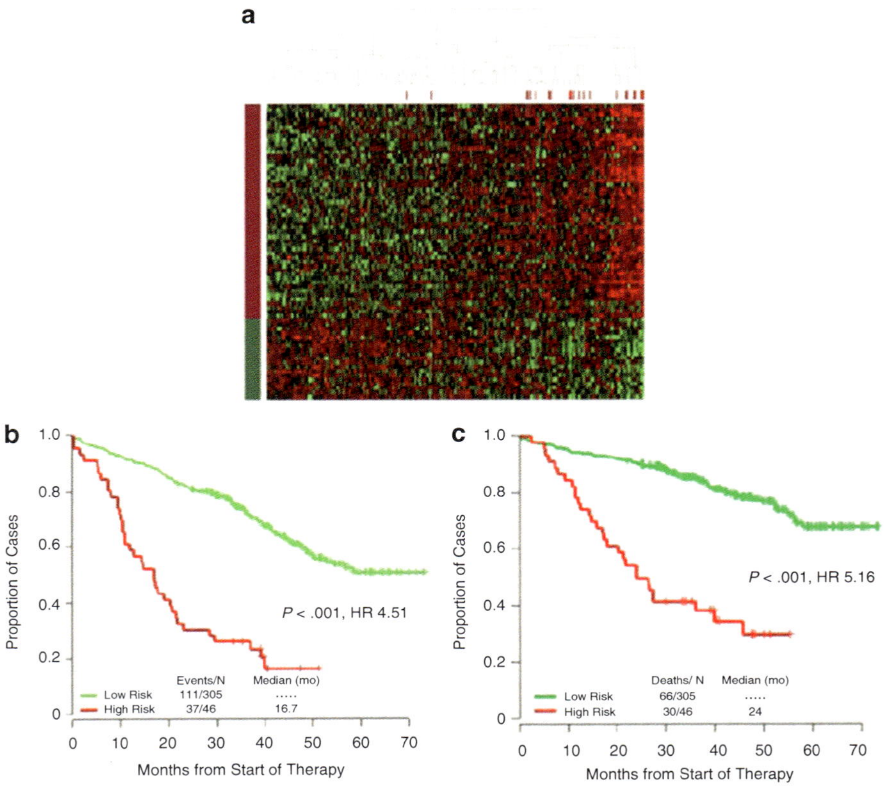

Fig. 5.2 70-gene signature risk model (GEP70) identified by Shaughnessy et al. [109]. (**a**) Heat map of 70 genes in the training cohort of 351 newly diagnosed patients from UARK 98-026 trial that were found associated with shorter survival parameters. The 51 upregulated genes are designated by *red bar* on the *left* and 19 downregulated genes are denoted by *green bar*. Kaplan Meier curves for (**b**) EFS and (**c**) OS in GEP70-defined high-risk myeloma (*red*) and low-risk myeloma (*green*)

define high-risk disease. Affymetrix U133 Plus 2.0 microarray-based analysis of tumor gene expression was used to identify a 70-gene signature (51 upregulated and 19 downregulated) in the training cohort that was found associated with shorter survival parameters in the training set and was also found associated with survival and hazard ratio in the independent validation test cohort (Fig. 5.2). The 70-gene risk-stratification model was also found predictive of post-relapse risk and survival in the 51 relapse samples of the training set. Furthermore, applying a stepwise multiple linear discriminant analysis (MSDA) on the 70 high-risk-associated genes to identify a minimum set of genes that could discriminate between low- and high-risk myeloma, a 17-gene model was obtained that could effectively substitute the 70-gene stratification model in predicting survival in both the training and validation sets with accuracy of over 95 %.

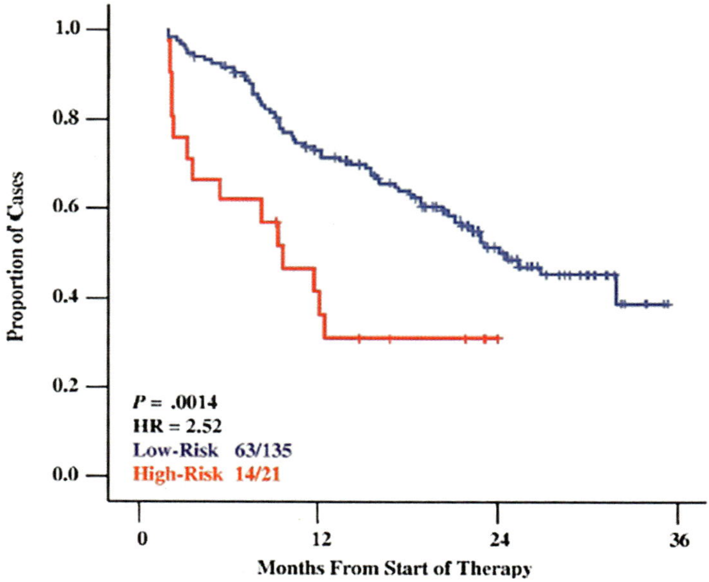

Fig. 5.3 Kaplan Meier survival plot of OS in APEX phase 3 clinical trial dataset stratified by a 16-gene signature-based model into high-risk (*red*) and low-risk (*blue*) disease [110]

Zhan et al. [110] reconstructed this 17-gene-based stratification model of high-risk MM using U133AB data on 144 newly diagnosed relapsed myeloma patients enrolled in the APEX phase 3 clinical trial that compared single-agent Bz (B) to high-dose dexamethasone (HD) and then used it to evaluate its utility as a prediction model for treatment outcome. Results showed that the 17-gene model was successful in identifying a high-risk group within the APEX trial having significantly shorter survival and most importantly, could predict high risk among patients undergoing Bz monotherapy (Fig. 5.3). It is quite intriguing to note that the gene expression patterns of the 17 genes related to outcome were similar in relapsed and newly diagnosed MM patients, independent of the platform used for GEP studies and most importantly was independent of specific therapeutic modality which raised a number of interesting unanswered questions.

Subsequently, Nair et al. [111] generated a GEP-derived 70-gene-based risk score from the patients enrolled in phase 3 Total Therapy 3 (TT3) clinical trial protocols 2003-33 (TT3A) and 2006-66 (TT3B) which incorporated Bz upfront to validate the finding that the use of a GEP-defined low-risk score in MM showed superior outcomes in the Bz-containing TT3 trials compared to its predecessor protocol Total Therapy 2 (TT2) trial [129–131]. Results showed that the eight GEP-defined molecular subgroups/entities could effectively present the prognostic impact on clinical outcomes of patients in the 2003-033 and 2006-066 trials when combined together. Multivariate analysis comparing adverse variables with clinical outcomes showed GEP-defined risk score affected OS, EFS, and complete response duration (CRD) adversely (Fig. 5.4).

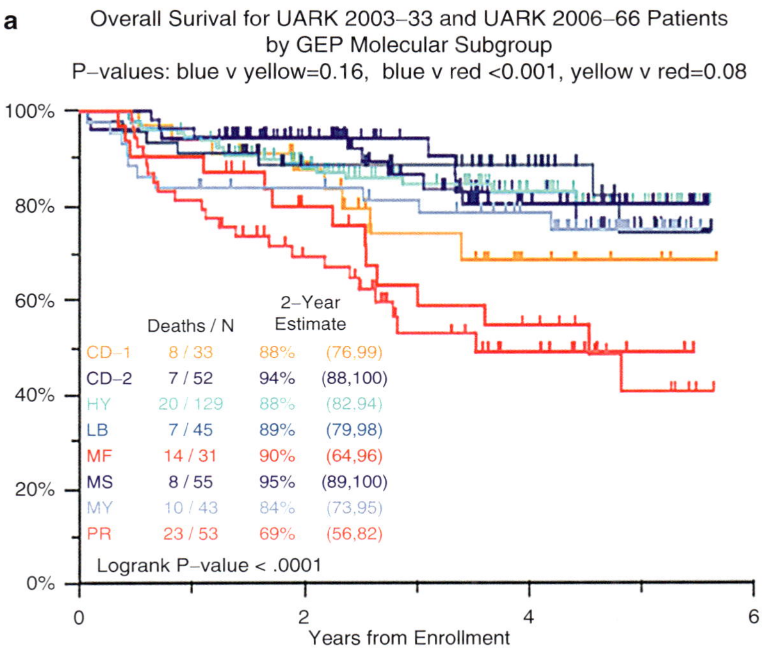

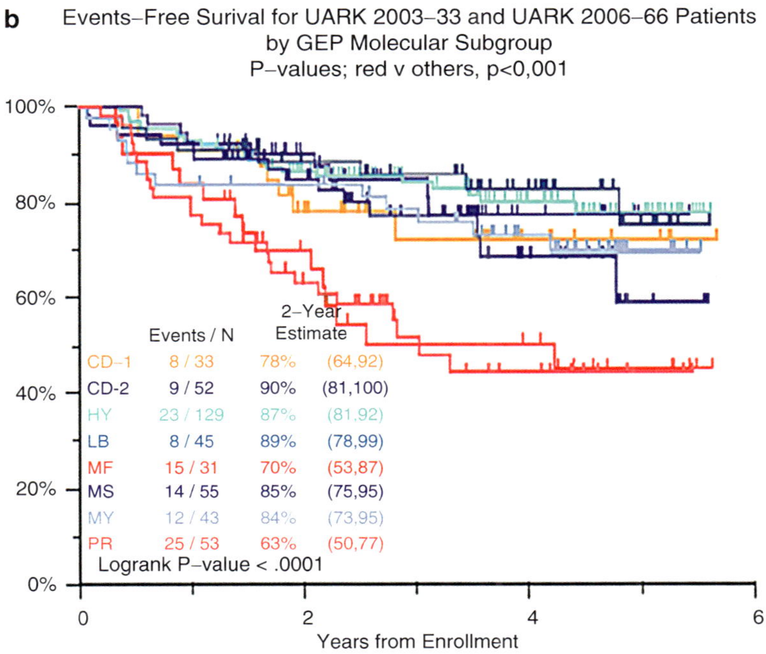

Fig. 5.4 Clinical outcomes in eight GEP-defined molecular subgroups in 2003-033 and 2006-066 trial patients when combined together [111]. The eight molecular subgroups were *CD-1* (CCND1 without CD20), *CD-2* (CCND1 with CD20 expression), *MS* (MMSET/FGFR3), *MF* (MAF/MAFB), *HY* (hyperdiploidy), *LB* (low bone disease), *MY* (myeloid), and *PR* (proliferation); favorable subgroups are represented by *blue*, unfavorable subgroups by *red*, and CD-1 by *yellow*. (**a**) OS; (**b**) EFS

The data from this study showed the superior results for GEP-defined low-risk myeloma in the Bz-containing TT3 study compared to the TT2 trial which further exemplified the importance of using a GEP-based signature to define low-risk myeloma that could help in predicting outcome and improving survival in clinical trials of MM.

However, most of these studies used only pretreatment patient samples. No GEP was performed on patient samples post-drug treatment, particularly those that relapsed with Bz-resistant disease. This is an important clinical consideration.

To further the findings of the earlier studies using the GEP-derived gene-based stratification model, Shaughnessy et al. [112] performed pharmacogenomic investigations of Bz in purified plasma cells from patients in the TT3 trials (TT3A and its successor trial TT3B) using Affymetrix U233 Plus 2.0 microarray-based gene expression analysis before and after 48-h intravenous test dosing with Bz (1 mg/m^2). GEP analysis of 142 patients from the TT3A trial identified a set of 80 differentially expressed genes (post-Bz GEP80) which could effectively discriminate between high-risk and low-risk disease. Multivariate analysis of the survival measures progression-free survival (PFS) and OS performed using the post-Bz GEP80 as one of the prognostic factors showed that GEP80-based risk score could be used as an independent prognostic parameter. Subsequently, the risk score for the validation set comprising gene expression data from 128 patients of the TT3B trial at baseline at 48 h after Bz treatment was calculated based on the GEP80 score obtained from the training set (Fig. 5.5).

Results demonstrated that the GEP80 model to baseline data [GEP80(BL)] showed significant discriminatory capability in terms of differences in survival (2-year PFS and OS) upon stratification among the GEP-based stratified high-risk

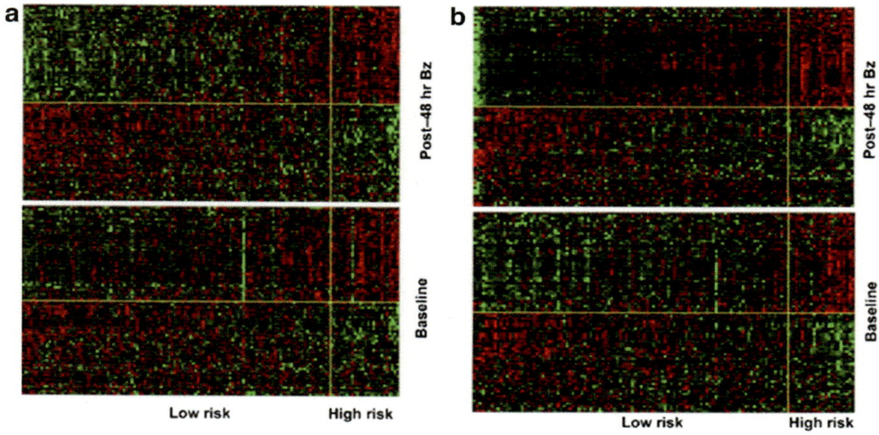

Fig. 5.5 GEP80 gene signature in training set (**a**) (TT3A trial) and (**b**) validation set (TT3B trial) 48 h after Bz treatment (*top*) and at baseline (*bottom*) [112]. Samples are represented in *columns* (each *column* represents one patient) and genes in *rows* (each *row* represents one gene). The favorable genes are separated from the unfavorable genes by the *horizontal yellow line*. *Vertical yellow lines* separate the low-risk and high-risk patients

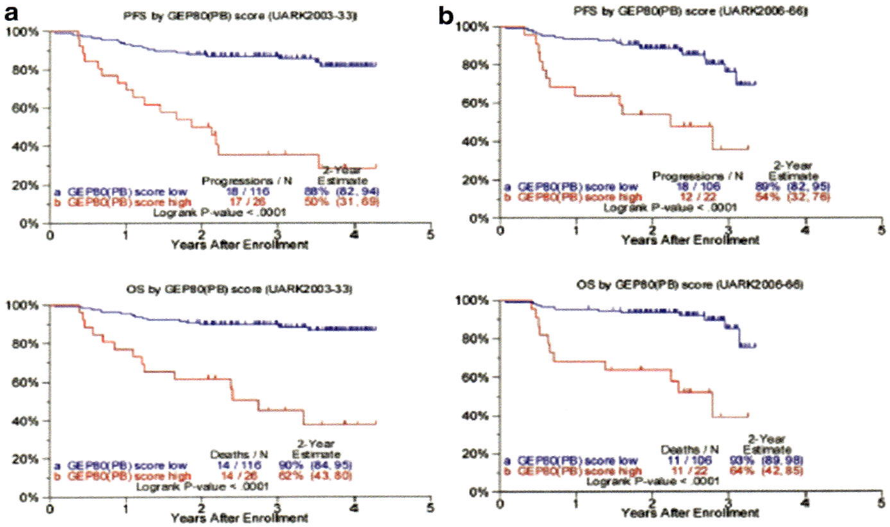

Fig. 5.6 Discriminatory power of post-Bz-GEP80 predictive model in training set (**a**) and test set (**b**) [112]. *Top* and *bottom panels* represent PFS and OS, respectively

and low-risk subgroups in both TT3 trials, training set TT3A and test set TT3B (Fig. 5.6). Furthermore, when the GEP80 model was applied to the TT2 trial, where the GEP70 risk-stratification model was used earlier, the GEP80 risk model increased and further refined the discriminatory power when applied to the GEP70-defined risk model in distinguishing survival outcomes between low- and high-risk disease. The TT2 trial randomly assigned thalidomide treatment in 668 patients between control and experimental arms with no Bz treatment. Similar refinement in the discriminatory power was also observed when the GEP80 model was applied to baseline samples. However, when applied to the GEP70-defined subgroups of the TT2 trial, the GEP80-defined model did not show such a significant discriminatory power. Comparison of the gene lists constituting the GEP70 and GEP80 gene models found three genes common to both models, including the PSM gene on chromosome 1q21. Upon successful use of the GEP signatures of Bz treatment from this study, GEP-defined risk-based assignments were performed for subsequent therapies in the TT4 and TT5 clinical trials.

In a recently published study, Stessman et al. [113] performed time-course-based analysis of kinetic gene expression profiles in a mouse model system to identify GEP signatures associated with response to Bz treatment in vitro. For the purpose of the study, clonally derived Bz-resistant mouse cell lines were created from Bz-sensitive cell lines. A 51-gene expression signature statistically distinguished sensitive and resistant responsiveness to Bz in the in vitro mouse model.

Subsequently, the GEP data on the genes that had human homologs was validated using GEP data on 210 patients from the University of Arkansas' TT3 trial described above. Finally, a 23-gene GEP signature was identified that was successful in

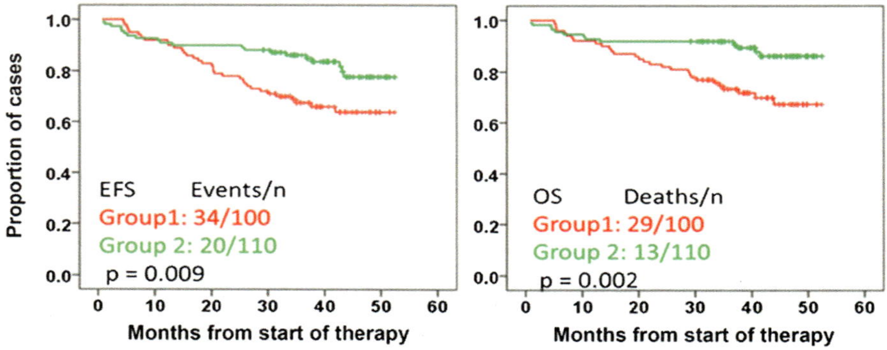

Fig. 5.7 Kaplan Meier curves for EFS (*left*) and OS (*right*) patients from MMTT3 clinical trial [113]. Patient samples were clustered based on mouse baseline GEP signature that most significantly distinguished between Bz-sensitive and Bz-resistant mouse cell lines

predicting/stratifying good versus poor outcomes (progression-free and overall survival) in human in vivo (patient) data from the MM TT3 trial (Fig. 5.7). Furthermore, combined analysis of the gene expression profiles of Bz-sensitive and Bz-resistant cell lines identified 219 genes that changed significantly in both groups in response to Bz treatment while 29 genes showed significant differential response to Bz between Bz-sensitive and Bz-resistant cell lines. The gene list of this 29-gene signature included components of the proteasome ubiquitination and the upregulation of downstream targets of the transcription factor NFE2L2 (NRF2), a transcription factor involved in oxidative stress response to proteasome inhibition, Hspb1, Dnajb1, Hspa1a, Hspa1b, and Ddit3 (CCAAT/enhancer-binding protein homologous protein (CHOP)) (Fig. 5.8). GSEA of the mouse Bz treatment-derived GEP signature showed significant enrichment for the GEP80 gene model defined by Shaughnessy et al. These results suggest that the in vitro mouse model of Bz resistance had predictive value in human MM drug trials which include Bz-based treatment regimen.

5.2.1.1 Analysis of GEP Signatures of Bz Resistance to Predict Potential Secondary Therapies

The differential gene expression signatures generated following Bz treatment of Bz-sensitive and Bz-resistant cell lines were queried against the connectivity map (CMAP) database to obtain connectivity scores to discover possible mechanisms of resistance and to predict novel secondary combination therapy approaches to evade Bz resistance based on common GEP signatures [113].

The CMAP database, based at The Broad Institute of MIT and Harvard in Cambridge, Massachusetts, is comprised of drug-induced gene expression signatures for 1,309 bioactive compounds from four (4) cultured human cell lines that help in the in silico discovery of drugs that have been previously used to identify cancer salvage therapies generating similar or dissimilar response compared to the

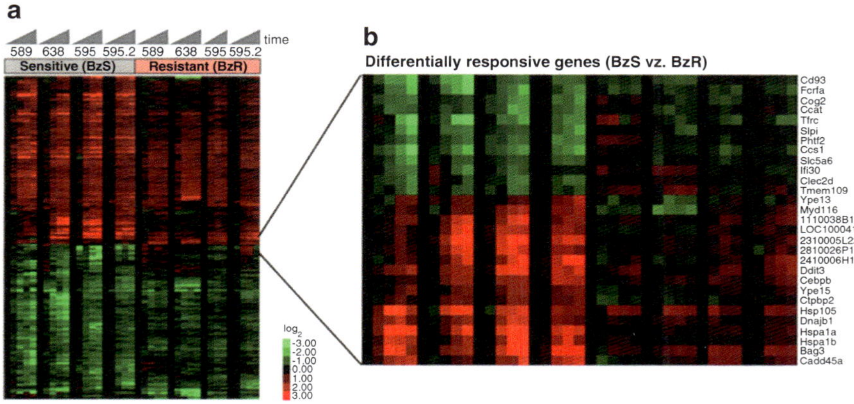

Fig. 5.8 Kinetic gene expression profiling to identify GEP signatures associated with Bz response [113]. (**a**) Heat map of Bz-responsive genes across the three Bz-sensitive mouse lines and clonally derived Bz-resistant counterparts (595 in duplicate) at 2, 8, 16, and 24 h following Bz (66 nmol/L) treatment compared to the 0-h time point. (**b**) Most significantly differentially responsive genes between Bz-sensitive and Bz-resistant mouse cell lines. *Columns*, ordered by sensitivity followed by sample, represent time points and *rows* represent genes ordered by hierarchical cluster analysis

drug of interest based on correlated gene expression changes [132, 133]. Gene expression signature of the drug of interest is used as input signature to query the database for correlated expression signature. A positive connectivity score indicates pathways that are likely targeted by the drug of interest used to create the input signature, while a negative connectivity score signifies either the pathway is inversely regulated by the drug of interest or the fact that there is a difference in pathway regulation between two disease states if a paired transcriptional analysis was used to create the input signature.

When the predicted compounds from Stessman et al.'s CMAP query [113] were ranked in ascending order of *p*-value, a number of compounds with signatures were predicted as significantly correlated (positive) or anticorrelated (negative) with the input signature for Bz-sensitive/Bz-resistant differential response. Several HDAC inhibitors (HDACis) were found significantly positively correlated, while topoisomerase inhibitors were significantly negatively correlated which might provide clues to design potential secondary therapies to overcome Bz resistance by either resensitizing resistant cells to Bz or effectively killing Bz-resistant cells.

As an alternative approach, a cell-based high-throughput drug screening was undertaken to screen for drugs that could overcome Bz resistance in Bz-resistant cell lines. Several chemical agents were identified with selective activity against Bz-resistant cells including topoisomerase inhibitors that were in concurrence with the CMAP findings. Additionally, a novel compound VRC2 (Velcade resensitizing compound 2) showed effective Bz resensitizing activity in combination with Bz which was further confirmed in multiple human and mouse cell lines. Further experimentation is ongoing to validate these initial in vitro findings within in vivo mouse models [134].

5.2.2 Epigenetic Profiling

Epigenetics, a term coined by Conrad Waddington, refers to chromatin-based modifications pertaining to histone and DNA modifications that regulate DNA-templated processes like transcription, DNA repair, and replication independent of the alterations in the nucleotide sequence.

Abnormal expression patterns or genomic alterations in chromatin may lead to the induction and maintenance of various cancers [135, 136]. Among the four different classes of DNA modifications [137, 138] and 16 classes of histone modifications [139, 140], histone methylation and DNA methylation are the best studied and most well characterized. Histone modifications pertaining to methylation of histones on the side chains of lysine, arginine, and histidine residues have a major influence, not just on transcription but in all DNA-templated processes [139]. The best-characterized sites on histones include the methylated lysine residues H3K4, H3K36, and H3K79 associated with active genes in euchromatin and H3K9, H3K27, and H4K20 associated with heterochromatic regions of the genome [141]. Enzymes involved in lysine methylation mostly contain a conserved SET domain, which performs histone lysine methyltransferases (KMT) activity. Cancer genomes have been shown to have recurrent translocations and/or coding mutations in a number of KMTs, including *MMSET*, *EZH2*, and *MLL* family members.

DNA methylation of 5-carbon on cytosine residues (5mC) of CpG dinucleotides is the most common heritable epigenetic modification present in around 70 % of all mammalian promoters that transcriptionally regulate the expression of both protein-coding genes and noncoding RNAs including microRNAs [137, 142]. Abnormal CpG promoter island methylation has been implicated in many cancers and is also the most commonly studied among epigenetic alterations [135, 137, 143]. DNA methylation analysis techniques have undergone a sea of evolution over the past decade with respect to both fashion (from qualitative to quantitative) and scale (locus specific to genome wide) [144–146]. Beginning from methods high-performance liquid chromatography (HPLC) and methylation-sensitive restriction enzyme-based analysis, DNA methylation analysis has come a long way [147, 148] with the most revolutionary change being the introduction of bisulfite conversion into DNA methylation research [149–151]. In bisulfite DNA conversion, DNA is chemically deaminated that modifies the unmethylated cytosine(C) to uracil (U). Thus, an epigenetic variation of methylated or unmethylated DNA is translated into a genetic difference of C to U change, a principle that is the fundamental basis of most of the subsequent methods beginning with the qualitative method locus-specific methylation-specific PCR (MSP) [152] and bisulfite genomic sequencing (BGS). Consequently, a number of quantitative epigenetic methods incorporated bisulfite conversion as the basic guiding procedure behind candidate gene-based DNA methylation analysis, including combined bisulfite restriction analysis (COBRA), methylation-sensitive single-nucleotide primer extension (Ms-SNuPE), MethyLight, pyrosequencing, and Sequenom's (Sequenom, San Diego, CA) MassARRAY-based EpiTYPER assay [143, 153–161]. More recently, the emergence of high-throughput genome-wide analysis technologies including DNA microarrays and deep sequencing technologies like the next-generation sequencing (NGS) platforms Infinium Methylation Assay (Illumina), Affymetrix, Agilent, and NimbleGen has led to the advent of modern sophisticated epigenetic profiling techniques like MeDIP-chip and MeDIP-seq which combines high-throughput genome-wide approaches with established chromatin techniques such as chromatin immunoprecipitation (ChIP-Seq) to map chromatin modifications [162–170]. This has brought about path-breaking improvements in understanding the complexity and plasticity of epigenetic regulation and its impact on the transcriptome.

DNA methylation analysis has been used in profiling MM to understand the epigenetic changes contributing towards the pathogenesis and disease progression both on a gene-by-gene basis and on a global genome scale [162, 171]. MSP identified hypermethylation of a number of genes including VHL, XAF1, IRF8, TP53, CDKN2A, CDKN2B, DAPK, SOCS1, CDH1, PTGS2, CCND2, DCC, *CDH1*, p16, INK4a, p15 INK4b, SHP1, ER and BNIP3, RARβ, DAPK, MGMT, and FHIT in MM [162, 171–183]. High methylation of the genes FHIT1, E-cadherin, DAPK, and TGFBR2 has been shown to be associated with lower overall survival, while the genes DKN2A and CDKN2B, TNF, and retinoblastoma pathways were found common in relapsed MM patients compared to untreated newly diagnosed patients [184].

However, research on the association of DNA methylation signature profile with Bz resistance is still at a very nascent stage with only one study so far analyzing the prognostic value of global and gene-specific DNA methylation patterns following Bz treatment. In this study by de Larrea et al. [114], global methylation was determined in total DNA from 75 patients with relapsed MM by the ELISA assay MethylFlash™ Methylated DNA Quantification Kit (Epigentek, Farmingdale, NY), which is based on recognition and quantification of the DNA methylated fraction by a 5-methylcytosine (5-mC) antibody. Thirty genes in pathways like cytokine network, apoptosis, tumor suppression, transcription factors, and cellular cycle were selected on the basis of association with hematological malignancies and treatment and availability of gene-specific commercial assays for CpG islands in each gene. Gene-specific CpG island DNA methylation profile of the 30 genes was then determined in 42 MM patients by a DNA methylation PCR system called Methyl-Profiler™ DNA Methylation PCR Array System (Qiagen, Germany) that is based on DNA digestion with methylation-sensitive and/or methylation-dependent restriction enzymes and investigated for association with PFS and overall survival (OS). Results showed that the patients with more than 3.95 % of globally methylated DNA had longer overall survival while gene-specific CpG island methylation analysis showed low methylation percentage of NF-KB1 and was associated with better response and higher overall survival following Bz treatment [114]. Unfortunately, no study so far focused on the comprehensive epigenetic profiling pertaining to differential modification in the DNA methylation status of promoter-associated CpG islands in response to treatment with Bz which may help to generate a predictive epigenetic signature-based stratification model to characterize the phenomenon interindividual variations in response to Bz treatment.

5.2.3 Genotypic Profiling

Single-nucleotide polymorphisms (SNPs or "snips") or point mutations in nuclear and mitochondrial DNA, whereby individuals differ in only a single base position, represent the most common types of variations in the human genome occurring in genes present within the regulatory regions, drug responding elements, drug metabolizing enzymes, drug transporters, drug receptors, proton pumps, and noncoding regions linked to disease susceptibility. SNPs can be distinguished from rare variations by a requirement for the least abundant allele to have a frequency of 1 % or more [185]. SNPs are considered best markers for association studies inhabiting the genome due to their wide prevalence, highly polymorphic and biallelic nature, codominance, low mutation rate, accessibility to high-throughput genotyping, easier automation for scoring, easy reproducibility, and their presence in both exonic as well as intronic regions of genes [186]. SNPs may serve as causative variations (causative SNPs) for simple and complex genetic diseases and drug resistance or can be indirectly associated to a diseased state by serving as markers genetically linked with the locus of interest on the human genome map associated with disease and/or drug response phenotypes.

Pharmacogenomics is the field of research that attempts to unravel the relationship between genetic variation affecting drug metabolism (pharmacokinetic level) or drug targets (pharmacodynamic level) and interindividual differences in pharmacoresponse. Therefore, generation of an SNP-based signature profile through high-throughput genome-wide SNP association studies and next-generation deep sequencing approaches may improve the biological understanding of the basis of Bz resistance and help in predicting response to Bz treatment and the development of more appropriate therapeutic measures. Studies on SNPs and treatment effect of Bz in MM have so far mostly undertaken candidate gene-based approaches focusing on pathway genes involved in Bz metabolism, drug action, and DNA repair. One such study involved the analysis of the loss-of-function variations CYP2C19*2, CYP2D6*3, CYP2D6*4, CYP2D6*5, and CYP2D6*6 and the gain-of-function polymorphism CYP2D6dup in the genes encoding the drug metabolizing enzymes CYP2C19 and CYP2D6 involved in the metabolism of cyclophosphamide, thalidomide, and Bz with treatment response in MM. Three hundred forty-eight (348) patients receiving high-dose cyclophosphamide and thalidomide or Bz at recurrence of disease were included in the study. One hundred seventy-seven (177) patients were treated with thalidomide at relapse, while 74 patients were treated with Bz. Results showed a trend ($p = 0.07$) towards a better time-to-next treatment (TNT) for Bz-treated patients having one or two mutant *CYP2D6* alleles, which means that this SNP could stratify the patients as intermediate metabolizers (IM) and poor metabolizers (PM). However, the data available for patients treated with Bz were very low [36, 117]. Another candidate gene-based study investigated the association of ABCB1/MDR1/P-glycoprotein 1 SNPs rs1045642 (3435C>T), rs2032582 (2677G>T or A), and rs1128503 (1236C>T) and the functional SNP in ABCC1/MRP1 gene rs4148356 (R723Q) with measures of treatment effect such as overall response rate, time to progression (TTP), PFS, and OS of pegylated liposomal doxorubicin (PLD) and Bz in a retrospective phase 3 clinical trial (DOXIL-MMY-3001) that compared PLD plus Bz with Bz alone in 646 Bz-naïve patients with MM. Results showed the MRP1/(PLZ+Bz) R723Q polymorphism was associated with a better TTP, progression-free survival, and overall survival, while the MDR1/3435 SNP (C>T) exhibited a trend ($0.05<p<0.1$) towards association with PFS, response rate, and TTP in the PLD+Bz arm, though no correlation was found in the Bz arm. The MDR1/3435 T allele was significantly associated with longer TTP and PFS in PLD+Bz patients when a recessive genetic model was considered [115]. Vangsted et al. [118] conducted a study on the association of promoter polymorphisms rs4848306, rs1143623, rs16944, and rs1143627 and functional haplotypes in IL-1B gene encoding the pro-inflammatory cytokine interleukin 1β (IL-1β) with TTF and OS in 243 patients who experienced relapse after HDT and were treated with thalidomide and Bz. However, no association was observed between IL-1B genotypes and outcome measures among relapse patients treated with thalidomide or Bz. Du et al. [116] analyzed 26 SNPs in the genes IKBα, NFKB2, and TRAF3 that regulate the NF-κB pathway using Sequenom's MassARRAY that uses matrix-assisted laser desorption ionization time-of-flight (MALDI-TOF) mass spectrometry for genotyping in 527 unrelated Chinese Han subjects comprising of 252 patients with MM and 275 age- and sex-matched controls following association studies with outcome in 83 patients treated with a Bz-containing regimen. Results showed that the SNPs rs11160707 (TRAF3), rs1056890, and rs12769316 (NFKB2) were significantly associated with outcome. Furthermore, a number of studies have also investigated the association of SNPs in candidate genes with the adverse effect of peripheral neuropathy (PN) in patients treated with Bz [119, 120]. However, no study has so far been performed that uses genome-wide SNP analysis for the purpose of genomic profiling and characterization of Bz resistance in MM.

5.2.4 *Immunophenotypic Profiling*

Recently, two notable studies used immunophenotyping involving antibody-based profiling of proteins expressed by cells to identify and validate predictive immunophenotypic signatures associated with Bz resistance in MM. Stessman et al. [122] identified the reduced expression of plasma cell maturation markers CD93, CD69, and CXCR4 associated with both acquired (Bz selected) and innate Bz resistance in cells derived from tumors of Bcl-X_L/Myc mouse model of plasma cell malignancy and with poorer survival in Bz-treated MM patients. This provided strong evidence that Bz resistance in MM could be due to Bz-induced and/or Bz-selected loss of plasma cell maturation markers resulting in reduced plasma cell commitment and less-differentiated phenotype. In a very elegant study, Leung-Hagesteijn et al. [123] demonstrated the presence of tumor progenitor subpopulations within primary MM which are responsible for Bz resistance, cytokine independence, and extramedullary growth resulting from decommitment to terminal plasma cell differentiation/maturation. The key factor demonstrated is a unique spliced form of XBP1 that was shown to

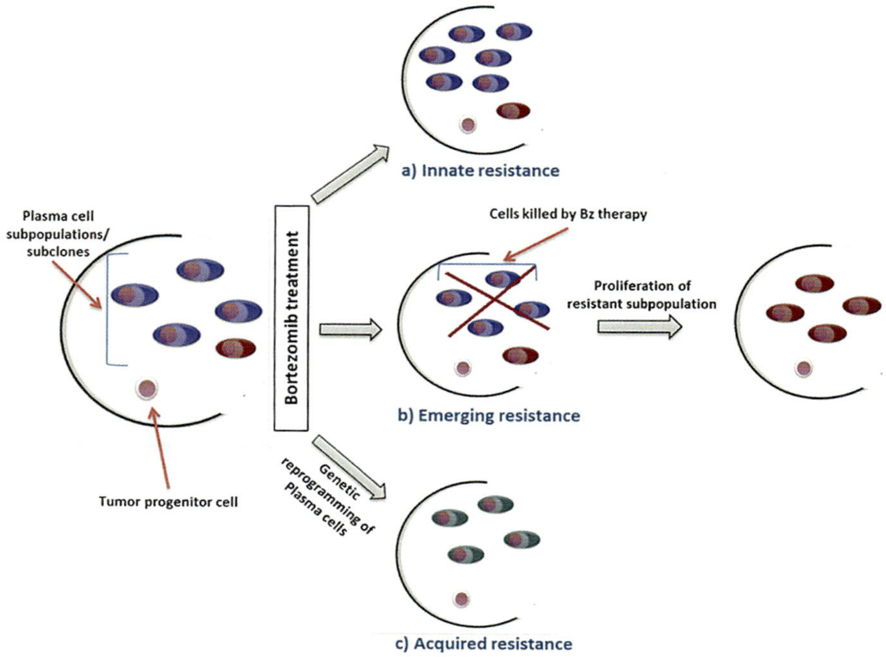

Fig. 5.9 Schema elucidating the potential mechanisms of resistance to Bz therapy. (**a**) Innate resistance: tumor cells never respond to Bz treatment (refractory disease). (**b**) Emerging resistance: presence and proliferation of tumor progenitor cells within primary MM tumors into Bz-resistant tumor cell subpopulation. (**c**) Acquired resistance: genetic reprogramming of plasma cells following Bz treatment leading to Bz resistance

induce the decommitment to plasma cell maturation and immunoglobulin production, which in turn reduces the endoplasmic reticulum loading of potential unfolded proteins. This then leads to decreased susceptibility to proteasome inhibitors. Stessman et al. [122] further showed that stimulation of plasma cell differentiation using lipopolysaccharide (LPS), a known inducer of B-cell differentiation, could reestablish the maturation markers and resensitize Bz-resistant cells to Bz treatment. These studies have potentially shepherded a paradigm shift in the understanding of the basis of resistance to proteasome inhibitors in MM and offered cues towards novel therapeutic approaches to treat Bz resistance (Fig. 5.9).

5.3 Perspectives and the Future

Tumor tissue and the bone marrow microenvironment encompass a wealth of genetic and epigenetic mysteries waiting to be unearthed. These complex genomic, transcriptomic, and epigenetic alterations associated with interindividual variations in

Bz response can be used for in-depth simultaneous large-scale transcriptomic (RNA-seq based gene expression analysis), genomic (genome wide association studies), and epigenomic (array-based DNA methylation analysis) signature profiling of innate (refractory) or acquired (relapsed) resistance to the proteasome inhibitor Bz in MM to generate an integrated pharmacogenomic signature profile qualitatively and quantitatively associated with resistance that can be further expanded to research on other drugs. Despite the considerable amount of interest in unraveling the signature profile of drug resistance in MM, strikingly few studies have been conducted so far that focus on generating a unique gene-based score to predict therapeutic response and particularly its use in guiding clinicians to more effective therapies.

Relapse and emerging drug resistance are unfortunately a common event, even in patients that may respond well to initial therapies like Bz. While profiling the first available sample from newly diagnosed patients has provided prognostic signatures that are particularly useful in identifying aggressive disease, the clinical utility in terms of designing individualized therapy has not been effectively demonstrated. There have been some recent approaches to develop predictive scoring systems, working first with cell lines representing some of the heterogeneity in tumor response. Using GEP, Moreaux et al. have developed sensitivity scores to histone deacetylases and methylase inhibitors [187, 188]. This may serve to guide clinical choices in the near future, although clinical trials will be needed to validate their effectiveness. Profiling tumors from refractory patients or relapse patients have demonstrated signatures that can distinguish response and resistance, but how to treat the refractory or resistant tumors once they occur had not been addressed. A large-scale RNAi screen-based study by Zhu et al. [121] identified a number of genes including *CDK5*, a regulator of the proteasome subunit PSMB5, which were found to be involved in the synergistic potentiation of the growth inhibitory effects of Bz and Cz in MM cells. Recently, Stessman et al. used the resistant GEP profiles to look for common elements in NCI available in CMAPs of drug response to identify potential secondary therapies [113]. Alternatively, efforts have been made to identify approaches that may resensitize emerging Bz resistance back to Bz response [122, 123]. These efforts represent potential applications of profiling to direct effective individualized therapies. Similar approaches to use profiles in identifying effective combinations will add to the personalization of therapies.

In recent studies, it has become very apparent that the initial diagnostic tumor sample likely contains a heterogeneous mix of tumor cells, which, while showing markers of common clonality, nevertheless show evidence of genetic heterogeneity [189]. Indeed, there is evidence in modeling systems that tumors may harbor subpopulations that are refractory to the therapy [190]. The consequence is an apparent initial response of the bulk population but with the selective outgrowth of a preexisting resistant population (Fig. 5.9). New technologies have been developed that allow profiling at the single cell level [191]; and one could imagine that signatures of response and resistance may be identified in such mixed tumor populations. If profiles are useful in predicting effective drug choices, combination therapies may serve two complementary purposes: (1) synergistic killing of tumor cells and (2) selective killing of mixed populations.

As described above, molecular profiling may include analysis of genomic variations, gene expression patterns, epigenetic patterns, protein patterns, or likely a combination of all to characterize each individual and their tumors. We conclude that robust approaches using multiple data types are of primary importance in profiling drug resistance in MM. The ultimate purpose of such an effort will be to create a pharmacogenomic profiling-guided therapeutic response score that can be cross-validated using clinical trials on MM patients undergoing Bz-based therapy or any chemotherapy, so that it can be routinely applied in clinical settings to improve selective response to available drugs, predict effective combinations, and identify secondary therapies to circumvent the challenges in the relapsed patient. This represents the future of pharmacogenomic profiling, which will result in more personalized treatments.

References

1. Kuehl WM, Bergsagel PL (2012) Molecular pathogenesis of multiple myeloma and its premalignant precursor. J Clin Invest 122(10):3456–3463
2. Herve AL, Florence M, Philippe M et al (2011) Molecular heterogeneity of multiple myeloma: pathogenesis, prognosis, and therapeutic implications. J Clin Oncol 29(14): 1893–1897
3. Raab MS, Podar K, Breitkreutz I, Richardson PG, Anderson KC (2009) Multiple myeloma. Lancet 374(9686):324–339
4. Rajkumar SV (2013) Multiple myeloma: 2013 update on diagnosis, risk-stratification, and management. Am J Hematol 88(3):226–235
5. Mahindra A, Hideshima T, Anderson KC (2010) Multiple myeloma: biology of the disease. Blood Rev 24(Suppl 1):S5–S11
6. Landgren O, Kyle RA, Pfeiffer RM et al (2009) Monoclonal gammopathy of undetermined significance (MGUS) consistently precedes multiple myeloma: a prospective study. Blood 113(22):5412–5417
7. International Myeloma Working Group (2003) Criteria for the classification of monoclonal gammopathies, multiple myeloma and related disorders: a report of the International Myeloma Working Group. Br J Haematol 121(5):749–757
8. Kyle RA, Rajkumar SV (2007) Monoclonal gammopathy of undetermined significance and smouldering multiple myeloma: emphasis on risk factors for progression. Br J Haematol 139(5):730–743
9. Kyle RA, Therneau TM, Rajkumar SV et al (2002) A long-term study of prognosis in monoclonal gammopathy of undetermined significance. N Engl J Med 346(8):564–569
10. Blade J, Rosinol L, Cibeira MT, de Larrea CF (2008) Pathogenesis and progression of monoclonal gammopathy of undetermined significance. Leukemia 22(9):1651–1657
11. Munshi NC, Anderson KC (2013) New strategies in the treatment of multiple myeloma. Clin Cancer Res 19(13):3337–3344
12. Hoogstraten B, Sheehe PR, Cuttner J et al (1967) Melphalan in multiple myeloma. Blood 30(1):74–83
13. Oken MM, Harrington DP, Abramson N, Kyle RA, Knospe W, Glick JH (1997) Comparison of melphalan and prednisone with vincristine, carmustine, melphalan, cyclophosphamide, and prednisone in the treatment of multiple myeloma: results of Eastern Cooperative Oncology Group Study E2479. Cancer 79(8):1561–1567
14. Alexanian R, Haut A, Khan AU et al (1969) Treatment for multiple myeloma. Combination chemotherapy with different melphalan dose regimens. JAMA 208(9):1680–1685

15. Anonymous (1998) Combination chemotherapy versus melphalan plus prednisone as treatment for multiple myeloma: an overview of 6,633 patients from 27 randomized trials. Myeloma Trialists' Collaborative Group. J Clin Oncol 16(12):3832–3842
16. Koreth J, Cutler CS, Djulbegovic B et al (2007) High-dose therapy with single autologous transplantation versus chemotherapy for newly diagnosed multiple myeloma: a systematic review and meta-analysis of randomized controlled trials. Biol Blood Marrow Transplant 13(2):183–196
17. Bensinger WI (2002) Allogeneic hematopoietic cell transplantation for multiple myeloma. Biomed Pharmacother 56(3):133–138
18. Maloney DG, Molina AJ, Sahebi F et al (2003) Allografting with nonmyeloablative conditioning following cytoreductive autografts for the treatment of patients with multiple myeloma. Blood 102(9):3447–3454
19. Samson D, Gaminara E, Newland A et al (1989) Infusion of vincristine and doxorubicin with oral dexamethasone as first-line therapy for multiple myeloma. Lancet 2(8668):882–885
20. Dimopoulos MA, San-Miguel JF, Anderson KC (2011) Emerging therapies for the treatment of relapsed or refractory multiple myeloma. Eur J Haematol 86(1):1–15
21. Mitsiades CS, Davies FE, Laubach JP et al (2011) Future directions of next-generation novel therapies, combination approaches, and the development of personalized medicine in myeloma. J Clin Oncol 29(14):1916–1923
22. Moreau P, Richardson PG, Cavo M et al (2012) Proteasome inhibitors in multiple myeloma: 10 years later. Blood 120(5):947–959
23. Kortuem KM, Stewart AK (2013) Carfilzomib. Blood 121(6):893–897
24. Potts BC, Albitar MX, Anderson KC et al (2011) Marizomib, a proteasome inhibitor for all seasons: preclinical profile and a framework for clinical trials. Curr Cancer Drug Targets 11(3):254–284
25. Hideshima T, Richardson P, Chauhan D et al (2001) The proteasome inhibitor PS-341 inhibits growth, induces apoptosis, and overcomes drug resistance in human multiple myeloma cells. Cancer Res 61(7):3071–3076
26. Hideshima T, Mitsiades C, Akiyama M et al (2003) Molecular mechanisms mediating anti-myeloma activity of proteasome inhibitor PS-341. Blood 101(4):1530–1534
27. Adams J, Palombella VJ, Sausville EA et al (1999) Proteasome inhibitors: a novel class of potent and effective antitumor agents. Cancer Res 59(11):2615–2622
28. Lightcap ES, McCormack TA, Pien CS, Chau V, Adams J, Elliott PJ (2000) Proteasome inhibition measurements: clinical application. Clin Chem 46(5):673–683
29. LeBlanc R, Catley LP, Hideshima T et al (2002) Proteasome inhibitor PS-341 inhibits human myeloma cell growth in vivo and prolongs survival in a murine model. Cancer Res 62(17): 4996–5000
30. Richardson PG, Sonneveld P, Schuster MW et al (2005) Bortezomib or high-dose dexamethasone for relapsed multiple myeloma. N Engl J Med 352(24):2487–2498
31. Dispenzieri A, Kyle RA (2005) Neurological aspects of multiple myeloma and related disorders. Best Pract Res Clin Haematol 18(4):673–688
32. Richardson PG, Briemberg H, Jagannath S et al (2006) Frequency, characteristics, and reversibility of peripheral neuropathy during treatment of advanced multiple myeloma with bortezomib. J Clin Oncol 24(19):3113–3120
33. Barlogie B, van Rhee F, Shaughnessy JD Jr et al (2008) Seven-year median time to progression with thalidomide for smoldering myeloma: partial response identifies subset requiring earlier salvage therapy for symptomatic disease. Blood 112(8):3122–3125
34. San Miguel JF, Schlag R, Khuageva NK et al (2008) Bortezomib plus melphalan and prednisone for initial treatment of multiple myeloma. N Engl J Med 359(9):906–917
35. Fonseca R, Bergsagel PL, Drach J et al (2009) International Myeloma Working Group molecular classification of multiple myeloma: spotlight review. Leukemia 23(12):2210–2221
36. Vangsted A, Klausen TW, Vogel U (2012) Genetic variations in multiple myeloma II: association with effect of treatment. Eur J Haematol 88(2):93–117

37. Richardson PG, Sonneveld P, Schuster MW et al (2007) Safety and efficacy of bortezomib in high-risk and elderly patients with relapsed multiple myeloma. Br J Haematol 137(5):429–435
38. Richardson PG, Sonneveld P, Schuster M et al (2007) Extended follow-up of a phase 3 trial in relapsed multiple myeloma: final time-to-event results of the APEX trial. Blood 110(10): 3557–3560
39. Laubach J, Richardson P, Anderson K (2011) Multiple myeloma. Annu Rev Med 62: 249–264
40. Kumar S, Rajkumar SV (2008) Many facets of bortezomib resistance/susceptibility. Blood 112(6):2177–2178
41. Grigorieva I, Thomas X, Epstein J (1998) The bone marrow stromal environment is a major factor in myeloma cell resistance to dexamethasone. Exp Hematol 26(7):597–603
42. Rowley M, Liu P, Van Ness B (2000) Heterogeneity in therapeutic response of genetically altered myeloma cell lines to interleukin 6, dexamethasone, doxorubicin, and melphalan. Blood 96(9):3175–3180
43. Mitsiades CS, Mitsiades N, Poulaki V et al (2002) Activation of NF-kappaB and upregulation of intracellular anti-apoptotic proteins via the IGF-1/Akt signaling in human multiple myeloma cells: therapeutic implications. Oncogene 21(37):5673–5683
44. Chauhan D, Uchiyama H, Akbarali Y et al (1996) Multiple myeloma cell adhesion-induced interleukin-6 expression in bone marrow stromal cells involves activation of NF-kappa B. Blood 87(3):1104–1112
45. Hideshima T, Chauhan D, Schlossman R, Richardson P, Anderson KC (2001) The role of tumor necrosis factor alpha in the pathophysiology of human multiple myeloma: therapeutic applications. Oncogene 20(33):4519–4527
46. Hideshima T, Mitsiades C, Tonon G, Richardson PG, Anderson KC (2007) Understanding multiple myeloma pathogenesis in the bone marrow to identify new therapeutic targets. Nat Rev Cancer 7(8):585–598
47. Caers J, Van Valckenborgh E, Menu E, Van Camp B, Vanderkerken K (2008) Unraveling the biology of multiple myeloma disease: cancer stem cells, acquired intracellular changes and interactions with the surrounding micro-environment. Bull Cancer 95(3):301–313
48. Urashima M, Chauhan D, Uchiyama H, Freeman GJ, Anderson KC (1995) CD40 ligand triggered interleukin-6 secretion in multiple myeloma. Blood 85(7):1903–1912
49. Hideshima T, Bergsagel PL, Kuehl WM, Anderson KC (2004) Advances in biology of multiple myeloma: clinical applications. Blood 104(3):607–618
50. Zang MR, Li F, An G et al (2012) Regulation of miRNA-15a/-16 expression on the drug resistance of myeloma cells. Zhonghua Yi Xue Za Zhi 92(16):1100–1103
51. Hao M, Zhang L, An G et al (2011) Bone marrow stromal cells protect myeloma cells from bortezomib induced apoptosis by suppressing microRNA-15a expression. Leuk Lymphoma 52(9):1787–1794
52. Wang X, Li C, Ju S, Wang Y, Wang H, Zhong R (2011) Myeloma cell adhesion to bone marrow stromal cells confers drug resistance by microRNA-21 up-regulation. Leuk Lymphoma 52(10):1991–1998
53. Kalitin NN, Kostyukova MN, Kakpakova ES, Tupitsyn NN, Karamysheva AF (2012) Expression of vascular endothelial growth factor receptors VEGFR1 in cultured multiple myeloma cells: correlation with immunophenotype and drug resistance. Bull Exp Biol Med 153(6):882–885
54. Kuhn DJ, Berkova Z, Jones RJ et al (2012) Targeting the insulin-like growth factor-1 receptor to overcome bortezomib resistance in preclinical models of multiple myeloma. Blood 120(16):3260–3270
55. Tai YT, Li XF, Catley L et al (2005) Immunomodulatory drug lenalidomide (CC-5013, IMiD3) augments anti-CD40 SGN-40-induced cytotoxicity in human multiple myeloma: clinical implications. Cancer Res 65(24):11712–11720
56. Azab AK, Runnels JM, Pitsillides C et al (2009) CXCR4 inhibitor AMD3100 disrupts the interaction of multiple myeloma cells with the bone marrow microenvironment and enhances their sensitivity to therapy. Blood 113(18):4341–4351

57. Adams J (2004) The proteasome: a suitable antineoplastic target. Nat Rev Cancer 4(5): 349–360
58. Lichter DI, Danaee H, Pickard MD et al (2012) Sequence analysis of beta-subunit genes of the 20S proteasome in patients with relapsed multiple myeloma treated with bortezomib or dexamethasone. Blood 120(23):4513–4516
59. Verbrugge SE, Al M, Assaraf YG et al (2013) Overcoming bortezomib resistance in human B cells by anti-CD20/rituximab-mediated complement-dependent cytotoxicity and epoxyketone-based irreversible proteasome inhibitors. Exp Hematol Oncol 2(1):2. doi:10.1186/2162-3619-2-2
60. Verbrugge SE, Assaraf YG, Dijkmans BA et al (2012) Inactivating PSMB5 mutations and P-glycoprotein (multidrug resistance-associated protein/ATP-binding cassette B1) mediate resistance to proteasome inhibitors: ex vivo efficacy of (immuno)proteasome inhibitors in mononuclear blood cells from patients with rheumatoid arthritis. J Pharmacol Exp Ther 341(1):174–182
61. Suzuki E, Demo S, Deu E et al (2011) Molecular mechanisms of bortezomib resistant adenocarcinoma cells. PLoS One 6(12):e27996
62. de Wilt LH, Jansen G, Assaraf YG et al (2012) Proteasome-based mechanisms of intrinsic and acquired bortezomib resistance in non-small cell lung cancer. Biochem Pharmacol 83(2):207–217
63. Li X, Wood TE, Sprangers R et al (2010) Effect of noncompetitive proteasome inhibition on bortezomib resistance. J Natl Cancer Inst 102(14):1069–1082
64. Franke NE, Niewerth D, Assaraf YG et al (2012) Impaired bortezomib binding to mutant beta5 subunit of the proteasome is the underlying basis for bortezomib resistance in leukemia cells. Leukemia 26(4):757–768
65. Lu SQ, Yang JM, Huang CM et al (2011) Comparison of protein expression profiles between bortezomib-resistant JurkatB cells with PSMB5 mutation and their parent cells. Zhongguo Shi Yan Xue Ye Xue Za Zhi 19(4):869–873
66. Ri M, Iida S, Nakashima T et al (2010) Bortezomib-resistant myeloma cell lines: a role for mutated PSMB5 in preventing the accumulation of unfolded proteins and fatal ER stress. Leukemia 24(8):1506–1512
67. Lu S, Chen Z, Yang J et al (2008) Overexpression of the PSMB5 gene contributes to bortezomib resistance in T-lymphoblastic lymphoma/leukemia cells derived from Jurkat line. Exp Hematol 36(10):1278–1284
68. Lu S, Yang J, Song X et al (2008) Point mutation of the proteasome beta5 subunit gene is an important mechanism of bortezomib resistance in bortezomib-selected variants of Jurkat T cell lymphoblastic lymphoma/leukemia line. J Pharmacol Exp Ther 326(2):423–431
69. Lu S, Yang J, Chen Z et al (2009) Different mutants of PSMB5 confer varying bortezomib resistance in T lymphoblastic lymphoma/leukemia cells derived from the Jurkat cell line. Exp Hematol 37(7):831–837
70. Oerlemans R, Franke NE, Assaraf YG et al (2008) Molecular basis of bortezomib resistance: proteasome subunit beta5 (PSMB5) gene mutation and overexpression of PSMB5 protein. Blood 112(6):2489–2499
71. Shuqing L, Jianmin Y, Chongmei H, Hui C, Wang J (2011) Upregulated expression of the PSMB5 gene may contribute to drug resistance in patient with multiple myeloma when treated with bortezomib-based regimen. Exp Hematol 39(12):1117–1118
72. Politou M, Karadimitris A, Terpos E, Kotsianidis I, Apperley JF, Rahemtulla A (2006) No evidence of mutations of the PSMB5 (beta-5 subunit of proteasome) in a case of myeloma with clinical resistance to bortezomib. Leuk Res 30(2):240–241
73. Wang L, Kumar S, Fridley BL et al (2008) Proteasome beta subunit pharmacogenomics: gene resequencing and functional genomics. Clin Cancer Res 14(11):3503–3513
74. Balsas P, Galan-Malo P, Marzo I, Naval J (2012) Bortezomib resistance in a myeloma cell line is associated to PSMbeta5 overexpression and polyploidy. Leuk Res 36(2):212–218
75. Barbone D, Cheung P, Battula S et al (2012) Vorinostat eliminates multicellular resistance of mesothelioma 3D spheroids via restoration of Noxa expression. PLoS One 7(12):e52753

76. Yeom SY, Lee SJ, Kim WS, Park C (2012) Rad knockdown induces mitochondrial apoptosis in bortezomib resistant leukemia and lymphoma cells. Leuk Res 36(9):1172–1178
77. Zhang L, Littlejohn JE, Cui Y, Cao X, Peddaboina C, Smythe WR (2010) Characterization of bortezomib-adapted I-45 mesothelioma cells. Mol Cancer 9:110. doi:10.1186/1476-4598-9-110
78. Ling X, Calinski D, Chanan-Khan AA, Zhou M, Li F (2010) Cancer cell sensitivity to bortezomib is associated with survivin expression and p53 status but not cancer cell types. J Exp Clin Cancer Res 29:8. doi:10.1186/1756-9966-29-8
79. Hu J, Dang N, Menu E et al (2012) Activation of ATF4 mediates unwanted Mcl-1 accumulation by proteasome inhibition. Blood 119(3):826–837
80. Smith AJ, Dai H, Correia C et al (2011) Noxa/Bcl-2 protein interactions contribute to bortezomib resistance in human lymphoid cells. J Biol Chem 286(20):17682–17692
81. Liu P, Xu B, Li J, Lu H (2009) BAG3 gene silencing sensitizes leukemic cells to bortezomib-induced apoptosis. FEBS Lett 583(2):401–406
82. Yang TM, Barbone D, Fennell DA, Broaddus VC (2009) Bcl-2 family proteins contribute to apoptotic resistance in lung cancer multicellular spheroids. Am J Respir Cell Mol Biol 41(1):14–23
83. Xu D, Hu J, De Bruyne E et al (2012) Dll1/Notch activation contributes to bortezomib resistance by upregulating CYP1A1 in multiple myeloma. Biochem Biophys Res Commun 428(4): 518–524
84. Kim A, Park S, Lee JE et al (2012) The dual PI3K and mTOR inhibitor NVP-BEZ235 exhibits anti-proliferative activity and overcomes bortezomib resistance in mantle cell lymphoma cells. Leuk Res 36(7):912–920
85. Hegde GV, Nordgren TM, Munger CM et al (2012) Novel therapy for therapy-resistant mantle cell lymphoma: multipronged approach with targeting of hedgehog signaling. Int J Cancer 131(12):2951–2960
86. Jung HJ, Chen Z, Wang M et al (2012) Calcium blockers decrease the bortezomib resistance in mantle cell lymphoma via manipulation of tissue transglutaminase activities. Blood 119(11):2568–2578
87. Markovina S, Callander NS, O'Connor SL et al (2008) Bortezomib-resistant nuclear factor-kappaB activity in multiple myeloma cells. Mol Cancer Res 6(8):1356–1364
88. Markovina S, Callander NS, O'Connor SL et al (2010) Bone marrow stromal cells from multiple myeloma patients uniquely induce bortezomib resistant NF-kappaB activity in myeloma cells. Mol Cancer 9:176. doi:10.1186/1476-4598-9-176
89. Yang DT, Young KH, Kahl BS, Markovina S, Miyamoto S (2008) Prevalence of bortezomib-resistant constitutive NF-kappaB activity in mantle cell lymphoma. Mol Cancer 7:40. doi:10.1186/1476-4598-7-40
90. Landowski TH, Olashaw NE, Agrawal D, Dalton WS (2003) Cell adhesion-mediated drug resistance (CAM-DR) is associated with activation of NF-kappa B (RelB/p50) in myeloma cells. Oncogene 22(16):2417–2421
91. Hazlehurst LA, Damiano JS, Buyuksal I, Pledger WJ, Dalton WS (2000) Adhesion to fibronectin via beta1 integrins regulates p27kip1 levels and contributes to cell adhesion mediated drug resistance (CAM-DR). Oncogene 19(38):4319–4327
92. Shi L, Wang S, Zangari M et al (2010) Over-expression of CKS1B activates both MEK/ERK and JAK/STAT3 signaling pathways and promotes myeloma cell drug-resistance. Oncotarget 1(1):22–33
93. Que W, Chen J, Chuang M, Jiang D (2012) Knockdown of c-Met enhances sensitivity to bortezomib in human multiple myeloma U266 cells via inhibiting Akt/mTOR activity. APMIS 120(3):195–203
94. Moriuchi M, Ohmachi K, Kojima M et al (2010) Three cases of bortezomib-resistant multiple myeloma with extramedullary masses. Tokai J Exp Clin Med 35(1):17–20
95. Pirrotta MT, Gozzetti A, Cerase A et al (2008) Unusual discordant responses in two multiple myeloma patients during bortezomib treatment. Onkologie 31(1–2):45–47
96. Filipczak PT, Piglowski W, Glowala-Kosinska M, Krawczyk Z, Scieglinska D (2012) HSPA2 overexpression protects V79 fibroblasts against bortezomib-induced apoptosis. Biochem Cell Biol 90(2):224–231

97. Mozos A, Roue G, Lopez-Guillermo A et al (2011) The expression of the endoplasmic reticulum stress sensor BiP/GRP78 predicts response to chemotherapy and determines the efficacy of proteasome inhibitors in diffuse large b-cell lymphoma. Am J Pathol 179(5):2601–2610
98. Rushworth SA, Bowles KM, MacEwan DJ (2011) High basal nuclear levels of Nrf2 in acute myeloid leukemia reduces sensitivity to proteasome inhibitors. Cancer Res 71(5): 1999–2009
99. Kern J, Untergasser G, Zenzmaier C et al (2009) GRP-78 secreted by tumor cells blocks the antiangiogenic activity of bortezomib. Blood 114(18):3960–3967
100. Du ZX, Zhang HY, Meng X, Guan Y, Wang HQ (2009) Role of oxidative stress and intracellular glutathione in the sensitivity to apoptosis induced by proteasome inhibitor in thyroid cancer cells. BMC Cancer 9:56. doi:10.1186/1471-2407-9-56
101. Chauhan D, Li G, Shringarpure R et al (2003) Blockade of Hsp27 overcomes bortezomib/proteasome inhibitor PS-341 resistance in lymphoma cells. Cancer Res 63(19):6174–6177
102. Shringarpure R, Catley L, Bhole D et al (2006) Gene expression analysis of B-lymphoma cells resistant and sensitive to bortezomib. Br J Haematol 134(2):145–156
103. Zhao M, Vuori K (2011) The docking protein p130Cas regulates cell sensitivity to proteasome inhibition. BMC Biol 9:73. doi:10.1186/1741-7007-9-73
104. Jia L, Gopinathan G, Sukumar JT, Gribben JG (2012) Blocking autophagy prevents bortezomib-induced NF-kappaB activation by reducing I-kappaB alpha degradation in lymphoma cells. PLoS One 7(2):e32584
105. Rzymski T, Milani M, Singleton DC, Harris AL (2009) Role of ATF4 in regulation of autophagy and resistance to drugs and hypoxia. Cell Cycle 8(23):3838–3847
106. Milani M, Rzymski T, Mellor HR et al (2009) The role of ATF4 stabilization and autophagy in resistance of breast cancer cells treated with bortezomib. Cancer Res 69(10):4415–4423
107. Nawrocki ST, Carew JS, Pino MS et al (2006) Aggresome disruption: a novel strategy to enhance bortezomib-induced apoptosis in pancreatic cancer cells. Cancer Res 66(7): 3773–3781
108. Mulligan G, Mitsiades C, Bryant B et al (2007) Gene expression profiling and correlation with outcome in clinical trials of the proteasome inhibitor bortezomib. Blood 109(8): 3177–3188
109. Shaughnessy JD Jr, Zhan F, Burington BE et al (2007) A validated gene expression model of high-risk multiple myeloma is defined by deregulated expression of genes mapping to chromosome 1. Blood 109(6):2276–2284
110. Zhan F, Barlogie B, Mulligan G, Shaughnessy JD Jr, Bryant B (2008) High-risk myeloma: a gene expression based risk-stratification model for newly diagnosed multiple myeloma treated with high-dose therapy is predictive of outcome in relapsed disease treated with single-agent bortezomib or high-dose dexamethasone. Blood 111(2):968–969
111. Nair B, van Rhee F, Shaughnessy JD Jr et al (2010) Superior results of total therapy 3 (2003-33) in gene expression profiling-defined low-risk multiple myeloma confirmed in subsequent trial 2006-66 with VRD maintenance. Blood 115(21):4168–4173
112. Shaughnessy JD Jr, Qu P, Usmani S et al (2011) Pharmacogenomics of bortezomib test-dosing identifies hyperexpression of proteasome genes, especially PSMD4, as novel high-risk feature in myeloma treated with total therapy 3. Blood 118(13):3512–3524
113. Stessman HA, Baughn LB, Sarver A et al (2013) Profiling bortezomib resistance identifies secondary therapies in a mouse myeloma model. Mol Cancer Ther 12(6):1140–1150
114. Fernandez de Larrea C, Martin-Antonio B, Cibeira MT et al (2013) Impact of global and gene-specific DNA methylation pattern in relapsed multiple myeloma patients treated with bortezomib. Leuk Res 37(6):641–646
115. Buda G, Ricci D, Huang CC et al (2010) Polymorphisms in the multiple drug resistance protein 1 and in P-glycoprotein 1 are associated with time to event outcomes in patients with advanced multiple myeloma treated with bortezomib and pegylated liposomal doxorubicin. Ann Hematol 89(11):1133–1140
116. Du J, Huo J, Shi J et al (2011) Polymorphisms of nuclear factor-kappaB family genes are associated with development of multiple myeloma and treatment outcome in patients receiving bortezomib-based regimens. Haematologica 96(5):729–737

117. Vangsted AJ, Soeby K, Klausen TW et al (2010) No influence of the polymorphisms CYP2C19 and CYP2D6 on the efficacy of cyclophosphamide, thalidomide, and bortezomib in patients with multiple myeloma. BMC Cancer 10:404. doi:10.1186/1471-2407-10-404
118. Vangsted AJ, Klausen TW, Abildgaard N et al (2011) Single nucleotide polymorphisms in the promoter region of the IL1B gene influence outcome in multiple myeloma patients treated with high-dose chemotherapy independently of relapse treatment with thalidomide and bortezomib. Ann Hematol 90(10):1173–1181
119. Broyl A, Corthals SL, Jongen JL et al (2010) Mechanisms of peripheral neuropathy associated with bortezomib and vincristine in patients with newly diagnosed multiple myeloma: a prospective analysis of data from the HOVON-65/GMMG-HD4 trial. Lancet Oncol 11(11): 1057–1065
120. Favis R, Sun Y, van de Velde H et al (2011) Genetic variation associated with bortezomib-induced peripheral neuropathy. Pharmacogenet Genomics 21(3):121–129
121. Zhu YX, Tiedemann R, Shi CX et al (2011) RNAi screen of the druggable genome identifies modulators of proteasome inhibitor sensitivity in myeloma including CDK5. Blood 117(14): 3847–3857
122. Stessman HA, Mansoor A, Zhan F, Linden MA, Van Ness B, Baughn LB (2013) Bortezomib resistance can be reversed by induced expression of plasma cell maturation markers in a mouse in vitro model of multiple myeloma. PLoS One 8(10):e77608
123. Leung-Hagesteijn C, Erdmann N, Cheung G et al (2013) Xbp1s-negative tumor B cells and pre-plasmablasts mediate therapeutic proteasome inhibitor resistance in multiple myeloma. Cancer Cell 24(3):289–304
124. Richardson PG, Barlogie B, Berenson J et al (2003) A phase 2 study of bortezomib in relapsed, refractory myeloma. N Engl J Med 348(26):2609–2617
125. Jagannath S, Barlogie B, Berenson J et al (2004) A phase 2 study of two doses of bortezomib in relapsed or refractory myeloma. Br J Haematol 127(2):165–172
126. Blade J, Samson D, Reece D et al (1998) Criteria for evaluating disease response and progression in patients with multiple myeloma treated by high-dose therapy and haemopoietic stem cell transplantation. Myeloma Subcommittee of the EBMT. European Group for Blood and Marrow Transplant. Br J Haematol 102(5):1115–1123
127. Subramanian A, Tamayo P, Mootha VK et al (2005) Gene set enrichment analysis: a knowledge-based approach for interpreting genome-wide expression profiles. Proc Natl Acad Sci U S A 102(43):15545–15550
128. Durie BG, Salmon SE (1975) A clinical staging system for multiple myeloma. Correlation of measured myeloma cell mass with presenting clinical features, response to treatment, and survival. Cancer 36(3):842–854
129. van Rhee F, Bolejack V, Hollmig K et al (2007) High serum-free light chain levels and their rapid reduction in response to therapy define an aggressive multiple myeloma subtype with poor prognosis. Blood 110(3):827–832
130. Barlogie B, Anaissie E, van Rhee F et al (2007) Incorporating bortezomib into upfront treatment for multiple myeloma: early results of total therapy 3. Br J Haematol 138(2):176–185
131. Pineda-Roman M, Zangari M, Haessler J et al (2008) Sustained complete remissions in multiple myeloma linked to bortezomib in total therapy 3: comparison with total therapy 2. Br J Haematol 140(6):625–634
132. Lamb J (2007) The connectivity map: a new tool for biomedical research. Nat Rev Cancer 7(1):54–60
133. Lamb J, Crawford ED, Peck D et al (2006) The connectivity map: using gene-expression signatures to connect small molecules, genes, and disease. Science 313(5795):1929–1935
134. Van Ness B, Stessman H, Baughn LB, et al (2013) Strategies to identify effective treatments for proteasome inhibitor resistant multiple myeloma [abstract]. ASH Abstract
135. Dawson MA, Kouzarides T (2012) Cancer epigenetics: from mechanism to therapy. Cell 150(1):12–27
136. Berger SL, Kouzarides T, Shiekhattar R, Shilatifard A (2009) An operational definition of epigenetics. Genes Dev 23(7):781–783

137. Baylin SB, Jones PA (2011) A decade of exploring the cancer epigenome—biological and translational implications. Nat Rev Cancer 11(10):726–734
138. Wu H, Zhang Y (2011) Mechanisms and functions of Tet protein-mediated 5-methylcytosine oxidation. Genes Dev 25(23):2436–2452
139. Kouzarides T (2007) Chromatin modifications and their function. Cell 128(4):693–705
140. Tan M, Luo H, Lee S et al (2011) Identification of 67 histone marks and histone lysine crotonylation as a new type of histone modification. Cell 146(6):1016–1028
141. Barski A, Cuddapah S, Cui K et al (2007) High-resolution profiling of histone methylations in the human genome. Cell 129(4):823–837
142. Robertson KD (2005) DNA methylation and human disease. Nat Rev Genet 6(8):597–610
143. Wong KY, Huang X, Chim CS (2012) DNA methylation of microRNA genes in multiple myeloma. Carcinogenesis 33(9):1629–1638
144. Dahl C, Guldberg P (2003) DNA methylation analysis techniques. Biogerontology 4(4): 233–250
145. Laird PW (2010) Principles and challenges of genome-wide DNA methylation analysis. Nat Rev Genet 11(3):191–203
146. Shen L, Waterland RA (2007) Methods of DNA methylation analysis. Curr Opin Clin Nutr Metab Care 10(5):576–581
147. Felsenfeld G, McGhee J (1982) Methylation and gene control. Nature 296(5858):602–603
148. Eick D, Fritz HJ, Doerfler W (1983) Quantitative determination of 5-methylcytosine in DNA by reverse-phase high-performance liquid chromatography. Anal Biochem 135(1):165–171
149. Frommer M, McDonald LE, Millar DS et al (1992) A genomic sequencing protocol that yields a positive display of 5-methylcytosine residues in individual DNA strands. Proc Natl Acad Sci U S A 89(5):1827–1831
150. Hayatsu H, Shiraishi M, Negishi K (2008) Bisulfite modification for analysis of DNA methylation. Curr Protoc Nucleic Acid Chem Chapter 6:Unit 6.10
151. Hayatsu H, Wataya Y, Kai K, Iida S (1970) Reaction of sodium bisulfite with uracil, cytosine, and their derivatives. Biochemistry 9(14):2858–2865
152. Herman JG, Graff JR, Myohanen S, Nelkin BD, Baylin SB (1996) Methylation-specific PCR: a novel PCR assay for methylation status of CpG islands. Proc Natl Acad Sci U S A 93(18):9821–9826
153. Xiong Z, Laird PW (1997) COBRA: a sensitive and quantitative DNA methylation assay. Nucleic Acids Res 25(12):2532–2534
154. Gonzalgo ML, Jones PA (1997) Rapid quantitation of methylation differences at specific sites using methylation-sensitive single nucleotide primer extension (Ms-SNuPE). Nucleic Acids Res 25(12):2529–2531
155. Eads CA, Danenberg KD, Kawakami K et al (2000) MethyLight: a high-throughput assay to measure DNA methylation. Nucleic Acids Res 28(8):E32
156. Colella S, Shen L, Baggerly KA, Issa JP, Krahe R (2003) Sensitive and quantitative universal pyrosequencing methylation analysis of CpG sites. Biotechniques 35(1):146–150
157. Ronaghi M, Karamohamed S, Pettersson B, Uhlen M, Nyren P (1996) Real-time DNA sequencing using detection of pyrophosphate release. Anal Biochem 242(1):84–89
158. Ehrich M, Nelson MR, Stanssens P et al (2005) Quantitative high-throughput analysis of DNA methylation patterns by base-specific cleavage and mass spectrometry. Proc Natl Acad Sci U S A 102(44):15785–15790
159. Zilberman D, Henikoff S (2007) Genome-wide analysis of DNA methylation patterns. Development 134(22):3959–3965
160. Kondo Y, Issa JP (2010) DNA methylation profiling in cancer. Expert Rev Mol Med 12:e23
161. Zuo T, Tycko B, Liu TM, Lin JJ, Huang TH (2009) Methods in DNA methylation profiling. Epigenomics 1(2):331–345
162. Walker BA, Wardell CP, Chiecchio L et al (2011) Aberrant global methylation patterns affect the molecular pathogenesis and prognosis of multiple myeloma. Blood 117(2):553–562
163. Amaral PP, Dinger ME, Mercer TR, Mattick JS (2008) The eukaryotic genome as an RNA machine. Science 319(5871):1787–1789

164. Tsai HC, Li H, Van Neste L et al (2012) Transient low doses of DNA-demethylating agents exert durable antitumor effects on hematological and epithelial tumor cells. Cancer Cell 21(3):430–446
165. Lister R, Pelizzola M, Dowen RH et al (2009) Human DNA methylomes at base resolution show widespread epigenomic differences. Nature 462(7271):315–322
166. Kim JH, Dhanasekaran SM, Prensner JR et al (2011) Deep sequencing reveals distinct patterns of DNA methylation in prostate cancer. Genome Res 21(7):1028–1041
167. Ordway JM, Bedell JA, Citek RW et al (2006) Comprehensive DNA methylation profiling in a human cancer genome identifies novel epigenetic targets. Carcinogenesis 27(12):2409–2423
168. Oda M, Glass JL, Thompson RF et al (2009) High-resolution genome-wide cytosine methylation profiling with simultaneous copy number analysis and optimization for limited cell numbers. Nucleic Acids Res 37(12):3829–3839
169. Ruike Y, Imanaka Y, Sato F, Shimizu K, Tsujimoto G (2010) Genome-wide analysis of aberrant methylation in human breast cancer cells using methyl-DNA immunoprecipitation combined with high-throughput sequencing. BMC Genomics 11:137. doi:10.1186/1471-2164-11-137
170. Cheung HH, Lee TL, Davis AJ, Taft DH, Rennert OM, Chan WY (2010) Genome-wide DNA methylation profiling reveals novel epigenetically regulated genes and non-coding RNAs in human testicular cancer. Br J Cancer 102(2):419–427
171. Bollati V, Fabris S, Pegoraro V et al (2009) Differential repetitive DNA methylation in multiple myeloma molecular subgroups. Carcinogenesis 30(8):1330–1335
172. Chen G, Wang Y, Huang H et al (2009) Combination of DNA methylation inhibitor 5-azacytidine and arsenic trioxide has synergistic activity in myeloma. Eur J Haematol 82(3):176–183
173. de Carvalho F, Colleoni GW, Almeida MS, Carvalho AL, Vettore AL (2009) TGFbetaR2 aberrant methylation is a potential prognostic marker and therapeutic target in multiple myeloma. Int J Cancer 125(8):1985–1991
174. Galm O, Yoshikawa H, Esteller M, Osieka R, Herman JG (2003) SOCS-1, a negative regulator of cytokine signaling, is frequently silenced by methylation in multiple myeloma. Blood 101(7):2784–2788
175. Hatzimichael E, Dranitsaris G, Dasoula A et al (2009) Von Hippel-Lindau methylation status in patients with multiple myeloma: a potential predictive factor for the development of bone disease. Clin Lymphoma Myeloma 9(3):239–242
176. Hodge DR, Peng B, Cherry JC et al (2005) Interleukin 6 supports the maintenance of p53 tumor suppressor gene promoter methylation. Cancer Res 65(11):4673–4682
177. Ng MH, Chung YF, Lo KW, Wickham NW, Lee JC, Huang DP (1997) Frequent hypermethylation of p16 and p15 genes in multiple myeloma. Blood 89(7):2500–2506
178. Seidl S, Ackermann J, Kaufmann H et al (2004) DNA-methylation analysis identifies the E-cadherin gene as a potential marker of disease progression in patients with monoclonal gammopathies. Cancer 100(12):2598–2606
179. Tshuikina M, Jernberg-Wiklund H, Nilsson K, Oberg F (2008) Epigenetic silencing of the interferon regulatory factor ICSBP/IRF8 in human multiple myeloma. Exp Hematol 36(12):1673–1681
180. Mateos MV, Garcia-Sanz R, Lopez-Perez R et al (2002) Methylation is an inactivating mechanism of the p16 gene in multiple myeloma associated with high plasma cell proliferation and short survival. Br J Haematol 118(4):1034–1040
181. Ribas C, Colleoni GW, Felix RS et al (2005) P16 gene methylation lacks correlation with angiogenesis and prognosis in multiple myeloma. Cancer Lett 222(2):247–254
182. Braggio E, Maiolino A, Gouveia ME et al (2010) Methylation status of nine tumor suppressor genes in multiple myeloma. Int J Hematol 91(1):87–96
183. Takada S, Morita K, Hayashi K et al (2005) Methylation status of fragile histidine triad (FHIT) gene and its clinical impact on prognosis of patients with multiple myeloma. Eur J Haematol 75(6):505–510
184. Sharma A, Heuck CJ, Fazzari MJ et al (2010) DNA methylation alterations in multiple myeloma as a model for epigenetic changes in cancer. Wiley Interdiscip Rev Syst Biol Med 2(6):654–669

185. Brookes AJ (1999) The essence of SNPs. Gene 234(2):177–186
186. Syvanen AC, Landegren U, Isaksson A, Gyllensten U, Brookes A (1999) First International SNP Meeting at Skokloster, Sweden, August 1998. Enthusiasm mixed with scepticism about single-nucleotide polymorphism markers for dissecting complex disorders. Eur J Hum Genet 7(1):98–101
187. Moreaux J, Reme T, Leonard W et al (2013) Gene expression-based prediction of myeloma cell sensitivity to histone deacetylase inhibitors. Br J Cancer 109(3):676–685
188. Moreaux J, Reme T, Leonard W et al (2012) Development of gene expression-based score to predict sensitivity of multiple myeloma cells to DNA methylation inhibitors. Mol Cancer Ther 11(12):2685–2692
189. Dick JE (2008) Stem cell concepts renew cancer research. Blood 112(13):4793–4807
190. Matsui W, Wang Q, Barber JP et al (2008) Clonogenic multiple myeloma progenitors, stem cell properties, and drug resistance. Cancer Res 68(1):190–197
191. Kalisky T, Quake SR (2011) Single-cell genomics. Nat Methods 8(4):311–314

Chapter 6
Targeting Mantle Cell Lymphoma with a Strategy of Combined Proteasome and Histone Deacetylase Inhibition

Michael Batalo*, Prithviraj Bose*, Beata Holkova, and Steven Grant

Abstract Although approved for over a decade, the clinical utility of proteasome inhibitors (PIs) remains largely restricted to the treatment of patients with multiple myeloma (MM) and mantle cell lymphoma (MCL). This has fueled interest in understanding mechanisms of resistance to their antineoplastic actions, leading to the development of new and improved PIs (e.g., carfilzomib, ixazomib, marizomib) and rational combinations with other novel classes of targeted agents. With respect to the latter, histone deacetylase inhibitors (HDACIs) represent one of the most extensively studied classes of agents. PIs and HDACIs interact at multiple levels to trigger synergistic cell killing in a variety of tumor types through multiple mechanisms, including induction of oxidative stress and DNA damage, PI-mediated inhibition of the cytoprotective NF-κB pathway activated by HDACIs, and promotion of proteotoxic stress through simultaneous proteasome inhibition and disruption of aggresome formation and chaperone proteins, leading to the accumulation of

---

*Author contributed equally with all other contributors.

M. Batalo
Department of Internal Medicine, Virginia Commonwealth University, Richmond, VA, USA

P. Bose • B. Holkova
Department of Internal Medicine, Virginia Commonwealth University, Richmond, VA, USA

Massey Cancer Center, Virginia Commonwealth University, Richmond, VA, USA

S. Grant, M.D. (✉)
Department of Internal Medicine, Virginia Commonwealth University, Richmond, VA, USA

Massey Cancer Center, Virginia Commonwealth University, Richmond, VA, USA

Department of Microbiology and Immunology, Virginia Commonwealth University, Richmond, VA, USA

Department of Biochemistry and Molecular Biology, Virginia Commonwealth University, Richmond, VA, USA

Department of Human and Molecular Genetics, Virginia Commonwealth University, Richmond, VA, USA

Institute of Molecular Medicine, Virginia Commonwealth University, Richmond, VA, USA
e-mail: stgrant@vcu.edu

Q.P. Dou (ed.), *Resistance to Proteasome Inhibitors in Cancer*, Resistance to Targeted Anti-Cancer Therapeutics, DOI 10.1007/978-3-319-06752-0_6

misfolded proteins. Clinically, this combination may be closest to regulatory approval in MM, but represents a promising avenue of investigation in MCL, a relatively uncommon but challenging disease that has been the focus of much recent attention given Food and Drug Administration approvals in 2013 for the immunomodulatory drug lenalidomide and the first-in-class Bruton's tyrosine kinase inhibitor, ibrutinib. In this chapter, we discuss the mechanisms of action of and interactions between PIs and HDACIs with an MCL focus and review the relevant preclinical and clinical data.

Keywords Mantle cell lymphoma • Proteasome inhibitor • Histone deacetylase inhibitor • Apoptosis • NF-κB • Aggresome • ER stress • Unfolded protein response • Hsp90 • Rational combinations • Targeted therapies • Clinical trials

Abbreviations

ABC	Activated B-cell
AML	Acute myeloid leukemia
ATM	Ataxia telangiectasia mutated
ATR	ATM and Rad3 related
BCR	B-cell receptor
BTK	Bruton's tyrosine kinase
CDK	Cyclin-dependent kinases
CDT1	Chromatin licensing and DNA replication factor-1
c-FLIP	Cellular FLICE-like inhibitory protein
CHOP	CAAT-/enhancer-binding protein homologous protein
CTCL	Cutaneous T-cell lymphoma
DDR	DNA damage response
DLBCL	Diffuse large B-cell lymphoma
DNMT1	DNA methyltransferase 1
DSB	Double-strand breaks
ER	Endoplasmic reticulum
ERK	Extracellular signal-regulated kinase
FL	Follicular lymphoma
FLICE	FADD-like IL-1β-converting enzyme
GC	Germinal center
GEP	Gene expression profiling
GSK3β	Glycogen synthase kinase-3-beta
HAT	Histone acetyl transferases
HDAC	Histone deacetylase
HDACI	Histone deacetylase inhibitor
HDM4	Human homolog of MDM4
Hsp90	Heat shock protein 90
IgVH	Immunoglobulin heavy chain variable region

IKK	IκB kinase
IκB	I kappa B
JAK	Janus kinase
JNK	Jun N-terminal kinase
MAPK	Mitogen-activated protein kinase
MCL	Mantle cell lymphoma
Mcl-1	Myeloid cell leukemia 1
MDM2	Murine double minute homolog 2
MIPI	Mantle cell lymphoma international prognostic index
MM	Multiple myeloma
mTOR	Mammalian target of rapamycin
NF-κB	Nuclear factor kappa B
NHEJ	Nonhomologous end joining
NHL	Non-Hodgkin lymphomas
ORR	Overall response rate
PERK	Protein kinase RNA-like ER kinase
PI	Proteasome inhibitor
PRDM1	PR domain zinc finger protein 1, Blimp1
Rb	Retinoblastoma protein
R-CHOP	Rituximab, cyclophosphamide, doxorubicin, vincristine prednisone
ROS	Reactive oxygen species
STAT	Signal transducer and activator of transcription
TTP	Time to progression
UPR	Unfolded protein response
UPS	Ubiquitin proteasome system
VEGF	Vascular endothelial growth factor
XIAP	X-linked inhibitor of apoptosis

6.1 Introduction

Comprising approximately 6 % of non-Hodgkin lymphomas (NHL), mantle cell lymphoma (MCL) represents a unique and difficult-to-treat mature B-cell neoplasm that shares features with both indolent and aggressive B-NHL [1]. Most patients present with advanced stages of disease, and extra-nodal, particularly bone marrow and gastrointestinal, involvement is common [2]. MCL is presently considered incurable and is generally characterized by aggressive behavior and high relapse rates that result in relatively short survival (median 5–7 years) despite initial responsiveness to conventional chemo-immunotherapy [1]. However, a subset of MCL, often associated with a low proliferative index, predominantly leukemic (non-nodal) presentation, low karyotypic complexity, hyper-mutated immunoglobulin heavy chain variable region (*IgVH*) genes, and absence of *SOX11* expression [1–4], frequently behaves in an indolent fashion. In these circumstances, observation may initially be appropriate for some patients [5]. MCL cells express CD20, surface

IgM/IgD, and the T-cell antigen CD5, and are usually negative for CD10, CD23 and Bcl-6 [2, 3]. The t(11;14)(q13;q32) translocation, leading to aberrant expression of cyclin D1, is the genetic hallmark of MCL [1, 2]. Treatment choices in MCL vary widely, and the mantle cell lymphoma international prognostic index (MIPI), with or without the Ki-67 proliferation index, may help inform therapeutic choices through improved risk stratification [2]. Recent advances in chemo-immunotherapy for this disease have included a role for rituximab maintenance in elderly patients, particularly following R-CHOP (rituximab, cyclophosphamide, doxorubicin, vincristine prednisone) [6], and the establishment of bendamustine plus rituximab as a preferred regimen over R-CHOP [7]. The US Food and Drug Administration (FDA) approval in 2006 of the first-in-class proteasome inhibitor (PI) bortezomib (Velcade®, Millennium) for relapsed MCL ushered in the era of molecularly targeted therapy for this disease [8]. More recently, the immunomodulatory drug lenalidomide (Revlimid®, Celgene) [9] and the first-in-class Bruton's tyrosine kinase (BTK) inhibitor ibrutinib (Imbruvica™, Janssen) [10] have received regulatory approval in the United States for relapsed/refractory MCL. Additionally, temsirolimus (Torisel®, Pfizer), a small-molecule inhibitor of mammalian target of rapamycin (mTOR), is approved in Europe [11]. Considering the central role of cyclin D1 in MCL pathogenesis, it is not surprising that PD0332991, a selective inhibitor of cyclin-dependent kinases (CDKs) 4 and 6, has shown promising activity in MCL [12]. Although histone deacetylase inhibitors (HDACIs) are not currently registered for the treatment of B-cell neoplasms and have limited single-agent activity, this class of agents interacts at multiple levels with PIs, and the mechanistic rationale for synergy, as well as the preclinical and clinical data supporting this combination of targeted agents, with a focus on MCL, will be reviewed in this chapter.

6.2 Pathogenesis of MCL

In addition to constitutive dysregulation of the cell cycle as a consequence of cyclin D1 overexpression resulting from the signature translocation event (t(11;14)(q13;q32)), a high degree of genetic instability, alterations in the DNA damage response (DDR) network, and activation of key survival pathways are integral to the pathogenesis of MCL [1, 3]. Cyclin D1 binds to CDKs 4 and 6 to phosphorylate the retinoblastoma protein (Rb), thus activating the E2F transcription factor and promoting S-phase entry through cyclin E/CDK2 activation [1, 3]. Additionally, cyclin D1/CDK4 complexes further promote cell cycle progression by binding the endogenous CDK inhibitor p27, thus removing its inhibitory influence on cyclin E/CDK2, and inhibiting the degradation of CDT1 (chromatin-licensing and DNA replication factor-1), the rate-limiting factor in DNA replication [1]. The latter phenomenon leads to increased numbers of DNA double-strand breaks (DSB) and activation of DDR checkpoints [1]. In S-phase, cyclin D1 is phosphorylated in a glycogen synthase kinase-3-beta (GSK3β)-dependent manner and undergoes proteasomal degradation [1]. Importantly, GSK3β is phosphorylated and inactivated by Akt and Wnt signaling, both key pathways in MCL pathogenesis [1, 3]. Cyclin D1 may also promote MCL cell survival by sequestering the proapoptotic protein Bax (itself a proteasomal substrate [13]) in the cytoplasm, potentiating the antiapoptotic function of Bcl-2 (B-cell lymphoma 2) [14]. Aside from cyclin D1 dysregulation, secondary genetic alterations in MCL frequently target the p16/CDK4/Rb, BMI1/ARF/MDM2 (murine double minute homolog 2), and ataxia telangiectasia mutated (ATM)/Chk1/Chk2 pathways, inactivating p53 and disrupting the DDR network [1, 3]. The phosphatidylinositol-3-kinase (PI3K)/Akt/mTOR, B-cell receptor (BCR), JAK/STAT (Janus kinase/signal transducer and activator of transcription), Wnt/β-catenin, and hedgehog pathways are activated in MCL [1, 3], and pharmacologic targeting of some of these pathways has been shown to be successful therapeutically [10, 11]. Constitutive nuclear factor kappa B (NF-κB) activation is a feature of MCL, with resultant overexpression of several target genes, such as those encoding the anti-apoptotic proteins Bcl-2, Bcl-xL, XIAP (X-linked inhibitor of apoptosis), and c-FLIP (cellular FLICE (FADD-like IL-1β-converting enzyme)-like inhibitory protein) [15–17]. The human homolog of MDM4 (HDM4) is overexpressed in MCL and, in addition to promoting proteasomal degradation of p21 and p53 in concert with HDM2, also inhibits p53-mediated transcriptional activation of p21 [18]. Interactions with the microenvironment are critical to the survival of MCL cells [19]. In the case of MM, expression of interleukin-6 (IL-6) in bone marrow stromal cells (BMSCs) induced by myeloma cell adhesion is an NF-κB-dependent process [20]. Finally, epigenetic silencing (through hypermethylation) as well as upregulation (via hypomethylation) of a number of genes is likely to play a pathogenetic role in MCL [21]. Oncogenic *c-myc* recruits histone deacetylases (HDACs) to repress key microRNAs in MCL and other B-NHLs, providing a target for histone modification in these diseases [22, 23].

6.3 The Proteasome and Proteasome Inhibitors

The intact 26S proteasome is the major site (~80 %) of protein degradation in eukaryotic cells, responsible primarily for degrading intracellular proteins [13, 24]. Present in both the nucleus and in the cytoplasm, it consists of a 20S cylindrical structure with a 19S regulatory "cap" at each end [24]. The β-subunits (β1, β2, and β5) of the 20S proteasome carry out the proteolytic activities of the organelle, which have been classified as "chymotrypsin-like," "trypsin-like," and "caspase-like" [13, 24]. Proteins marked for degradation are recognized by the proteasome by their polyubiquitin "tag," after which the tag is removed and the protein unfolded and linearized by an ATP-dependent mechanism, followed by entry into the catalytic central chamber (formed by the two inner rings of the cylinder composed of β-subunits; the α subunits form the top and bottom rings) of the 20S proteasome [24]. Proteins destined for proteasomal degradation become polyubiquitinated through the sequential action of ubiquitin-activating (E1), ubiquitin-conjugating (E2), and ubiquitin-ligating (E3) enzymes [24]. Among the multitude of proteasomal substrates are key cell cycle regulatory proteins, e.g., cyclins, the endogenous CDK inhibitors p21 and p27, and the CDC25 family of phosphatases; the tumor suppressor p53 (the negative regulator of p53, MDM2, is itself an E3 ubiquitin ligase that targets p53 for proteasomal degradation); several pro- and antiapoptotic proteins of the Bcl-2 family; oncoproteins such as c-fos, c-jun, and N-myc; and I kappa B (IκB), the inhibitor protein that maintains the transcription factor NF-κB in an inactivated state in the cytoplasm under normal conditions [13, 24]. In addition, cell adhesion molecules, stress response enzymes, proinflammatory cytokines, proangiogenic factors, and the unfolded protein response (UPR, reviewed in [25]) are some of the many cellular processes affected by proteasomal activity [13, 24].

Proteasome inhibition induces apoptosis in a wide range of tumor types, both hematologic [16, 26–31] and solid tumor malignancies [32–38]. While some studies have demonstrated marked apoptosis induction in proliferating but not in quiescent cells [28, 39], others have shown considerable activity against tumor types with low proliferative indices [30, 33]. In fact, in preclinical studies, the combination of the proteasome inhibitor MG-132 and idarubicin was shown to preferentially target acute myeloid leukemia (AML) stem cells while sparing normal stem cells [40], findings that served as the basis of a clinical trial of bortezomib and "7 + 3" in newly diagnosed patients with AML [41].

Mechanisms of PI lethality include stabilization of p21, p27, and p53 [35, 37, 38, 42]; of c-jun N-terminal kinase (JNK) [43–46], reactive oxygen species (ROS) generation [46–48], and inhibition of NF-κB activation [29, 49–51]; and of extracellular signal-regulated kinase (ERK) signaling [46, 52] and disruption of the UPR, thereby leading to endoplasmic reticulum (ER) stress [53–55], interference with tumor-microenvironment interactions [29], inhibition of DNA repair [56], upregulation/activation of proapoptotic Bcl-2 family proteins [44, 48, 57], downregulation of several antiapoptotic proteins [44], and antiangiogenic effects [36, 58–60], among others (Fig. 6.1). The complex regulation of apoptosis proteins in cancer cells by the ubiquitin proteasome system (UPS) has been reviewed [61]. Although long regarded as a central mechanism of PI lethality, the notion that PIs inhibit NF-κB activation in cancer cells has recently been called into question, at least in multiple myeloma (MM) [62] and to some extent also in MCL [63, 64]. In MM cells, it has been appreciated for some time that the effects of PIs cannot solely be ascribed to suppression of NF-κB activity, as inhibitors of IκB kinase (IKK) produce apoptosis to a significantly lesser degree [50]. However, it is clear that in certain tumor types characterized by constitutive activation of NF-κB, such as the activated B-cell (ABC) subtype of diffuse large B-cell lymphoma (DLBCL), bortezomib can significantly reverse resistance to chemotherapy [65]. The lethal effects of proteasome inhibition appear to be primarily confined to transformed cells [30, 42, 66], a somewhat unexpected finding that has been attributed to diminished tolerance of the accumulation of misfolded or damaged proteins in rapidly proliferating tumors, leading to elicitation of the UPR which, though initially cytoprotective, subsequently becomes proapoptotic [53, 67]; increased susceptibility to the stress imposed by proteasome inhibition in cancer cells with defective cell cycle checkpoints; and dependence of some tumors on proteasome-dependent NF-κB activation for survival [13, 24].

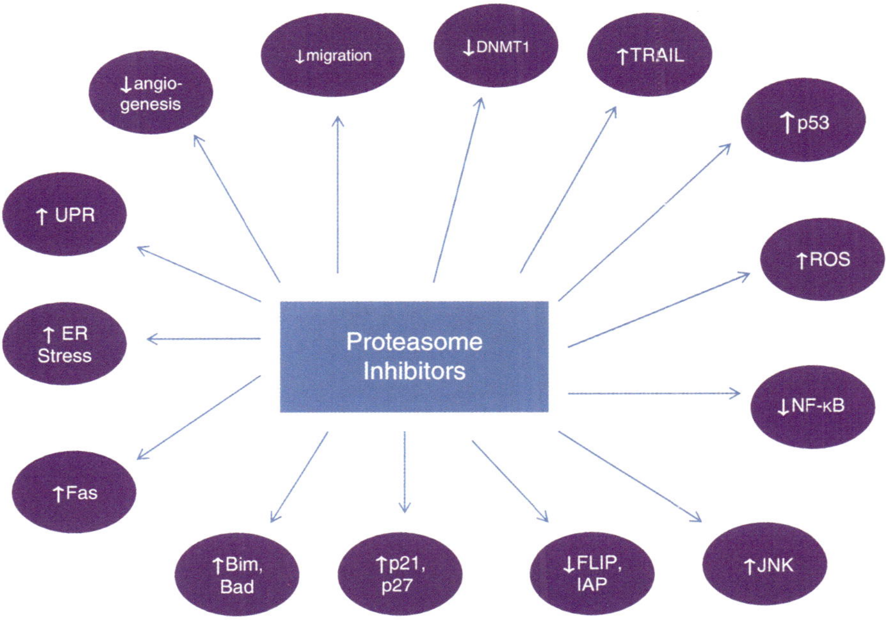

Fig. 6.1 Mechanisms of proteasome inhibitor lethality. *Bad* Bcl-2-associated death promoter, *Bim* Bcl-2-interacting mediator of cell death, *DNMT1* DNA methyltransferase 1, *ER* endoplasmic reticulum, *FLIP FLICE-like inhibitory protein*, *IAP* inhibitor of apoptosis, *JNK* c-Jun N-terminal kinase, *NF-κB* nuclear factor kappa B, *ROS* reactive oxygen species, *TRAIL TNF-related apoptosis-inducing ligand*, *UPR* unfolded protein response. Modified, with permission, from: Holkova B, Grant S. Proteasome inhibitors in mantle cell lymphoma. *Best Pract Res Clin Haematol.* 2012 Jun;25 (2):133-141. Epub 2012 May 16

Bortezomib (formerly PS-341) is a dipeptidyl boronic acid PI that was selected for further study after it demonstrated promising cytotoxic activity in an in vitro screen against a standard National Cancer Institute (NCI) panel of 60 human tumor cell lines [68]. It received first accelerated (in 2003) and then regular approval (in 2005) from the FDA for the treatment of relapsed/refractory MM based on substantial clinical efficacy in phase II and III trials [69, 70], providing proof of principle and validating the proteasome as a rational therapeutic target in cancer. The studies that led to FDA approval for bortezomib in 2006 for MCL [8] are summarized below. Importantly, PIs, and in particular bortezomib, sensitize cells from a variety of tumor types to the lethal effects of chemotherapy [29, 32, 45, 49, 71–74], monoclonal antibodies [31], glucocorticoids [75], and radiation [74, 76], in large part by blocking the effects of NF-κB activation, a physiologic response to cellular stress (reviewed in [77]) that leads to activation of transcription of genes for growth factors, stress response enzymes, cell adhesion molecules, and apoptosis inhibitors [78–80], although other mechanisms exist [45, 81]. In particular, the ability of PIs to phosphorylate and cleave the antiapoptotic protein Bcl-2 into proapoptotic fragments [34] and to inhibit the maturation of P-glycoprotein (multidrug resistance

(MDR) protein) [82, 83], an NF-κB-dependent process [84], exemplify the important role these agents can play in circumventing common mechanisms employed by tumors to acquire resistance to chemotherapy. In MM, these findings have been successfully translated to the clinic, and combination regimens involving bortezomib and conventional chemotherapeutic agents such as melphalan and pegylated liposomal doxorubicin are widely used in patients today [85, 86].

In 2012, the FDA granted accelerated approval to carfilzomib (Kyprolis™, Onyx, formerly PR-171), a cell-permeable tetrapeptide epoxyketone that irreversibly and selectively inhibits the chymotrypsin-like site of the proteasome, for the treatment of patients with relapsed/refractory MM [87]. Their large protein load makes MM cells particularly sensitive to proteasome inhibition [88]. Carfilzomib retains efficacy in patients with relapsed and/or refractory MM who have previously been treated with bortezomib [89]. A number of other PIs, some reversible and others irreversible, administered via oral or intravenous (IV) routes, are currently in various phases of development in an effort to overcome mechanisms of resistance to bortezomib inherent to the proteasome itself (reviewed in [90]).

6.4 Proteasome Inhibitors in MCL

Proteasome inhibition induces cell cycle arrest and apoptosis in MCL cells [26]. Increased proteasomal degradation of p27 is associated with decreased overall survival (OS) in MCL [91]. As noted above, MCL is characterized by constitutive activation of the NF-κB pathway [1, 3]. The ability of IKK inhibitors to induce apoptosis in MCL cells in vitro validated NF-κB as a therapeutic target in this disease [16, 17]. However, although initially believed to be the major mechanism of bortezomib-induced apoptosis in MCL, inhibition of the NF-κB pathway may not represent the predominant mechanism of PI lethality in this disease [63, 64]. Indeed, it has been demonstrated that bortezomib induces apoptosis in MCL cells through ROS generation and upregulation of the BH3-only proapoptotic protein Noxa, which displaces the apoptosis effector Bak from the antiapoptotic protein myeloid cell leukemia 1 (Mcl-1) [48, 92], potentially counteracting bortezomib-induced accumulation of the latter [93, 94]. In accordance with the E3 ligase function of HDM2, sequence-dependent synergistic, antiproliferative effects of inhibitors of the p53/HDM2 interaction and bortezomib in MCL cells have been observed [95]. Bortezomib also exhibits sequence-dependent synergism with cytarabine in MCL [96]. Constitutive activation of Akt and mTOR has distinct functional consequences in MCL cells, and their inhibition downregulates cyclin D1 via GSK3-mediated proteasomal degradation and causes nuclear accumulation of p27 [97]; additionally, proteasome inhibition leads to dephosphorylation and downregulation of protein expression of members of the Akt/mTOR pathway in MCL [98], arguing for the combination of PIs with inhibitors of the PI3K/Akt/mTOR pathway as a therapeutic strategy in MCL [99]. The transcriptional repressor PRDM1 (PR domain zinc finger protein 1, Blimp1) appears to be a key mediator of bortezomib activity in MCL [100].

Finally, constitutive and BCR-induced activation of STAT3 are important signaling pathways targeted by bortezomib in leukemic MCL [101].

In a phase II study of bortezomib in 26 patients with previously treated indolent B-NHL and MCL that included 11 patients with MCL, one patient with MCL achieved an unconfirmed complete response (CRu), four partial response (PR), and four stable disease (SD) [102]. Another phase II study reported a 41 % overall response rate (ORR) in 29 evaluable patients with relapsed or refractory MCL [103]. In the pivotal multicenter phase II PINNACLE trial, bortezomib produced a 33 % ORR in 141 assessable patients (out of 155 treated) with MCL and one to three prior therapies and exhibited a safety profile similar to that seen in patients with MM [104]. Median time to progression (TTP) was 6.7 months in the overall study population and 12.4 months in responding patients. Median OS was 23.5 months in the study population as a whole and 35.4 months in responders, with 1-year OS rates of 69 % and 91 %, respectively [105]. A smaller study conducted in Canada enrolled 29 patients with MCL, 13 of whom had not received prior chemotherapy [106]. There were 13 responders (46.4 %) to bortezomib, including one CRu, and the median duration of response (DOR) was 10 months [106]. Response rates were similar in previously untreated (46.2 %) and treated (46.7 %) patients [106]. In contrast, among 11 patients with MCL treated on two phase I trials of carfilzomib, only 1 responded (with a CRu) [107, 108]. The combination of bortezomib, bendamustine, and rituximab was investigated in a multicenter phase II study in 30 patients with relapsed or refractory indolent NHL and MCL ($n=7$) [109]. Of 29 patients evaluable for efficacy, the ORR was 83 %, with 51.7 % achieving a complete response (CR) [109]. With median follow-up of 24 months, 2-year progression-free survival (PFS) was 47 % [109].

6.5 HDACs and HDACIs

DNA (chromatin) is wrapped around histone octamers to form nucleosomes, and these histones can be reversibly modified in various ways in order to render DNA accessible to transcription factors, the best characterized of which is acetylation [110, 111]. Acetylation of histones is reciprocally regulated by histone acetyl transferases (HATs) and HDACs [110, 111]. Acetylation of positively charged N-terminal lysine residues in the histone tails interferes with their binding to negatively charged DNA, allowing a more open or relaxed chromatin configuration that favors gene transcription [110]. Conversely, deacetylation of histones favors compaction of chromatin, which is generally associated with gene silencing [110], although some genes can be downregulated by histone acetylation, depending on the cellular context [112]. HDACs, which are frequently dysregulated in cancer, represent the products of 18 genes, which can be subdivided into 4 classes [111]. Classes I (HDACs 1, 2, 3, and 8), II (HDACs 4, 5, 6, 7, 9, and 10), and IV (HDAC 11) are zinc-dependent enzymes, whereas the class III enzymes (sirtuins) are zinc independent but nicotinamide adenine dinucleotide (NAD) dependent [110].

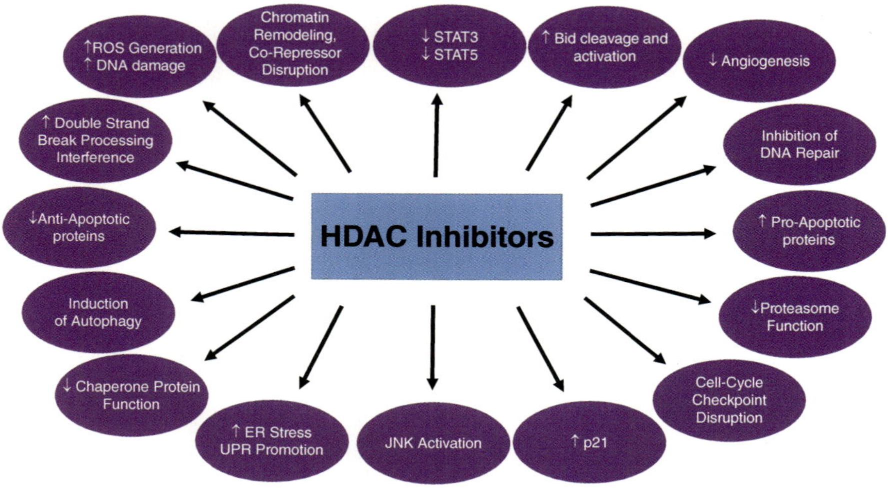

Fig. 6.2 Mechanisms of HDAC inhibitor lethality. *Bid* BH3-interacting domain death agonist, *ER* endoplasmic reticulum, *JNK* c-Jun N-terminal kinase, *ROS* reactive oxygen species, *STAT* signal transducer and activator of transcription, *UPR* unfolded protein response

The class IIb HDAC, HDAC6, is distinguished by its ability to deacetylate tubulin, which has important mechanistic implications related to disruption of aggresome formation and downregulation of chaperone proteins by HDAC6 inhibitors [110, 111]. Clinically relevant HDACIs represent different chemical classes, e.g., hydroxamic acids (vorinostat, dacinostat, panobinostat, belinostat), benzamides (entinostat, mocetinostat), and cyclic tetrapeptides (romidepsin) [110, 111]. Some of these (the hydroxamic acids) act as pan-HDACIs, whereas others predominantly target the class I (entinostat, mocetinostat) or class IIb (e.g., ACY-1215) enzymes [110, 111].

Although initially viewed as acting primarily as epigenetic agents, it has become increasingly apparent in recent years that HDACIs exert diverse cytotoxic actions, in large part owing to acetylation of a plethora of nonhistone proteins; indeed, determining which of their multiple mechanisms of lethality are primarily responsible for their antitumor activity and relative selectivity for transformed cells remains a formidable challenge [110, 111]. Key determinants of HDACI lethality (Fig. 6.2) include downregulation of antiapoptotic proteins such as caspase inhibitors (e.g., XIAP, survivin, and c-FLIP) [113–117], Bcl-w [117], and Mcl-1 (through reversal of microRNA silencing) [118]; upregulation of proapoptotic proteins such as Bim, Bmf, and Noxa (through acetylation of p53) [119–126]; activation of the death receptor pathway [127–129]; induction of Bid cleavage and activation [130–132]; induction of the endogenous CDK inhibitors p21 [117, 131, 133–136] and p16 [110]; ROS generation [117] and induction of DNA damage [132, 137–147]; and disruption of chaperone protein (in particular, heat shock protein 90 (Hsp90)) function (via acetylation) [148], an effect that has been attributed to HDAC6 inhibition [149].

This inhibition leads to Hsp70-mediated proteasomal degradation of Hsp90 "client" oncoproteins [150] and inhibition of DNA repair through acetylation of Ku70 [142, 151, 152]; downregulation of the DNA repair proteins Ku86, BRCA1, CHEK1, RAD50, RAD51, and MRE11 [142, 153]; interference with the S-phase checkpoint through loss of HDAC3 function [154]; disruption of both the homologous [155] and nonhomologous end-joining (NHEJ) [156] processes of DNA repair; and interference with HDAC-mediated coordination of ATR (ATM and Rad3-related) checkpoint function, DSB processing, and autophagy [157, 158]. The pleiotropic actions of HDACIs (Fig. 6.2) also include interference with the function of corepressors (e.g., Bcl-6 in DLBCL [159]) and cofactors (e.g., the NCOR1/SMRT axis, critical for maintaining chromatin structure and genomic stability [154, 160]); promotion of proteotoxic (UPR) and endoplasmic reticulum (ER) stress via disruption of aggresome formation via HDAC6 inhibition and acetylation of glucose-regulated protein 78 kDa (GRP78), a critical sensor of the ER stress response [134, 161–165], as well as through inhibition of class I HDACs [166]; disruption of cell cycle (especially mitotic spindle assembly) checkpoints [167–170], dysregulation of which is frequent in neoplastic cells; JNK activation [146, 147, 171, 172]; STAT5 and STAT3 inhibition [173–175]; interference with proteasome function [114, 176]; antiangiogenic effects [177, 178]; generation of the proapoptotic lipid second messenger ceramide [179]; and induction of autophagy, possibly through acetylation of the autophagy signaling component Atg3 [180]; however, autophagy induced by HDACIs can be cytoprotective [181, 182], as can induction of p21 by these agents [183], providing a basis for synergism with agents that block these phenomena [181–183]. The selective toxicity of HDACIs toward transformed cells may be explained in part by the ability of normal but not neoplastic cells to escape HDACI-induced oxidative injury by upregulating thioredoxin [139] and to repair HDACI-induced DNA damage [153] and by the activation of death receptor pathways in transformed cells [128, 129].

6.6 HDACIs in MCL

At present, the only two FDA-approved HDACIs, vorinostat (Zolinza®, Merck) and romidepsin (Istodax®, Celgene), are indicated for the treatment of patients with cutaneous or peripheral T-cell lymphoma (romidepsin) who have received one (romidepsin) or two (vorinostat) prior therapies [184]. However, several preclinical studies support investigation of this class of agents in MCL. Vorinostat suppresses the translation of cyclin D1 in MCL cells by inhibiting the PI3K/Akt/mTOR/eIF4E-BP pathway [185]. HDACIs upregulate p21 and p27, reduce vascular endothelial growth factor (VEGF) production, and induce growth suppression and apoptosis in human MCL cells [186]. In MCL cell lines and patient-derived cells, vorinostat caused caspase-dependent cell death by activating the mitochondrial pathway of apoptosis, as evidenced by Bax and Bak conformational changes, mitochondrial depolarization, and ROS generation, accompanied by histone H4 hyperacetylation on promoter regions and consequent transcriptional activation of genes for the proapoptotic BH3-only proteins Bim, Bmf, and Noxa [126]. Adhesion of MCL and other NHL cells to stromal cells triggers a c-Myc/miR-548m feed-forward loop, linking sustained c-Myc activation, miR-548m downregulation, and subsequent HDAC6 upregulation and stroma-mediated cell survival and lymphoma progression [187]. Furthermore, treatment with an HDAC6-selective inhibitor, both alone and in combination with a c-Myc inhibitor, enhanced cell death, abolished cell adhesion-mediated drug resistance, and suppressed clonogenicity and lymphoma growth in vitro and in vivo [187]. A phase I trial of vorinostat in Japanese patients with NHL provided a signal of activity in MCL and follicular lymphoma (FL) [188]. There were, however, no formal responders among nine patients with MCL in a phase II trial of vorinostat, although one patient maintained SD for 26 months [189]. Similarly, tumor shrinkage of between 43 and 49 % was reported after two cycles in two MCL patients participating in a phase I clinical trial of oral belinostat (J Clin Oncol 27:15 s, 2009 (suppl; abstr 8580).

6.7 Rationale for the Combination of PIs and HDACIs as a Therapeutic Strategy

In many respects, PIs and HDACIs have overlapping actions in malignant cells. These include stabilization/induction of endogenous CDK inhibitors, ROS generation, JNK activation, inhibition of DNA repair mechanisms, upregulation of pro-apoptotic proteins and downregulation of antiapoptotic proteins (the upregulation by PIs of the antiapoptotic protein, Mcl-1 is a notable exception), interference with tumor–microenvironment interactions, and antiangiogenic effects (see above sections). Given their pleiotropic actions and selectivity for transformed cells, it is not surprising that both these classes of agents lend themselves particularly well to rational combinatorial strategies with a large number of cytotoxic and targeted agents [111, 190]. However, for a number of reasons aside from the overlapping actions mentioned above, the combination of PIs and HDACIs has inherent appeal as in several instances, one of these classes of agents can counteract compensatory cellular survival mechanisms activated by the other. For example, it is well-established that HDACIs activate NF-κB, which diminishes the lethality of this class of agents [191, 192]. In human leukemia cells, this has been shown to stem from oxidative injury and induction of NF-κB by the atypical, inside-out ATM/NEMO (NF-κB essential modulator)/SUMOylation DNA damage pathway [143]. It had previously been shown that in leukemia cells, HDACI-induced NF-κB activation is associated with hyperacetylation and nuclear translocation of RelA/p65 [138]. Blockade of the latter events and of the inhibitory association of RelA/p65 with IκBα by an inhibitor of IκBα phosphorylation markedly potentiated HDACI-induced apoptosis through enhanced oxidative damage, JNK activation, and down-regulation of NF-κB-dependent antiapoptotic proteins [138]. Similar observations have been made in MM cells, where it has been demonstrated that IKKβ-mediated RelA phosphorylation promotes RelA acetylation, inducing NF-κB activation and limiting HDACI lethality [193]. These events could be blocked by either pan-IKK or IKKβ-selective inhibitors, resulting in marked apoptosis [193]. In AML cells, NF-κB inhibition can convert HDACI-induced cell cycle arrest and maturation into apoptosis [172, 194]. As PIs such as bortezomib, carfilzomib, and marizomib block IκBα degradation, inhibiting NF-κB activation and diminishing the expression of NF-κB target genes, they are expected to synergize with HDACIs in triggering apoptosis, and this has indeed proved to be the case in preclinical studies in MM [195, 196], CLL [122], MCL [147, 197, 198], DLBCL [146], cutaneous T-cell lymphoma (CTCL) [199], T-cell leukemia/lymphoma [200], AML/ALL [123, 201], and Bcr-Abl$^+$ [202] cells. In general, synergistic enhancement of apoptosis in these studies has been accompanied by abrogation of HDACI-mediated NF-κB activation; accumulation of phosphorylated IκBα; diminished hyperacetylation of RelA/p65; downregulation of antiapoptotic proteins (i.e., Bcl-2, Bcl-xL, Mcl-1, and XIAP); upregulation of the proapoptotic proteins Bim and Noxa; JNK and p38 mitogen-activated protein kinase (MAPK) activation; ERK1/2 and Akt inactivation; induction of p53, p21, and p27; cyclin D1 downregulation; ROS generation; and induction of DNA damage [122, 123, 146, 147, 195, 197–202]. Several of these observations have resulted in early-phase clinical trials [203–207]. The studies in MCL, both preclinical and clinical, are discussed in detail below.

Another major mechanism of synergy between PIs and HDACIs relates to simultaneous inhibition of proteasome function and disruption of aggresome formation, which leads to massive accumulation of polyubiquitinated proteins within the cell, and resultant increased cellular and ER stress and induction of apoptosis [29, 190, 208]. Aggresome formation is dependent on the interaction of HDAC6 with tubulin and dynein and is induced as a cytoprotective response to the increasing burden of misfolded proteins created by proteasome inhibition in cancer cells [190, 208]. Targeting HDAC6 with tubacin or panobinostat hyperacetylates α-tubulin and inhibits this interaction, inducing marked accumulation of ubiquitinated proteins and synergistically augmenting bortezomib-induced cytotoxicity through JNK and caspase activation in MM cells, including those adherent to BMSCs [162, 209]. These findings have been recapitulated in pancreatic cancer cells in vitro and in vivo but not in immortalized normal human pancreatic epithelial cells in vitro or in murine pancreatic epithelial cells in vivo, suggesting selectivity of this phenomenon for tumor cells [163]. Induction of ER stress and a terminal UPR in cancer cells is a well-established consequence of proteasome inhibition [45, 53, 55]. Acetylation of GRP78, a critical sensor of the ER stress response, by HDAC6 inhibitors diminishes its binding to the ER stress mediator PERK (protein kinase RNA-like ER kinase) and activates a lethal UPR in human breast cancer cells [165]. With respect to clinical development, the PI-HDACI concept has advanced furthest in MM [210]. In addition, a selective HDAC6 inhibitor, ACY-1215, has demonstrated promising anti-myeloma activity in combination with bortezomib at the preclinical level both in vitro and in vivo [211].

The chaperone protein Hsp90 is also deacetylated by the class IIB HDAC, HDAC6, and targeted inhibition of HDAC6 leads to acetylation of HSP90 and disruption of its chaperone function, resulting in polyubiquitination and depletion of pro-growth and pro-survival HSP90 client proteins such as Akt and c-Raf [149]. Depletion of HDAC6 sensitized human leukemia cells to proteasome inhibitors [149]. Interestingly, there is some evidence that similar downregulation of Hsp90 client proteins can be achieved by the class I selective HDACI entinostat [212]. Hsp inhibition may directly lead to induction of ER stress and the UPR and cell death [213]. However, the Hsp90 inhibitor IPI-504 has been reported to overcome resistance to bortezomib and synergistically induce apoptosis in MCL cells, both in vitro and in vivo, by provoking the dissociation of Hsp90/BiP complexes, leading to depletion of the pro-survival ER chaperone BiP/Grp78, inhibition of the UPR, and promotion of NOXA-mediated mitochondrial depolarization [214]. In MCL cells, panobinostat acetylates Hsp90 and depletes the levels of Hsp90 client proteins such as CDK4, c-Raf, and Akt and abrogates bortezomib-induced aggresome formation [164]. Panobinostat also induces a lethal UPR, associated with induction of CAAT-/enhancer-binding protein homologous protein (CHOP) [164]. Co-treatment with panobinostat increased bortezomib-induced expression of CHOP and Noxa, as well as increased bortezomib-induced UPR and apoptosis of cultured and primary MCL cells [164]. Blockade of Hsp27 has also been shown to overcome bortezomib resistance in lymphoma cells [215].

Preclinical studies in AML have demonstrated that abrogation of the Sp1/NF-κB complex by bortezomib causes transcriptional repression of the *DNMT1* (DNA methyltransferase 1) gene and downregulation of DNMT1 protein, which in turn induces global DNA hypomethylation in vitro and in vivo and re-expression of epigenetically silenced genes, adding epigenetic modification to the long list of possible mechanisms of action of this agent [216]. Dual epigenetic targeting using HDACIs and DNMT inhibitors has been a popular rational combination strategy in the targeted therapy of cancer [217, 218]. In human hepatoma cells but not in primary human hepatocytes, vorinostat induced the extrinsic apoptotic pathway and Bid cleavage, upregulation of Bim, and dephosphorylation and inactivation of Akt, and stimulated alternative splicing of the Bcl-X transcript with expression of the proapoptotic Bcl-Xs isoform, resulting in apoptosis induction via both the intrinsic and extrinsic pathways, and synergized with bortezomib [219]. Finally, in MM cells, it has been shown that bortezomib specifically downregulates the expression of class I HDACs [220], while the pan-HDACI dacinostat inhibits proteasome function [221], suggesting that at least in MM, PIs might themselves serve as HDACIs and vice versa [114]. Dysregulated proteasome activity has been identified as a contributor to the anticancer activity of HDACIs in a genome-wide loss-of-function screen [176] and HDACI-induced downregulation of genes encoding proteasome components specifically demonstrated by gene expression profiling (GEP) in NHL cell lines [222]. Figure 6.3 schematically depicts the many levels at which PIs and HDACIs interact to enhance each other's toxicity toward malignant cells.

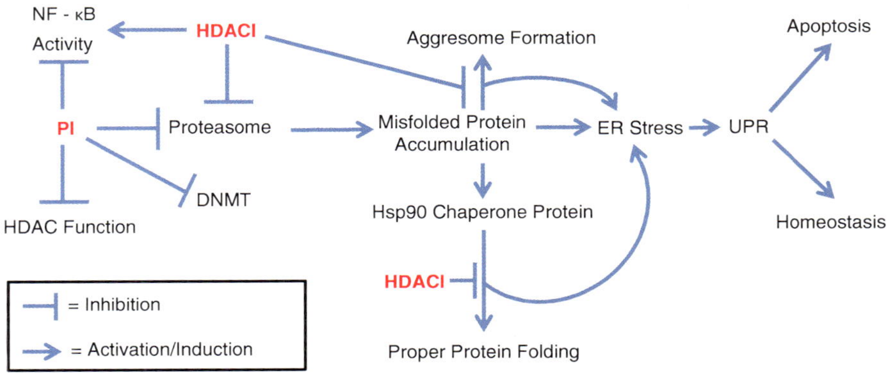

Fig. 6.3 Synergistic interactions between HDAC and proteasome inhibitors. HDAC inhibitors (HDACIs) and proteasome inhibitors (PIs) represent a rational drug combination in which synergism is mediated by multiple overlapping actions (not shown), as well as complementary, disabling activities that disable cellular safeguards and compensatory protective responses resulting from each drug's direct activities. HDACIs disrupt the compensatory effects of aggresome formation and Hsp90 chaperone function that guard against PI-induced misfolded protein accumulation. The latter event leads to increased ER stress and activation of the unfolded protein response (UPR), an adaptive cellular response to proteotoxic stress that beyond a certain point may promote cell death. PI and HDACI synergism could reflect potentiating the UPR past a critical point, culminating in apoptosis. PIs also block NF-κB, which can be activated by HDACIs and which limits HDACI lethality. PIs can inhibit DNMT, possibly recapitulating the established synergism between hypomethylating agents and HDACIs. Finally, PIs and HDACI can exert reciprocal actions, e.g., PIs may inhibit HDACs and HDACI inhibition may disrupt proteasome function. *DNMT* DNA methyltransferase, *ER* endoplasmic reticulum, *HDAC* histone deacetylase, *HDACI* histone deacetylase inhibitor, *Hsp90* heat shock protein 90, *NF-κB* nuclear factor kappa B, *PI* proteasome inhibitor, *UPR* unfolded protein response

6.8 PI-HDACI Combinations in MCL: Preclinical and Clinical Studies

Synergistic induction of apoptosis in MCL cells by the combination of vorinostat and bortezomib was first reported by Heider et al. [197]. In these studies, ROS generation was a major determinant of lethality, and marked reduction of proteasome activity, inhibition of NF-κB, and caspase [3, 8, 9] activation were documented, suggesting activation of both the intrinsic and extrinsic pathways of apoptosis [197]. Subsequently, both romidepsin and belinostat were demonstrated to synergize with bortezomib in MCL cell lines, whereas no significant apoptosis was observed in peripheral blood mononuclear cells (PBMCs) from healthy donors with the combination [198]. These events were associated with a decrease in cyclin D1 and Bcl-xL and accumulation of acetylated histone H3, acetylated α-tubulin, and Noxa in the MCL cell lines [198].

Similar effects were observed using the antihistamine cyproheptadine, which acts as an HDACI in this context [223]. As discussed above, panobinostat induced Hsp90 acetylation and downregulation of Hsp90 client proteins CDK4, c-Raf, and Akt in human, cultured, and primary MCL cells, as well as disruption of bortezomib-induced aggresome formation, triggering a lethal UPR in these cells [164]. Panobinostat potentiated bortezomib-induced expression of Noxa and CHOP, as well as the UPR and apoptosis in this setting [164]. Most recently, the second generation, irreversible PI carfilzomib has also been shown to interact synergistically with both vorinostat and entinostat in MCL cells in vitro and in vivo [147]. Striking synergism was observed, even at marginally toxic concentrations of both carfilzomib and the HDACIs, and activity was observed in bortezomib-resistant MCL cells [147]. Enhanced lethality was associated with JNK activation, increased DNA damage, ERK1/2 and Akt inactivation, and a marked increase in ROS generation [147]. Very similar findings were reported with these regimens in both germinal center (GC)- and ABC-subtype DLBCL cells and in a murine xenograft model [146]. The combination of carfilzomib and vorinostat only minimally affected normal $CD34^+$ hematopoietic cells, while retaining dramatic efficacy against bortezomib-resistant GC- and ABC-subtype DLBCL cells [146]. Strongly synergistic induction of ROS- and caspase-dependent apoptosis was observed in all NHL cell lines tested in preclinical studies of the combination of bortezomib and the broad spectrum HDACI PCI-24781 [222]. The PCI-24781-bortezomib combination resulted in increased caspase cleavage, mitochondrial depolarization, and histone acetylation compared with either agent alone [222]. GEP showed that PCI-24781 alone significantly downregulated several antioxidant genes, proteasome components, and NF-κB pathway genes, effects that were enhanced further by bortezomib [222].

A phase I clinical trial (NCT01276717) of carfilzomib and vorinostat in patients with relapsed/refractory B-NHLs has recently completed accrual, and preliminary results were presented at the 2013 annual meeting of the American Society of Hematology [207]. Of 20 treated patients, 10 had MCL. The combination was found to be reasonably tolerable in a heavily pretreated patient population, and the recommended phase II doses of vorinostat were 100 or 200 mg twice daily, depending on whether or not carfilzomib dosing was escalated from 20 to 27 mg/m^2 in cycle 2 (as currently FDA-approved) [207]. NCT00703664 is an ongoing phase II clinical trial of bortezomib and vorinostat in treatment-naïve or previously treated patients with MCL and patients with DLBCL who have received at least one prior systemic therapy. Currently, prior exposure to bortezomib is not allowed in either cohort in this trial, which uses a Simon 2-stage design. Preliminary results from this trial were presented at the 2011 annual meeting of the American Society of Hematology [205]. The cohort of bortezomib-exposed MCL patients was closed early, owing to limited accrual [205]. At the time of presentation, the ORR in the MCL cohort was 47 % and that in the DLBCL cohort was 12 %, allowing both cohorts to proceed to stage 2 of enrollment [205].

6.9 Conclusion

The number of possible rational combinations of targeted agents involving PIs or HDACIs is extremely large. As reviewed in this chapter, the combination of PIs with HDACIs is based on a sound theoretical foundation and appears particularly promising in MM and in MCL. However, of the many other rational combinations possible, a few deserve mention. For example, the CDK inhibitors, particularly pan-CDK inhibitors such as flavopiridol (alvocidib), interact synergistically with both PIs (e.g., bortezomib) [224] and HDACIs (e.g., vorinostat) [115, 183], including in MCL [225]. These findings have led to several clinical trials in a number of hematologic malignancies, including MCL [226–228]. Combinatorial drug screening has identified synergistic co-targeting of BTK and the proteasome in MCL [229]. Indeed, the BTK inhibitor ibrutinib was recently shown to synergistically increase bortezomib lethality in DLBCL and MCL cells sensitive or resistant to bortezomib [230]. Finally, a particularly promising combination in MCL is that of PIs with BH3 mimetics [231, 232], although thus far, evidence of clinical efficacy is limited to obatoclax [233] and navitoclax [234], neither of which is currently in development. Additionally, this class of agents also synergizes with HDACIs [121, 235]. These topics are outside the scope of the present chapter and are therefore not discussed here.

Acknowledgements This work was supported in part by the following awards to Dr. Grant: R01 CA167708-01A1 and R01 CA100866-09 from the National Institutes of Health, an award from the Leukemia and Lymphoma Society, and an award from Onyx Pharmaceuticals, Inc.

References

1. Perez-Galan P, Dreyling M, Wiestner A (2011) Mantle cell lymphoma: biology, pathogenesis, and the molecular basis of treatment in the genomic era. Blood 117:26–38
2. Vose JM (2013) Mantle cell lymphoma: 2013 update on diagnosis, risk-stratification, and clinical management. Am J Hematol 88:1082–1088
3. Jares P, Colomer D, Campo E (2012) Molecular pathogenesis of mantle cell lymphoma. J Clin Invest 122:3416–3423
4. Navarro A, Clot G, Royo C, Jares P, Hadzidimitriou A, Agathangelidis A, Bikos V, Darzentas N, Papadaki T, Salaverria I et al (2012) Molecular subsets of mantle cell lymphoma defined by the IGHV mutational status and SOX11 expression have distinct biologic and clinical features. Cancer Res 72:5307–5316
5. Martin P, Chadburn A, Christos P, Weil K, Furman RR, Ruan J, Elstrom R, Niesvizky R, Ely S, Diliberto M et al (2009) Outcome of deferred initial therapy in mantle-cell lymphoma. J Clin Oncol 27:1209–1213
6. Kluin-Nelemans HC, Hoster E, Hermine O, Walewski J, Trneny M, Geisler CH, Stilgenbauer S, Thieblemont C, Vehling-Kaiser U, Doorduijn JK et al (2012) Treatment of older patients with mantle-cell lymphoma. N Engl J Med 367:520–531
7. Rummel MJ, Niederle N, Maschmeyer G, Banat GA, von Grunhagen U, Losem C, Kofahl-Krause D, Heil G, Welslau M, Balser C et al (2013) Bendamustine plus rituximab versus CHOP plus rituximab as first-line treatment for patients with indolent and mantle-cell lymphomas: an open-label, multicentre, randomised, phase 3 non-inferiority trial. Lancet 381:1203–1210

8. Kane RC, Dagher R, Farrell A, Ko CW, Sridhara R, Justice R, Pazdur R (2007) Bortezomib for the treatment of mantle cell lymphoma. Clin Cancer Res 13:5291–5294
9. Goy A, Sinha R, Williams ME, Kalayoglu Besisik S, Drach J, Ramchandren R, Zhang L, Cicero S, Fu T, Witzig TE (2013) Single-agent lenalidomide in patients with mantle-cell lymphoma who relapsed or progressed after or were refractory to bortezomib: phase II MCL-001 (EMERGE) study. J Clin Oncol 31:3688–3695
10. Wang ML, Rule S, Martin P, Goy A, Auer R, Kahl BS, Jurczak W, Advani RH, Romaguera JE, Williams ME et al (2013) Targeting BTK with ibrutinib in relapsed or refractory mantle-cell lymphoma. N Engl J Med 369:507–516
11. Hess G, Herbrecht R, Romaguera J, Verhoef G, Crump M, Gisselbrecht C, Laurell A, Offner F, Strahs A, Berkenblit A et al (2009) Phase III study to evaluate temsirolimus compared with investigator's choice therapy for the treatment of relapsed or refractory mantle cell lymphoma. J Clin Oncol 27:3822–3829
12. Leonard JP, LaCasce AS, Smith MR, Noy A, Chirieac LR, Rodig SJ, Yu JQ, Vallabhajosula S, Schoder H, English P et al (2012) Selective CDK4/6 inhibition with tumor responses by PD0332991 in patients with mantle cell lymphoma. Blood 119:4597–4607
13. Adams J (2004) The development of proteasome inhibitors as anticancer drugs. Cancer Cell 5:417–421
14. Beltran E, Fresquet V, Martinez-Useros J, Richter-Larrea JA, Sagardoy A, Sesma I, Almada LL, Montes-Moreno S, Siebert R, Gesk S et al (2011) A cyclin-D1 interaction with BAX underlies its oncogenic role and potential as a therapeutic target in mantle cell lymphoma. Proc Natl Acad Sci U S A 108:12461–12466
15. Martinez N, Camacho FI, Algara P, Rodriguez A, Dopazo A, Ruiz-Ballesteros E, Martin P, Martinez-Climent JA, Garcia-Conde J, Menarguez J et al (2003) The molecular signature of mantle cell lymphoma reveals multiple signals favoring cell survival. Cancer Res 63:8226–8232
16. Pham LV, Tamayo AT, Yoshimura LC, Lo P, Ford RJ (2003) Inhibition of constitutive NF-kappa B activation in mantle cell lymphoma B cells leads to induction of cell cycle arrest and apoptosis. J Immunol 171:88–95
17. Roue G, Perez-Galan P, Lopez-Guerra M, Villamor N, Campo E, Colomer D (2007) Selective inhibition of IkappaB kinase sensitizes mantle cell lymphoma B cells to TRAIL by decreasing cellular FLIP level. J Immunol 178:1923–1930
18. Liang M, Han X, Vadhan-Raj S, Nguyen M, Zhang YH, Fernandez M, Drakos E, Konoplev SN, Yin CC, Miranda RN et al (2010) HDM4 is overexpressed in mantle cell lymphoma and its inhibition induces p21 expression and apoptosis. Mod Pathol 23:381–391
19. Kurtova AV, Tamayo AT, Ford RJ, Burger JA (2009) Mantle cell lymphoma cells express high levels of CXCR4, CXCR5, and VLA-4 (CD49d): importance for interactions with the stromal microenvironment and specific targeting. Blood 113:4604–4613
20. Chauhan D, Uchiyama H, Akbarali Y, Urashima M, Yamamoto K, Libermann TA, Anderson KC (1996) Multiple myeloma cell adhesion-induced interleukin-6 expression in bone marrow stromal cells involves activation of NF-kappa B. Blood 87:1104–1112
21. Leshchenko VV, Kuo PY, Shaknovich R, Yang DT, Gellen T, Petrich A, Yu Y, Remache Y, Weniger MA, Rafiq S et al (2010) Genome wide DNA methylation analysis reveals novel targets for drug development in mantle cell lymphoma. Blood 116:1025–1034
22. Zhang X, Chen X, Lin J, Lwin T, Wright G, Moscinski LC, Dalton WS, Seto E, Wright K, Sotomayor E et al (2012) Myc represses miR-15a/miR-16-1 expression through recruitment of HDAC3 in mantle cell and other non-Hodgkin B-cell lymphomas. Oncogene 31:3002–3008
23. Zhang X, Zhao X, Fiskus W, Lin J, Lwin T, Rao R, Zhang Y, Chan JC, Fu K, Marquez VE et al (2012) Coordinated silencing of MYC-mediated miR-29 by HDAC3 and EZH2 as a therapeutic target of histone modification in aggressive B-Cell lymphomas. Cancer Cell 22:506–523
24. Adams J (2004) The proteasome: a suitable antineoplastic target. Nat Rev Cancer 4:349–360
25. Walter P, Ron D (2011) The unfolded protein response: from stress pathway to homeostatic regulation. Science 334:1081–1086

26. Bogner C, Ringshausen I, Schneller F, Fend F, Quintanilla-Martinez L, Hacker G, Goetze K, Oostendorp R, Peschel C, Decker T (2003) Inhibition of the proteasome induces cell cycle arrest and apoptosis in mantle cell lymphoma cells. Br J Haematol 122:260–268
27. Bogner C, Schneller F, Hipp S, Ringshausen I, Peschel C, Decker T (2003) Cycling B-CLL cells are highly susceptible to inhibition of the proteasome: involvement of p27, early D-type cyclins, Bax, and caspase-dependent and -independent pathways. Exp Hematol 31:218–225
28. Drexler HC (1997) Activation of the cell death program by inhibition of proteasome function. Proc Natl Acad Sci U S A 94:855–860
29. Hideshima T, Richardson P, Chauhan D, Palombella VJ, Elliott PJ, Adams J, Anderson KC (2001) The proteasome inhibitor PS-341 inhibits growth, induces apoptosis, and overcomes drug resistance in human multiple myeloma cells. Cancer Res 61:3071–3076
30. Masdehors P, Merle-Beral H, Maloum K, Omura S, Magdelenat H, Delic J (2000) Deregulation of the ubiquitin system and p53 proteolysis modify the apoptotic response in B-CLL lymphocytes. Blood 96:269–274
31. Tan C, Waldmann TA (2002) Proteasome inhibitor PS-341, a potential therapeutic agent for adult T-cell leukemia. Cancer Res 62:1083–1086
32. Bold RJ, Virudachalam S, McConkey DJ (2001) Chemosensitization of pancreatic cancer by inhibition of the 26S proteasome. J Surg Res 100:11–17
33. Frankel A, Man S, Elliott P, Adams J, Kerbel RS (2000) Lack of multicellular drug resistance observed in human ovarian and prostate carcinoma treated with the proteasome inhibitor PS-341. Clin Cancer Res 6:3719–3728
34. Ling YH, Liebes L, Ng B, Buckley M, Elliott PJ, Adams J, Jiang JD, Muggia FM, Perez-Soler R (2002) PS-341, a novel proteasome inhibitor, induces Bcl-2 phosphorylation and cleavage in association with G2-M phase arrest and apoptosis. Mol Cancer Ther 1: 841–849
35. Shah SA, Potter MW, McDade TP, Ricciardi R, Perugini RA, Elliott PJ, Adams J, Callery MP (2001) 26S proteasome inhibition induces apoptosis and limits growth of human pancreatic cancer. J Cell Biochem 82:110–122
36. Sunwoo JB, Chen Z, Dong G, Yeh N, Crowl Bancroft C, Sausville E, Adams J, Elliott P, Van Waes C (2001) Novel proteasome inhibitor PS-341 inhibits activation of nuclear factor-kappa B, cell survival, tumor growth, and angiogenesis in squamous cell carcinoma. Clin Cancer Res 7:1419–1428
37. MacLaren AP, Chapman RS, Wyllie AH, Watson CJ (2001) P53-dependent apoptosis induced by proteasome inhibition in mammary epithelial cells. Cell Death Differ 8:210–218
38. Kudo Y, Takata T, Ogawa I, Kaneda T, Sato S, Takekoshi T, Zhao M, Miyauchi M, Nikai H (2000) p27Kip1 accumulation by inhibition of proteasome function induces apoptosis in oral squamous cell carcinoma cells. Clin Cancer Res 6:916–923
39. Drexler HC, Risau W, Konerding MA (2000) Inhibition of proteasome function induces programmed cell death in proliferating endothelial cells. FASEB J 14:65–77
40. Guzman ML, Swiderski CF, Howard DS, Grimes BA, Rossi RM, Szilvassy SJ, Jordan CT (2002) Preferential induction of apoptosis for primary human leukemic stem cells. Proc Natl Acad Sci U S A 99:16220–16225
41. Attar EC, Johnson JL, Amrein PC, Lozanski G, Wadleigh M, DeAngelo DJ, Kolitz JE, Powell BL, Voorhees P, Wang ES et al (2013) Bortezomib added to daunorubicin and cytarabine during induction therapy and to intermediate-dose cytarabine for consolidation in patients with previously untreated acute myeloid leukemia age 60 to 75 years: CALGB (Alliance) study 10502. J Clin Oncol 31:923–929
42. An B, Goldfarb RH, Siman R, Dou QP (1998) Novel dipeptidyl proteasome inhibitors overcome Bcl-2 protective function and selectively accumulate the cyclin-dependent kinase inhibitor p27 and induce apoptosis in transformed, but not normal, human fibroblasts. Cell Death Differ 5:1062–1075
43. Hideshima T, Mitsiades C, Akiyama M, Hayashi T, Chauhan D, Richardson P, Schlossman R, Podar K, Munshi NC, Mitsiades N et al (2003) Molecular mechanisms mediating antimyeloma activity of proteasome inhibitor PS-341. Blood 101:1530–1534

44. Mitsiades N, Mitsiades CS, Poulaki V, Chauhan D, Fanourakis G, Gu X, Bailey C, Joseph M, Libermann TA, Treon SP et al (2002) Molecular sequelae of proteasome inhibition in human multiple myeloma cells. Proc Natl Acad Sci U S A 99:14374–14379
45. Nawrocki ST, Carew JS, Pino MS, Highshaw RA, Dunner K Jr, Huang P, Abbruzzese JL, McConkey DJ (2005) Bortezomib sensitizes pancreatic cancer cells to endoplasmic reticulum stress-mediated apoptosis. Cancer Res 65:11658–11666
46. Yu C, Rahmani M, Dent P, Grant S (2004) The hierarchical relationship between MAPK signaling and ROS generation in human leukemia cells undergoing apoptosis in response to the proteasome inhibitor Bortezomib. Exp Cell Res 295:555–566
47. Ling YH, Liebes L, Zou Y, Perez-Soler R (2003) Reactive oxygen species generation and mitochondrial dysfunction in the apoptotic response to Bortezomib, a novel proteasome inhibitor, in human H460 non-small cell lung cancer cells. J Biol Chem 278:33714–33723
48. Perez-Galan P, Roue G, Villamor N, Montserrat E, Campo E, Colomer D (2006) The proteasome inhibitor bortezomib induces apoptosis in mantle-cell lymphoma through generation of ROS and Noxa activation independent of p53 status. Blood 107:257–264
49. Cusack JC Jr, Liu R, Houston M, Abendroth K, Elliott PJ, Adams J, Baldwin AS Jr (2001) Enhanced chemosensitivity to CPT-11 with proteasome inhibitor PS-341: implications for systemic nuclear factor-kappaB inhibition. Cancer Res 61:3535–3540
50. Hideshima T, Chauhan D, Richardson P, Mitsiades C, Mitsiades N, Hayashi T, Munshi N, Dang L, Castro A, Palombella V et al (2002) NF-kappa B as a therapeutic target in multiple myeloma. J Biol Chem 277:16639–16647
51. Jeremias I, Kupatt C, Baumann B, Herr I, Wirth T, Debatin KM (1998) Inhibition of nuclear factor kappaB activation attenuates apoptosis resistance in lymphoid cells. Blood 91:4624–4631
52. Orlowski RZ, Small GW, Shi YY (2002) Evidence that inhibition of p44/42 mitogen-activated protein kinase signaling is a factor in proteasome inhibitor-mediated apoptosis. J Biol Chem 277:27864–27871
53. Obeng EA, Carlson LM, Gutman DM, Harrington WJ Jr, Lee KP, Boise LH (2006) Proteasome inhibitors induce a terminal unfolded protein response in multiple myeloma cells. Blood 107:4907–4916
54. Lee AH, Iwakoshi NN, Anderson KC, Glimcher LH (2003) Proteasome inhibitors disrupt the unfolded protein response in myeloma cells. Proc Natl Acad Sci U S A 100:9946–9951
55. Nawrocki ST, Carew JS, Dunner K Jr, Boise LH, Chiao PJ, Huang P, Abbruzzese JL, McConkey DJ (2005) Bortezomib inhibits PKR-like endoplasmic reticulum (ER) kinase and induces apoptosis via ER stress in human pancreatic cancer cells. Cancer Res 65: 11510–11519
56. Vaziri SA, Hill J, Chikamori K, Grabowski DR, Takigawa N, Chawla-Sarkar M, Rybicki LR, Gudkov AV, Mekhail T, Bukowski RM et al (2005) Sensitization of DNA damage-induced apoptosis by the proteasome inhibitor PS-341 is p53 dependent and involves target proteins 14-3-3sigma and survivin. Mol Cancer Ther 4:1880–1890
57. Luciano F, Jacquel A, Colosetti P, Herrant M, Cagnol S, Pages G, Auberger P (2003) Phosphorylation of Bim-EL by Erk1/2 on serine 69 promotes its degradation via the proteasome pathway and regulates its proapoptotic function. Oncogene 22:6785–6793
58. Roccaro AM, Hideshima T, Raje N, Kumar S, Ishitsuka K, Yasui H, Shiraishi N, Ribatti D, Nico B, Vacca A et al (2006) Bortezomib mediates antiangiogenesis in multiple myeloma via direct and indirect effects on endothelial cells. Cancer Res 66:184–191
59. LeBlanc R, Catley LP, Hideshima T, Lentzsch S, Mitsiades CS, Mitsiades N, Neuberg D, Goloubeva O, Pien CS, Adams J et al (2002) Proteasome inhibitor PS-341 inhibits human myeloma cell growth in vivo and prolongs survival in a murine model. Cancer Res 62: 4996–5000
60. Williams S, Pettaway C, Song R, Papandreou C, Logothetis C, McConkey DJ (2003) Differential effects of the proteasome inhibitor bortezomib on apoptosis and angiogenesis in human prostate tumor xenografts. Mol Cancer Ther 2:835–843
61. Zhang HG, Wang J, Yang X, Hsu HC, Mountz JD (2004) Regulation of apoptosis proteins in cancer cells by ubiquitin. Oncogene 23:2009–2015

62. Hideshima T, Ikeda H, Chauhan D, Okawa Y, Raje N, Podar K, Mitsiades C, Munshi NC, Richardson PG, Carrasco RD et al (2009) Bortezomib induces canonical nuclear factor-kappaB activation in multiple myeloma cells. Blood 114:1046–1052
63. Yang DT, Young KH, Kahl BS, Markovina S, Miyamoto S (2008) Prevalence of bortezomib-resistant constitutive NF-kappaB activity in mantle cell lymphoma. Mol Cancer 7:40
64. Rizzatti EG, Mora-Jensen H, Weniger MA, Gibellini F, Lee E, Daibata M, Lai R, Wiestner A (2008) Noxa mediates bortezomib induced apoptosis in both sensitive and intrinsically resistant mantle cell lymphoma cells and this effect is independent of constitutive activity of the AKT and NF-kappaB pathways. Leuk Lymphoma 49:798–808
65. Dunleavy K, Pittaluga S, Czuczman MS, Dave SS, Wright G, Grant N, Shovlin M, Jaffe ES, Janik JE, Staudt LM et al (2009) Differential efficacy of bortezomib plus chemotherapy within molecular subtypes of diffuse large B-cell lymphoma. Blood 113:6069–6076
66. Orlowski RZ, Eswara JR, Lafond-Walker A, Grever MR, Orlowski M, Dang CV (1998) Tumor growth inhibition induced in a murine model of human Burkitt's lymphoma by a proteasome inhibitor. Cancer Res 58:4342–4348
67. Lin JH, Li H, Yasumura D, Cohen HR, Zhang C, Panning B, Shokat KM, Lavail MM, Walter P (2007) IRE1 signaling affects cell fate during the unfolded protein response. Science 318:944–949
68. Adams J, Palombella VJ, Sausville EA, Johnson J, Destree A, Lazarus DD, Maas J, Pien CS, Prakash S, Elliott PJ (1999) Proteasome inhibitors: a novel class of potent and effective antitumor agents. Cancer Res 59:2615–2622
69. Richardson PG, Barlogie B, Berenson J, Singhal S, Jagannath S, Irwin D, Rajkumar SV, Srkalovic G, Alsina M, Alexanian R et al (2003) A phase 2 study of bortezomib in relapsed, refractory myeloma. N Engl J Med 348:2609–2617
70. Richardson PG, Sonneveld P, Schuster MW, Irwin D, Stadtmauer EA, Facon T, Harousseau JL, Ben-Yehuda D, Lonial S, Goldschmidt H et al (2005) Bortezomib or high-dose dexamethasone for relapsed multiple myeloma. N Engl J Med 352:2487–2498
71. Ma MH, Yang HH, Parker K, Manyak S, Friedman JM, Altamirano C, Wu ZQ, Borad MJ, Frantzen M, Roussos E et al (2003) The proteasome inhibitor PS-341 markedly enhances sensitivity of multiple myeloma tumor cells to chemotherapeutic agents. Clin Cancer Res 9:1136–1144
72. Mitsiades N, Mitsiades CS, Richardson PG, Poulaki V, Tai YT, Chauhan D, Fanourakis G, Gu X, Bailey C, Joseph M et al (2003) The proteasome inhibitor PS-341 potentiates sensitivity of multiple myeloma cells to conventional chemotherapeutic agents: therapeutic applications. Blood 101:2377–2380
73. Ogiso Y, Tomida A, Lei S, Omura S, Tsuruo T (2000) Proteasome inhibition circumvents solid tumor resistance to topoisomerase II-directed drugs. Cancer Res 60:2429–2434
74. Teicher BA, Ara G, Herbst R, Palombella VJ, Adams J (1999) The proteasome inhibitor PS-341 in cancer therapy. Clin Cancer Res 5:2638–2645
75. Chandra J, Niemer I, Gilbreath J, Kliche KO, Andreeff M, Freireich EJ, Keating M, McConkey DJ (1998) Proteasome inhibitors induce apoptosis in glucocorticoid-resistant chronic lymphocytic leukemic lymphocytes. Blood 92:4220–4229
76. Russo SM, Tepper JE, Baldwin AS Jr, Liu R, Adams J, Elliott P, Cusack JC Jr (2001) Enhancement of radiosensitivity by proteasome inhibition: implications for a role of NF-kappaB. Int J Radiat Oncol Biol Phys 50:183–193
77. Karin M (2006) Nuclear factor-kappaB in cancer development and progression. Nature 441:431–436
78. Wang CY, Mayo MW, Baldwin AS Jr (1996) TNF- and cancer therapy-induced apoptosis: potentiation by inhibition of NF-kappaB. Science 274:784–787
79. Wang CY, Mayo MW, Korneluk RG, Goeddel DV, Baldwin AS Jr (1998) NF-kappaB antiapoptosis: induction of TRAF1 and TRAF2 and c-IAP1 and c-IAP2 to suppress caspase-8 activation. Science 281:1680–1683
80. Wang CY, Cusack JC Jr, Liu R, Baldwin AS Jr (1999) Control of inducible chemoresistance: enhanced anti-tumor therapy through increased apoptosis by inhibition of NF-kappaB. Nat Med 5:412–417

81. Desai SD, Li TK, Rodriguez-Bauman A, Rubin EH, Liu LF (2001) Ubiquitin/26S proteasome-mediated degradation of topoisomerase I as a resistance mechanism to camptothecin in tumor cells. Cancer Res 61:5926–5932
82. Loo TW, Clarke DM (1999) The human multidrug resistance P-glycoprotein is inactive when its maturation is inhibited: potential for a role in cancer chemotherapy. FASEB J 13:1724–1732
83. Loo TW, Clarke DM (1998) Superfolding of the partially unfolded core-glycosylated intermediate of human P-glycoprotein into the mature enzyme is promoted by substrate-induced transmembrane domain interactions. J Biol Chem 273:14671–14674
84. Bentires-Alj M, Barbu V, Fillet M, Chariot A, Relic B, Jacobs N, Gielen J, Merville MP, Bours V (2003) NF-kappaB transcription factor induces drug resistance through MDR1 expression in cancer cells. Oncogene 22:90–97
85. San Miguel JF, Schlag R, Khuageva NK, Dimopoulos MA, Shpilberg O, Kropff M, Spicka I, Petrucci MT, Palumbo A, Samoilova OS et al (2008) Bortezomib plus melphalan and prednisone for initial treatment of multiple myeloma. N Engl J Med 359:906–917
86. Orlowski RZ, Nagler A, Sonneveld P, Blade J, Hajek R, Spencer A, San Miguel J, Robak T, Dmoszynska A, Horvath N et al (2007) Randomized phase III study of pegylated liposomal doxorubicin plus bortezomib compared with bortezomib alone in relapsed or refractory multiple myeloma: combination therapy improves time to progression. J Clin Oncol 25:3892–3901
87. Kortuem KM, Stewart AK (2013) Carfilzomib. Blood 121:893–897
88. Meister S, Schubert U, Neubert K, Herrmann K, Burger R, Gramatzki M, Hahn S, Schreiber S, Wilhelm S, Herrmann M et al (2007) Extensive immunoglobulin production sensitizes myeloma cells for proteasome inhibition. Cancer Res 67:1783–1792
89. Vij R, Siegel DS, Jagannath S, Jakubowiak AJ, Stewart AK, McDonagh K, Bahlis N, Belch A, Kunkel LA, Wear S et al (2012) An open-label, single-arm, phase 2 study of single-agent carfilzomib in patients with relapsed and/or refractory multiple myeloma who have been previously treated with bortezomib. Br J Haematol 158:739–748
90. Ruschak AM, Slassi M, Kay LE, Schimmer AD (2011) Novel proteasome inhibitors to overcome bortezomib resistance. J Natl Cancer Inst 103:1007–1017
91. Chiarle R, Budel LM, Skolnik J, Frizzera G, Chilosi M, Corato A, Pizzolo G, Magidson J, Montagnoli A, Pagano M et al (2000) Increased proteasome degradation of cyclin-dependent kinase inhibitor p27 is associated with a decreased overall survival in mantle cell lymphoma. Blood 95:619–626
92. Weniger MA, Rizzatti EG, Perez-Galan P, Liu D, Wang Q, Munson PJ, Raghavachari N, White T, Tweito MM, Dunleavy K et al (2011) Treatment-induced oxidative stress and cellular antioxidant capacity determine response to bortezomib in mantle cell lymphoma. Clin Cancer Res 17:5101–5112
93. Derouet M, Thomas L, Cross A, Moots RJ, Edwards SW (2004) Granulocyte macrophage colony-stimulating factor signaling and proteasome inhibition delay neutrophil apoptosis by increasing the stability of Mcl-1. J Biol Chem 279:26915–26921
94. Nencioni A, Hua F, Dillon CP, Yokoo R, Scheiermann C, Cardone MH, Barbieri E, Rocco I, Garuti A, Wesselborg S et al (2005) Evidence for a protective role of Mcl-1 in proteasome inhibitor-induced apoptosis. Blood 105:3255–3262
95. Jones RJ, Chen Q, Voorhees PM, Young KH, Bruey-Sedano N, Yang D, Orlowski RZ (2008) Inhibition of the p53 E3 ligase HDM-2 induces apoptosis and DNA damage-independent p53 phosphorylation in mantle cell lymphoma. Clin Cancer Res 14:5416–5425
96. Weigert O, Pastore A, Rieken M, Lang N, Hiddemann W, Dreyling M (2007) Sequence-dependent synergy of the proteasome inhibitor bortezomib and cytarabine in mantle cell lymphoma. Leukemia 21:524–528
97. Dal Col J, Zancai P, Terrin L, Guidoboni M, Ponzoni M, Pavan A, Spina M, Bergamin S, Rizzo S, Tirelli U et al (2008) Distinct functional significance of Akt and mTOR constitutive activation in mantle cell lymphoma. Blood 111:5142–5151
98. Hutter G, Zimmermann Y, Rieken M, Hartmann E, Rosenwald A, Hiddemann W, Dreyling M (2012) Proteasome inhibition leads to dephosphorylation and downregulation of protein expression of members of the Akt/mTOR pathway in MCL. Leukemia 26:2442–2444

99. Shanks JC, Fauble V, Lobocki CA, Terebelo H (2008) Dual proteasome and mTOR inhibition promotes apoptosis in non-Hodgkin lymphoma cell lines. ASH Annual Meeting Abstracts 112:5039
100. Desai S, Maurin M, Smith MA, Bolick SC, Dessureault S, Tao J, Sotomayor E, Wright KL (2010) PRDM1 is required for mantle cell lymphoma response to bortezomib. Mol Cancer Res 8:907–918
101. Baran-Marszak F, Boukhiar M, Harel S, Laguillier C, Roger C, Gressin R, Martin A, Fagard R, Varin-Blank N, Ajchenbaum-Cymbalista F et al (2010) Constitutive and B-cell receptor-induced activation of STAT3 are important signaling pathways targeted by bortezomib in leukemic mantle cell lymphoma. Haematologica 95:1865–1872
102. O'Connor OA, Wright J, Moskowitz C, Muzzy J, MacGregor-Cortelli B, Stubblefield M, Straus D, Portlock C, Hamlin P, Choi E et al (2005) Phase II clinical experience with the novel proteasome inhibitor bortezomib in patients with indolent non-Hodgkin's lymphoma and mantle cell lymphoma. J Clin Oncol 23:676–684
103. Goy A, Younes A, McLaughlin P, Pro B, Romaguera JE, Hagemeister F, Fayad L, Dang NH, Samaniego F, Wang M et al (2005) Phase II study of proteasome inhibitor bortezomib in relapsed or refractory B-cell non-Hodgkin's lymphoma. J Clin Oncol 23:667–675
104. Fisher RI, Bernstein SH, Kahl BS, Djulbegovic B, Robertson MJ, de Vos S, Epner E, Krishnan A, Leonard JP, Lonial S et al (2006) Multicenter phase II study of bortezomib in patients with relapsed or refractory mantle cell lymphoma. J Clin Oncol 24:4867–4874
105. Goy A, Bernstein SH, Kahl BS, Djulbegovic B, Robertson MJ, de Vos S, Epner E, Krishnan A, Leonard JP, Lonial S et al (2009) Bortezomib in patients with relapsed or refractory mantle cell lymphoma: updated time-to-event analyses of the multicenter phase 2 PINNACLE study. Ann Oncol 20:520–525
106. Belch A, Kouroukis CT, Crump M, Sehn L, Gascoyne RD, Klasa R, Powers J, Wright J, Eisenhauer EA (2007) A phase II study of bortezomib in mantle cell lymphoma: the National Cancer Institute of Canada Clinical Trials Group trial IND.150. Ann Oncol 18:116–121
107. O'Connor OA, Stewart AK, Vallone M, Molineaux CJ, Kunkel LA, Gerecitano JF, Orlowski RZ (2009) A phase 1 dose escalation study of the safety and pharmacokinetics of the novel proteasome inhibitor carfilzomib (PR-171) in patients with hematologic malignancies. Clin Cancer Res 15:7085–7091
108. Alsina M, Trudel S, Furman RR, Rosen PJ, O'Connor OA, Comenzo RL, Wong A, Kunkel LA, Molineaux CJ, Goy A (2012) A phase I single-agent study of twice-weekly consecutive-day dosing of the proteasome inhibitor carfilzomib in patients with relapsed or refractory multiple myeloma or lymphoma. Clin Cancer Res 18:4830–4840
109. Friedberg JW, Vose JM, Kelly JL, Young F, Bernstein SH, Peterson D, Rich L, Blumel S, Proia NK, Liesveld J et al (2011) The combination of bendamustine, bortezomib, and rituximab for patients with relapsed/refractory indolent and mantle cell non-Hodgkin lymphoma. Blood 117:2807–2812
110. Rosato RR, Grant S (2005) Histone deacetylase inhibitors: insights into mechanisms of lethality. Expert Opin Ther Targets 9:809–824
111. Grant S, Dai Y (2012) Histone deacetylase inhibitors and rational combination therapies. Adv Cancer Res 116:199–237
112. Peart MJ, Smyth GK, van Laar RK, Bowtell DD, Richon VM, Marks PA, Holloway AJ, Johnstone RW (2005) Identification and functional significance of genes regulated by structurally different histone deacetylase inhibitors. Proc Natl Acad Sci U S A 102:3697–3702
113. Aron JL, Parthun MR, Marcucci G, Kitada S, Mone AP, Davis ME, Shen T, Murphy T, Wickham J, Kanakry C et al (2003) Depsipeptide (FR901228) induces histone acetylation and inhibition of histone deacetylase in chronic lymphocytic leukemia cells concurrent with activation of caspase 8-mediated apoptosis and down-regulation of c-FLIP protein. Blood 102:652–658
114. Mitsiades CS, Mitsiades NS, McMullan CJ, Poulaki V, Shringarpure R, Hideshima T, Akiyama M, Chauhan D, Munshi N, Gu X et al (2004) Transcriptional signature of histone deacetylase inhibition in multiple myeloma: biological and clinical implications. Proc Natl Acad Sci U S A 101:540–545

115. Rosato RR, Almenara JA, Kolla SS, Maggio SC, Coe S, Gimenez MS, Dent P, Grant S (2007) Mechanism and functional role of XIAP and Mcl-1 down-regulation in flavopiridol/vorinostat antileukemic interactions. Mol Cancer Ther 6:692–702
116. Rosato RR, Maggio SC, Almenara JA, Payne SG, Atadja P, Spiegel S, Dent P, Grant S (2006) The histone deacetylase inhibitor LAQ824 induces human leukemia cell death through a process involving XIAP down-regulation, oxidative injury, and the acid sphingomyelinase-dependent generation of ceramide. Mol Pharmacol 69:216–225
117. Sanda T, Okamoto T, Uchida Y, Nakagawa H, Iida S, Kayukawa S, Suzuki T, Oshizawa T, Suzuki T, Miyata N et al (2007) Proteome analyses of the growth inhibitory effects of NCH-51, a novel histone deacetylase inhibitor, on lymphoid malignant cells. Leukemia 21:2344–2353
118. Sampath D, Liu C, Vasan K, Sulda M, Puduvalli VK, Wierda WG, Keating MJ (2012) Histone deacetylases mediate the silencing of miR-15a, miR-16, and miR-29b in chronic lymphocytic leukemia. Blood 119:1162–1172
119. Zhao Y, Tan J, Zhuang L, Jiang X, Liu ET, Yu Q (2005) Inhibitors of histone deacetylases target the Rb-E2F1 pathway for apoptosis induction through activation of proapoptotic protein Bim. Proc Natl Acad Sci U S A 102:16090–16095
120. Tan J, Zhuang L, Jiang X, Yang KK, Karuturi KM, Yu Q (2006) Apoptosis signal-regulating kinase 1 is a direct target of E2F1 and contributes to histone deacetylase inhibitor-induced apoptosis through positive feedback regulation of E2F1 apoptotic activity. J Biol Chem 281:10508–10515
121. Chen S, Dai Y, Pei XY, Grant S (2009) Bim upregulation by histone deacetylase inhibitors mediates interactions with the Bcl-2 antagonist ABT-737: evidence for distinct roles for Bcl-2, Bcl-xL, and Mcl-1. Mol Cell Biol 29:6149–6169
122. Dai Y, Chen S, Kramer LB, Funk VL, Dent P, Grant S (2008) Interactions between bortezomib and romidepsin and belinostat in chronic lymphocytic leukemia cells. Clin Cancer Res 14:549–558
123. Dai Y, Chen S, Wang L, Pei XY, Kramer LB, Dent P, Grant S (2011) Bortezomib interacts synergistically with belinostat in human acute myeloid leukaemia and acute lymphoblastic leukaemia cells in association with perturbations in NF-kappaB and Bim. Br J Haematol 153:222–235
124. Inoue S, Riley J, Gant TW, Dyer MJ, Cohen GM (2007) Apoptosis induced by histone deacetylase inhibitors in leukemic cells is mediated by Bim and Noxa. Leukemia 21:1773–1782
125. Terui T, Murakami K, Takimoto R, Takahashi M, Takada K, Murakami T, Minami S, Matsunaga T, Takayama T, Kato J et al (2003) Induction of PIG3 and NOXA through acetylation of p53 at 320 and 373 lysine residues as a mechanism for apoptotic cell death by histone deacetylase inhibitors. Cancer Res 63:8948–8954
126. Xargay-Torrent S, Lopez-Guerra M, Saborit-Villarroya I, Rosich L, Campo E, Roue G, Colomer D (2011) Vorinostat-induced apoptosis in mantle cell lymphoma is mediated by acetylation of proapoptotic BH3-only gene promoters. Clin Cancer Res 17:3956–3968
127. Glick RD, Swendeman SL, Coffey DC, Rifkind RA, Marks PA, Richon VM, La Quaglia MP (1999) Hybrid polar histone deacetylase inhibitor induces apoptosis and CD95/CD95 ligand expression in human neuroblastoma. Cancer Res 59:4392–4399
128. Insinga A, Monestiroli S, Ronzoni S, Gelmetti V, Marchesi F, Viale A, Altucci L, Nervi C, Minucci S, Pelicci PG (2005) Inhibitors of histone deacetylases induce tumor-selective apoptosis through activation of the death receptor pathway. Nat Med 11:71–76
129. Nebbioso A, Clarke N, Voltz E, Germain E, Ambrosino C, Bontempo P, Alvarez R, Schiavone EM, Ferrara F, Bresciani F et al (2005) Tumor-selective action of HDAC inhibitors involves TRAIL induction in acute myeloid leukemia cells. Nat Med 11:77–84
130. Lindemann RK, Newbold A, Whitecross KF, Cluse LA, Frew AJ, Ellis L, Williams S, Wiegmans AP, Dear AE, Scott CL et al (2007) Analysis of the apoptotic and therapeutic activities of histone deacetylase inhibitors by using a mouse model of B cell lymphoma. Proc Natl Acad Sci U S A 104:8071–8076
131. Mitsiades N, Mitsiades CS, Richardson PG, McMullan C, Poulaki V, Fanourakis G, Schlossman R, Chauhan D, Munshi NC, Hideshima T et al (2003) Molecular sequelae of histone deacetylase inhibition in human malignant B cells. Blood 101:4055–4062

132. Ruefli AA, Ausserlechner MJ, Bernhard D, Sutton VR, Tainton KM, Kofler R, Smyth MJ, Johnstone RW (2001) The histone deacetylase inhibitor and chemotherapeutic agent suberoylanilide hydroxamic acid (SAHA) induces a cell-death pathway characterized by cleavage of Bid and production of reactive oxygen species. Proc Natl Acad Sci U S A 98:10833–10838
133. Li H, Wu X (2004) Histone deacetylase inhibitor, Trichostatin A, activates p21WAF1/CIP1 expression through downregulation of c-myc and release of the repression of c-myc from the promoter in human cervical cancer cells. Biochem Biophys Res Commun 324:860–867
134. Nawrocki ST, Carew JS, Douglas L, Cleveland JL, Humphreys R, Houghton JA (2007) Histone deacetylase inhibitors enhance lexatumumab-induced apoptosis via a p21Cip1-dependent decrease in survivin levels. Cancer Res 67:6987–6994
135. Richon VM, Sandhoff TW, Rifkind RA, Marks PA (2000) Histone deacetylase inhibitor selectively induces p21WAF1 expression and gene-associated histone acetylation. Proc Natl Acad Sci U S A 97:10014–10019
136. Wang H, Zhou W, Zheng Z, Zhang P, Tu B, He Q, Zhu WG (2012) The HDAC inhibitor depsipeptide transactivates the p53/p21 pathway by inducing DNA damage. DNA Repair (Amst) 11:146–156
137. Rosato RR, Almenara JA, Grant S (2003) The histone deacetylase inhibitor MS-275 promotes differentiation or apoptosis in human leukemia cells through a process regulated by generation of reactive oxygen species and induction of p21CIP1/WAF1 1. Cancer Res 63:3637–3645
138. Dai Y, Rahmani M, Dent P, Grant S (2005) Blockade of histone deacetylase inhibitor-induced RelA/p65 acetylation and NF-kappaB activation potentiates apoptosis in leukemia cells through a process mediated by oxidative damage, XIAP downregulation, and c-Jun N-terminal kinase 1 activation. Mol Cell Biol 25:5429–5444
139. Ungerstedt JS, Sowa Y, Xu WS, Shao Y, Dokmanovic M, Perez G, Ngo L, Holmgren A, Jiang X, Marks PA (2005) Role of thioredoxin in the response of normal and transformed cells to histone deacetylase inhibitors. Proc Natl Acad Sci U S A 102:673–678
140. Xu W, Ngo L, Perez G, Dokmanovic M, Marks PA (2006) Intrinsic apoptotic and thioredoxin pathways in human prostate cancer cell response to histone deacetylase inhibitor. Proc Natl Acad Sci U S A 103:15540–15545
141. Petruccelli LA, Dupere-Richer D, Pettersson F, Retrouvey H, Skoulikas S, Miller WH Jr (2011) Vorinostat induces reactive oxygen species and DNA damage in acute myeloid leukemia cells. PLoS One 6:e20987
142. Rosato RR, Almenara JA, Maggio SC, Coe S, Atadja P, Dent P, Grant S (2008) Role of histone deacetylase inhibitor-induced reactive oxygen species and DNA damage in LAQ-824/fludarabine antileukemic interactions. Mol Cancer Ther 7:3285–3297
143. Rosato RR, Kolla SS, Hock SK, Almenara JA, Patel A, Amin S, Atadja P, Fisher PB, Dent P, Grant S (2010) Histone deacetylase inhibitors activate NF-kappaB in human leukemia cells through an ATM/NEMO-related pathway. J Biol Chem 285:10064–10077
144. Gaymes TJ, Padua RA, Pla M, Orr S, Omidvar N, Chomienne C, Mufti GJ, Rassool FV (2006) Histone deacetylase inhibitors (HDI) cause DNA damage in leukemia cells: a mechanism for leukemia-specific HDI-dependent apoptosis? Mol Cancer Res 4:563–573
145. Hu Y, Lu W, Chen G, Zhang H, Jia Y, Wei Y, Yang H, Zhang W, Fiskus W, Bhalla K et al (2010) Overcoming resistance to histone deacetylase inhibitors in human leukemia with the redox modulating compound beta-phenylethyl isothiocyanate. Blood 116:2732–2741
146. Dasmahapatra G, Lembersky D, Kramer L, Fisher RI, Friedberg J, Dent P, Grant S (2010) The pan-HDAC inhibitor vorinostat potentiates the activity of the proteasome inhibitor carfilzomib in human DLBCL cells in vitro and in vivo. Blood 115:4478–4487
147. Dasmahapatra G, Lembersky D, Son MP, Attkisson E, Dent P, Fisher RI, Friedberg JW, Grant S (2011) Carfilzomib interacts synergistically with histone deacetylase inhibitors in mantle cell lymphoma cells in vitro and in vivo. Mol Cancer Ther 10:1686–1697
148. Yu X, Guo ZS, Marcu MG, Neckers L, Nguyen DM, Chen GA, Schrump DS (2002) Modulation of p53, ErbB1, ErbB2, and Raf-1 expression in lung cancer cells by depsipeptide FR901228. J Natl Cancer Inst 94:504–513

149. Bali P, Pranpat M, Bradner J, Balasis M, Fiskus W, Guo F, Rocha K, Kumaraswamy S, Boyapalle S, Atadja P et al (2005) Inhibition of histone deacetylase 6 acetylates and disrupts the chaperone function of heat shock protein 90: a novel basis for antileukemia activity of histone deacetylase inhibitors. J Biol Chem 280:26729–26734
150. Nimmanapalli R, Fuino L, Bali P, Gasparetto M, Glozak M, Tao J, Moscinski L, Smith C, Wu J, Jove R et al (2003) Histone deacetylase inhibitor LAQ824 both lowers expression and promotes proteasomal degradation of Bcr-Abl and induces apoptosis of imatinib mesylate-sensitive or -refractory chronic myelogenous leukemia-blast crisis cells. Cancer Res 63: 5126–5135
151. Cohen HY, Lavu S, Bitterman KJ, Hekking B, Imahiyerobo TA, Miller C, Frye R, Ploegh H, Kessler BM, Sinclair DA (2004) Acetylation of the C terminus of Ku70 by CBP and PCAF controls Bax-mediated apoptosis. Mol Cell 13:627–638
152. Subramanian C, Opipari AW Jr, Bian X, Castle VP, Kwok RP (2005) Ku70 acetylation mediates neuroblastoma cell death induced by histone deacetylase inhibitors. Proc Natl Acad Sci U S A 102:4842–4847
153. Lee JH, Choy ML, Ngo L, Foster SS, Marks PA (2010) Histone deacetylase inhibitor induces DNA damage, which normal but not transformed cells can repair. Proc Natl Acad Sci U S A 107:14639–14644
154. Bhaskara S, Chyla BJ, Amann JM, Knutson SK, Cortez D, Sun ZW, Hiebert SW (2008) Deletion of histone deacetylase 3 reveals critical roles in S phase progression and DNA damage control. Mol Cell 30:61–72
155. Kachhap SK, Rosmus N, Collis SJ, Kortenhorst MS, Wissing MD, Hedayati M, Shabbeer S, Mendonca J, Deangelis J, Marchionni L et al (2010) Downregulation of homologous recombination DNA repair genes by HDAC inhibition in prostate cancer is mediated through the E2F1 transcription factor. PLoS One 5:e11208
156. Miller KM, Tjeertes JV, Coates J, Legube G, Polo SE, Britton S, Jackson SP (2010) Human HDAC1 and HDAC2 function in the DNA-damage response to promote DNA nonhomologous end-joining. Nat Struct Mol Biol 17:1144–1151
157. Robert T, Vanoli F, Chiolo I, Shubassi G, Bernstein KA, Rothstein R, Botrugno OA, Parazzoli D, Oldani A, Minucci S et al (2011) HDACs link the DNA damage response, processing of double-strand breaks and autophagy. Nature 471:74–79
158. Shubassi G, Robert T, Vanoli F, Minucci S, Foiani M (2012) Acetylation: a novel link between double-strand break repair and autophagy. Cancer Res 72:1332–1335
159. Cerchietti LC, Hatzi K, Caldas-Lopes E, Yang SN, Figueroa ME, Morin RD, Hirst M, Mendez L, Shaknovich R, Cole PA et al (2010) BCL6 repression of EP300 in human diffuse large B cell lymphoma cells provides a basis for rational combinatorial therapy. J Clin Invest. doi:10.1172/JCI42869
160. Bhaskara S, Knutson SK, Jiang G, Chandrasekharan MB, Wilson AJ, Zheng S, Yenamandra A, Locke K, Yuan JL, Bonine-Summers AR et al (2010) Hdac3 is essential for the maintenance of chromatin structure and genome stability. Cancer Cell 18:436–447
161. Kawaguchi Y, Kovacs JJ, McLaurin A, Vance JM, Ito A, Yao TP (2003) The deacetylase HDAC6 regulates aggresome formation and cell viability in response to misfolded protein stress. Cell 115:727–738
162. Hideshima T, Bradner JE, Wong J, Chauhan D, Richardson P, Schreiber SL, Anderson KC (2005) Small-molecule inhibition of proteasome and aggresome function induces synergistic antitumor activity in multiple myeloma. Proc Natl Acad Sci U S A 102:8567–8572
163. Nawrocki ST, Carew JS, Pino MS, Highshaw RA, Andtbacka RH, Dunner K Jr, Pal A, Bornmann WG, Chiao PJ, Huang P et al (2006) Aggresome disruption: a novel strategy to enhance bortezomib-induced apoptosis in pancreatic cancer cells. Cancer Res 66: 3773–3781
164. Rao R, Nalluri S, Fiskus W, Savoie A, Buckley KM, Ha K, Balusu R, Joshi A, Coothankandaswamy V, Tao J et al (2010) Role of CAAT/enhancer binding protein homologous protein in panobinostat-mediated potentiation of bortezomib-induced lethal endoplasmic reticulum stress in mantle cell lymphoma cells. Clin Cancer Res 16:4742–4754

165. Rao R, Nalluri S, Kolhe R, Yang Y, Fiskus W, Chen J, Ha K, Buckley KM, Balusu R, Coothankandaswamy V et al (2010) Treatment with panobinostat induces glucose-regulated protein 78 acetylation and endoplasmic reticulum stress in breast cancer cells. Mol Cancer Ther 9:942–952
166. Kahali S, Sarcar B, Prabhu A, Seto E, Chinnaiyan P (2012) Class I histone deacetylases localize to the endoplasmic reticulum and modulate the unfolded protein response. FASEB J 26:2437–2445
167. Warrener R, Beamish H, Burgess A, Waterhouse NJ, Giles N, Fairlie D, Gabrielli B (2003) Tumor cell-selective cytotoxicity by targeting cell cycle checkpoints. FASEB J 17:1550–1552
168. Stevens FE, Beamish H, Warrener R, Gabrielli B (2008) Histone deacetylase inhibitors induce mitotic slippage. Oncogene 27:1345–1354
169. Magnaghi-Jaulin L, Eot-Houllier G, Fulcrand G, Jaulin C (2007) Histone deacetylase inhibitors induce premature sister chromatid separation and override the mitotic spindle assembly checkpoint. Cancer Res 67:6360–6367
170. Ishii S, Kurasawa Y, Wong J, Yu-Lee LY (2008) Histone deacetylase 3 localizes to the mitotic spindle and is required for kinetochore-microtubule attachment. Proc Natl Acad Sci U S A 105:4179–4184
171. Vrana JA, Decker RH, Johnson CR, Wang Z, Jarvis WD, Richon VM, Ehinger M, Fisher PB, Grant S (1999) Induction of apoptosis in U937 human leukemia cells by suberoylanilide hydroxamic acid (SAHA) proceeds through pathways that are regulated by Bcl-2/Bcl-XL, c-Jun, and p21CIP1, but independent of p53. Oncogene 18:7016–7025
172. Dai Y, Guzman ML, Chen S, Wang L, Yeung SK, Pei XY, Dent P, Jordan CT, Grant S (2010) The NF (Nuclear factor)-kappaB inhibitor parthenolide interacts with histone deacetylase inhibitors to induce MKK7/JNK1-dependent apoptosis in human acute myeloid leukaemia cells. Br J Haematol 151:70–83
173. Rascle A, Johnston JA, Amati B (2003) Deacetylase activity is required for recruitment of the basal transcription machinery and transactivation by STAT5. Mol Cell Biol 23:4162–4173
174. Nguyen T, Dai Y, Attkisson E, Kramer L, Jordan N, Nguyen N, Kolluri N, Muschen M, Grant S (2011) HDAC inhibitors potentiate the activity of the BCR/ABL kinase inhibitor KW-2449 in imatinib-sensitive or -resistant BCR/ABL + leukemia cells in vitro and in vivo. Clin Cancer Res 17:3219–3232
175. Shao W, Growney JD, Feng Y, O'Connor G, Pu M, Zhu W, Yao YM, Kwon P, Fawell S, Atadja P (2010) Activity of deacetylase inhibitor panobinostat (LBH589) in cutaneous T-cell lymphoma models: Defining molecular mechanisms of resistance. Int J Cancer 127:2199–2208
176. Fotheringham S, Epping MT, Stimson L, Khan O, Wood V, Pezzella F, Bernards R, La Thangue NB (2009) Genome-wide loss-of-function screen reveals an important role for the proteasome in HDAC inhibitor-induced apoptosis. Cancer Cell 15:57–66
177. Deroanne CF, Bonjean K, Servotte S, Devy L, Colige A, Clausse N, Blacher S, Verdin E, Foidart JM, Nusgens BV et al (2002) Histone deacetylases inhibitors as anti-angiogenic agents altering vascular endothelial growth factor signaling. Oncogene 21:427–436
178. Qian DZ, Wang X, Kachhap SK, Kato Y, Wei Y, Zhang L, Atadja P, Pili R (2004) The histone deacetylase inhibitor NVP-LAQ824 inhibits angiogenesis and has a greater antitumor effect in combination with the vascular endothelial growth factor receptor tyrosine kinase inhibitor PTK787/ZK222584. Cancer Res 64:6626–6634
179. Maggio SC, Rosato RR, Kramer LB, Dai Y, Rahmani M, Paik DS, Czarnik AC, Payne SG, Spiegel S, Grant S (2004) The histone deacetylase inhibitor MS-275 interacts synergistically with fludarabine to induce apoptosis in human leukemia cells. Cancer Res 64:2590–2600
180. Yi C, Ma M, Ran L, Zheng J, Tong J, Zhu J, Ma C, Sun Y, Zhang S, Feng W et al (2012) Function and molecular mechanism of acetylation in autophagy regulation. Science 336: 474–477
181. Carew JS, Nawrocki ST, Kahue CN, Zhang H, Yang C, Chung L, Houghton JA, Huang P, Giles FJ, Cleveland JL (2007) Targeting autophagy augments the anticancer activity of the histone deacetylase inhibitor SAHA to overcome Bcr-Abl-mediated drug resistance. Blood 110:313–322

182. Gammoh N, Lam D, Puente C, Ganley I, Marks PA, Jiang X (2012) Role of autophagy in histone deacetylase inhibitor-induced apoptotic and nonapoptotic cell death. Proc Natl Acad Sci U S A 109:6561–6565
183. Almenara J, Rosato R, Grant S (2002) Synergistic induction of mitochondrial damage and apoptosis in human leukemia cells by flavopiridol and the histone deacetylase inhibitor suberoylanilide hydroxamic acid (SAHA). Leukemia 16:1331–1343
184. Watanabe T (2010) Investigational histone deacetylase inhibitors for non-Hodgkin lymphomas. Expert Opin Investig Drugs 19:1113–1127
185. Kawamata N, Chen J, Koeffler HP (2007) Suberoylanilide hydroxamic acid (SAHA; vorinostat) suppresses translation of cyclin D1 in mantle cell lymphoma cells. Blood 110:2667–2673
186. Heider U, Kaiser M, Sterz J, Zavrski I, Jakob C, Fleissner C, Eucker J, Possinger K, Sezer O (2006) Histone deacetylase inhibitors reduce VEGF production and induce growth suppression and apoptosis in human mantle cell lymphoma. Eur J Haematol 76:42–50
187. Lwin T, Zhao X, Cheng F, Zhang X, Huang A, Shah B, Zhang Y, Moscinski LC, Choi YS, Kozikowski AP et al (2013) A microenvironment-mediated c-Myc/miR-548m/HDAC6 amplification loop in non-Hodgkin B cell lymphomas. J Clin Invest 123:4612–26
188. Watanabe T, Kato H, Kobayashi Y, Yamasaki S, Morita-Hoshi Y, Yokoyama H, Morishima Y, Ricker JL, Otsuki T, Miyagi-Maesima A et al (2010) Potential efficacy of the oral histone deacetylase inhibitor vorinostat in a phase I trial in follicular and mantle cell lymphoma. Cancer Sci 101:196–200
189. Kirschbaum M, Frankel P, Popplewell L, Zain J, Delioukina M, Pullarkat V, Matsuoka D, Pulone B, Rotter AJ, Espinoza-Delgado I et al (2011) Phase II study of vorinostat for treatment of relapsed or refractory indolent non-Hodgkin's lymphoma and mantle cell lymphoma. J Clin Oncol 29:1198–1203
190. Wright JJ (2010) Combination therapy of bortezomib with novel targeted agents: an emerging treatment strategy. Clin Cancer Res 16:4094–4104
191. Mayo MW, Denlinger CE, Broad RM, Yeung F, Reilly ET, Shi Y, Jones DR (2003) Ineffectiveness of histone deacetylase inhibitors to induce apoptosis involves the transcriptional activation of NF-kappa B through the Akt pathway. J Biol Chem 278:18980–18989
192. Roychowdhury S, Baiocchi RA, Vourganti S, Bhatt D, Blaser BW, Freud AG, Chou J, Chen CS, Xiao JJ, Parthun M et al (2004) Selective efficacy of depsipeptide in a xenograft model of Epstein-Barr virus-positive lymphoproliferative disorder. J Natl Cancer Inst 96:1447–1457
193. Dai Y, Chen S, Wang L, Pei XY, Funk VL, Kramer LB, Dent P, Grant S (2011) Disruption of IkappaB kinase (IKK)-mediated RelA serine 536 phosphorylation sensitizes human multiple myeloma cells to histone deacetylase (HDAC) inhibitors. J Biol Chem 286:34036–34050
194. Dai Y, Rahmani M, Grant S (2003) An intact NF-kappaB pathway is required for histone deacetylase inhibitor-induced G1 arrest and maturation in U937 human myeloid leukemia cells. Cell Cycle 2:467–472
195. Pei XY, Dai Y, Grant S (2004) Synergistic induction of oxidative injury and apoptosis in human multiple myeloma cells by the proteasome inhibitor bortezomib and histone deacetylase inhibitors. Clin Cancer Res 10:3839–3852
196. Campbell RA, Sanchez E, Steinberg J, Shalitin D, Li ZW, Chen H, Berenson JR (2010) Vorinostat enhances the antimyeloma effects of melphalan and bortezomib. Eur J Haematol 84:201–211
197. Heider U, von Metzler I, Kaiser M, Rosche M, Sterz J, Rotzer S, Rademacher J, Jakob C, Fleissner C, Kuckelkorn U et al (2008) Synergistic interaction of the histone deacetylase inhibitor SAHA with the proteasome inhibitor bortezomib in mantle cell lymphoma. Eur J Haematol 80:133–142
198. Paoluzzi L, Scotto L, Marchi E, Zain J, Seshan VE, O'Connor OA (2010) Romidepsin and belinostat synergize the antineoplastic effect of bortezomib in mantle cell lymphoma. Clin Cancer Res 16:554–565
199. Heider U, Rademacher J, Lamottke B, Mieth M, Moebs M, von Metzler I, Assaf C, Sezer O (2009) Synergistic interaction of the histone deacetylase inhibitor SAHA with the proteasome inhibitor bortezomib in cutaneous T cell lymphoma. Eur J Haematol 82:440–449

200. Zhang QL, Wang L, Zhang YW, Jiang XX, Yang F, Wu WL, Janin A, Chen Z, Shen ZX, Chen SJ et al (2009) The proteasome inhibitor bortezomib interacts synergistically with the histone deacetylase inhibitor suberoylanilide hydroxamic acid to induce T-leukemia/lymphoma cells apoptosis. Leukemia 23:1507–1514
201. Miller CP, Ban K, Dujka ME, McConkey DJ, Munsell M, Palladino M, Chandra J (2007) NPI-0052, a novel proteasome inhibitor, induces caspase-8 and ROS-dependent apoptosis alone and in combination with HDAC inhibitors in leukemia cells. Blood 110:267–277
202. Yu C, Rahmani M, Conrad D, Subler M, Dent P, Grant S (2003) The proteasome inhibitor bortezomib interacts synergistically with histone deacetylase inhibitors to induce apoptosis in Bcr/Abl + cells sensitive and resistant to STI571. Blood 102:3765–3774
203. Badros A, Burger AM, Philip S, Niesvizky R, Kolla SS, Goloubeva O, Harris C, Zwiebel J, Wright JJ, Espinoza-Delgado I et al (2009) Phase I study of vorinostat in combination with bortezomib for relapsed and refractory multiple myeloma. Clin Cancer Res 15:5250–5257
204. Holkova B, Bose P, Tombes MB, Shrader E, Wan W, Weir-Wiggins C, Stoddert E, Sankala H, Kmieciak M, Roberts JD et al (2012) Phase I trial of belinostat and bortezomib in patients with relapsed or refractory acute leukemia, myelodysplastic syndrome, or chronic myelogenous leukemia in blast crisis—one year update. ASH Annual Meeting Abstracts 120:3588
205. Holkova B, Perkins EB, Sokol L, Richards KL, Parekh S, Elstrom R, Badros AZ, Espinoza-Delgado I, Schell MJ, Kimball A et al (2011) A phase II trial of bortezomib and vorinostat in mantle cell lymphoma and diffuse large B-cell lymphoma. ASH Annual Meeting Abstracts 118:779
206. Holkova B, Shea TC, Bose P, Tombes MB, Shrader E, Wan W, Weir-Wiggins C, Stoddert E, Sankala H, Kmieciak M et al (2012) Phase I study of bortezomib and romidepsin in patients with chronic lymphocytic leukemia/small lymphocytic lymphoma, indolent B-cell lymphoma, or peripheral T-cell lymphoma. ASH Annual Meeting Abstracts 120:1794
207. Holkova B, Kmieciak M, Bose P, Barr PM, Tombes MB, Shrader E, Cebula E, Pierce E, Herr MM, Sankala H, Feng C et al (2013) Phase I trial of carfilzomib in combination with vorinostat (SAHA) in patients with relapsed/refractory B-cell lymphomas. Blood 122:4375
208. Hideshima T, Richardson PG, Anderson KC (2011) Mechanism of action of proteasome inhibitors and deacetylase inhibitors and the biological basis of synergy in multiple myeloma. Mol Cancer Ther 10:2034–2042
209. Catley L, Weisberg E, Kiziltepe T, Tai YT, Hideshima T, Neri P, Tassone P, Atadja P, Chauhan D, Munshi NC et al (2006) Aggresome induction by proteasome inhibitor bortezomib and alpha-tubulin hyperacetylation by tubulin deacetylase (TDAC) inhibitor LBH589 are synergistic in myeloma cells. Blood 108:3441–3449
210. Richardson PG, Schlossman RL, Alsina M, Weber DM, Coutre SE, Gasparetto C, Mukhopadhyay S, Ondovik MS, Khan M, Paley CS et al (2013) PANORAMA 2: panobinostat in combination with bortezomib and dexamethasone in patients with relapsed and bortezomib-refractory myeloma. Blood 122:2331–2337
211. Santo L, Hideshima T, Kung AL, Tseng JC, Tamang D, Yang M, Jarpe M, van Duzer JH, Mazitschek R, Ogier WC et al (2012) Preclinical activity, pharmacodynamic, and pharmacokinetic properties of a selective HDAC6 inhibitor, ACY-1215, in combination with bortezomib in multiple myeloma. Blood 119:2579–2589
212. Nishioka C, Ikezoe T, Yang J, Takeuchi S, Koeffler HP, Yokoyama A (2008) MS-275, a novel histone deacetylase inhibitor with selectivity against HDAC1, induces degradation of FLT3 via inhibition of chaperone function of heat shock protein 90 in AML cells. Leuk Res 32:1382–1392
213. Davenport EL, Moore HE, Dunlop AS, Sharp SY, Workman P, Morgan GJ, Davies FE (2007) Heat shock protein inhibition is associated with activation of the unfolded protein response pathway in myeloma plasma cells. Blood 110:2641–2649
214. Roue G, Perez-Galan P, Mozos A, Lopez-Guerra M, Xargay-Torrent S, Rosich L, Saborit-Villarroya I, Normant E, Campo E, Colomer D (2011) The Hsp90 inhibitor IPI-504 overcomes bortezomib resistance in mantle cell lymphoma in vitro and in vivo by down-regulation of the prosurvival ER chaperone BiP/Grp78. Blood 117:1270–1279

215. Chauhan D, Li G, Shringarpure R, Podar K, Ohtake Y, Hideshima T, Anderson KC (2003) Blockade of Hsp27 overcomes Bortezomib/proteasome inhibitor PS-341 resistance in lymphoma cells. Cancer Res 63:6174–6177
216. Liu S, Liu Z, Xie Z, Pang J, Yu J, Lehmann E, Huynh L, Vukosavljevic T, Takeki M, Klisovic RB et al (2008) Bortezomib induces DNA hypomethylation and silenced gene transcription by interfering with Sp1/NF-kappaB-dependent DNA methyltransferase activity in acute myeloid leukemia. Blood 111:2364–2373
217. Baylin SB, Jones PA (2011) A decade of exploring the cancer epigenome—biological and translational implications. Nat Rev Cancer 11:726–734
218. Jones PA, Baylin SB (2007) The epigenomics of cancer. Cell 128:683–692
219. Emanuele S, Lauricella M, Carlisi D, Vassallo B, D'Anneo A, Di Fazio P, Vento R, Tesoriere G (2007) SAHA induces apoptosis in hepatoma cells and synergistically interacts with the proteasome inhibitor Bortezomib. Apoptosis 12:1327–1338
220. Kikuchi J, Wada T, Shimizu R, Izumi T, Akutsu M, Mitsunaga K, Noborio-Hatano K, Nobuyoshi M, Ozawa K, Kano Y et al (2010) Histone deacetylases are critical targets of bortezomib-induced cytotoxicity in multiple myeloma. Blood 116:406–417
221. Catley L, Weisberg E, Tai YT, Atadja P, Remiszewski S, Hideshima T, Mitsiades N, Shringarpure R, LeBlanc R, Chauhan D et al (2003) NVP-LAQ824 is a potent novel histone deacetylase inhibitor with significant activity against multiple myeloma. Blood 102:2615–2622
222. Bhalla S, Balasubramanian S, David K, Sirisawad M, Buggy J, Mauro L, Prachand S, Miller R, Gordon LI, Evens AM (2009) PCI-24781 induces caspase and reactive oxygen species-dependent apoptosis through NF-kappaB mechanisms and is synergistic with bortezomib in lymphoma cells. Clin Cancer Res 15:3354–3365
223. Paoluzzi L, Scotto L, Marchi E, Seshan VE, O'Connor OA (2009) The anti-histaminic cyproheptadine synergizes the antineoplastic activity of bortezomib in mantle cell lymphoma through its effects as a histone deacetylase inhibitor. Br J Haematol 146:656–659
224. Dai Y, Rahmani M, Grant S (2003) Proteasome inhibitors potentiate leukemic cell apoptosis induced by the cyclin-dependent kinase inhibitor flavopiridol through a SAPK/JNK- and NF-kappaB-dependent process. Oncogene 22:7108–7122
225. Kapanen A, Tucker C, Chikh G, Bally M, Klasa R (2005) Cell based assays completed with the mantle cell lymphoma cell lines Z138 and NCEB-1 indicate that combinations of bortezomid and flavopiridol interact to achieve synergistic activity. ASH Annual Meeting Abstracts 106:2410
226. Holkova B, Perkins EB, Ramakrishnan V, Tombes MB, Shrader E, Talreja N, Wellons MD, Hogan KT, Roodman GD, Coppola D et al (2011) Phase I trial of bortezomib (PS-341; NSC 681239) and alvocidib (flavopiridol; NSC 649890) in patients with recurrent or refractory B-cell neoplasms. Clin Cancer Res 17:3388–3397
227. Holkova B, Perkins EB, Bose P, Sullivan DM, Baz R, Tombes MB, Shrader E, Ramakrishnan V, Wan W, Sankala H et al (2012) Phase I trial of bortezomib (PS-341; NSC 681239) and alvocidib (flavopiridol; NSC 649890) in patients with recurrent or refractory indolent B-cell neoplasms—update of the "bolus" infusion schedule of alvocidib. ASH Annual Meeting Abstracts 120:2959
228. Holkova B, Supko JG, Ames MM, Reid JM, Shapiro GI, Perkins EB, Ramakrishnan V, Tombes MB, Honeycutt C, McGovern RM et al (2013) A phase I trial of vorinostat and alvocidib in patients with relapsed, refractory, or poor prognosis acute leukemia, or refractory anemia with excess blasts-2. Clin Cancer Res 19:1873–1883
229. Axelrod M, Ou Z, Brett LK, Zhang L, Lopez ER, Tamayo AT, Gordon V, Ford RJ, Williams ME, Pham LV et al (2014) Combinatorial drug screening identifies synergistic co-targeting of Bruton's tyrosine kinase and the proteasome in mantle cell lymphoma. Leukemia 28:407–410
230. Dasmahapatra G, Patel H, Dent P, Fisher RI, Friedberg J, Grant S (2013) The Bruton tyrosine kinase (BTK) inhibitor PCI-32765 synergistically increases proteasome inhibitor activity in diffuse large-B cell lymphoma (DLBCL) and mantle cell lymphoma (MCL) cells sensitive or resistant to bortezomib. Br J Haematol 161:43–56

231. Paoluzzi L, Gonen M, Bhagat G, Furman RR, Gardner JR, Scotto L, Gueorguiev VD, Heaney ML, Manova K, O'Connor OA (2008) The BH3-only mimetic ABT-737 synergizes the antineoplastic activity of proteasome inhibitors in lymphoid malignancies. Blood 112:2906–2916
232. Perez-Galan P, Roue G, Villamor N, Campo E, Colomer D (2007) The BH3-mimetic GX15-070 synergizes with bortezomib in mantle cell lymphoma by enhancing Noxa-mediated activation of Bak. Blood 109:4441–4449
233. Goy A, Ford P, Feldman T, Pecora A, Goldberg S, Donato M, Siegel D, Panush D, Berger MS (2007) A phase 1 trial of the Pan Bcl-2 family inhibitor obatoclax mesylate (GX15-070) in combination with bortezomib in patients with relapsed/refractory mantle cell lymphoma. ASH Annual Meeting Abstracts 110:2569
234. Wilson WH, O'Connor OA, Czuczman MS, LaCasce AS, Gerecitano JF, Leonard JP, Tulpule A, Dunleavy K, Xiong H, Chiu YL et al (2010) Navitoclax, a targeted high-affinity inhibitor of BCL-2, in lymphoid malignancies: a phase 1 dose-escalation study of safety, pharmacokinetics, pharmacodynamics, and antitumour activity. Lancet Oncol 11:1149–1159
235. Whitecross KF, Alsop AE, Cluse LA, Wiegmans A, Banks KM, Coomans C, Peart MJ, Newbold A, Lindemann RK, Johnstone RW (2009) Defining the target specificity of ABT-737 and synergistic antitumor activities in combination with histone deacetylase inhibitors. Blood 113:1982–1991

Chapter 7
Preclinical Studies on the Molecular Basis of Bortezomib Resistance and Modalities to Overcome Resistance in Hematological Malignancies

Jacqueline Cloos, Denise Niewerth, and Gerrit Jansen

Abstract The success of the proteasome inhibitor bortezomib for the treatment of multiple myeloma has encouraged its broader use for other hematological malignancies such as lymphomas and acute leukemia. An important feature for the successful implementation of bortezomib in the treatment of acute leukemia would rely on the selection of patients that will benefit. In order to achieve this goal, preclinical studies can help to establish the mechanism(s) of action underlying proteasome inhibition in leukemic cells and recognize possible mechanisms of acquired resistance. This chapter presents an overview about the current knowledge of these mechanisms based on in vitro and ex vivo studies. Moreover, strategies are discussed that have been set up to overcome resistance, e.g., by novel proteasome inhibitors and combinations of bortezomib with other chemotherapeutic drugs. Finally, an update is provided of the ongoing clinical trials investigating the potential benefits of proteasome inhibitors in acute leukemia.

Keywords Acute leukemia • Bortezomib • Proteasome inhibition • Immunoproteasome • Drug resistance

J. Cloos, Ph.D. (✉) • D. Niewerth, Ph.D.
Department of Pediatric Oncology/Hematology, VU University Medical Center, de Boelelaan 1117, 1081 HV, Amsterdam, The Netherlands

Department of Hematology, VU University Medical Center, Amsterdam, The Netherlands
e-mail: j.cloos@vumc.nl; d.niewerth@vumc.nl

G. Jansen, Ph.D.
Department of Rheumatology, VU University Medical Center, Amsterdam, The Netherlands
e-mail: g.jansen@vumc.nl

Q.P. Dou (ed.), *Resistance to Proteasome Inhibitors in Cancer*, Resistance to Targeted Anti-Cancer Therapeutics, DOI 10.1007/978-3-319-06752-0_7

Abbreviations

5AHQ	5-Amino-8-hydroxyquinole
ABC	ATP-binding cassette
ALL	Acute lymphoblastic leukemia
AML	Acute myeloid leukemia
BCRP	Breast cancer resistance protein
BTZ	Bortezomib
CFZ	Carfilzomib
C-L	Caspase-like
cP	Constitutive proteasome
CR	Complete remission
CT-L	Chymotrypsin-like
ER	Endoplasmic reticulum
IGFR	Insulin-like growth factor receptor
iP	Immunoproteasome
IRF4	Interferon regulating factor 4
MDR	Multidrug resistance
MHC	Major histocompatibility complex
MM	Multiple myeloma
MRP	Multidrug resistance-associated protein
MTT-assay	MTT (3-(4,5-dimethylthiazol-2-yl)-2,5-diphenyltetrazolium bromide) tetrazolium reduction assay
Pgp	P-glycoprotein
SEM	Standard error of the mean
T-L	Trypsin-like
TRAF	TNF activating factor
WT	Wild type

7.1 Introduction

In the last decades, considerable improvements have been accomplished in the prognosis of patients suffering from acute leukemia. This can be attributed to better supportive care and risk group tailored-treatment strategies. In particular for childhood acute lymphoblastic leukemia (ALL), the prognosis is very good with 5-year survival rates of about 85 %. For adult ALL patients, however, the survival is currently still unsatisfactorily low with 5-year survival ranging from 50 % for younger adults and only 20 % for patients older than 45 years of age [1]. These survival rates are achieved by intensive chemotherapy (combination treatment including glucocorticoids, vincristine, and asparaginase for remission induction) and risk stratification among others based on minimal residual disease measurements.

Especially patients with a poor initial response to glucocorticoids are classified as belonging to an unfavorable risk group, and novel treatment strategies are warranted for these treatment-refractory patients.

In comparison to ALL patients, those suffering from acute myeloid leukemia (AML) have a dismal prognosis. Children with AML treated with cytarabine and anthracycline-based regimens currently experience a probability of long-term survival of about 70 %, while again adult patients experience an even worse outcome with 5-year survival rates of around 40 %, which further decline with age to approximately 4 % for patients >75 years [2, 3]. The main reason why survival rates lack further improvement is largely due to recurrence of the disease. Although the majority of AML patients achieve initial complete remission (CR), 30–40 % of these patients will experience a relapse. Recent studies revealed that leukemic cells from relapsed patients differ from the initial AML cells with regard to the mutational status and the immunophenotype [4, 5]. Beyond these, there is evidence that clonal selection of a small subpopulation within the heterogeneous stem cell population at diagnosis is responsible for the development of relapse [6]. Overall, resistance to conventional chemotherapeutics is a critical factor in the poor outcome from patients with relapsed acute leukemia [7]. Thus, new treatment strategies are required which may include new-generation antileukemic drugs with novel mechanisms of action or those that can (re)sensitize leukemia cells for conventional chemotherapeutics. From this perspective, proteasome inhibitors are attractive candidates given their proven track record in the treatment of several hematological malignancies, including multiple myeloma (MM) and mantle cell lymphoma [8].

In this chapter, we will discuss preclinical data addressing the composition and function of proteasomes in leukemic cells and the impact of proteasome inhibition to elicit antileukemic effects. Another important issue relates to the acquisition of resistance to proteasome inhibitors in leukemic cells, delineation of the molecular mechanisms of resistance, and referring to modalities to overcome resistance to proteasome inhibition. Lastly, an overview is presented of ongoing and completed clinical trials using proteasome inhibitors in acute leukemia.

7.2 Role of the Proteasome in the Leukemic Cell

In order to retain cellular homeostasis, proteins marked for degradation are ubiquitin tagged and proteolyzed by the proteasome. Peptides generated by this process can be further hydrolyzed by aminopeptidases to generate amino acids which can be reutilized for new protein synthesis or processed for antigen presentation by major histocompatibility complex (MHC) class I molecules [9].

Proteasomal protein degradation is facilitated by at least two types of proteasome harboring different catalytic activities. The constitutive 26S proteasome represents a commonly expressed proteasome subtype that consists of two outer 19S regulatory particles and an inner 20S core particle with two identical rings of seven α-subunits

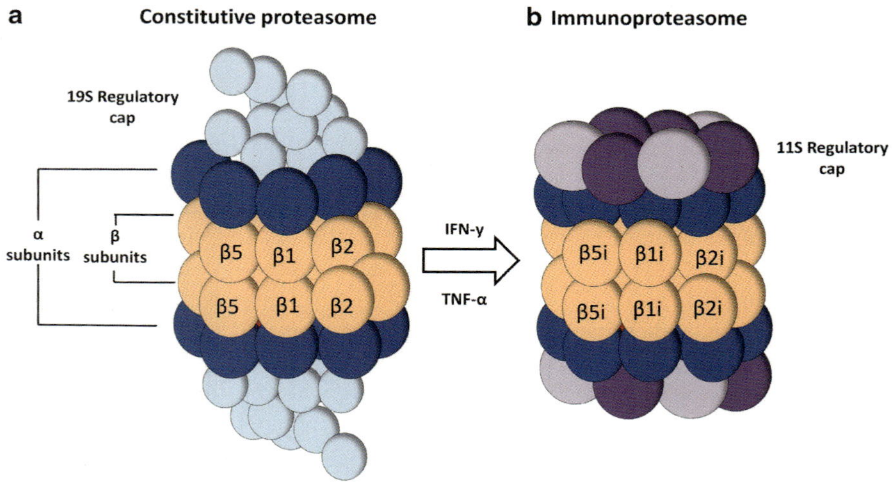

Fig. 7.1 Assembly of constitutive- and immunoproteasome. (**a**) The commonly expressed proteasome subtype is the constitutive proteasome, which is composed of an 20S core with 2α- and 2β-rings and a 19S regulatory cap on each site and β1, β2, and β5 as dominant catalytic subunits. (**b**) The immunoproteasome is predominantly expressed in hematopoietic cells and can be markedly induced upon stimulation of inflammatory cytokines such as IFNγ and to a lesser extent TNF-α. It consists of 11S regulatory caps and the catalytically active β-subunits β1i, β2i, and β5i

and two identical rings of seven β-subunits. The α-subunits are responsible for recognizing and unfolding the ubiquitin-bound proteins and the three catalytically active β-subunits; β1 (*PSMB6*, caspase-like (C-L) activity), β2 (*PSMB7*, trypsin-like (T-L) activity), and β5 (*PSMB5*, chymotrypsin-like (CT-L) activity) facilitate proteolysis of peptide bonds after acidic, basic, and hydrophobic amino acids, respectively (Fig. 7.1a). In hematological cells, another subtype, i.e., the immunoproteasome, is most abundantly expressed. This subtype has 11S regulatory particles and is assembled by other catalytically active β-subunits: β1i (*PSMB9*), β2i (*PSMB10*), and β5i (*PSMB8*) (Fig. 7.1b). Recently, an additional complexity was indicated by the identification of hybrid proteasomes consisting of both constitutive and immune subunits [10, 11]. Therefore, proteasome assembly may also be of importance for the regulation of protein degradation by the proteasome [12] (Fig. 7.1).

Immunoproteasome expression is markedly induced in response to inflammatory cytokines such as IFNγ and to a lesser extent TNF-α [13–15]. For a long time, the dominant function of immunoproteasomes was assigned for the provision of antigenic peptides for presentation on MHC class I molecules. Recently, Seifert et al. described an alternative function of the immunoproteasome in facilitating efficient clearance of protein aggregates that arise upon IFN-induced oxidative stress, thereby preventing cell death [16]. However, this function was disputed by Nathan et al. who reported that immunoproteasomes did not degrade ubiquitinated proteins more efficiently than constitutive proteasomes [17]. Nonetheless, the notion that in leukemic cells, immunoproteasome expression outweighs constitutive proteasome expression may have implications for proteasome inhibitor targeting. Recently, we showed that in ALL cells, the immunoproteasome subunits are relatively highly expressed compared to AML cells, but still the expression of the immunoproteasomes is most pronounced in both leukemic cell types and their expression dictate the total amount of proteasomes [18].

7.3 Effect of Proteasome Inhibition

Since proteasomal degradation of ubiquitinated proteins is pivotal for cellular homeostasis, it is recognized as an attractive therapeutic target. It is obvious that this is in particular important for MM cells since these antibody-producing cells are highly dependent on their protein turnover and rely on a tight balance between proteasome workload and catalytic capacity [19]. However, it is conceivable that cells of other hematological malignancies also critically rely on proteasome-dependent protein turnover and antigen presentation via MHC class I to elicit immune responses. These considerations support further investigations into the clinical application of proteasome inhibitors in other hematological malignancies, including acute leukemias [20]. Bortezomib (BTZ) is the first proteasome inhibitor that entered clinical practice and is now routinely used for the treatment of relapsed/refractory MM and mantle cell lymphoma [21, 22]. BTZ is a reversible proteasome inhibitor which mainly targets the CT-L activity (of both constitutive- and immunoproteasome) and to lesser extent the C-L proteasomal activity. Several mechanisms have been identified that are involved in the apoptosis induction and targeting of leukemic cells by proteasome inhibition [23]. The most prototypical mechanism is the accumulation of ubiquitinated proteins, which can be regulatory proteins that should be broken down for appropriate signal transduction and cell cycle regulation. An important example in this respect is the transcription and pro-survival factor NF-κB, whose natural inhibitory protein IκB regulates NF-κB nuclear translocation and activation following phosphorylation, ubiquitination, and degradation of IκB. Proteasome inhibition impairs IκB degradation and, thus, obstructs activation of NF-κB. It is well accepted that particularly AML cells rely on the activation of the NF-κB pathway for cell survival and this may underlie a relevant mechanism for their sensitivity to BTZ [24]. Other regulatory proteins that have been shown to be stabilized by proteasome inhibition are cell cycle regulation proteins (p21 and p27) and p53 [25, 26]. The accumulation of ubiquitinated proteins, irrespective of the type of proteins, results in the formation of aggresomes, which induce endoplasmic reticulum stress leading to apoptosis induction [27]. It has been suggested that the overload of proteins can also be relieved by autophagy [28]. In BTZ-resistant leukemic cell lines, however, no obvious changes were observed in the expression of proteins related to autophagy. Proteasome inhibition does introduce an impaired antigen presentation by MHC class I molecules [29, 30], an effect that is also observed in BTZ-resistant leukemic cell lines [18].

7.4 Mechanisms of Resistance to Bortezomib

Although the first results of the antileukemic effects of proteasome inhibition are very encouraging, clinical studies in MM patients indicate that there are patients refractory to BTZ and that some patients acquire BTZ resistance [8]. Therefore, in order to optimally implement proteasome inhibitors as treatment modality for acute leukemia, it would be of importance to select patients that will benefit to proteasome inhibitor-based therapy and also recognize onset of resistance upon prolonged treatment. To this end, we and others performed preclinical in vitro studies to explore possible resistance modalities to BTZ. As an experimental approach, we followed a classical procedure of culturing leukemic cells in stepwise increasing dosages of BTZ as a mimic for repeated administration in the clinical setting. This procedure provoked acquired resistance to BTZ in 3 hematological cell lines of various backgrounds: one ALL (CEM-C7), one AML (THP-1), and one MM cell line (8226) [31, 32] (Fig. 7.2). Remarkably, however, there were considerable differences between these 3 cell lines in the time period to acquire an appreciable level of BTZ resistance. As shown in Fig. 7.2a, for CEM high levels of BTZ could be achieved within 2 months, whereas for 8226 cells, this took much longer (>6 months). In addition, the highest level of resistance obtained for 8226 cells was reached when culturing the cells at 100 nM BTZ, whereas CEM cells could be cultured to withstand up to 500 nM BTZ. This is also illustrated by the resistance factors calculated from IC50 values for BTZ growth inhibition in BTZ-resistant sublines compared to parental cells (Table insert in Fig. 7.2). Notably, BTZ-resistant lines were cross-resistant to other proteasome inhibitors which also primarily target the β5 subunit (e.g., carfilzomib (CFZ) and to a lesser extent MG132) (Table 7.1).

Interestingly, BTZ-resistant cells were still sensitive to proteasome inhibitors targeting the α7 subunits of the proteasome such as 5-amino-8-hydroxyquinole (5AHQ) [32, 33]. These results underscore the importance of alterations in the β5 proteasome subunit in relation to BTZ resistance. Further detailed characterization of the molecular defects underlying BTZ resistance in hematological cells, as investigated by our laboratory and others, is discussed below.

7.4.1 Impact of the β5 Subunit Expression

Drug resistance mechanisms often reveal the Achilles heel of targeted therapies. With respect to BTZ, characterization of multiple BTZ-adapted or BTZ-resistant hematological cell lines exposed to relatively low concentrations of BTZ (up to 50 nM) revealed upregulated expression of proteasome subunits and in particular β5 subunits as primary target of BTZ [34–37]. Conceivably, β5 induction puts up a first line of defense to compensate for the inhibition of catalytic activity imposed by BTZ and to retain proficient residual catalytic activity to process polyubiquinated proteins and maintain cellular homeostasis. In a clinical setting, Lu et al. [38] reported that β5 induction was also observed in a small-sized study in MM patients and could be a contributing factor in diminished BTZ efficacy return.

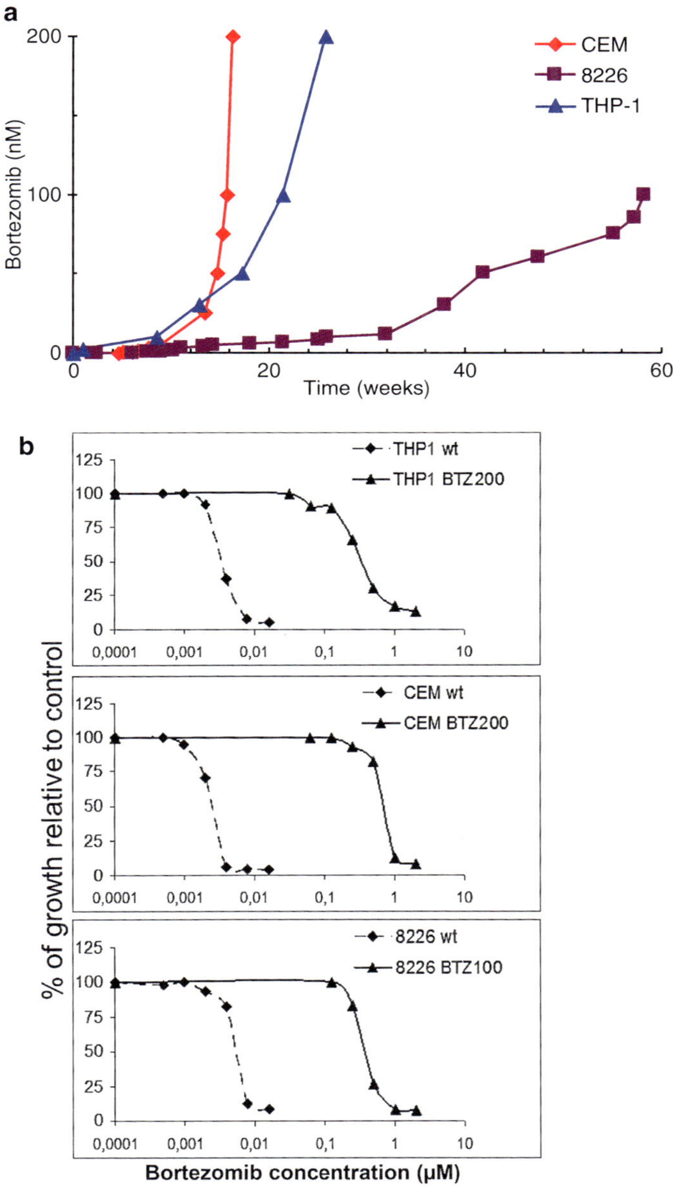

Fig. 7.2 Dynamics of bortezomib resistance induction in human leukemic cell lines. (**a**) Timeline of the generation of BTZ-resistant human monocytic/macrophage THP-1 cells, human T-acute lymphoblastic leukemia CEM cells, and human multiple myeloma 8226 cells. The timeline depicts dose increments of BTZ during the acquisition of resistance. For CEM and THP-1, cells were challenged to withstand 200 nM BTZ, for 8226; 100 nM. (**b**) Dose–response curve for BTZ-induced growth inhibition of wild-type (WT) and BTZ-resistant variants of CEM, THP-1, and 8226. Results depicted are the mean of 3–6 separate experiments, measured after 96 h drug exposure by MTT cytotoxicity assay. The table insert presents the resistance factors to proteasome inhibitors in a series of BTZ-resistant hematological cell lines as determined on the basis of the IC50 ratio compared to the parental (WT) cells. For comparison, resistance factors are shown for CEM cells overexpressing the multidrug resistance drug efflux transporter P-glycoprotein (Pgp) in the absence or presence of an agent blocking Pgp activity

Resistance factors compared to parental (WT) cells

Cell line		Directed to β subunits			Directed to α subunits
		BTZ	CFZ	MG132	5AHQ
CEM	BTZ200	170	38.8	122	1.1
THP-1	BTZ200	73.6	22.3	15.8	1.2
8226	BTZ100	14.9	9.7	12.6	1.3
JY	BTZ100	10.4	1.3	2.2	
CEM	PgP	4.5	114		
	+ Pgp blocker	1.5	4.8		

Fig. 7.2 (continued)

Table 7.1 Overview of mutations in exon 2 of the *PSMB5* gene in hematological bortezomib-resistant cell lines

Cell type	Cell line	Selective concentration	Sequence change	Protein change	Reference
T-ALL	CEM: first selection	7 nM	G332T	Cys52Phe	[32]
	second selection	200 nM	G332T and C323T	Cys52Phe and Ala49Val	
		7–100 nM	G322A	Ala49Thr	
	Jurkat: B2	1,000 nM	G322A	Ala49Thr	[40]
	B3	1,000 nM	C323T	Ala49Val	
	B5	1,000 nM	G322A and C326T	Ala49Thr and Ala50Val	
EBV-transformed B lymphocytes	JY	35–100 nM	G311T	Met45Ile	[47]
AML (monocytic)	THP-1: first selection	7 nM	G322A	Ala49Thr	[31]
	second selection	500 nM	G322A and G311T	Ala49Thr and Met45Iso	
		7–100 nM	A310G	Met45Val	
Multiple myeloma	8226	7 nM	A247G	Thr21Ala	[32]
		100 nM	G322A	Ala49Thr	
	KSM-11	NA (24.7)		Ala49Thr	[41]
	OPM-2	NA (16.6)		Ala49Thr	[41]

Rather than absolute levels of β5 expression, Niewerth et al. [18] showed that the increased ratio of immunoproteasome β5i over constitutive β5 could serve as an indicator of ex vivo proteasome inhibitor sensitivity of BTZ and other proteasome inhibitors in primary pediatric ALL and AML clinical samples.

7.4.2 *Impact of PSMB5/Beta 5 Subunit Mutations*

Beyond β5 subunit induction, a growing body of studies has identified point mutations in the *PSMB5* gene as an underlying cause of acquired resistance to BTZ in hematological cell lines [31, 32, 39–43] as well as solid tumor cells [44, 45]. A common feature for all these BTZ-resistant cell lines is that the mutations reside in exon 2 encoding for the highly conserved S1 binding pocket region for BTZ within the β5 protein [46, 47] (Fig. 7.3).

In the functional β5 subunit protein, these mutations introduce substitutions at amino acid positions in the conserved substrate/inhibitor pocket binding domain of the β5 subunit. Computational biology analysis revealed that these mutations lead to impaired BTZ-binding efficiency but probably did not affect catalytic activity [32]. An overview of these mutations and amino acid substitutions in various BTZ-resistant hematological cell lines is presented in Table 7.1. Strikingly, these mutations cluster around nucleotide position 310/311 and critical amino acid position Ala49 and Met 45 in the β5 protein (Fig. 7.3). Interestingly, Table 7.1 illustrates that when the same parental cells were exposed for a second independent round of BTZ resistance development, again mutations were found in the indicated hot spots, even though amino

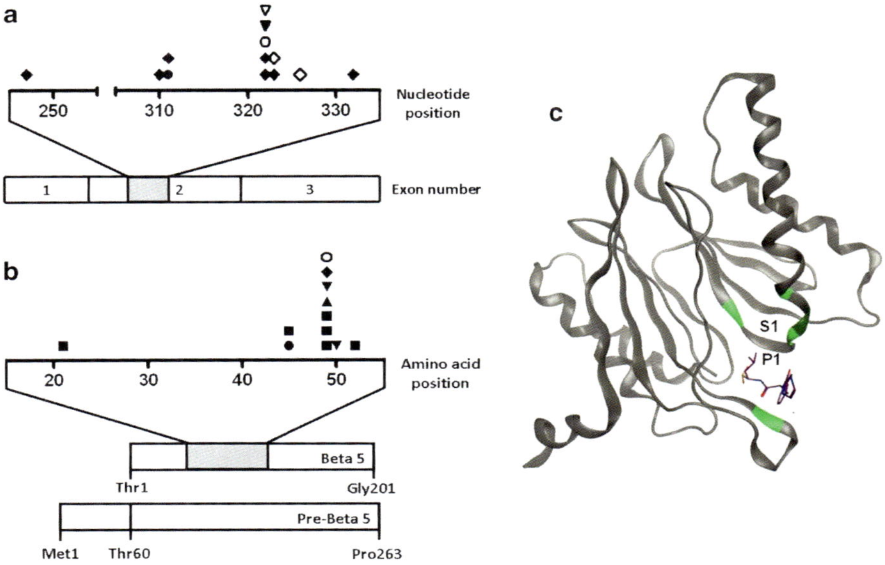

Fig. 7.3 Clustering of mutations in the *PSMB5* gene (β5 subunit) in bortezomib-resistant hematological cell lines. (**a**) Mutations cluster together in DNA of exon 2 of *PSMB5* and (**b**) in protein sequence. Represented mutations are described in: (*filled diamond*) Franke et al. [32], (*filled inverted triangle*) Oerlemans et al. [31], (*open diamond*) Lu et al. [41], (*inverted triangle*) Lu et al. [40], (*open circle*) Ri et al. [42], and (*filled circle*) Verbrugge et al. [43]. (**c**) Graphic representation of the 3D protein-backbone structure of the β5 subunit. Mutations are depicted in *green*. P1, substrate side chain 1; S1, specificity binding pocket 1. Figure adapted from Franke et al. [32]

acid substitutions were not necessarily the same. This indicates that the mutations did not emerge from a preexisting clone harboring growth advantage during drug selection but that the de novo mutations were acquired. It should be emphasized that mutations in *PSMB5* were not (yet) observed in clinical specimens of patients, either from therapy-naïve patients or those receiving BTZ-containing therapies. It remains to be investigated whether *PSMB5* mutations may emerge in leukemic cells from patients who received multiple rounds of BTZ therapy and became therapy refractory. It should be mentioned that *PSMB5* mutations similar to those in leukemia cells were observed in human BTZ-resistant EBV-transformed JY lymphoblastoid cells [43], suggesting that also nonmalignant cells may acquire these mutations. Moreover, it is of interest to note that *PSMB5* mutations were also observed in the marine bacterium *Salinispora tropica* as a self-protective mechanism against the proteasome inhibitor salinosporamide A (NPI-0052/marizomib); it produces as defense modus against other microbes [48, 49]. Lastly, in hematological malignancies, polymorphic variations in the *PSMB5* gene have been described, but these were not implicated in variations in drug response or BTZ efficacy [50].

Together, *PSMB5* mutations can contribute to BTZ resistance but may not be accountable for the complete resistance phenotype. Currently, BTZ-resistant CEM, THP-1, and 8226 cells are subjected to genome-wide studies aimed to investigate additional mechanisms of resistance. As a preliminary account, it was remarkable to note that with respect to differential expression of genes, miRNA and/or proteins between the parental and BTZ-resistant cells, there were little overlap features between the three different types of hematological cell lines. Hence, this warrants further analyses in each cell type separately.

7.4.3 Role of Immunoproteasome in Bortezomib Resistance

Where BTZ resistance can be due to upregulation of constitutive β5 proteasome subunits expression and acquisition of mutations in the *PSMB5* gene, it is of interest to note that the immunoproteasome counterpart β5i was not subject to upregulation and/or acquisition of mutations during chronic BTZ exposure. In fact, in BTZ-resistant CEM, THP-1 and 8226 cells displayed a marked downregulation of immunoproteasome levels, including β5i, as compared to BTZ-sensitive parental cells [18, 31, 32]. Such a response may serve as an escape mechanism to undergo apoptosis by targeting of (non-mutated) β5i by BTZ. In this context, it is of interest to note that other than malignant BTZ-resistant cells, BTZ-resistant JY lymphoblastoid cells did not display a downregulation of β5i, which supports observations that JY/BTZ cells largely retain drug sensitivity to CFZ and immunoproteasome inhibitors [43].

7.4.4 Role of Drug Efflux Transporters

Drug efflux transporters belonging to the superfamily of ATP-binding cassette (ABC) proteins have an established role in conferring a multidrug-resistant (MDR) phenotype by facilitating drug extrusion from cancer cells [51]. Several studies have examined whether or not BTZ and other proteasome inhibitors may serve as potential substrates for MDR-related drug efflux transporters. Initial studies by Minderman et al. [52] showed that BTZ can be exported by the drug efflux transporter P-glycoprotein (Pgp), but this was not accompanied by conferring high levels of BTZ resistance. These observations were confirmed by Verbrugge et al. [53], who showed that BTZ was a modest Pgp substrate, whose activity could be enhanced by blocking of Pgp function (see Table in Fig. 7.2). Recent studies by O'Connor et al. [54] demonstrated that BTZ exposure suppressed Pgp expression, which may contribute to self-potentiation of BTZ activity. Other than BTZ, studies by Verbrugge et al. [53] showed that epoxyketone peptide-based proteasome inhibitors such as CFZ, ONX0912, and ONX0914 were bona fide substrates for Pgp, conferring high levels of resistance in Pgp overexpression cells, being reversible by blocking of Pgp function. Consistent with a role for Pgp in resistance to epoxyketone-based proteasome inhibitors, acquired resistance to CFZ [55] and epoxomicin [56] was found to be mediated by upregulation of Pgp. Medicinal chemistry of epoxyketone-based drugs showed that modifications of the N-cap of the peptide epoxyketone backbone, in particular introducing (5-Me)-3-isoxazole or 2-(S)-tetrahydrofuran, retained CT-L proteasome inhibitory activity while the Pgp substrate activity was abolished [57]. Lastly, Verbrugge et al. [53] showed that BTZ and epoxyketone-based proteasome inhibitors lacked substrate affinity for ABC transporters other than Pgp, e.g., multidrug resistance-associated protein 1–5 (MRP1–5) or breast cancer resistance protein (BCRP), suggesting that these drug efflux transporters are no major contributors to proteasome inhibitor resistance.

7.4.5 Other Mechanisms of Bortezomib Resistance

At least three other mechanisms were recently identified to contribute to BTZ resistance. In multiple myeloma, increased activation of insulin-like growth factor-1 receptor signaling served as a pro-survival modality to overcome cytotoxic effects of BTZ [58]. In mantle cell lymphoma, BTZ resistance could be induced by plasmacytic differentiation associated with upregulation of interferon regulatory factor 4 (IRF4) and increased expression of CD38 and CD138 [59]. High tumor necrosis factor activating factor (TRAF6) is related to MM cell survival via activation of the pro-survival NF-κB pathway. In this respect, TRAF6 inhibition is an interesting novel treatment strategy [60] which also can resensitize BTZ-resistant AML cells [61].

Together, multifactorial mechanisms may contribute in conferring acquired resistance to BTZ in in vitro model systems of leukemic cells (summarized in

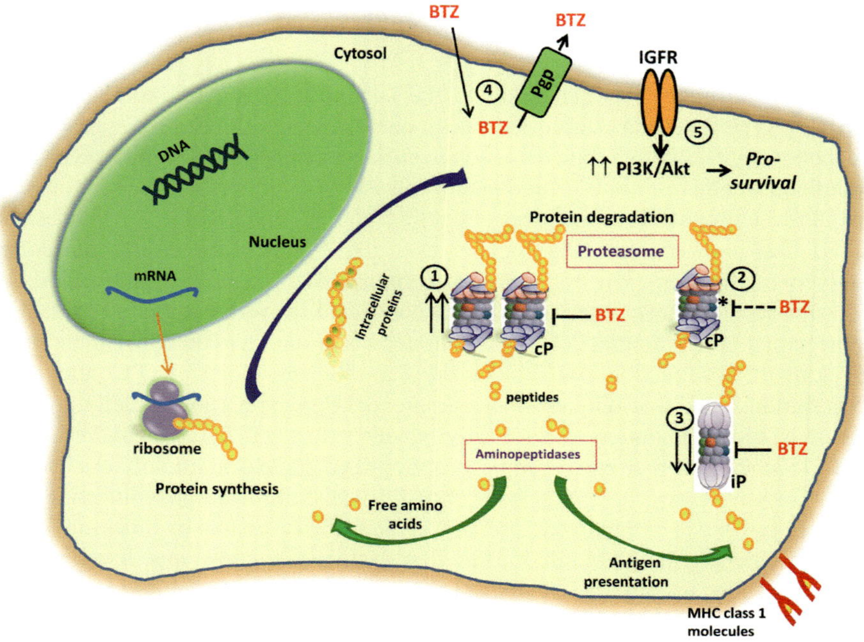

Fig. 7.4 Overview of molecular mechanisms contributing to acquired resistance to bortezomib in in vitro model systems of hematological malignancies. Resistance mechanisms depicted include (1) upregulation of constitutive proteasome (cP) subunit expression, in particular β5, requiring increased concentrations of BTZ to achieve sufficient inhibition of chymotrypsin-like proteasome catalytic activity; (2) point mutations in the *PSMB5* gene introducing amino acid substitutions in critical positions of the BTZ-binding pocket of the β5 subunit; (3) downregulation of immunoproteasome (iP) subunit β5i to escape inhibitory activity of BTZ; (4) cellular extrusion of BTZ facilitated by the drug efflux transporter P-glycoprotein (this mechanism may be more relevant for epoxyketone-based proteasome inhibitors); and (5) activation of PI3K/Akt pro-survival pathways, through insulin-like growth factor-1 receptor (IGFR) signaling. * denotes β5 subunit mutation

Fig. 7.4). Which mechanism would appear dominant in clinical specimen of therapy refractory patients warrants further investigations but may depend on cell types, type of the proteasome inhibitor, and duration of drug administration (Fig. 7.4).

7.5 New Strategies to Overcome Bortezomib Resistance

Despite the encouraging results of BTZ in several hematological malignancies, emergence of BTZ resistance as well as side effects are factors that limit its long-term efficacy [8]. Several reviews discussed the rationale and design of new generation of proteasome inhibitors that may help to overcome BTZ resistance in minimize toxic side effects [20, 62–66].

7.5.1 Next-Generation Proteasome Inhibitors

Late July 2012, the FDA approved the proteasome inhibitor CFZ, which is a potent, more selective, and irreversible inhibitor of the CT-L activity (both constitutive- and immunoproteasome). A beneficial property over BTZ is that CFZ has minimal off-target effects on other proteases, which may underlie the fewer side effects [55, 67, 68]. In a recent study including primary human AML and ALL patient samples, we established their ex vivo sensitivity for BTZ and CFZ, revealing both IC50s in the nanomolar range, but CFZ being slightly more potent [18, 69].

Another active site irreversible proteasome inhibitor is marizomib (salinosporamide A/NPI-0052), a potent proteasome inhibitor with a natural β-lactone active group. Marizomib differs from the other proteasome inhibitors in that it predominantly inhibits the CT-L and T-L activities of the proteasome and to some extent also the C-L activity [70, 71].

The abovementioned proteasome inhibitors exhibit their most potent inhibitory activity towards constitutive proteasome subunits, but recently also inhibitors with greater specificity to immunoproteasome subunits have been developed. ONX 0914 is a prototypical β5i-specific irreversible proteasome inhibitor with 40-fold greater specificity for β5i over β5 [72, 73] based on efficiency of immunoproteasome inhibition in rats. ONX 0914 activity has been evaluated in a T-ALL cell line where it shows immunoproteasome inhibitory capacity in the nanomolar concentration range, although its cell growth inhibitory potency was 30-fold and 55-fold less than BTZ and CFZ, respectively. Despite the different specificity for β5 and β5i subunits, it remains to be established whether ONX 0914 may be useful in a clinical setting of BTZ-resistant patients, since cross-resistance to ONX 0914 was observed in BTZ-resistant ALL cell lines [32].

The epoxyketone-based tripeptide PR924 is a novel proteasome inhibitor designed to be more selective for human immunoproteasome targeting. PR-924 is 130-fold more selective for β5i than β5 [74]. Remarkably, despite complete β5i inhibition, the antileukemic effects of the immunoproteasome inhibitors ONX 0914 and PR924 only arise at concentrations that also inhibit the constitutive β5 subunit.

5AHQ [33] represents a novel class of noncompetitive proteasome inhibitors that primarily targets the α7 subunits of the (immune)proteasome rather than the β-subunits targeted by BTZ. 5AHQ displays antileukemic activity at low micromolar drug concentrations and displays full sensitivity towards BTZ-resistant leukemia cells [32].

7.5.2 Oral Availability

Clinically relevant disadvantages of BTZ relate to its inability of oral administration and its toxicity profile, let alone the emergence of resistance discussed above. One other drawback of BTZ includes its binding to red blood cells and slow dissociation rate thereof. To overcome these limitations, the orally available boronate MLN9708 (ixazomib) was designed, which is a reversible inhibitor of the proteasomal CT-L activity and at higher concentrations also C-L and T-L catalytic activities. MLN9708 is featured by a faster proteasome dissociation rate from red blood cells, which should improve tissue distribution compared to BTZ [75]. MLN9708 is the first orally available inhibitor to enter clinical trials in MM [76]. In addition, ONX 0912 (oprozomib) has been developed as an orally available analog of CFZ. This drug is currently tested in hematological malignancies [77].

7.5.3 Protein Degradation Inhibition More Upstream from the Proteasome

Proteins prone for degradation by the proteasome require tagging with multiple ubiquitin moieties. This ubiquitination process upstream of the proteasome is accomplished by the chronological action of four enzyme families (E1, E2, E3, and E4). Currently, several compounds have been developed that inhibit key steps in this process leading to disruption of the cellular protein homeostasis [78]. In particular in normal hematopoiesis, this pathway is crucial for control of quiescence, self-renewal, and differentiation of normal hematopoietic stem cells. This implies that disruption of this control may lead to leukemogenesis and knowledge of this process will lead to novel targeted therapies [79, 80]. An example of a recently developed inhibitor is MLN 4924, directed against the NEDD8 activating enzyme. This enzyme is important for the activation of cullin-RING-dependent ubiquitin E3 ligases, which are crucial for the protein cascade responsible for the poly-ubiquitination of proteins marked for degradation by the proteasome. In preclinical studies, MLN4924 showed promising results as antileukemic drug [81, 82].

7.5.4 Combinations of Bortezomib with Conventional Chemotherapeutics

Knowledge about the shortcomings in BTZ efficacy and mechanisms of BTZ resistance can set the stage for exploring drug combinations that may (re)sensitize leukemic cells for BTZ-induced cytotoxicity. In leukemic cell lines, BTZ was shown to interact in an additive or synergistic way when combined with traditional antileukemic drugs, including glucocorticoids [83]. Furthermore, BTZ and CFZ combined with idarubicin or cytarabine showed additive antiproliferative and proapoptotic effects on primary AML blasts [69]. Together, these results demonstrate the potential of incorporating proteasome inhibitors in conventional chemotherapeutic regimens for hematological malignancies, thereby paving the way to limit off-target effects and limit toxicity.

7.5.5 *Combinations of Bortezomib with Other Proteasome Inhibitors*

Since changes in the β5 subunit are implicated with BTZ resistance, combinations with other proteasome inhibitors that display inhibitory activities to other subunits serve as a plausible rationalized option. In MM cells, combinations of CEP-18770 with BTZ [84] and ONX 0912 combined with BTZ showed synergistic effects [77]. Combinations of BTZ and marizomib below their individual IC50 concentrations showed synergistic effects in MM, leukemia, and lymphoma cell lines [85].

7.5.6 *Combinations of Bortezomib with HDAC Inhibitors*

Another approach is to combine BTZ with histone deacetylase inhibitors (HDACi), which can be highly beneficial given that HDACs, in particular HDAC6, are relevant for the formation of protein aggregates [86]. Several preclinical studies have been performed to explore the added value of HDACi in BTZ combination therapy. Combining BTZ with the HDACi trichostatin A displayed synergistic or additive effects in both ALL and AML cell lines [83]. Furthermore, combining BTZ and valproic acid showed additivity in an AML cell line and synergism in a therapy-resistant AML subline [87]. Consistently, greater inhibition of proliferation of AML blasts was noted when BTZ was combined with vorinostat compared to each drug alone [69]. Also marizomib was found to synergistically induce apoptosis with HDACi MS-275, even with greater potency than for BTZ combined with MS-275 [71]. In the CEM, THP-1, and 8226 cells and their BTZ-resistant counterparts, vorinostat was combined with BTZ in a viability (MTT) assay in a wide dose range (0.09–1 μM vorinostat and 0.005–0.5 μM BTZ). Interestingly, BTZ-resistant 8226 cells were twofold more sensitive for vorinostat compared to the parental cells. All cells, in particular the resistant cells, could be sensitized for BTZ by co-incubation with vorinostat. The combination indexes ranged from 0.05 in the higher concentrations to 0.7 in the lower concentration range (Calcusyn analysis) indicating synergy between these two drugs (unpublished observations).

7.6 Translational Implications

One novel feature emerging from characterization of BTZ-resistant leukemia cell line models, i.e., upregulation of the constitutive and concomitant downregulation of the immunoproteasome, was examined in further detail in relation to diminished proteasome inhibitor sensitivity of primary pediatric ALL and AML cells. Ex vivo data showed that pediatric ALL patient samples were significantly more sensitive than AML samples for BTZ, CFZ, ONX 0912, ONX 0914, and dexamethasone [18]. For proteasome inhibitors, this may be explained by the fact that although total proteasome levels in ALL and AML cells did not differ significantly, the ratio of immunoproteasome over constitutive proteasome was markedly higher in the relative BTZ-sensitive ALL cells compared to AML cells. Additionally, both in ALL and AML, increased ratios of β5i/β5, β1i/β1, and β2i/β2 correlated with increased sensitivity to BTZ as measured with a cell viability (MTT) assay [18]. Hence, this ratio deserves further exploration as potential biomarker to select patients that will benefit from BTZ treatment and may facilitate the monitoring of acquired resistance during BTZ treatment. Currently, patient samples from cohorts of children treated with BTZ in recent Children's Oncology Group protocols for refractory and relapsed ALL and AML are collected for further validation. Proteasome subunit expression of these samples will be related to response to BTZ treatment in order to confirm the relevance of the proteasome β5i/β5 ratio to predict which patients are eligible for BTZ treatment.

The relative resistance to BTZ in ex vivo leukemia patient samples with relative low immunoproteasome suggests that upregulation of the immunoproteasome is a promising option to sensitize leukemic cells for proteasome inhibitors. Indeed, as a proof of concept, we noted that upregulation of immunoproteasomes in BTZ-resistant hematological cell lines by IFNγ pretreatment partially resensitized cells to BTZ [88]. Since clinical application of IFNγ administration may face safety limitations, other approaches to upregulate immunoproteasomes levels deserve further exploration.

7.7 Current Clinical Trials in Acute Leukemia

Based on the promising results in MM, BTZ also has been subject of clinical evaluation in patients with leukemia, with currently 16 studies recruiting patients (as assessed from http://www.clinicaltrials.gov and http://www.trialregister.nl). A summary of ongoing clinical trials of proteasome inhibitors in acute leukemia is presented in Table 7.2.

Studies published so far showed modest single-agent activity in children [89] and adults [90–92]. However, phase I studies in which BTZ was combined with conventional chemotherapeutics showed promising clinical activity in both adult AML patients [93–95] and pediatric ALL patients [96, 97]. Conversely, a phase II study of BTZ combined with reinduction chemotherapy in relapsed pediatric AML patients did not show improved CR rates or overall survival [98]. Szczepanek et al. [99] showed that BTZ was even more potent in T-ALL patient samples compared to common/pre-B ALL. This notion that BTZ appeared to be a potent drug for this relatively therapy-resistant subgroup of ALL should not be overinterpreted as the two T-ALL patients included in the phase II clinical trial did not reach a CR [97]. In this context, it should also be taken into account that the recent clinical trials include heavily pretreated patients.

One of the main challenges in chemotherapeutic interventions is to find optimal conditions for single drugs or drug combinations that selectively target malignant cells while sparing normal cells to limit drug-induced toxicities. For BTZ, modest clinical activity was noted as single agent in hematological malignancies, whereas combination therapies were clearly superior [100]. In fact, for the treatment of leu-

Table 7.2 Summary of ongoing clinical trials of proteasome inhibitors in acute leukemia

Study	Time period	*N*	Phase	Cohort	Age group (year)	Sponsor	Reference
Bortezomib + belinostat	May 2010–February 2014	24	Phase 1	Relapsed/refractory acute leukemias	>18	Virginia Commonwealth University	NCT01075425
Bortezomib + mitoxantrone + etoposide + cytarabine	January 2006–January 2014	55	Phase 1/2	Relapsed/refractory acute leukemias	>18	Thomas Jefferson University	NCT00410423
Decitabine vs. bortezomib + decitabine	November 2011–November 2013	172	Phase 2	AML	>60	National Cancer Institute	NCT01420926
Bortezomib + combination chemotherapy	March 2013–March 2014	17	Phase 2	Relapsed/refractory ALL	>18	Stanford University	NCT01769209
Bortezomib + EPOCH chemotherapy	September 2010–April 2018	20	Phase 1/2	Adult T-cell leukemia/lymphoma	>18	Washington University School of Medicine	NCT01000285
Bortezomib	November 2011–September 2013	35	Phase 2	AML in remission	>18	Fred Hutchinson Cancer Research Center/University of Washington Cancer Consortium	NCT01465386
Bortezomib + mitoxantrone + etoposide + cytarabine	July 2010–February 2014	24	Phase 1	Relapsed/refractory AML	18–70	Case Comprehensive Cancer Center	NCT01127009
Bortezomib + midostaurin vs. Bortezomib + midostaurin + mitoxantrone + etoposide + cytarabine	August 2010–August 2014	42	Phase 1	Relapsed/refractory AML	>18	Ohio State University Comprehensive Cancer Center	NCT01174888
Bortezomib + vorinostat + sorafenib	February 2010–February 2015	38	Phase 1/2	AML	>18	Indiana University	NCT01534260

(continued)

Table 7.2 (continued)

Study	Time period	*N*	Phase	Cohort	Age group (year)	Sponsor	Reference
Bortezomib ± several chemotherapeutic drugs in randomization arms	June 2011–February 2015	1,250	Phase 3	Initial AML	>29	National Cancer Institute	NCT01371981
Bortezomib + Doxil (doxorubicin)	March 2013–March 2017	30	Phase 2	AML	18–80	University of California, Davis	NCT01736943
Bortezomib + vorinostat + dexamethasone + methotrexate	June 2011–June 2013	33	Phase 2	Relapsed/refractory ALL	2–30	Masonic Cancer Center, University of Minnesota	NCT01312818
Bortezomib + intensive reinduction chemotherapy	March 2009–September 2014	151	Phase 2	Relapsed ALL	1–31	Children's Oncology Group	NCT00873093
Bortezomib + nelfinavir mesylate	July 2010–March 2013	24	Phase 1	Relapsed or progressive advanced hematologic cancer	>18	Swiss Group for Clinical Cancer Research	NCT01164709
Bortezomib + dexamethasone + vincristine + methotrexate	September 2009–September 2012	24	Phase 2	Relapsed/refractory ALL	0.5–19	Erasmus Medical Center	NTR1881
Carfilzomib	October 2010–August 2013	36	Phase 1	Relapsed/refractory CLL, SLL (small), PLL (pro)	>18	Ohio State University Comprehensive Cancer Center	NCT01212380
Carfilzomib	October 2010–October 2013	18	Phase 1	Relapsed/refractory ALL and AML	>18	Washington University School of Medicine	NCT01137747
NPI-0052 (marizomib)	July 2007–December 2012	50	Phase 1	Advanced malignancies	>18	Nereus Pharmaceuticals, Inc.	NCT00629473

AML acute myeloid leukemia, *ALL* acute lymphoblastic leukemia, *CLL* chronic lymphocytic leukemia, *SLL* small lymphocytic leukemia, *PLL* prolymphocytic leukemia

kemia, there is growing consensus that BTZ should be tested only in combination with the standard use of intensive combined chemotherapeutic agents.

Currently, 13 clinical trials are combining BTZ and HDACi (mostly vorinostat) in hematological malignancies, of which 2 in leukemia. The first phase II trial (NCT01312818) examines BTZ, vorinostat, and DEX in patients with relapsed or refractory ALL from 2 to 30 years of age. The second phase I/II study (NCT01534260) evaluates BTZ, vorinostat, and sorafenib in a subgroup of adult patients with AML [27]. Despite all encouraging preclinical data, a recent study (NCT00818649) combining vorinostat (400 mg daily on days 1–14) and BTZ (1.3 mg/m^2 IV on days 1, 4, 8, and 11 of a 21-day cycle) in relapsed/refractory acute myeloid leukemia (AML) and high-risk myelodysplastic syndrome was aborted prematurely due to toxicity [101]. Other ongoing combination clinical trials of BTZ include those with HDACi, tyrosine kinase inhibitors, farnesyltransferase inhibitors, Bcl-2 family inhibitors, and heat shock protein inhibitors [102]. Accumulating data indicated that most combinations were tolerable and supported interest for studying combinations with next-generation proteasome inhibitors (e.g., CFZ), both for MM and leukemia.

Together, the known toxicity profile of BTZ invites for further optimization of combination therapies to achieve a broader proteasome inhibition at lower and probably safer doses. The majority of the combinations involving BTZ in MM and lymphoma patients showed synergistic antitumor efficacy in preclinical studies and therefore provide the rationale for future design of new clinical trials.

7.8 Concluding Remarks

In vitro studies were useful in identifying multifactorial mechanisms of acquired resistance to BTZ. While some of these mechanisms are unique for BTZ, others may also apply to new-generation proteasome inhibitors. By no means this list of mechanisms is considered complete. Future challenges will be to integrate the expanding knowledge of clinical, molecular, and biochemical data into the design of new clinical studies to aid hematologists/oncologists in identifying patients who will or will not respond to proteasome inhibitor-based therapies or those who are prone to develop resistance to these drugs. The reported laboratory studies set the first steps into this direction but definitely require further follow-up studies.

References

1. Inaba H, Greaves M, Mullighan CG (2013) Acute lymphoblastic leukaemia. Lancet 381:1943–1955
2. Creutzig U, van den Heuvel-Eibrink MM, Gibson B et al (2012) Diagnosis and management of acute myeloid leukemia in children and adolescents: recommendations from an international expert panel. Blood 120:3187–3205
3. Kumar CC (2011) Genetic abnormalities and challenges in the treatment of acute myeloid leukemia. Genes Cancer 2:95–107

4. Bachas C, Schuurhuis GJ, Hollink IHIM et al (2010) High-frequency type I/II mutational shifts between diagnosis and relapse are associated with outcome in pediatric AML: implications for personalized medicine. Blood 116:2752–2758
5. Bachas C, Schuurhuis GJ, Assaraf YG et al (2012) The role of minor subpopulations within the leukemic blast compartment of AML patients at initial diagnosis in the development of relapse. Leukemia 26:1313–1320
6. Welch JS, Ley TJ, Link DC et al (2012) The origin and evolution of mutations in acute myeloid leukemia. Cell 150:264–278
7. Kaspers GJL, Zimmermann M, Reinhardt D et al (2013) Improved outcome in pediatric relapsed acute myeloid leukemia: results of a randomized trial on liposomal daunorubicin by the International BFM Study Group. J Clin Oncol 31:599–607
8. Moreau P, Richardson PG, Cavo M et al (2012) Proteasome inhibitors in multiple myeloma: 10 years later. Blood 120:947–959
9. Saric T, Graef CI, Goldberg AL (2004) Pathway for degradation of peptides generated by proteasomes: a key role for thimet oligopeptidase and other metallopeptidases. J Biol Chem 279:46723–46732
10. Drews O, Wildgruber R, Zong C et al (2007) Mammalian proteasome subpopulations with distinct molecular compositions and proteolytic activities. Mol Cell Proteomics 6:2021–2031
11. Guillaume B, Chapiro J, Stroobant V et al (2010) Two abundant proteasome subtypes that uniquely process some antigens presented by HLA class I molecules. Proc Natl Acad Sci U S A 107:18599–18604
12. Kunjappu MJ, Hochstrasser M (2014) Assembly of the 20S proteasome. Biochim Biophys Acta 1843(1):2–12
13. Groettrup M, Khan S, Schwarz K, Schmidtke G (2001) Interferon-gamma inducible exchanges of 20S proteasome active site subunits: why? Biochimie 83:367–372
14. Aki M, Shimbara N, Takashina M et al (1994) Interferon-gamma induces different subunit organizations and functional diversity of proteasomes. J Biochem 115:257–269
15. Altun M, Galardy PJ, Shringarpure R et al (2005) Effects of PS-341 on the activity and composition of proteasomes in multiple myeloma cells. Cancer Res 65:7896–7901
16. Seifert U, Bialy LP, Ebstein F et al (2010) Immunoproteasomes preserve protein homeostasis upon interferon-induced oxidative stress. Cell 142:613–624
17. Nathan J, Spinnenhirn V, Schmidtke G et al (2013) Immuno- and constitutive proteasomes do not differ in their abilities to degrade ubiquitinated proteins. Cell 152:1184–1194
18. Niewerth D, Franke NE, Jansen G et al (2013) Higher ratio immune vs. constitutive proteasome level as novel indicator of sensitivity of pediatric acute leukemia cells to proteasome inhibitors. Haematologica 98(12):1896–1904
19. Bianchi G, Oliva L, Cascio P et al (2009) The proteasome load versus capacity balance determines apoptotic sensitivity of multiple myeloma cells to proteasome inhibition. Blood 113:3040–3049
20. Niewerth D, Dingjan I, Cloos J et al (2013) Proteasome inhibitors in acute leukemia. Expert Rev Anticancer Ther 13:327–337
21. Kane RC, Farrell AT, Sridhara R, Pazdur R (2006) United States Food and Drug Administration approval summary: bortezomib for the treatment of progressive multiple myeloma after one prior therapy. Clin Cancer Res 12:2955–2960
22. Kane RC, Dagher R, Farrell A et al (2007) Bortezomib for the treatment of mantle cell lymphoma. Clin Cancer Res 13:5291–5294
23. Frankland-Searby S, Bhaumik SR (2012) The 26S proteasome complex: an attractive target for cancer therapy. Biochim Biophys Acta 1825:64–76
24. McConkey DJ, Zhu K (2008) Mechanisms of proteasome inhibitor action and resistance in cancer. Drug Resist Updat 11:164–179
25. Naujokat C, Sezer O, Zinke H et al (2000) Proteasome inhibitors induce caspase-dependent apoptosis and accumulation leukemic cells. Eur J Hematol 65:221–236
26. Nasr R, El-Sabban ME, Karam J-A et al (2005) Efficacy and mechanism of action of the proteasome inhibitor PS-341 in T-cell lymphomas and HTLV-I associated adult T-cell leukemia/lymphoma. Oncogene 24:419–430

27. Martinon F (2012) Targeting endoplasmic reticulum signaling pathways in cancer. Acta Oncol 51:822–830
28. Driscoll JJ, De Chowdhury R (2012) Molecular crosstalk between the proteasome, aggresomes and autophagy: translational potential and clinical implications. Cancer Lett 325:147–154
29. Kincaid EZ, Che JW, York I et al (2012) Mice completely lacking immunoproteasomes show major changes in antigen presentation. Nat Immunol 13:129–135
30. Vigneron N, Van den Eynde BJ (2012) Proteasome subtypes and the processing of tumor antigens: increasing antigenic diversity. Curr Opin Hematol 24:84–91
31. Oerlemans R, Franke NE, Assaraf YG et al (2008) Molecular basis of bortezomib resistance: proteasome subunit beta5 (PSMB5) gene mutation and overexpression of PSMB5 protein. Blood 112:2489–2499
32. Franke NE, Niewerth D, Assaraf YG et al (2012) Impaired bortezomib binding to mutant beta5 subunit of the proteasome is the underlying basis for bortezomib resistance in leukemia cells. Leukemia 26:757–768
33. Li X, Wood TE, Sprangers R et al (2010) Effect of noncompetitive proteasome inhibition on bortezomib resistance. J Natl Cancer Inst 102:1069–1082
34. Ruckrich T, Kraus M, Gogel J et al (2009) Characterization of the ubiquitin-proteasome system in bortezomib-adapted cells. Leukemia 23:1098–1105
35. Kraus M, Ruckrich T, Reich M et al (2007) Activity patterns of proteasome subunits reflect bortezomib sensitivity of hematologic malignancies and are variable in primary human leukemia cells. Leukemia 21:84–92
36. Busse A, Kraus M, Na IK et al (2008) Sensitivity of tumor cells to proteasome inhibitors is associated with expression levels and composition of proteasome subunits. Cancer 112:659–670
37. Balsas P, Galan-Malo P, Marzo I, Naval J (2012) Bortezomib resistance in a myeloma cell line is associated to PSMβ5 overexpression and polyploidy. Leuk Res 36:212–218
38. Lu S, Yang J, Huang C et al (2011) Upregulated expression of the PSMB5 gene may contribute to drug resistance in patient with multiple myeloma when treated with bortezomib-based regimen. Exp Hematol 39:1117–1118
39. Lü S-Q, Yang J-M, Huang C-M et al (2011) Comparison of protein expression profiles between bortezomib-resistant Jurkat B cells with PSMB5 mutation and their parent cells. J Exp Hematol 19:869–873
40. Lu S, Chen Z, Yang J et al (2008) Overexpression of the PSMB5 gene contributes to bortezomib resistance in T-lymphoblastic lymphoma/leukemia cells derived from Jurkat line. Exp Hematol 36:1278–1284
41. Lu S, Yang J, Chen Z et al (2009) Different mutants of PSMB5 confer varying bortezomib resistance in T lymphoblastic lymphoma/leukemia cells derived from the Jurkat cell line. Exp Hematol 37:831–837
42. Ri M, Iida S, Nakashima T et al (2010) Bortezomib-resistant myeloma cell lines: a role for mutated PSMB5 in preventing the accumulation of unfolded proteins and fatal ER stress. Leukemia 24:1506–1512
43. Verbrugge SE, Al M, Assaraf YG et al (2013) Overcoming bortezomib resistance in human B cells by anti-CD20/rituximab-mediated complement-dependent cytotoxicity and epoxyketone-based irreversible proteasome inhibitors. Exp Hematol Oncol 2:2
44. De Wilt LH, Jansen G, Assaraf YG et al (2012) Proteasome-based mechanisms of intrinsic and acquired bortezomib resistance in non-small cell lung cancer. Biochem Pharmacol 83:207–217
45. Suzuki E, Demo S, Deu E et al (2011) Molecular mechanisms of bortezomib resistant adenocarcinoma cells. PLoS One 6:e27996
46. Groll M, Berkers CR, Ploegh HL, Ovaa H (2006) Crystal structure of the boronic acid-based proteasome inhibitor bortezomib in complex with the yeast 20S proteasome. Structure 14:451–456

47. Borissenko L, Groll M (2007) Diversity of proteasomal missions: fine tuning of the immune response. Biol Chem 388:947–955
48. Kale AJ, McGlinchey RP, Lechner A, Moore BS (2011) Bacterial self-resistance to the natural proteasome inhibitor salinosporamide A. ACS Chem Biol 6:1257–1264
49. Kale AJ, Moore BS (2012) Molecular mechanisms of acquired proteasome inhibitor resistance. J Med Chem 55:10317–10327
50. Lichter DI, Danaee H, Pickard MD et al (2012) Sequence analysis of β-subunit genes of the 20S proteasome in patients with relapsed multiple myeloma treated with bortezomib or dexamethasone. Blood 120:4513–4516
51. Gillet J-P, Gottesman MM (2012) Overcoming multidrug resistance in cancer: 35 years after the discovery of ABCB1. Drug Resist Updat 15:2–4
52. Minderman H, Zhou Y, O'Loughlin KL, Baer MR (2007) Bortezomib activity and in vitro interactions with anthracyclines and cytarabine in acute myeloid leukemia cells are independent of multidrug resistance mechanisms and p53 status. Cancer Chemother Pharmacol 60:245–255
53. Verbrugge SE, Assaraf YG, Dijkmans BC et al (2012) Inactivating PSMB5 mutations and P-glycoprotein (multidrug resistance-associated protein/ATP-binding cassette B1) mediate resistance to proteasome inhibitors: ex vivo efficacy of (immuno)proteasome inhibitors in mononuclear blood cells from patients with. J Pharmacol Exp Ther 341:174–182
54. O'Connor R, Ooi MG, Meiller J et al (2013) The interaction of bortezomib with multidrug transporters: implications for therapeutic applications in advanced multiple myeloma and other neoplasias. Cancer Chemother Pharmacol 71:1357–1368
55. Ao L, Wu Y, Kim D et al (2012) Development of peptide-based reversing agents for p-glycoprotein-mediated resistance to carfilzomib. Mol Pharm 9(8):2197–2205
56. Gutman D, Morales A, Boise LH (2009) Acquisition of a multidrug-resistant phenotype with a proteasome inhibitor in multiple myeloma. Leukemia 23:2181–2183
57. Zhou H-J, Aujay M, Bennett MK et al (2009) Design and synthesis of an orally bioavailable and selective peptide epoxyketone proteasome inhibitor (PR-047). J Med Chem 52: 3028–3038
58. Kuhn DJ, Berkova Z, Jones RJ et al (2012) Targeting the insulin-like growth factor-1 receptor to overcome bortezomib resistance in preclinical models of multiple myeloma. Blood 120:3260–3270
59. Pérez-Galán P, Mora-Jensen H, Weniger MA et al (2011) Bortezomib resistance in mantle cell lymphoma is associated with plasmacytic differentiation. Blood 117:542–552
60. Liu H, Tamashiro S, Baritaki S et al (2012) TRAF6 activation in multiple myeloma: a potential therapeutic target. Clin Lymphoma Myeloma Leuk 12:155–163
61. Fang J, Rhyasen G, Bolanos L et al (2012) Cytotoxic effects of bortezomib in myelodysplastic syndrome/acute myeloid leukemia depend on autophagy-mediated lysosomal degradation of TRAF6 and repression of PSMA1. Blood 120:858–867
62. Dick LR, Fleming PE (2010) Building on bortezomib: second-generation proteasome inhibitors as anti-cancer therapy. Drug Discov Today 15:243–249
63. Kortuem KM, Stewart K (2013) Carfilzomib. Blood 121:893–897
64. Kisselev AF, van der Linden WA, Overkleeft HS (2012) Proteasome inhibitors: an expanding army attacking a unique target. Chem Biol 19:99–115
65. Orlowski RZ, Kuhn DJ (2008) Proteasome inhibitors in cancer therapy: lessons from the first decade. Clin Cancer Res 14:1649–1657
66. Ruschak AM, Slassi M, Kay LE, Schimmer AD (2011) Novel proteasome inhibitors to overcome bortezomib resistance. J Natl Cancer Inst 103:1007–1017
67. Parlati F, Lee SJ, Aujay M et al (2009) Carfilzomib can induce tumor cell death through selective inhibition of the chymotrypsin-like activity of the proteasome. Blood 114: 3439–3447
68. Kuhn DJ, Chen Q, Voorhees PM et al (2007) Potent activity of carfilzomib, a novel, irreversible inhibitor of the ubiquitin-proteasome pathway, against preclinical models of multiple myeloma. Blood 110:3281–3290

69. Stapnes C, Doskeland AP, Hatfield K et al (2007) The proteasome inhibitors bortezomib and PR-171 have antiproliferative and proapoptotic effects on primary human acute myeloid leukaemia cells. Br J Haematol 136:814–828
70. Chauhan D, Catley L, Li G et al (2005) A novel orally active proteasome inhibitor induces apoptosis in multiple myeloma cells with mechanisms distinct from Bortezomib. Cancer Cell 8:407–419
71. Miller CP, Ban K, Dujka ME et al (2007) NPI-0052, a novel proteasome inhibitor, induces caspase-8 and ROS-dependent apoptosis alone and in combination with HDAC inhibitors in leukemia cells. Blood 110:267–277
72. Kuhn DJ, Orlowski RZ (2012) The immunoproteasome as a target in hematologic malignancies. Semin Hematol 49:258–262
73. Muchamuel T, Basler M, Aujay MA et al (2009) A selective inhibitor of the immunoproteasome subunit LMP7 blocks cytokine production and attenuates progression of experimental arthritis. Nat Med 15:781–787
74. Singh AV, Bandi M, Aujay MA et al (2011) PR-924, a selective inhibitor of the immunoproteasome subunit LMP-7, blocks multiple myeloma cell growth both in vitro and in vivo. Br J Haematol 152:155–163
75. Chauhan D, Tian Z, Zhou B et al (2011) In vitro and in vivo selective antitumor activity of a novel orally bioavailable proteasome inhibitor MLN9708 against multiple myeloma cells. Clin Cancer Res 17:5311–5321
76. Assouline S, Chang JE, Cheson BD et al (2012) Results of a phase 1 dose-escalation study of once-weekly MLN9708, an investigational proteasome inhibitor, in patients with relapsed/refractory lymphoma. ASH annual meeting 120:3646
77. Chauhan D, Singh AV, Aujay M et al (2010) A novel orally active proteasome inhibitor ONX 0912 triggers in vitro and in vivo cytotoxicity in multiple myeloma. Blood 116:4906–4915
78. Micel LN, Tentler JJ, Smith PG, Eckhardt GS (2013) Role of ubiquitin ligases and the proteasome in oncogenesis: novel targets for anticancer therapies. J Clin Oncol 31:1231–1238
79. Moran-Crusio K, Reavie LB, Aifantis I (2012) Regulation of hematopoietic stem cell fate by the ubiquitin proteasome system. Trends Immunol 33:357–363
80. Krämer OH, Stauber RH, Bug G et al (2013) SIAH proteins: critical roles in leukemogenesis. Leukemia 27:792–802
81. Swords RT, Kelly KR, Smith PG et al (2010) Brief report Inhibition of NEDD8-activating enzyme: a novel approach for the treatment of acute myeloid leukemia. Blood 115: 3796–3800
82. Smith MA, Maris JM, Gorlick R et al (2012) Initial testing of the investigational NEDD8-activating enzyme inhibitor MLN4924 by the pediatric preclinical testing program. Pediatr Blood Cancer 59:246–253
83. Horton TM, Gannavarapu A, Blaney SM et al (2006) Bortezomib interactions with chemotherapy agents in acute leukemia in vitro. Cancer Chemother Pharmacol 58:13–23
84. Sanchez E, Li M, Li J et al (2012) CEP-18770 (delanzomib) in combination with dexamethasone and lenalidomide inhibits the growth of multiple myeloma. Leuk Res 36:1422–1427
85. Chauhan D, Singh A, Brahmandam M et al (2008) Combination of proteasome inhibitors bortezomib and NPI-0052 trigger in vivo synergistic cytotoxicity in multiple myeloma. Blood 111:1654–1664
86. Kawaguchi Y, Kovacs JJ, McLaurin A et al (2003) The deacetylase HDAC6 regulates aggresome formation and cell viability in response to misfolded protein stress. Cell 115:727–738
87. Nie D, Huang K, Yin S et al (2012) Synergistic/additive interaction of valproic acid with bortezomib on proliferation and apoptosis of acute myeloid leukemia cells. Leuk Lymphoma 53:2487–2495
88. Niewerth D, Franke N, Jansen G et al (2012) Interferon-y-induced upregulation of immunoproteasome subunit assembly overcomes bortezomib resistance of leukemia cell lines har-

bouring bortezomib-induced mutations in constitutive PSMB5. ASH annual meeting abstracts 120:1346
89. Horton TM, Pati D, Plon SE et al (2007) A phase 1 study of the proteasome inhibitor bortezomib in pediatric patients with refractory leukemia: a Children's Oncology Group study. Clin Cancer Res 13:1516–1522
90. Cortes J, Thomas D, Koller C et al (2004) Phase I study of bortezomib in refractory or relapsed acute leukemias. Clin Cancer Res 10:3371–3376
91. Faderl S, Rai K, Gribben J et al (2006) Phase II study of single-agent bortezomib for the treatment of patients with fludarabine-refractory B-cell chronic lymphocytic leukemia. Cancer 107:916–924
92. Santos FP, Kantarjian H, McConkey D et al (2011) Pilot study of bortezomib for patients with imatinib-refractory chronic myeloid leukemia in chronic or accelerated phase. Clin Lymphoma Myeloma Leuk 11:355–360
93. Attar EC, De Angelo DJ, Supko JG et al (2008) Phase I and pharmacokinetic study of bortezomib in combination with idarubicin and cytarabine in patients with acute myelogenous leukemia. Clin Cancer Res 14:1446–1454
94. Blum W, Schwind S, Tarighat SS et al (2012) Clinical and pharmacodynamic activity of bortezomib and decitabine in acute myeloid leukemia. Blood 119:6025–6031
95. Orlowski RZ, Voorhees PM, Garcia RA et al (2005) Phase 1 trial of the proteasome inhibitor bortezomib and pegylated liposomal doxorubicin in patients with advanced hematologic malignancies. Blood 105:3058–3065
96. Brown RE, Bostrom B, Zhang PL (2004) Morphoproteomics and bortezomib/dexamethasone-induced response in relapsed acute lymphoblastic leukemia. Ann Clin Lab Sci 34:203–205
97. Messinger YH, Gaynon PS, Sposto R et al (2012) Bortezomib with chemotherapy is highly active in advanced B-precursor acute lymphoblastic leukemia: Therapeutic Advances in Childhood Leukemia & Lymphoma (TACL) Study. Blood 120:285–290
98. Horton TM, Perentesis J, Gamis AS et al (2012) A phase 2 study of bortezomib combined with reinduction chemotherapy in children and young adults with recurrent, refractory or secondary acute myeloid leukemia: a Children's Oncology Group (COG) study. ASH annual meeting 120:3580
99. Szczepanek J, Pogorzala M, Konatkowska B et al (2010) Differential ex vivo activity of bortezomib in newly diagnosed paediatric acute lymphoblastic and myeloblastic leukaemia. Anticancer Res 30:2119–2124
100. Kapoor P, Ramakrishnan V, Rajkumar SV (2012) Bortezomib combination therapy in multiple myeloma. Semin Hematol 49:228–242
101. Warlick ED, Cao Q, Miller J (2013) Bortezomib and vorinostat in refractory acute myelogenous leukemia and high-risk myelodysplastic syndromes: produces stable disease but at the cost of high toxicity. Leukemia 27:1789–1791
102. Wright JJ (2010) Combination therapy of bortezomib with novel targeted agents: an emerging treatment strategy. Clin Cancer Res 16:4094–4104

Chapter 8
Overcoming Inherent Resistance to Proteasome Inhibitors in Head and Neck Cancer: Challenges and New Approaches

Jason I. Kass, Jennifer R. Grandis, and Daniel E. Johnson

Abstract Advanced stage head and neck squamous cell carcinoma (HNSCC) is a relatively common human malignancy that generally carries a poor prognosis. Despite the in vitro sensitivity of HNSCC cells to proteasome inhibitors, clinical testing of bortezomib in HNSCC patients has encountered obstacles of inherent resistance and adverse toxicities. To combat these difficulties, current efforts are focused on developing strategies that co-target the proteasome and other key signaling pathways. In addition, new proteasome inhibitors are being developed which exhibit reduced side effects in patients. This chapter will review our current understanding of the pathology and biology of HNSCC, findings from preclinical studies of proteasome inhibitors in HNSCC models, results from early-stage clinical testing of proteasome inhibitors in HNSCC patients, and the unique opportunities for proteasome targeting in human papillomavirus-positive HNSCC.

Keywords Head and neck cancer • HNSCC • Bortezomib • Carfilzomib • Oprozomib • HPV • Apoptosis • Autophagy

---

J.I. Kass
Department of Otolaryngology, University of Pittsburgh School of Medicine,
Eye & Ear Building, Suite 500, 200 Lothrop Street, Pittsburgh, PA 15213, USA
e-mail: kassji@upmc.edu

J.R. Grandis
Departments of Otolaryngology and Pharmacology & Chemical Biology,
University of Pittsburgh School of Medicine, and The University of Pittsburgh Cancer
Institute Eye & Ear Building, Suite 500, 200 Lothrop Street, Pittsburgh, PA 15213, USA
e-mail: jgrandis@pitt.edu

D.E. Johnson (✉)
Departments of Medicine and Pharmacology & Chemical Biology,
University of Pittsburgh School of Medicine, and The University of Pittsburgh
Cancer Institute, Hillman Cancer Center, Room 2.18c, 5117 Centre Avenue, Pittsburgh,
PA 15213, USA
e-mail: johnsond@pitt.edu

Q.P. Dou (ed.), *Resistance to Proteasome Inhibitors in Cancer*, Resistance to Targeted Anti-Cancer Therapeutics, DOI 10.1007/978-3-319-06752-0_8

Abbreviations

HNSCC	Head and neck squamous cell carcinoma
HPV	Human papillomavirus
BMI	Body mass index
RT	Radiation therapy
CRT	Chemoradiation
FDA	Food and Drug Administration
EGFR	Epidermal growth factor receptor
PARP	Poly(ADP-ribose) polymerase
MTD	Maximum tolerated dose
ROS	Reactive oxygen species
HDAC	Histone deacetylase
PR	Partial response
SD	Stable disease
PD	Progressive disease

8.1 Introduction

Head and neck cancer is a major disease burden in humans. Although there are over 100 specific cancer subtypes than can occur in the head and neck, squamous cell cancer (HNSCC) comprises the vast majority, with estimates of 90 %. HNSCC is currently the seventh leading cause for cancer-related mortality worldwide with recent estimates of 600,000 new cases each year and 300,000 annual deaths [1]. Traditionally, men with heavy smoking and alcohol use have been largely affected; however, the demographics are now changing as risk factors and human behaviors are shifting [2, 3]. Unique to HNSCC is the morbidity this disease can cause because of its destruction of normal head and neck anatomy. Patients surviving HNSCC are often cosmetically disfigured, either as a result of the primary disease process or following surgical and chemoradioactive therapies. Extirpation of disease can require sacrifice of portions of the oral cavity, pharynx and larynx. This results in significant impairment in overall quality of life with respect to speaking, swallowing, taste, and smell.

8.2 Scope of the Problem

Of the estimated 600,000 new cases of HNSCC worldwide, about 10 % will originate in the USA [4]. A high rate of disease is observed in South East Asia, Western Pacific (including Australia), and Europe, with South East Asia accounting for over 40 % of new cancers. Overall mortality of head and neck cancer is also very high with rates that vary from 60 % in North America to 80 % in South East Asia [1]. Men are at a greater risk than women with ratios varying from 2:1 to 15:1 based on site of disease.

8.3 Risk Factors for HNSCC (Tobacco, Alcohol, HPV, and Others)

HNSCC occurs in the wide variety of anatomical subsites of the head and neck, including the oral cavity, oropharynx, larynx, and nasal and paranasal sinuses. While these are all mucosal-lined surfaces, they have unique incidence, response rates to treatment, mechanisms of spread, and susceptibility to carcinogens. Approximately 65 % of HNSCC occurs in the oral cavity, 25 % is laryngeal, 10 % is pharyngeal, and the remaining 5 % from the nasal and paranasal sinuses [1]. Traditional risk factors include tobacco and alcohol. Genetics play a role with increased prevalence if a first-degree relative has had HNSCC. More recently, it has been recognized that certain subtypes of the human papillomavirus, HPV, cause HNSCC, particularly in the oropharynx, and accounts for the changing demographics of the disease. Additional risk factors such as dental hygiene, body mass index (BMI), and diet have also been identified.

8.3.1 Tobacco and Alcohol as Risk Factors for HNSCC

Tobacco and alcohol are the major risk factors for disease in all subsites, except the nasal and paranasal sinuses. They alone are estimated to be responsible for approximately 75 % of oral cavity and oropharyngeal cases [5]. Both are independent risk factors and together their risk is multiplicative. For tobacco, smoking and smokeless products are associated with HNSCC. In a study of nearly 10,000 cases of HNSCC, cigarette smokers who never drank alcohol were twice as likely to have HNSCC than nonsmokers [6]. The number of daily cigarettes, duration, and number of pack-years of cigarette smoking all demonstrated a dose-response relationship. There was also variability based on site with laryngeal cancers having upwards of sevenfold increase in risk. In addition, smoking methods do not appear to make a difference as both cigar and pipe smoking also carry a twofold increased risk [7]. Smokeless tobacco products including betel quid, a combination of the betel leaf and tobacco widely used in South and Southeast Asia, are also major risk factors for oral cavity HNSCC [8].

Alcohol consumption of three or more drinks per day in never smokers carries twice the risk of cancer when compared to nondrinkers [6]. This increases to approximately fivefold with consumption of over thirty drinks per week regardless of whether the alcohol is either beer or liquor [9]. When alcohol and tobacco use are combined, there is a multiplicative increase in risk upwards of 15-fold depending on site.

8.3.2 Human Papillomavirus and HNSCC

The remaining 25 % of HNSCC not caused by smoking and alcohol is largely attributable to HPV-related disease. This has caused a dramatic change in patient demographics with a shifting burden from the more traditional risk factors of smoking and alcohol [2, 3]. HPV prevalence in oropharyngeal cancers has increased nearly 50 % in the USA over the last 30 years (16 % in the 1980s to over 70 % in cases from 2000 to 2004) [3]. This rise in oropharyngeal cancer has also been documented in Sweden and has been associated with increased HPV exposure [10]. If the trends in the USA continue, HPV-positive oropharyngeal cancers are estimated to exceed the incidence of cervical cancer in 2020 [3]. In the USA, younger people, aged 20–44, are exhibiting the largest annual increase in tonsil cancer [11].

Many consider HPV-associated HNSCC to be a distinct entity, and HPV-associated oropharyngeal cancer has unique biology with early metastasis to the neck and improved responsiveness to chemoradiation. HPV is a DNA virus with over 100 subtypes. Certain high-risk subtypes, including HPV-16 and HPV-18, cause cervical cancer, while lower-risk subtypes cause papillomas and genital warts. HPV has a relatively small genome; however, two of its genes, E6 and E7, have wide-ranging effects on cell growth, death, and immortalization [12]. Two of the best-characterized mechanisms for driving cellular replication are through tight binding and inactivation of the tumor-suppressor genes p53 and pRb (see Sect. 8.9).

8.3.3 Dental Hygiene, BMI, Diet, and Other Risk Factors for HNSCC

A number of additional risk factors have been associated with HNSCC including dental hygiene, gender, BMI, and diet. With regard to poor dental hygiene, a study of never smokers and never or former drinkers in Japan showed an increased risk of oral cavity HNSCC in edentulous individuals [13]. This has been supported by a recent meta-analysis of eight studies showing an odds ratio between 1.3 and 3 of tooth loss and HNSCC [14]. Periodontal disease with chronic bacterial infections and chronic inflammation has been posited as a potential mechanism for disease. Diet and BMI have both been associated with risks for HNSCC albeit in opposing directions. People with a healthier diet of increased fruits and vegetables have a lower risk of cancer [15]. This would suggest that thinner people may be at a lower risk. However, pooled data from 17 case-controlled studies recently showed that low BMI (18–25) is associated with an increased risk when compared to overweight individuals (BMI >25) [16]. The mechanism that underlies this increased risk is currently unknown and proposed theories relate to thinner people having increased cellular metabolism and higher levels of oxidative stress.

As mentioned above, squamous cell cancer of the nose and paranasal sinuses are not caused by the traditional risk factors. Most causes are unknown; however, risk factors that have been identified include industrial exposure to heavy metals (nickel, radium, chromium), softwood dust, and leather tanning [17].

8.4 Current Treatment Paradigms

State-of-the-art treatment for HNSCC involves a multidisciplinary collaborative decision-making process with head and neck surgeons and medical and radiation oncologists. Treatment decisions are typically based on stage and site of disease. In general, single modality therapy, whether radiation or surgery, is reserved for early-stage disease (stages I/II). Currently there is no chemotherapy approved as a single modality therapy. Advanced disease (stages III/IV) involves multimodality therapy with a combination of surgery, radiation, and chemotherapy.

8.4.1 Surgical Treatment as Single Modality Therapy

Surgical excision as a primary modality is used for early-stage cancers in the oral cavity and larynx. In the mouth, small lesions on the tongue, floor of mouth, buccal mucosa, and palate can be entirely excised with adequate margins, and the patient is disease-free. The same is true with small, early-stage laryngeal cancers either on the true vocal folds or supraglottis. Direct visualization and surgical excision, often using a laser, is all that is required for treatment. In many early laryngeal cancers, radiation is also a well-accepted alternative for treatment. However, in the oral cavity, surgery is generally preferred because of the proximity of the mandible. Treatment doses greater than 50 Gy place the mandible at risk for late radiation side effects including osteoradionecrosis [18].

8.4.2 Radiation Treatment as a Single Modality Therapy

Radiation as a single treatment option is largely restricted to small early laryngeal lesions. Here the balance between surgery and radiation as treatment options centers around voice preservation. If the cancer is superficial and located on only one true vocal fold (away from the anterior commissure), radiation and surgery are equally good options with equivalent local control and overall survival [19]. In these cancers, voice outcomes have also been shown to be equivalent [20]. If the mass, however, extends deeper into the true vocal fold or extends to the contralateral side across the commissure, then surgical excision is likely to have poorer voice outcomes and radiation is often the preferred option. Although there are consequences to radiation exposure including mucositis, destruction of mucous secreting glands, fibrosis, and scarring, voice outcomes are better without sacrificing local control or overall survival. Radiation therapy (RT) alone is also used as palliative therapy for unresectable HNSCC [21] or as adjunctive therapy following surgical excision of advanced disease.

8.4.3 Treatment of HNSCC with Chemoradiation

Chemotherapy alone is currently an ineffective treatment strategy for curative intent. Combined chemoradiation (CRT), however, is the current treatment strategy of choice with respect to many oropharyngeal and advanced laryngeal cancers. Tumors of the oropharynx including the tonsils and base of tongue can be excised surgically, but traditional surgical approaches have been quite morbid, often requiring a mandibulotomy and lip splitting incision. These approaches have not proven to provide better outcomes over CRT with respect to either local control or overall survival. With newer robotic-assisted techniques, a role for surgery in HPV-associated oropharyngeal cancers is an active area of discussion [22].

Similarly, surgical laryngectomy is an option for advanced laryngeal cancers, but this carries significant morbidity, eliminating normal speech and diverting the trachea to the neck as a stoma. The Veteran Affairs prospective study of advanced laryngeal cancer demonstrated that patients with advanced laryngeal cancer treated with CRT had similar overall survival as those with an upfront laryngectomy [23]. This ushered in an era of nonsurgical "voice preservation" treatment. Treatment of advanced laryngeal cancer continues to be actively debated because the consequences of CRT on the larynx must be weighed against the morbidity of a total laryngectomy. Patients may ultimately undergo salvage laryngectomy after CRT for a cancer-free but nonfunctional larynx secondary to aspiration and chondroradionecrosis [24].

Chemotherapeutics can be generally separated into two categories: nontargeted and targeted drugs. Nontargeting drugs approved by the FDA include platinum-based compounds (cisplatinum, carboplatinum), taxane-derived drugs (paclitaxel, docetaxel), and the antimetabolite 5-fluorouracil. The only targeted drug approved by the FDA is cetuximab, an epidermal growth factor receptor (EGFR) inhibitor. Clinical trials have established that CRT, incorporation of either platinum or platinum plus a taxane, is better than radiotherapy (RT) alone [25, 26]. Additionally, timing of chemotherapy is important, with concurrent chemotherapy during RT having better outcomes than induction chemotherapy [27, 28].

Cetuximab, a chimeric monoclonal mouse/human antibody, has been approved for the treatment of HSNCC since 2006. Four phase III trials have evaluated its effectiveness with either radiation- or platinum-based treatment in advanced disease [29–32]. In the Bonner trial, which led to the FDA approval, the addition of cetuximab to radiation led to a prolonged survival of nearly 20 months [30]. Interestingly, one of the side effects of cetuximab use, a prominent acneiform rash, also predicts its effectiveness. In the 5-year follow-up to the Bonner study, subgroup analysis of the patients who displayed the rash determined that the severity of the rash was associated with prolonged survival. Unfortunately, cetuximab as monotherapy has a modest response, and many patients develop resistance to the therapy [33].

8.5 Proteasome Inhibition in Preclinical In Vitro and In Vivo Models of HNSCC

The application of proteasome inhibitors to solid tumor malignancies, including HNSCC, follows impressive clinical results using bortezomib (Velcade/PS-341) in certain hematologic malignancies. Bortezomib is a potent and reversible inhibitor of the chymotrypsin-like and caspase-like activities of the proteasome and has been approved by the United States Food and Drug Administration (FDA) for the treatment of multiple myeloma and mantle cell lymphoma [34–36]. In general, preclinical and clinical testing of bortezomib against solid tumor malignancies has produced less promising results than those obtained in multiple myeloma and mantle cell lymphoma. However, apoptosis-inducing activity of bortezomib has been observed in a number of different solid tumor models, including those representing melanoma, non-small cell lung cancer, renal cell carcinoma, prostate cancer, and colon cancer [37–45]. Moreover, as discussed later, the activity of bortezomib can be markedly enhanced by co-targeting additional key regulatory proteins in the cell. Thus, the full potential of proteasome inhibition as a therapeutic approach in solid tumors has yet to be fully explored.

Preclinical evaluation of bortezomib against HNSCC was first reported by Sunwoo et al. in 2001 [46]. Cytotoxicity of bortezomib was observed at concentrations of roughly 100 nM in 4 murine SCC cell lines and 2 human HNSCC cell lines [46]. Subsequently, several different investigators have demonstrated potent induction of cell death by bortezomib in multiple HNSCC cell lines, with IC_{50} values as low as 1 nM [47–51]. The ability of bortezomib to kill HNSCC cell lines is associated with induction of hallmark features of apoptosis. In particular, bortezomib treatment of HNSCC cells leads to activation of the intrinsic apoptosis pathway, characterized by the release of mitochondrial cytochrome c into the cytosol, activation of caspase-9 and caspase-3, and cleavage of the caspase-3 substrate protein poly(ADP-ribose) polymerase (PARP) [46, 47, 49]. In addition, bortezomib treatment also has the capacity to induce cell cycle arrest when used at nontoxic concentrations. As has been seen in other cancer cell types, bortezomib treatment of HNSCC cells can activate either the G1/S or the G2/M cell cycle checkpoints [52–55]. Thus, an important aspect of the therapeutic potential of bortezomib lies in its ability to either kill HNSCC cells via apoptosis or slow the growth of the cells by promoting cell cycle arrest.

Lorch et al. have shown that bortezomib also acts to inhibit cell-cell adhesion and cell migration [56]. Treatment of two oral squamous cell carcinoma cell lines with bortezomib led to reduction in the levels of desmoglein 2 and accompanying reduction in the strength of mechanical cell-cell adhesion [56]. Further, bortezomib stimulated recruitment of phospho(Tyr397)-focal adhesion kinase to the cell periphery and concurrent inhibition of cell migration [56]. While inhibition of HNSCC migration would have clear therapeutic benefit, it is unknown whether bortezomib inhibition of cell-cell contact would be beneficial. Disruption of HNSCC cell–cell contact would be useful therapeutically if it were to lead to activation of anoikis. On the other hand, this disruption could be detrimental if it promoted metastasis or development of anchorage independence.

The impact of bortezomib treatment on HNSCC tumor growth has been evaluated in subcutaneous xenograft models. Intraperitoneal bortezomib doses of 1.0 or 2.0 mg/kg, thrice weekly, demonstrated significant growth inhibition of tumors derived from UM-SCC-11B HNSCC cells [46]. The inhibition of tumor growth was accompanied by dramatic reduction in tumor blood vessel densities [46]. The maximum tolerated dose (MTD) of bortezomib appeared to be reached using the 2.0 mg/kg dose in these experiments [46, 48]. In a different study, twice-weekly doses of 1 mg/kg were found to inhibit the growth of tumors derived from SAS HNSCC cells [50]. Together, these studies have demonstrated in vivo activity of bortezomib against HNSCC tumors.

A serious drawback to the use of bortezomib in patients is the high frequency and severity of side effects. In particular is the development of peripheral neuropathy, a painful condition that affects the mobility of patients. Roughly 35–52 % of multiple myeloma patients treated with bortezomib have been reported to develop peripheral neuropathy [57–60]. Careful examination of the specificity of bortezomib has revealed that side effects such as peripheral neuropathy may be due to inhibition of serine proteases, including chymase, HtrA2/Omi, dipeptidyl peptidase II, and cathepsins A and G [61]. For this, and other reasons, a considerable amount of effort has been invested in the development of next-generation proteasome inhibitors with heightened potencies and fewer off-target activities. Among the new compounds that have been developed, only two, carfilzomib and oprozomib, have been evaluated against HNSCC [62, 63].

Carfilzomib is a well-tolerated, irreversible inhibitor of the proteasome that demonstrates greater specificity than bortezomib for the chymotrypsin-like activity of the proteasome [64–66]. The heightened specificity of carfilzomib is likely responsible for the reduced rates of peripheral neuropathy that have been observed in early clinical testing [61]. Moreover, because carfilzomib acts as an irreversible inhibitor, its effects may be more lasting, perhaps requiring less frequent administration. However, neither carfilzomib nor bortezomib are orally bioavailable. Oprozomib is a derivative of carfilzomib and offers the distinct advantage of being orally bioavailable [67]. Importantly, both carfilzomib and oprozomib have been shown to promote apoptosis in multiple myeloma cells that have become resistant to bortezomib [66, 68]. Thus, treatment with these next-generation proteasome inhibitors may offer a valuable means for overcoming bortezomib resistance in other cancers as well. In HNSCC subcutaneous xenograft models (tumors from Cal33 cells), twice-weekly intraperitoneal administration of 3 or 5 mg/kg led to dose-dependent inhibition of tumor growth [62]. Similarly, twice-weekly oral administration of 30 mg/kg oprozomib led to highly significant inhibition of HNSCC tumor growth [62]. The antitumor effects of oprozomib were shown to be accompanied by inhibition of chymotrypsin-like proteasome activity in blood, liver, and tumor tissues [62]. These studies raise hope that more selective proteasome inhibitors, with reduced cytotoxic side effects, can be applied in the treatment of patients with HNSCC.

8.6 Molecular Mechanisms of Proteasome Inhibitor-Induced HNSCC Cell Death

The proteasome is responsible for the degradation of a wide variety of cellular proteins. This is true whether the cell is operating under basal conditions or is responding to some extracellular stimulus [69]. Because of this, inhibition of the proteasome impacts multiple different signaling pathways that are important for cellular survival, proliferation, or differentiation (Fig. 8.1).

One key pathway that is altered upon proteasome inhibition is the NF-KB signaling pathway (Fig. 8.1). NF-KB is a transcription which, following activation, translocates to the nucleus and induces the expression of genes that promote cellular proliferation and survival, as well as genes encoding pro-inflammatory cytokines and angiogenesis-inducing chemokines/growth factors [70]. The activity of NF-KB is negatively regulated by an endogenous inhibitor, IKB, that acts to sequester the NF-KB protein in the cytoplasm [71]. However, IKB is routinely subjected to ubiquitination and proteasomal degradation, allowing NF-KB activation and migration to the nucleus [71, 72]. Moreover, in a large number of hematologic and solid tumor malignancies, negative regulation of NF-KB appears deficient and the NF-KB protein is constitutively activated [73, 74]. Such is the case in HNSCC, where constitutive activation of NF-KB is seen in a large percentage of tumor specimens and correlates with poor prognosis [75–80]. Importantly, because IKB is routinely degraded by the proteasome, inhibition of the proteasome results in marked elevation of IKB levels and resultant sequestration/inhibition of NF-KB [81]. The ability of proteasome inhibitors, including bortezomib, to inhibit signaling by NF-KB is well established in numerous cell types. Bortezomib inhibition of NF-KB has been demonstrated in HNSCC cell lines in vitro,

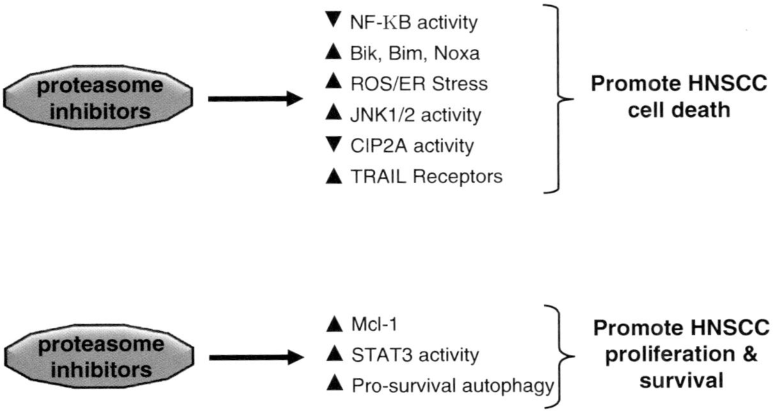

Fig. 8.1 Proteasome inhibitors promote both cell death and cell survival pathways in HNSCC cells. Treatment of HNSCC cells with proteasome inhibitors leads to inhibition of cell survival pathways and induction of proapoptotic proteins, resulting in cell death. At the same time, proteasome inhibition also induces the expression or activation of pathways and processes that promote HNSCC cell survival. A key to overcoming inherent resistance to proteasome inhibitors in HNSCC will involve co-targeting of cell survival pathways and processes that are activated by proteasome inhibition

as well as in specimens from HNSCC patients administered with bortezomib in clinical testing [46, 48, 82, 83]. The administration of bortezomib to HNSCC patients also resulted in tumor downregulation of several NF-KB target genes that encode proteins regulating the cell cycle, apoptosis, and angiogenesis, including cyclin A, cyclin B, cyclin D1, IAP-1, Bcl-X_L, IL-6, and VEGF [82]. Thus, proteasome inhibition represents a viable means for inhibiting NF-KB and the growth-promoting effects of this transcription factor, in HNSCC tumors.

In addition to promoting cancer cell death via inhibition of NF-KB signaling, proteasome inhibitors also impact apoptosis by modulating the expression of key members of the Bcl-2 protein family. Several members of the Bcl-2 protein family have been shown to be actively degraded via the proteasome, including proapoptotic Bik, Bim, Puma, and Noxa, and antiapoptotic Mcl-1 (Fig. 8.1). Treatment of SCC cells with bortezomib has been shown to modestly induce Puma and dramatically induce Noxa [84]. Suppression of Noxa using siRNAs markedly attenuated bortezomib-induced apoptosis, while suppression of Puma expression had little effect. Importantly, bortezomib induction of Noxa was found to occur in cisplatin-resistant SCC cells and was sufficient to induce apoptosis in these resistant cells [84]. In other studies, treatment of HNSCC cell lines with bortezomib was found to induce both Bik and Bim [49], while treatment with carfilzomib or oprozomib led to potent Bik induction [62, 63]. Suppression of either Bik or Bim attenuated apoptosis induction by these agents [62]. Collectively, these experiments have revealed the importance of Noxa, Bik, and Bim induction for driving apoptotic cell death caused by proteasome inhibitors. On the other hand, bortezomib, carfilzomib, and oprozomib have each been shown to induce expression of a key inhibitor of apoptosis, the Mcl-1 protein [49, 62]. Furthermore, siRNA-mediated suppression of Mcl-1 expression enhances the killing activity of proteasome inhibitors [49, 62]. This demonstrates that proteasome inhibitors not only induce the expression of proteins that drive cell death but also induce the expression of proteins (e.g., Mcl-1) that blunt their proapoptotic activities (Fig. 8.1). Selective co-targeting of molecules such as Mcl-1 with small molecule inhibitors may represent an important avenue for enhancing the therapeutic efficacies of proteasome inhibitors.

The induction of reactive oxygen species (ROS) and endoplasmic reticulum (ER) stress also appears to play a role in proteasome inhibitor-induced HNSCC cell death (Fig. 8.1). Treatment of HNSCC cell lines with bortezomib results in elevated levels of ROS [47, 51]. Moreover, the cell-permeable ROS scavengers Tiron or *N*-acetyl-L-cysteine diminish cell death resulting from proteasome inhibition, demonstrating the significance ROS elevation [47, 51]. As might be expected, bortezomib treatment leads to the accumulation of unfolded proteins in HNSCC cells and concomitant activation of ER stress. Specifically, bortezomib induces the phosphorylation of PERK and upregulation of ATF-4, GRP-78, and GADD-34 associated with the ER stress response [47].

Other mechanisms of cell death induction by proteasome inhibitors are likely to be discovered in the future. For example, in other model systems, proteasome inhibitors have been shown to activate JNK enzymes [85, 86], which have the potential to drive apoptosis (Fig. 8.1). Also, recent studies have shown that bortezomib treatment of HNSCC cells leads to inhibition of cancerous inhibitor of protein phosphatase 2A (CIP2A) (Fig. 8.1), leading to activation of PP2A phosphatase, and dephosphorylation and inactivation of the pro-survival kinase Akt [50]. In view of the diverse number of substrates that are routinely and rapidly subjected to degradation by the proteasome, it is not surprising that multiple different mechanisms contribute to the proapoptotic action of proteasome inhibitors.

8.7 Enhancing Sensitivity to Proteasome Inhibitors in HNSCC by Co-targeting Key Signaling Proteins and Pathways

Proteasome inhibitors have been combined with a wide variety of agents, including both nonselective and selective targeting agents, in preclinical studies with HNSCC models (Table 8.1; clinical studies involving co-targeting are described in Sect. 8.8). Some of these studies have been purely empirical, aiming to identify synergistic drug combinations that may have therapeutic value. Other co-targeting efforts have been driven by an understanding of the signaling pathways regulated by the proteasome and have sought to use this information to develop rationale strategies for improving the anticancer efficacies of proteasome inhibitors. Successes have been achieved using both approaches and hold promise for more effective treatment of patients with HNSCC.

Table 8.1 Preclinical combination of proteasome inhibitors (PIs) and other agents (bortezomib, BTZ; carfilzomib, CFZ; oprozomib, OPZ; MG, MG132)

PI	Other agent	In vitro	In vivo	Ref.
BTZ	Cisplatin	+		[49, 87]
BTZ	Docetaxel	+		[87]
BTZ	Radiation	+	+	[88, 89]
BTZ, CFZ, OPZ	Mcl-1 siRNA	+		[49, 62]
BTZ	STAT3 decoy	+		[90]
BTZ	Guggulsterone	+		[90]
CFZ, OPZ	Chloroquine	+		[62, 63]
BTZ	Cetuximab	+		[91, 92]
MG	TRAIL	+		[93]
BTZ	TRAIL	+		[94]
BTZ	Trichostatin A	+	+	[95, 96]
BTZ	PXD101	+	+	[96]
BTZ	Dexamethasone	+		[97]
BTZ	PLK-1 inhibitor (BI2536)	+		[31]
BTZ	JNK inhibitor (SP600125)	+		[48]
BTZ	p38 inhibitor (SB203580)	+		[48]

Information gleaned from co-targeting experiments also may assist in identifying strategies for overcoming resistance to proteasome inhibitors. In the case of HNSCC, models of acquired proteasome inhibitor resistance have not yet been developed. Thus, all preclinical studies done to date in HNSCC models are relevant primarily to inherent resistance mechanisms. Nonetheless, the opportunity to counter inherent resistance to proteasome inhibitors (via co-targeting strategies) is particularly valuable, as this may allow the development of therapeutic regimens incorporating lower doses of the cytotoxic drugs, thereby limiting undesirable side effects.

As discussed earlier, the primary chemotherapy drugs used in the treatment of HNSCC are platinum-based or taxane compounds. Wagenblast et al. showed that bortezomib alone demonstrates significant antiproliferative activity against eight different SCC cell lines and that this activity was enhanced by the addition of either cisplatin or docetaxel [87]. Using rigorous algorithms for determination of synergism, Li et al. showed that bortezomib potently synergizes with cisplatin in the killing of two HNSCC cell lines [49]. This synergistic cell killing was associated with synergistic induction of apoptosis signaling, as assessed by caspase-3 activation and cleavage of PARP [49]. Radiation therapy also represents a mainstay of therapy for HNSCC patients. In vitro and in vivo studies have shown that bortezomib substantially enhances the sensitivity of HNSCC cells and tumors to radiation therapy [88, 89]. This enhancement was found to be associated with suppression of NF-KB, enhanced PARP cleavage, decreased production of angiogenic factors, and reduced numbers of tumor blood vessels [89].

Although proteasome inhibitors are relatively potent (nM range) at inducing cell death in HNSCC cells, the effectiveness of these agents is limited by the fact that proteasome inhibition leads to the upregulation of certain proteins and processes that support HNSCC cell survival. In particular, proteasome inhibition has been shown to upregulate expression of Mcl-1, STAT3, and pro-survival autophagy in HNSCC cells [49, 62, 90, 91] (Fig. 8.1). Thus, studies have been performed to determine whether specific targeting of these proteins, or the process of autophagy, can be used to further diminish inherent resistance to proteasome inhibitors. As mentioned earlier, targeting of Mcl-1 using siRNAs has been found to enhance the abilities of bortezomib, carfilzomib, and oprozomib to promote cell death in HNSCC cell lines [49, 62]. In the case of STAT3, bortezomib treatment of three HNSCC cell lines was shown to induce expression levels of the phosphorylated/activated form of STAT3, which was accompanied by induced expression from a luciferase-based STAT3 reporter construct [90]. In further experiments, selective targeting of the active form of STAT3 was achieved via expression of a dominant-negative STAT3 mutant or treatment with a STAT3 decoy oligonucleotide or the naturally occurring inhibitor guggulsterone [90]. Co-targeting of STAT3 dramatically improved the potency of bortezomib against HNSCC cells, as assessed by enhanced apoptosis signaling and loss of cell viability and by decreased clonogenic survival. Targeting of autophagy has been accomplished using the relatively non-specific agent chloroquine. Induction of HNSCC cell autophagy has been demonstrated following treatment with bortezomib, carfilzomib, or oprozomib and is partially dependent on activation of JNK enzymes as well as activation of the unfolded protein response pathway [62, 91]. Co-treatment with chloroquine enhanced the sensitivities of HNSCC cells to proteasome inhibitors, indicating that the autophagy induced by proteasome inhibitors is acting to promote HNSCC cell survival [62]. Since chloroquine is a well-tolerated agent in humans, co-treatment with chloroquine and a proteasome inhibitor may be therapeutically beneficial.

Another co-targeting approach attracting interest involves targeting of the EGFR. Overexpression of EGFR is found in a majority of HNSCC patient tumors and in preclinical models correlates with resistance to radiation and chemotherapy [92, 93]. HNSCC tumors also commonly overexpress the EGFR ligand TGFα, leading to autocrine activation of EGFR [92, 94, 95]. Overexpression of either EGFR or TGFα has been shown to correlate with poor survival in HNSCC patients [92, 96]. In clinical trials, addition of the EGFR-neutralizing antibody cetuximab has been shown to modestly enhance the responsiveness of HNSCC tumors to radiation therapy or conventional chemotherapies, leading to FDA approval of cetuximab in this disease [30, 31, 97, 98]. Preclinical studies in HNSCC have shown that cetuximab enhances the antiproliferative and cell death-inducing activities of bortezomib [99, 100]. However, it should be noted (as discussed in Sect. 8.8) that a recent clinical trial raises concerns about combining bortezomib with cetuximab and radiation therapy [101].

Co-treatment with proteasome inhibitor and activators of the death receptor-mediated extrinsic apoptosis pathway represents another possible therapeutic strategy. Most HNSCC cell lines, as well as esophageal SCC cell lines, are relatively resistant to death receptor-mediated apoptosis, including apoptosis activated by TRAIL or agonistic anti-Fas antibody. Low levels of death receptor expression, or high levels of the extrinsic pathway inhibitor c-FLIP, may partly account for the low sensitivities of these cells. However, treatment of HNSCC or esophageal SCC cells lines with proteasome inhibitor has been shown to upregulate expression of DR4 and DR5, the cell surface receptors for TRAIL [102, 103] (Fig. 8.1). Downregulation of the apoptosis inhibitors cIAP-1, XIAP, and survivin was also noted [102]. Importantly, treatment with proteasome inhibitor markedly enhances TRAIL-induced cell death in both HNSCC and esophageal SCC cells [102, 103]. Thus, inhibition of the proteasome may prove effective for restoring tumor cell sensitivity to death ligands.

Synergistic induction of HNSCC cell apoptosis has been reported using the combination of bortezomib and the histone deacetylase (HDAC) inhibitor trichostatin A (TSA) [104]. This in vitro synergism was found to be partially dependent on the upregulation of proapoptotic Noxa protein [104]. In vivo, the addition of TSA significantly enhanced bortezomib inhibition of HNSCC xenograft tumor growth [104]. In a separate in vivo study, a combination of bortezomib with the HDAC inhibitor PXD101 resulted in growth inhibition of xenograft tumors derived from bortezomib-resistant UMSCC-11A HNSCC cells [105]. However, enhanced gastrointestinal side effects and weight loss were also observed using the combination. Nonetheless, targeting of HDACs may present an opportunity for overcoming proteasome inhibitor resistance in HNSCC tumors.

Additional studies have shown that the ability of bortezomib to kill HNSCC cells in vitro can be enhanced by co-treatment with dexamethasone [106], or inhibitors of polo-like-kinase-1 [107], JNKs [48], or p38 [48]. It remains unclear whether in vivo studies will confirm these findings or whether enhanced cytotoxic side effects may be observed using these combinations.

8.8 Clinical Trials in HNSCC Incorporating Proteasome Inhibitors

The impact of proteasome inhibition has been evaluated in several early-stage clinical trials of HNSCC patients (see Table 8.2). In each case, bortezomib has been used as the proteasome inhibitor, and patients have had either advanced stage, recurrent, or metastatic disease. These trials have examined bortezomib alone, or bortezomib in combination with radiation therapy (RT), conventional chemotherapy, or cetuximab.

Allen et al. examined tumor biopsies from patients with recurrent HNSCC who received low-dose bortezomib (0.6 mg/m^2) prior to reirradiation [83]. They observed inhibition of canonical NF-KB signaling and induction of apoptosis in three of four evaluable tumors. Gilbert et al. treated a total of 48 recurrent or metastatic HNSCC patients with bortezomib alone and observed a partial response (PR) in 1 patient, stable disease (SD) in 10 patients, and progressive disease (PD) in 27 patients; 10 patients were unevaluable [108]. Thus, in these clinical trials, bortezomib was capable of inducing a pharmacodynamic effect in HNSCC patient tumors, but did not appreciably improve clinical outcomes.

The combination of bortezomib with RT (50–70 Gy) in nine HNSCC patients was found to exceed the MTD of bortezomib at 0.6 mg/m^2 [82]. However, analysis of blood and serum from these patients demonstrated differences in proteasome activity, NF-KB localization, expression of NF-KB target genes, and induction of apoptosis. Two of the nine patients exhibited minor reductions in tumor size [82]. By contrast, in another study, concurrent RT and weekly bortezomib at 1.6 mg/m^2 was well tolerated in patients with metastatic solid tumors, including three patients with HNSCC [109]. A phase I trial of bortezomib and concurrent chemoradiotherapy (cisplatin) by Kubicek et al. enrolled a total of 27 HNSCC patients and concluded that the combination therapy was safe, with a bortezomib MTD of 1.0 mg/m^2 in previously treated patients and 1.3 mg/m^2 in radiation-naïve patients [110].

In a phase II trial of recurrent or metastatic HNSCC patients, Gilbert et al. combined bortezomib with irinotecan [108]. Of 23 patients, 3 exhibited a PR, 5 achieved SD, 11 showed PD, and 4 were unevaluable. These results suggested only minimal

Table 8.2 Clinical trials in HNSCC incorporating bortezomib

Patient population	Treatment	Ref.
Recurrent HNSCC (phase I)	BTZ alone	[83]
Recurrent or metastatic HNSCC (phase II)	BTZ alone	[108]
Advanced HNSCC (phase I)	BTZ+RT	[109]
Recurrent HNSCC (phase I)	BTZ+RT	[82]
Recurrent HNSCC (phase I)	BTZ+RT+cisplatin	[110]
Recurrent or metastatic HNSCC (phase II)	BTZ+irinotecan	[108]
Recurrent or metastatic HNSCC (phase II)	BTZ+docetaxel	[111]
Advanced HNSCC expressing EGFR (phase I)	BTZ+cetuximab	[112]
RT-naïve stage IV or recurrent HNSCC (phase I)	BTZ+RT+cetuximab	[107]

benefit of adding bortezomib to irinotecan. In a different phase II trial, bortezomib (1.6 mg/m^2) was combined with docetaxel (40 mg/m^2) on days 1 and 8 of a 21-day cycle. This regimen was found to be well tolerated [111]. Of 21 evaluable patients, 1 had a PR, 10 had SD, and 10 exhibited PD. Correlative studies revealed that patients with PD had higher expression levels of NF-KB and EGFR-associated genes, indicating that these may provide molecular markers for resistance to this drug combination [111].

In vitro studies with HNSCC and renal cell lines have indicated that inhibition of EGFR enhances the cell killing activity of bortezomib [99, 100, 112]. Thus, two phase I trials have added bortezomib to cetuximab-containing regimens in HNSCC. Dudek et al. combined bortezomib and cetuximab in patients with solid tumors expressing EGFR [113]. The regimen was well tolerated and MTD was not reached at the bortezomib dose of 2.0 mg/m^2. The study concluded that bortezomib plus cetuximab was moderately effective at inducing SD in patients with HNSCC or non-small cell lung cancer [113]. Argiris et al. set out to evaluate bortezomib in combination with cetuximab and RT in patients with radiation-naïve stage IV or recurrent HNSCC [101]. Seven patients were enrolled; however, the trial was terminated early when five of six patients with favorable prognosis oropharyngeal cancer underwent early progression (within 1 year). The authors concluded that bortezomib antagonized the effects of the cetuximab/RT combination and cautioned against the use of this triple combination [101].

Although modest glimmers of bortezomib activity in HNSCC clinical trials have been observed, in general, the impact of bortezomib has been only minimal. These results underscore the importance of identifying mechanisms that contribute to the inherent resistance of HNSCC tumors to proteasome inhibitors. The testing of novel combinations of targeting agents will also be important. Furthermore, in view of the toxicities associated with bortezomib use, the evaluation of proteasome inhibitors with reduced adverse toxicities (e.g., carfilzomib/oprozomib) will be important.

8.9 The Potential Utility of Proteasome Inhibitors in HPV-Positive HNSCC

As discussed in Sect. 8.3, infection with HPV represents a major risk factor for development of HNSCC [114–116]. The incidence of HPV-positive HNSCC is steadily increasing, particularly among younger adults [3, 11, 117, 118]. HPV-positive HNSCC represents a distinct disease entity from HPV-negative HNSCC [119] and generally exhibits better prognosis [120–126]. Importantly, the unique molecular nature of HPV-positive HNSCC offers potential opportunities for therapeutic intervention with proteasome inhibitors. In contrast to HPV-negative HNSCCs, which are primarily p53 mutant or deficient, HPV-positive HNSCCs almost always harbor wild-type p53 [127–129]. However, as is the case in HPV-positive cervical cancer, the HPV E6 protein promotes the continuous ubiquitination and proteasomal degradation of the wild-type p53 protein (Fig. 8.2) [130, 131].

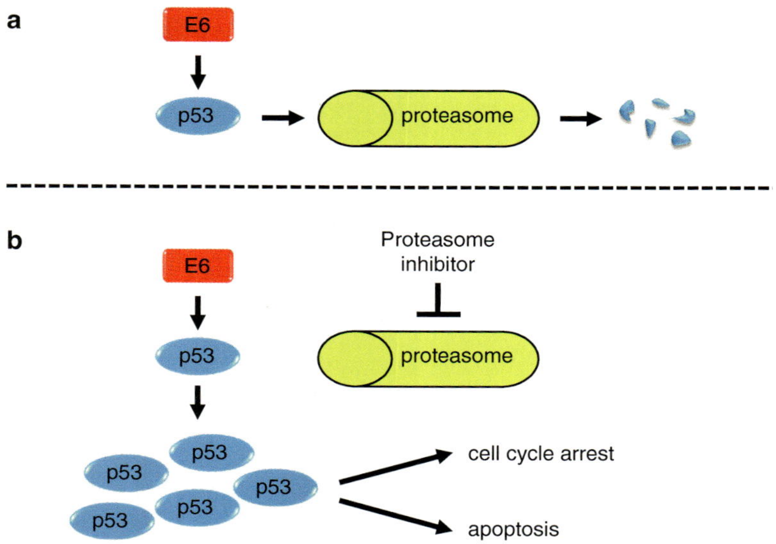

Fig. 8.2 Proteasome inhibition results in elevated expression of wild-type p53 in HPV-positive HNSCC cells. (**a**) In HPV-positive HNSCC cells, the HPV E6 protein continuously promotes ubiquitination and proteasomal degradation of wild-type p53. (**b**) Inhibition of the proteasome in HPV-positive HNSCC cells prevents p53 degradation, resulting in marked induction of the wild-type p53 protein

Thus, the expression of the wild-type p53 protein is maintained at very low levels in HPV-positive disease, and there is very little selective pressure to mutate or delete the *p53* gene. Since p53 is degraded via the proteasome in HPV-positive HNSCC, the use of proteasome inhibitors has the potential to upregulate p53 expression in these cells (Fig. 8.2). The upregulation of wild-type p53 would likely be beneficial from a therapeutic perspective. The p53 protein can promote cell cycle arrest through the induction of the cell cycle regulator p21 (Fig. 8.2). Alternatively, p53 can induce the expression of proapoptotic Puma and Noxa proteins, leading to Bax- and Bak-dependent activation of the intrinsic apoptosis pathway (Fig. 8.3). In either scenario, the induction of wild-type p53 in HPV-positive HNSCC is likely to promote antitumor effects.

Studies by Ferris et al. and Rampias et al. have shown that siRNA or shRNA directed against HPV E6/E7 bicistronic mRNA results in the upregulation of p53 protein in HPV-positive HNSCC cell lines [132, 133]. Coincident with the upregulation of wild-type p53, suppression of E6/E7 expression also led to induction of p53 target genes and activation of apoptotic cell death. These studies supported the idea that expression of wild-type p53 by HPV-positive HNSCC tumor cells may, in part, explain the better prognosis of HPV-positive HNSCC patients. In further support, Kimple et al. have recently shown that HPV-positive HNSCC cell lines exhibit enhanced sensitivity to radiation [134]. The impact of the proteasome inhibitor bortezomib on HPV-positive HNSCC has also been recently evaluated. Bortezomib treatment led to the upregulation of functional p53 and p53 target

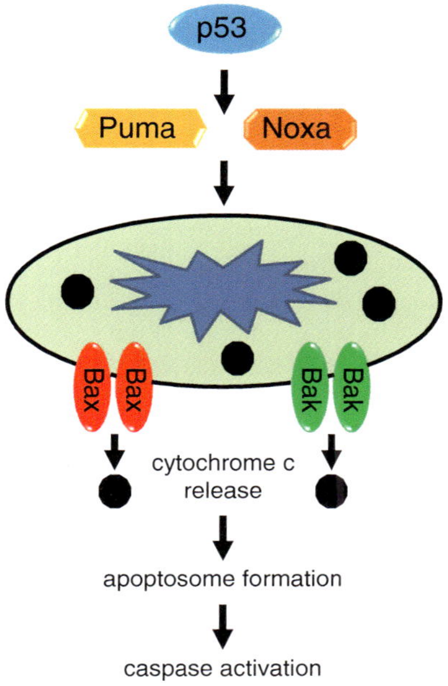

Fig. 8.3 Wild-type p53 in HPV-positive HNSCC cells promotes activation of the intrinsic apoptosis pathway. Wild-type p53 protein activates apoptosis signaling by directly inducing the expression of proapoptotic Puma and Noxa proteins. Puma and Noxa migrate to the mitochondria where they induce oligomerization of Bax and Bak, allowing cytochrome c to be released from the mitochondria into the cytosol. The cytosolic cytochrome c binds to Apaf-1 and procaspase-9 protein forming a complex referred to as the apoptosome. Formation of the apoptosome results in processing/activation of caspase-9, followed by caspase-9-mediated processing/activation of the executioner caspase, caspase-3

genes in HPV-positive, but not HPV-negative, HNSCC cell lines [52]. Morevoer, subtoxic doses of bortezomib promoted p21-dependent cell cycle arrest in HPV-positive HNSCC cells [52]. These experiments directly demonstrate the potential value of treating HPV-positive disease with proteasome inhibitors. However, a cautionary note must be added. As mentioned earlier, a phase I clinical trial of bortezomib in combination with cetuximab and radiation was prematurely terminated due to early progression in patients with favorable prognosis HPV-positive HNSCC [101]. The reasons for this early progression are unclear but may be due to bortezomib stabilization of the EGFR [101]. Therefore, the application of proteasome inhibitors to HPV-positive HNSCC should be closely monitored.

8.10 Conclusions

HNSCC remains a prevalent and difficult to treat cancer. Conventional chemoradiation regimens carry considerable adverse toxicities and are often ineffective. Targeted therapy using FDA-approved cetuximab benefits only a minority of

HNSCC patients. The proteasome inhibitor bortezomib has demonstrated considerable therapeutic efficacy in certain hematologic malignancies, and application of proteasome inhibitors to the treatment of HNSCC holds promise. However, early clinical testing of bortezomib in HNSCC, as well as other solid tumor malignancies, has revealed only modest, or minimal, benefit to adding this agent to current conventional regimens. Despite the relative sensitivity of HNSCC cell line models to proteasome inhibitors, more work is needed to develop strategies for further lowering the inherent resistance of HNSCC tumor cells. In this regard, multiple preclinical studies have now demonstrated the value of co-targeting the proteasome and other signaling pathways. Indeed, synergy of proteasome inhibitors with other molecular targeting agents has been demonstrated in vitro. Further development of these co-targeting strategies will be essential for improving the success of proteasome inhibitors in HNSCC patients. Moreover, these co-targeting studies have the potential to reveal key mechanisms that contribute to inherent, and acquired, resistance to proteasome inhibitors. Continued efforts are also needed to develop next-generation proteasome inhibitors with reduced side effects. Already, highly selective proteasome inhibitors such as carfilzomib and oprozomib are showing reduced rates of peripheral neuropathy relative to those seen with bortezomib. Further refinement and the identification of new inhibitors will allow higher doses to be applied, along with improved methods of delivery (e.g., orally bioavailable drugs). Collectively, the development of novel co-targeting strategies, the identification of molecular mechanisms contributing to proteasome inhibitor resistance, and the generation of orally available proteasome inhibitors with reduced adverse toxicities, is likely to lead to useful application of these agents in the treatment of patients with HNSCC.

Acknowledgements We apologize to those authors whose work we have been unable to cite. This work was supported by National Institutes of Health grants R01 CA137260 and P50 CA097190.

References

1. Mehanna H, Paleri V, West CML, Nutting C (2010) Head and neck cancer—Part 1: Epidemiology, presentation, and prevention. BMJ 341:c4684–c4684
2. Sturgis EM, Ang KK (2011) The epidemic of HPV-associated oropharyngeal cancer is here: is it time to change our treatment paradigms? Journal of the National Comprehensive Cancer Network : JNCCN 9(6):665–673
3. Chaturvedi AK, Engels EA, Pfeiffer RM, Hernandez BY, Xiao W, Kim E, Jiang B, Goodman MT, Sibug-Saber M, Cozen W, Liu L, Lynch CF, Wentzensen N, Jordan RC, Altekruse S, Anderson WF, Rosenberg PS, Gillison ML (2011) Human papillomavirus and rising oropharyngeal cancer incidence in the United States. J Clin Oncol 29(32):4294–4301
4. Sturgis EM, Cinciripini PM (2007) Trends in head and neck cancer incidence in relation to smoking prevalence: an emerging epidemic of human papillomavirus-associated cancers? Cancer 110:1429–1435
5. Blot WJ, Mclaughlin JK, Winn DM, Austin DF, Greenberg RS, Bernstein L, Schoenberg JB, Stemhagen A, Fraumeni JF (1988) smoking and drinking in relation to oral and pharyngeal cancer smoking and drinking in relation to oral and pharyngeal cancer. Cancer Res. 48(11): 3282-7.

6. Hashibe M, Brennan P, Benhamou S, Castellsague X, Chen C, Curado MP, Dal Maso L, Daudt AW, Fabianova E, Fernandez L, Wünsch-Filho V, Franceschi S, Hayes RB, Herrero R, Koifman S, La Vecchia C, Lazarus P, Levi F, Mates D, Matos E, Menezes A, Muscat J, Eluf-Neto J, Olshan AF, Rudnai P, Schwartz SM, Smith E, Sturgis EM, Szeszenia-Dabrowska N, Talamini R, Wei Q, Winn DM, Zaridze D, Zatonski W, Zhang Z-F, Berthiller J, Boffetta P (2007) Alcohol drinking in never users of tobacco, cigarette smoking in never drinkers, and the risk of head and neck cancer: pooled analysis in the International Head and Neck Cancer Epidemiology Consortium. J Natl Cancer Inst 99:777–789
7. Wyss A, Hashibe M, Chuang S-C, Amy Lee Y-C, Zhang Z-F, Yu G-P, Winn DM, Wei Q, Talamini R, Szeszenia-Dabrowska N, Sturgis EM, Smith E, Shangina O, Schwartz SM, Schantz S, Rudnai P, Purdue MP, Eluf-Neto J, Muscat J, Morgenstern H, Michaluart P, Menezes A, Matos E, Mates IN, Lissowska J, Levi F, Lazarus P, La Vecchia C, Koifman S, Herrero R, Hayes RB, Franceschi S, Wünsch-Filho V, Fernandez L, Fabianova E, Daudt AW, Dal Maso L, Curado MP, Chen C, Castellsague X, de Carvalho MB, Cadoni G, Boccia S, Brennan P, Boffetta P, Olshan AF (2013) Cigarette, Cigar, and Pipe Smoking and the Risk of Head and Neck Cancers: Pooled Analysis in the International Head and Neck Cancer Epidemiology Consortium. American journal of epidemiology:1-12
8. Sharan RN, Mehrotra R, Choudhury Y, Asotra K (2012) Association of betel nut with carcinogenesis: revisit with a clinical perspective. PLoS One 7:e42759
9. Purdue MP, Hashibe M, Berthiller J, La Vecchia C, Dal Maso L, Herrero R, Franceschi S, Castellsague X, Wei Q, Sturgis EM, Morgenstern H, Zhang Z-F, Levi F, Talamini R, Smith E, Muscat J, Lazarus P, Schwartz SM, Chen C, Neto JE, Wünsch-Filho V, Zaridze D, Koifman S, Curado MP, Benhamou S, Matos E, Szeszenia-Dabrowska N, Olshan AF, Lence J, Menezes A, Daudt AW, Mates IN, Pilarska A, Fabianova E, Rudnai P, Winn D, Ferro G, Brennan P, Boffetta P, Hayes RB (2009) Type of alcoholic beverage and risk of head and neck cancer—a pooled analysis within the INHANCE Consortium. Am J Epidemiol 169:132–142
10. Hammarstedt L, Lindquist D, Dahlstrand H, Romanitan M, Dahlgren LO, Joneberg J, Creson N, Lindholm J, Ye W, Dalianis T, Munck-Wikland E (2006) Human papillomavirus as a risk factor for the increase in incidence of tonsillar cancer. International journal of cancer Journal international du cancer 119:2620–2623
11. Shiboski CH, Schmidt BL, Jordan RC (2005) Tongue and tonsil carcinoma: increasing trends in the U.S. population ages 20-44 years. Cancer 103(9):1843–1849
12. Ca M, La L (2010) Human papillomavirus oncoproteins: pathways to transformation. Nat Rev Cancer 10:550–560
13. Hiraki A, Matsuo K, Suzuki T, Kawase T, Tajima K (2008) Teeth loss and risk of cancer at 14 common sites in Japanese. Cancer epidemiology biomarkers prevention a publication of the American Association for Cancer Research cosponsored by the American Society of Preventive Oncology 17:1222–1227
14. Wang R-S, Hu X-Y, Gu W-J, Hu Z, Wei B (2013) Tooth loss and risk of head and neck cancer: a meta-analysis. PLoS One 8:e71122
15. Freedman ND, Park Y, Subar AF, Hollenbeck AR, Leitzmann MF, Schatzkin A, Abnet CC (2008) Fruit and vegetable intake and head and neck cancer risk in a large United States prospective cohort study. International journal of cancer Journal international du cancer 122:2330–2336
16. Gaudet MM, Olshan AF, Chuang S-C, Berthiller J, Zhang Z-F, Lissowska J, Zaridze D, Winn DM, Wei Q, Talamini R, Szeszenia-Dabrowska N, Sturgis EM, Schwartz SM, Rudnai P, Eluf-Neto J, Muscat J, Morgenstern H, Menezes A, Matos E, Bucur A, Levi F, Lazarus P, La Vecchia C, Koifman S, Kelsey K, Herrero R, Hayes RB, Franceschi S, Wunsch-Filho V, Fernandez L, Fabianova E, Daudt AW, Dal Maso L, Curado MP, Chen C, Castellsague X, Benhamou S, Boffetta P, Brennan P, Hashibe M (2010) Body mass index and risk of head and neck cancer in a pooled analysis of case-control studies in the International Head and Neck Cancer Epidemiology (INHANCE) Consortium. Int J Epidemiol 39:1091–1102
17. Carrau R, Zimmer L, Myers EN (2006) Neoplasm of the nose and paranasal sinuses. Lippincott-Raven, Philadelphia

18. Tsai CJ, Hofstede TM, Sturgis EM, Garden AS, Lindberg ME, Wei Q, Tucker SL, Dong L (2013) Osteoradionecrosis and radiation dose to the mandible in patients with oropharyngeal cancer. Int J Radiat Oncol Biol Phys 85(2):415–420
19. Higgins KM (2011) What treatment for early-stage glottic carcinoma among adult patients: CO2 endolaryngeal laser excision versus standard fractionated external beam radiation is superior in terms of cost utility? Laryngoscope 121(1):116–134
20. Peeters AJ, van Gogh CD, Goor KM, Verdonck-de Leeuw IM, Langendijk JA, Mahieu HF (2004) Health status and voice outcome after treatment for T1a glottic carcinoma. Eur Arch Otorhinolaryngol 261(10):534–540
21. Chen AM, Vaughan A, Narayan S, Vijayakumar S (2008) Palliative radiation therapy for head and neck cancer: toward an optimal fractionation scheme. Head Neck 30(12):1586–1591
22. Genden EM (2012) The role for surgical management of HPV-related oropharyngeal carcinoma. Head Neck Pathol 6(Suppl 1):S98–103
23. Wolf G, Hong W, Fisher S, Urba S (1991) Induction chemotherapy plus radiation compared with surgery plus radiation in patients with advanced laryngeal cancer. N Engl J Med 324:1685
24. Raol N, Hutcheson KA, Lewin JS, Kupferman ME (2013) Surgical management of the nonfunctional larynx after organ preservation therapy. J Otol Rhinol 2(1)
25. Bernier J, Domenge C, Ozsahin M, Matuszewska K, Lefèbvre J-L, Greiner RH, Giralt J, Maingon P, Rolland F, Bolla M, Cognetti F, Bourhis J, Kirkpatrick A, van Glabbeke M (2004) Postoperative irradiation with or without concomitant chemotherapy for locally advanced head and neck cancer. N Engl J Med 350:1945–1952
26. Zhang L, Zhao C, Peng PJ, Lu LX, Huang PY, Han F, Wu SX (2005) Phase III study comparing standard radiotherapy with or without weekly oxaliplatin in treatment of locoregionally advanced nasopharyngeal carcinoma: preliminary results. J Clin Oncol 23(33):8461–8468
27. Argiris A, Karamouzis MV, Raben D, Ferris RL (2008) Head and neck cancer. Lancet 371:1695–1709
28. Pignon J-P, le Maître A, Maillard E, Bourhis J (2009) Meta-analysis of chemotherapy in head and neck cancer (MACH-NC): an update on 93 randomised trials and 17,346 patients. Radiotherapy and oncology : journal of the European Society for Therapeutic Radiology and Oncology 92:4–14
29. Burtness B, Ma G, Flood W, Mattar B, Aa F (2005) Phase III randomized trial of cisplatin plus placebo compared with cisplatin plus cetuximab in metastatic/recurrent head and neck cancer: an Eastern Cooperative Oncology Group study. J Clin Oncol 23:8646–8654
30. Bonner JA, Harari PM, Giralt J, Azarnia N, Shin DM, Cohen RB, Jones CU, Sur R, Raben D, Jassem J, Ove R, Kies MS, Baselga J, Youssoufian H, Amellal N, Rowinsky EK, Ang KK (2006) Radiotherapy plus cetuximab for squamous-cell carcinoma of the head and neck. N Engl J Med 354(6):567–578
31. Vermorken JB, Mesia R, Rivera F, Remenar E, Kawecki A, Rottey S, Erfan J, Zabolotnyy D, Kienzer H-R, Cupissol D, Peyrade F, Benasso M, Vynnychenko I, De Raucourt D, Bokemeyer C, Schueler A, Amellal N, Hitt R (2008) Platinum-based chemotherapy plus cetuximab in head and neck cancer. N Engl J Med 359:1116–1127
32. Ang KK ZQ, Rosenthal DI, Nguyen-Tan P, Sherman EJ, Weber RS, Galvin JM, Schwartz DL, El-Naggar AK, Gillison ML, Jordan R, List MA, Konski AA, Thorstad WL, Trotti A, BeitlerJJ, Garden AS, Spanos WJ, Yom SS and RS Alelrod (2011) A randomized phase III trial (RTOG 0522) of concurrent accelerated radiation plus cisplatin with or without cetuximab for stage III-IV head and neck squamous cell carcinomas (HNC).
33. Chen LF, Cohen EE, Grandis JR (2010) New strategies in head and neck cancer: understanding resistance to epidermal growth factor receptor inhibitors. Clin Cancer Res 16(9):2489–2495
34. Adams J, Kauffman M (2004) Development of the proteasome inhibitor Velcade (Bortezomib). Cancer Invest 22(2):304–311
35. Bross PF, Kane R, Farrell AT, Abraham S, Benson K, Brower ME, Bradley S, Gobburu JV, Goheer A, Lee SL, Leighton J, Liang CY, Lostritto RT, McGuinn WD, Morse DE, Rahman A, Rosario LA, Verbois SL, Williams G, Wang YC, Pazdur R (2004) Approval summary for

bortezomib for injection in the treatment of multiple myeloma. Clin Cancer Res 10(12 Pt 1): 3954–3964
36. Richardson PG, Mitsiades C, Hideshima T, Anderson KC (2006) Bortezomib: proteasome inhibition as an effective anticancer therapy. Annu Rev Med 57:33–47
37. Sayers TJ, Brooks AD, Koh CY, Ma W, Seki N, Raziuddin A, Blazar BR, Zhang X, Elliott PJ, Murphy WJ (2003) The proteasome inhibitor PS-341 sensitizes neoplastic cells to TRAIL-mediated apoptosis by reducing levels of c-FLIP. Blood 102(1):303–310
38. Nikrad M, Johnson T, Puthalalath H, Coultas L, Adams J, Kraft AS (2005) The proteasome inhibitor bortezomib sensitizes cells to killing by death receptor ligand TRAIL via BH3-only proteins Bik and Bim. Mol Cancer Ther 4(3):443–449
39. Qin JZ, Ziffra J, Stennett L, Bodner B, Bonish BK, Chaturvedi V, Bennett F, Pollock PM, Trent JM, Hendrix MJ, Rizzo P, Miele L, Nickoloff BJ (2005) Proteasome inhibitors trigger NOXA-mediated apoptosis in melanoma and myeloma cells. Cancer Res 65(14): 6282–6293
40. Zhu H, Guo W, Zhang L, Wu S, Teraishi F, Davis JJ, Dong F, Fang B (2005) Proteasome inhibitors-mediated TRAIL resensitization and Bik accumulation. Cancer Biol Ther 4(7): 781–786
41. Zhu H, Zhang L, Dong F, Guo W, Wu S, Teraishi F, Davis JJ, Chiao PJ, Fang B (2005) Bik/NBK accumulation correlates with apoptosis-induction by bortezomib (PS-341, Velcade) and other proteasome inhibitors. Oncogene 24(31):4993–4999
42. Perez-Galan P, Roue G, Villamor N, Montserrat E, Campo E, Colomer D (2006) The proteasome inhibitor bortezomib induces apoptosis in mantle-cell lymphoma through generation of ROS and Noxa activation independent of p53 status. Blood 107(1):257–264
43. Liu X, Yue P, Chen S, Hu L, Lonial S, Khuri FR, Sun SY (2007) The proteasome inhibitor PS-341 (bortezomib) up-regulates DR5 expression leading to induction of apoptosis and enhancement of TRAIL-induced apoptosis despite up-regulation of c-FLIP and survivin expression in human NSCLC cells. Cancer Res 67(10):4981–4988
44. Perez-Galan P, Roue G, Villamor N, Campo E, Colomer D (2007) The BH3-mimetic GX15-070 synergizes with bortezomib in mantle cell lymphoma by enhancing Noxa-mediated activation of Bak. Blood 109(10):4441–4449
45. Voortman J, Checinska A, Giaccone G, Rodriguez JA, Kruyt FA (2007) Bortezomib, but not cisplatin, induces mitochondria-dependent apoptosis accompanied by up-regulation of noxa in the non-small cell lung cancer cell line NCI-H460. Mol Cancer Ther 6(3):1046–1053
46. Sunwoo JB, Chen Z, Dong G, Yeh N, Crowl Bancroft C, Sausville E, Adams J, Elliott P, Van Waes C (2001) Novel proteasome inhibitor PS-341 inhibits activation of nuclear factor-kappa B, cell survival, tumor growth, and angiogenesis in squamous cell carcinoma. Clin Cancer Res 7(5):1419–1428
47. Fribley A, Zeng Q, Wang CY (2004) Proteasome inhibitor PS-341 induces apoptosis through induction of endoplasmic reticulum stress-reactive oxygen species in head and neck squamous cell carcinoma cells. Mol Cell Biol 24(22):9695–9704
48. Chen Z, Ricker JL, Malhotra PS, Nottingham L, Bagain L, Lee TL, Yeh NT, Van Waes C (2008) Differential bortezomib sensitivity in head and neck cancer lines corresponds to proteasome, nuclear factor-kappaB and activator protein-1 related mechanisms. Mol Cancer Ther 7(7):1949–1960
49. Li C, Li R, Grandis JR, Johnson DE (2008) Bortezomib induces apoptosis via Bim and Bik up-regulation and synergizes with cisplatin in the killing of head and neck squamous cell carcinoma cells. Mol Cancer Ther 7(6):1647–1655
50. Lin YC, Chen KC, Chen CC, Cheng AL, Chen KF (2012) CIP2A-mediated Akt activation plays a role in bortezomib-induced apoptosis in head and neck squamous cell carcinoma cells. Oral Oncol 48(7):585–593
51. Yang X (2012) Proteasome inhibitor bortezomi-induced the apoptosis of laryngeal squamous cell carcinoma Hep-2 cell line via disrupting redox equilibrium. Biomedicine & pharmacotherapy = Biomedecine & pharmacotherapie 66(8):607–611
52. Li C, Johnson DE (2013) Liberation of functional p53 by proteasome inhibition in human papilloma virus-positive head and neck squamous cell carcinoma cells promotes apoptosis and cell cycle arrest. Cell Cycle 12(6):923–934

53. Yin D, Zhou H, Kumagai T, Liu G, Ong JM, Black KL, Koeffler HP (2005) Proteasome inhibitor PS-341 causes cell growth arrest and apoptosis in human glioblastoma multiforme (GBM). Oncogene 24(3):344–354
54. Huang C, Hu X, Wang L, Lu S, Cheng H, Song X, Wang J, Yang J (2012) Bortezomib suppresses the growth of leukemia cells with Notch1 overexpression in vivo and in vitro. Cancer Chemother Pharmacol 70(6):801–809
55. Hutter G, Rieken M, Pastore A, Weigert O, Zimmermann Y, Weinkauf M, Hiddemann W, Dreyling M (2012) The proteasome inhibitor bortezomib targets cell cycle and apoptosis and acts synergistically in a sequence-dependent way with chemotherapeutic agents in mantle cell lymphoma. Ann Hematol 91(6):847–856
56. Lorch JH, Thomas TO, Schmoll HJ (2007) Bortezomib inhibits cell-cell adhesion and cell migration and enhances epidermal growth factor receptor inhibitor-induced cell death in squamous cell cancer. Cancer Res 67(2):727–734
57. Orlowski RZ, Nagler A, Sonneveld P, Blade J, Hajek R, Spencer A, San Miguel J, Robak T, Dmoszynska A, Horvath N, Spicka I, Sutherland HJ, Suvorov AN, Zhuang SH, Parekh T, Xiu L, Yuan Z, Rackoff W, Harousseau JL (2007) Randomized phase III study of pegylated liposomal doxorubicin plus bortezomib compared with bortezomib alone in relapsed or refractory multiple myeloma: combination therapy improves time to progression. J Clin Oncol 25(25):3892–3901
58. Richardson PG, Briemberg H, Jagannath S, Wen PY, Barlogie B, Berenson J, Singhal S, Siegel DS, Irwin D, Schuster M, Srkalovic G, Alexanian R, Rajkumar SV, Limentani S, Alsina M, Orlowski RZ, Najarian K, Esseltine D, Anderson KC, Amato AA (2006) Frequency, characteristics, and reversibility of peripheral neuropathy during treatment of advanced multiple myeloma with bortezomib. J Clin Oncol 24(19):3113–3120
59. Cavaletti G, Jakubowiak AJ Peripheral neuropathy during bortezomib treatment of multiple myeloma: a review of recent studies. Leuk Lymphoma 51 (7):1178-1187
60. Corso A, Mangiacavalli S, Varettoni M, Pascutto C, Zappasodi P, Lazzarino M Bortezomib-induced peripheral neuropathy in multiple myeloma: a comparison between previously treated and untreated patients. Leuk Res 34 (4):471-474
61. Arastu-Kapur S, Anderl JL, Kraus M, Parlati F, Shenk KD, Lee SJ, Muchamuel T, Bennett MK, Driessen C, Ball AJ, Kirk CJ Nonproteasomal targets of the proteasome inhibitors bortezomib and carfilzomib: a link to clinical adverse events. Clin Cancer Res 17 (9):2734-2743
62. Zang Y, Thomas SM, Chan ET, Kirk CJ, Freilino ML, DeLancey HM, Grandis JR, Li C, Johnson DE (2012) Carfilzomib and ONX 0912 inhibit cell survival and tumor growth of head and neck cancer and their activities are enhanced by suppression of Mcl-1 or autophagy. Clin Cancer Res 18(20):5639–5649
63. Zang Y, Thomas SM, Chan ET, Kirk CJ, Freilino ML, DeLancey HM, Grandis JR, Li C, Johnson DE (2012) The next generation proteasome inhibitors carfilzomib and oprozomib activate prosurvival autophagy via induction of the unfolded protein response and ATF4. Autophagy 8(12):1873–1874
64. Demo SD, Kirk CJ, Aujay MA, Buchholz TJ, Dajee M, Ho MN, Jiang J, Laidig GJ, Lewis ER, Parlati F, Shenk KD, Smyth MS, Sun CM, Vallone MK, Woo TM, Molineaux CJ, Bennett MK (2007) Antitumor activity of PR-171, a novel irreversible inhibitor of the proteasome. Cancer Res 67(13):6383–6391
65. O'Connor OA, Stewart AK, Vallone M, Molineaux CJ, Kunkel LA, Gerecitano JF, Orlowski RZ (2009) A phase 1 dose escalation study of the safety and pharmacokinetics of the novel proteasome inhibitor carfilzomib (PR-171) in patients with hematologic malignancies. Clin Cancer Res 15(22):7085–7091
66. Kuhn DJ, Chen Q, Voorhees PM, Strader JS, Shenk KD, Sun CM, Demo SD, Bennett MK, van Leeuwen FW, Chanan-Khan AA, Orlowski RZ (2007) Potent activity of carfilzomib, a novel, irreversible inhibitor of the ubiquitin-proteasome pathway, against preclinical models of multiple myeloma. Blood 110(9):3281–3290

67. Zhou HJ, Aujay MA, Bennett MK, Dajee M, Demo SD, Fang Y, Ho MN, Jiang J, Kirk CJ, Laidig GJ, Lewis ER, Lu Y, Muchamuel T, Parlati F, Ring E, Shenk KD, Shields J, Shwonek PJ, Stanton T, Sun CM, Sylvain C, Woo TM, Yang J (2009) Design and synthesis of an orally bioavailable and selective peptide epoxyketone proteasome inhibitor (PR-047). J Med Chem 52(9):3028–3038
68. Chauhan D, Singh AV, Aujay M, Kirk CJ, Bandi M, Ciccarelli B, Raje N, Richardson P, Anderson KC (2010) A novel orally active proteasome inhibitor ONX 0912 triggers in vitro and in vivo cytotoxicity in multiple myeloma. Blood 116(23):4906–4915
69. Ciechanover A (2005) Proteolysis: from the lysosome to ubiquitin and the proteasome. Nat Rev Mol Cell Biol 6(1):79–87
70. Ghosh S, Karin M (2002) Missing pieces in the NF-kappaB puzzle. Cell 109(Suppl):S81–96
71. Ghosh S, Baltimore D (1990) Activation in vitro of NF-kappa B by phosphorylation of its inhibitor I kappa B. Nature 344(6267):678–682
72. Traenckner EB, Pahl HL, Henkel T, Schmidt KN, Wilk S, Baeuerle PA (1995) Phosphorylation of human I kappa B-alpha on serines 32 and 36 controls I kappa B-alpha proteolysis and NF-kappa B activation in response to diverse stimuli. EMBO J 14(12):2876–2883
73. Aggarwal BB (2004) Nuclear factor-kappaB: the enemy within. Cancer Cell 6(3):203–208
74. Van Waes C (2007) Nuclear factor-kappaB in development, prevention, and therapy of cancer. Clin Cancer Res 13(4):1076–1082
75. Ondrey FG, Dong G, Sunwoo J, Chen Z, Wolf JS, Crowl-Bancroft CV, Mukaida N, Van Waes C (1999) Constitutive activation of transcription factors NF-(kappa)B, AP-1, and NF-IL6 in human head and neck squamous cell carcinoma cell lines that express pro-inflammatory and pro-angiogenic cytokines. Mol Carcinog 26(2):119–129
76. Allen CT, Ricker JL, Chen Z, Van Waes C (2007) Role of activated nuclear factor-kappaB in the pathogenesis and therapy of squamous cell carcinoma of the head and neck. Head Neck 29(10):959–971
77. Druzgal CH, Chen Z, Yeh NT, Thomas GR, Ondrey FG, Duffey DC, Vilela RJ, Ende K, McCullagh L, Rudy SF, Muir C, Herscher LL, Morris JC, Albert PS, Van Waes C (2005) A pilot study of longitudinal serum cytokine and angiogenesis factor levels as markers of therapeutic response and survival in patients with head and neck squamous cell carcinoma. Head Neck 27(9):771–784
78. Zhang PL, Pellitteri PK, Law A, Gilroy PA, Wood GC, Kennedy TL, Blasick TM, Lun M, Schuerch C 3rd, Brown RE (2005) Overexpression of phosphorylated nuclear factor-kappa B in tonsillar squamous cell carcinoma and high-grade dysplasia is associated with poor prognosis. Mod Pathol 18(7):924–932
79. Chung CH, Parker JS, Ely K, Carter J, Yi Y, Murphy BA, Ang KK, El-Naggar AK, Zanation AM, Cmelak AJ, Levy S, Slebos RJ, Yarbrough WG (2006) Gene expression profiles identify epithelial-to-mesenchymal transition and activation of nuclear factor-kappaB signaling as characteristics of a high-risk head and neck squamous cell carcinoma. Cancer Res 66(16):8210–8218
80. Allen C, Duffy S, Teknos T, Islam M, Chen Z, Albert PS, Wolf G, Van Waes C (2007) Nuclear factor-kappaB-related serum factors as longitudinal biomarkers of response and survival in advanced oropharyngeal carcinoma. Clin Cancer Res 13(11):3182–3190
81. Traenckner EB, Wilk S, Baeuerle PA (1994) A proteasome inhibitor prevents activation of NF-kappa B and stabilizes a newly phosphorylated form of I kappa B-alpha that is still bound to NF-kappa B. EMBO J 13(22):5433–5441
82. Van Waes C, Chang AA, Lebowitz PF, Druzgal CH, Chen Z, Elsayed YA, Sunwoo JB, Rudy SF, Morris JC, Mitchell JB, Camphausen K, Gius D, Adams J, Sausville EA, Conley BA (2005) Inhibition of nuclear factor-kappaB and target genes during combined therapy with proteasome inhibitor bortezomib and reirradiation in patients with recurrent head-and-neck squamous cell carcinoma. Int J Radiat Oncol Biol Phys 63(5):1400–1412
83. Allen C, Saigal K, Nottingham L, Arun P, Chen Z, Van Waes C (2008) Bortezomib-induced apoptosis with limited clinical response is accompanied by inhibition of canonical but not alternative nuclear factor-{kappa}B subunits in head and neck cancer. Clin Cancer Res 14(13):4175–4185

84. Fribley AM, Evenchik B, Zeng Q, Park BK, Guan JY, Zhang H, Hale TJ, Soengas MS, Kaufman RJ, Wang CY (2006) Proteasome inhibitor PS-341 induces apoptosis in cisplatin-resistant squamous cell carcinoma cells by induction of Noxa. J Biol Chem 281(42): 31440–31447
85. Yang Y, Ikezoe T, Saito T, Kobayashi M, Koeffler HP, Taguchi H (2004) Proteasome inhibitor PS-341 induces growth arrest and apoptosis of non-small cell lung cancer cells via the JNK/c-Jun/AP-1 signaling. Cancer Sci 95(2):176–180
86. Dai Y, Rahmani M, Pei XY, Dent P, Grant S (2004) Bortezomib and flavopiridol interact synergistically to induce apoptosis in chronic myeloid leukemia cells resistant to imatinib mesylate through both Bcr/Abl-dependent and -independent mechanisms. Blood 104(2): 509–518
87. Wagenblast J, Hambek M, Baghi M, Gstottner W, Strebhardt K, Ackermann H, Knecht R (2008) Antiproliferative activity of bortezomib alone and in combination with cisplatin or docetaxel in head and neck squamous cell carcinoma cell lines. J Cancer Res Clin Oncol 134(3):323–330
88. Weber CN, Cerniglia GJ, Maity A, Gupta AK (2007) Bortezomib sensitizes human head and neck carcinoma cells SQ20B to radiation. Cancer Biol Ther 6(2):156–159
89. Tamatani T, Takamaru N, Hara K, Kinouchi M, Kuribayashi N, Ohe G, Uchida D, Fujisawa K, Nagai H, Miyamoto Y (2013) Bortezomib-enhanced radiosensitization through the suppression of radiation-induced nuclear factor-kappaB activity in human oral cancer cells. Int J Oncol 42(3):935–944
90. Li C, Zang Y, Sen M, Leeman-Neill RJ, Man DS, Grandis JR, Johnson DE (2009) Bortezomib up-regulates activated signal transducer and activator of transcription-3 and synergizes with inhibitors of signal transducer and activator of transcription-3 to promote head and neck squamous cell carcinoma cell death. Mol Cancer Ther 8(8):2211–2220
91. Li C, Johnson DE (2012) Bortezomib induces autophagy in head and neck squamous cell carcinoma cells via JNK activation. Cancer Lett 314(1):102–107
92. Grandis JR, Tweardy DJ (1993) Elevated levels of transforming growth factor alpha and epidermal growth factor receptor messenger RNA are early markers of carcinogenesis in head and neck cancer. Cancer Res 53(15):3579–3584
93. Fung C, Grandis JR (2010) Emerging drugs to treat squamous cell carcinomas of the head and neck. Expert Opin Emerg Drugs 15(3):355–373
94. Rubin Grandis J, Zeng Q, Tweardy DJ (1996) Retinoic acid normalizes the increased gene transcription rate of TGF-alpha and EGFR in head and neck cancer cell lines. Nat Med 2(2):237–240
95. Sheu JJ, Hua CH, Wan L, Lin YJ, Lai MT, Tseng HC, Jinawath N, Tsai MH, Chang NW, Lin CF, Lin CC, Hsieh LJ, Wang TL, Shih Ie M, Tsai FJ (2009) Functional genomic analysis identified epidermal growth factor receptor activation as the most common genetic event in oral squamous cell carcinoma. Cancer Res 69(6):2568–2576. doi:10.1158/0008-5472.CAN-08-3199
96. Rubin Grandis J, Melhem MF, Gooding WE, Day R, Holst VA, Wagener MM, Drenning SD, Tweardy DJ (1998) Levels of TGF-alpha and EGFR protein in head and neck squamous cell carcinoma and patient survival. J Natl Cancer Inst 90(11):824–832
97. Rivera F, Garcia-Castano A, Vega N, Vega-Villegas ME, Gutierrez-Sanz L (2009) Cetuximab in metastatic or recurrent head and neck cancer: the EXTREME trial. Expert Rev Anticancer Ther 9(10):1421–1428
98. Bonner JA, Harari PM, Giralt J, Cohen RB, Jones CU, Sur RK, Raben D, Baselga J, Spencer SA, Zhu J, Youssoufian H, Rowinsky EK, Ang KK (2010) Radiotherapy plus cetuximab for locoregionally advanced head and neck cancer: 5-year survival data from a phase 3 randomised trial, and relation between cetuximab-induced rash and survival. Lancet Oncol 11(1):21–28. doi:10.1016/S1470-2045(09)70311-0
99. Wagenblast J, Baghi M, Arnoldner C, Bisdas S, Gstottner W, Ackermann H, May A, Knecht R, Hambek M (2008) Effect of bortezomib and cetuximab in EGF-stimulated HNSCC. Anticancer Res 28(4B):2239–2243

100. Wagenblast J, Baghi M, Arnoldner C, Bisdas S, Gstottner W, Ackermann H, May A, Hambek M, Knecht R (2009) Cetuximab enhances the efficacy of bortezomib in squamous cell carcinoma cell lines. J Cancer Res Clin Oncol 135(3):387–393
101. Argiris A, Duffy AG, Kummar S, Simone NL, Arai Y, Kim SW, Rudy SF, Kannabiran VR, Yang X, Jang M, Chen Z, Suksta N, Cooley-Zgela T, Ramanand SG, Ahsan A, Nyati MK, Wright JJ, Van Waes C (2011) Early tumor progression associated with enhanced EGFR signaling with bortezomib, cetuximab, and radiotherapy for head and neck cancer. Clin Cancer Res 17(17):5755–5764
102. Yoshiba S, Iwase M, Kurihara S, Uchida M, Kurihara Y, Watanabe H, Shintani S (2011) Proteasome inhibitor sensitizes oral squamous cell carcinoma cells to TRAIL-mediated apoptosis. Oncol Rep 25(3):645–652
103. Seki N, Toh U, Sayers TJ, Fujii T, Miyagi M, Akagi Y, Kusukawa J, Kage M, Shirouzu K, Yamana H (2010) Bortezomib sensitizes human esophageal squamous cell carcinoma cells to TRAIL-mediated apoptosis via activation of both extrinsic and intrinsic apoptosis pathways. Mol Cancer Ther 9(6):1842–1851
104. Kim J, Guan J, Chang I, Chen X, Han D, Wang CY (2010) PS-341 and histone deacetylase inhibitor synergistically induce apoptosis in head and neck squamous cell carcinoma cells. Mol Cancer Ther 9(7):1977–1984
105. Duan J, Friedman J, Nottingham L, Chen Z, Ara G, Van Waes C (2007) Nuclear factor-kappaB p65 small interfering RNA or proteasome inhibitor bortezomib sensitizes head and neck squamous cell carcinomas to classic histone deacetylase inhibitors and novel histone deacetylase inhibitor PXD101. Mol Cancer Ther 6(1):37–50
106. Wagenblast J, Baghi M, Arnoldner C, Bisdas S, Gstottner W, May A, Knecht R, Hambek M (2008) Effects of combination treatment of bortezomib and dexamethasone in SCCHN cell lines depend on tumor cell specificity. Oncol Rep 20(5):1207–1211
107. Leinung M, Hirth D, Tahtali A, Diensthuber M, Stover T, Wagenblast J (2012) Fighting cancer from different signalling pathways: Effects of the proteasome inhibitor Bortezomib in combination with the polo-like-kinase-1-inhibitor BI2536 in SCCHN. Oncol Lett 4(6): 1305–1308
108. Gilbert J, Lee JW, Argiris A, Haigentz M Jr, Feldman LE, Jang M, Arun P, Van Waes C, Forastiere AA (2013) Phase II 2-arm trial of the proteasome inhibitor, PS-341 (bortezomib) in combination with irinotecan or PS-341 alone followed by the addition of irinotecan at time of progression in patients with locally recurrent or metastatic squamous cell carcinoma of the head and neck (E1304): a trial of the Eastern Cooperative Oncology Group. Head Neck 35(7):942–948
109. Pugh TJ, Chen C, Rabinovitch R, Eckhardt SG, Rusthoven KE, Swing R, Raben D (2010) Phase I trial of bortezomib and concurrent external beam radiation in patients with advanced solid malignancies. Int J Radiat Oncol Biol Phys 78(2):521–526
110. Kubicek GJ, Axelrod RS, Machtay M, Ahn PH, Anne PR, Fogh S, Cognetti D, Myers TJ, Curran WJ Jr, Dicker AP (2012) Phase I trial using the proteasome inhibitor bortezomib and concurrent chemoradiotherapy for head-and-neck malignancies. Int J Radiat Oncol Biol Phys 83(4):1192–1197
111. Chung CH, Aulino J, Muldowney NJ, Hatakeyama H, Baumann J, Burkey B, Netterville J, Sinard R, Yarbrough WG, Cmelak AJ, Slebos RJ, Shyr Y, Parker J, Gilbert J, Murphy BA (2010) Nuclear factor-kappa B pathway and response in a phase II trial of bortezomib and docetaxel in patients with recurrent and/or metastatic head and neck squamous cell carcinoma. Ann Oncol 21(4):864–870
112. An J, Rettig MB (2007) Epidermal growth factor receptor inhibition sensitizes renal cell carcinoma cells to the cytotoxic effects of bortezomib. Mol Cancer Ther 6(1):61–69
113. Dudek AZ, Lesniewski-Kmak K, Shehadeh NJ, Pandey ON, Franklin M, Kratzke RA, Greeno EW, Kumar P (2009) Phase I study of bortezomib and cetuximab in patients with solid tumours expressing epidermal growth factor receptor. Br J Cancer 100(9):1379–1384
114. Mork J, Lie AK, Glattre E, Hallmans G, Jellum E, Koskela P, Moller B, Pukkala E, Schiller JT, Youngman L, Lehtinen M, Dillner J (2001) Human papillomavirus infection as a risk factor for squamous-cell carcinoma of the head and neck. N Engl J Med 344(15):1125–1131

115. Herrero R, Castellsague X, Pawlita M, Lissowska J, Kee F, Balaram P, Rajkumar T, Sridhar H, Rose B, Pintos J, Fernandez L, Idris A, Sanchez MJ, Nieto A, Talamini R, Tavani A, Bosch FX, Reidel U, Snijders PJ, Meijer CJ, Viscidi R, Munoz N, Franceschi S (2003) Human papillomavirus and oral cancer: the International Agency for Research on Cancer multicenter study. J Natl Cancer Inst 95(23):1772–1783
116. Gillison ML, Koch WM, Capone RB, Spafford M, Westra WH, Wu L, Zahurak ML, Daniel RW, Viglione M, Symer DE, Shah KV, Sidransky D (2000) Evidence for a causal association between human papillomavirus and a subset of head and neck cancers. J Natl Cancer Inst 92(9):709–720
117. Chaturvedi AK, Engels EA, Anderson WF, Gillison ML (2008) Incidence trends for human papillomavirus-related and -unrelated oral squamous cell carcinomas in the United States. J Clin Oncol 26(4):612–619
118. Nasman A, Attner P, Hammarstedt L, Du J, Eriksson M, Giraud G, Ahrlund-Richter S, Marklund L, Romanitan M, Lindquist D, Ramqvist T, Lindholm J, Sparen P, Ye W, Dahlstrand H, Munck-Wikland E, Dalianis T (2009) Incidence of human papillomavirus (HPV) positive tonsillar carcinoma in Stockholm, Sweden: an epidemic of viral-induced carcinoma? Int J Cancer 125(2):362–366
119. Gillison ML (2004) Human papillomavirus-associated head and neck cancer is a distinct epidemiologic, clinical, and molecular entity. Semin Oncol 31(6):744–754
120. Lindel K, Beer KT, Laissue J, Greiner RH, Aebersold DM (2001) Human papillomavirus positive squamous cell carcinoma of the oropharynx: a radiosensitive subgroup of head and neck carcinoma. Cancer 92(4):805–813
121. Li W, Thompson CH, O'Brien CJ, McNeil EB, Scolyer RA, Cossart YE, Veness MJ, Walker DM, Morgan GJ, Rose BR (2003) Human papillomavirus positivity predicts favourable outcome for squamous carcinoma of the tonsil. Int J Cancer 106(4):553–558
122. Weinberger PM, Yu Z, Haffty BG, Kowalski D, Harigopal M, Brandsma J, Sasaki C, Joe J, Camp RL, Rimm DL, Psyrri A (2006) Molecular classification identifies a subset of human papillomavirus-associated oropharyngeal cancers with favorable prognosis. J Clin Oncol 24(5):736–747
123. Licitra L, Perrone F, Bossi P, Suardi S, Mariani L, Artusi R, Oggionni M, Rossini C, Cantu G, Squadrelli M, Quattrone P, Locati LD, Bergamini C, Olmi P, Pierotti MA, Pilotti S (2006) High-risk human papillomavirus affects prognosis in patients with surgically treated oropharyngeal squamous cell carcinoma. J Clin Oncol 24(36):5630–5636
124. Fakhry C, Westra WH, Li S, Cmelak A, Ridge JA, Pinto H, Forastiere A, Gillison ML (2008) Improved survival of patients with human papillomavirus-positive head and neck squamous cell carcinoma in a prospective clinical trial. J Natl Cancer Inst 100(4):261–269
125. Gillison ML, D'Souza G, Westra W, Sugar E, Xiao W, Begum S, Viscidi R (2008) Distinct risk factor profiles for human papillomavirus type 16-positive and human papillomavirus type 16-negative head and neck cancers. J Natl Cancer Inst 100(6):407–420
126. Psyrri A, Gouveris P, Vermorken JB (2009) Human papillomavirus-related head and neck tumors: clinical and research implication. Curr Opin Oncol 21(3):201–205
127. Balz V, Scheckenbach K, Gotte K, Bockmuhl U, Petersen I, Bier H (2003) Is the p53 inactivation frequency in squamous cell carcinomas of the head and neck underestimated? Analysis of p53 exons 2-11 and human papillomavirus 16/18 E6 transcripts in 123 unselected tumor specimens. Cancer Res 63(6):1188–1191
128. Poeta ML, Manola J, Goldwasser MA, Forastiere A, Benoit N, Califano JA, Ridge JA, Goodwin J, Kenady D, Saunders J, Westra W, Sidransky D, Koch WM (2007) TP53 mutations and survival in squamous-cell carcinoma of the head and neck. N Engl J Med 357(25):2552–2561
129. Westra WH, Taube JM, Poeta ML, Begum S, Sidransky D, Koch WM (2008) Inverse relationship between human papillomavirus-16 infection and disruptive p53 gene mutations in squamous cell carcinoma of the head and neck. Clin Cancer Res 14(2):366–369
130. Scheffner M, Huibregtse JM, Vierstra RD, Howley PM (1993) The HPV-16 E6 and E6-AP complex functions as a ubiquitin-protein ligase in the ubiquitination of p53. Cell 75(3): 495–505

131. Munger K, Basile JR, Duensing S, Eichten A, Gonzalez SL, Grace M, Zacny VL (2001) Biological activities and molecular targets of the human papillomavirus E7 oncoprotein. Oncogene 20(54):7888–7898
132. Ferris RL, Martinez I, Sirianni N, Wang J, Lopez-Albaitero A, Gollin SM, Johnson JT, Khan S (2005) Human papillomavirus-16 associated squamous cell carcinoma of the head and neck (SCCHN): a natural disease model provides insights into viral carcinogenesis. Eur J Cancer 41(5):807–815
133. Rampias T, Sasaki C, Weinberger P, Psyrri A (2009) E6 and e7 gene silencing and transformed phenotype of human papillomavirus 16-positive oropharyngeal cancer cells. J Natl Cancer Inst 101(6):412–423
134. Kimple RJ, Smith MA, Blitzer GC, Torres AD, Martin JA, Yang RZ, Peet CR, Lorenz LD, Nickel KP, Klingelhutz AJ, Lambert PF, Harari PM (2013) Enhanced Radiation Sensitivity in HPV-Positive Head and Neck Cancer. Cancer Res 73(15):4791–4800

Chapter 9
Targeting the Proteasome Pathway for the Treatment of Solid Tumors

Nisar Ahmad, Elias Anaissie, Mohamed A.Y. Abdel Malek, and James J. Driscoll

Abstract The ubiquitin-proteasome system (UPS) is a highly complex protein network that maintains proteostasis and cell viability through the targeted and timely turnover of selected substrates. The proteasome serves as the catalytic core of the UPS to precisely recognize and efficiently execute the rapid ATP-dependent removal of ubiquitinated proteins. Small-molecule pharmacologic inhibitors exploit the pivotal role of the proteasome in cellular metabolism as a molecular vulnerability in cancer cells to promote the selective cytotoxicity of tumor cells. Proteasome inhibitors (PIs) have yielded durable clinically responses that dramatically improve the survival of patients diagnosed with the invariably fatal hematologic malignancy multiple myeloma (MM). Success of the PI bortezomib in the treatment of the hematologic malignancy MM has emerged as the standard of care and catapulted the UPS into a position of prominence as a model system in cancer biology and drug

N. Ahmad
Division of Hematology & Oncology, Department of Internal Medicine, University of Cincinnati College of Medicine, Cincinnati, OH 45267, USA

E. Anaissie
Division of Hematology & Oncology, Hematologic Malignancies and Bone Marrow Transplant, Department of Internal Medicine, University of Cincinnati College of Medicine, Cincinnati, OH 45267, USA

M.A.Y.A. Malek
University of Cincinnati College of Medicine, Division of Hematology & Oncology, Department of Internal Medicine, Cincinnati, OH 45267, USA

J.J. Driscoll (✉)
Division of Hematology & Oncology, Hematologic Malignancies and Bone Marrow Transplant, Department of Internal Medicine, University of Cincinnati College of Medicine, Cincinnati, OH 45267, USA
e-mail: driscojs@ucmail.uc.edu

Q.P. Dou (ed.), *Resistance to Proteasome Inhibitors in Cancer*, Resistance to Targeted Anti-Cancer Therapeutics, DOI 10.1007/978-3-319-06752-0_9

development. However, advancement of PIs to improve the treatment of patients with solid tumors has been far more challenging and less successful. Clinical assessment of second-generation PIs progresses as well as pharmacologics to intervene at other points within the UPS is being explored for both hematologic and solid tumors. Agents to target non-proteolytic activities associated with the proteasome are emerging as are agents to inhibit Ub-binding proteins. New approaches to unravel the UPS should advance its utilization as a drug development platform in mechanism-based anticancer strategies that include PIs as monotherapy or in synergistic combinations that improve the outcome of patients with solid tumors.

Keywords Proteasome • Ubiquitin • Bortezomib • Carfilzomib

Abbreviations

ATP	Adenosine triphosphate
CP	Catalytic particle
CR	Complete response
Ct-L	Chymotryptic-like
DLT	Dose limiting toxicities
EGFR	Epidermal growth factor receptor
ER	Endoplasmic reticulum
FDA	Federal Drug Administration
γ-IFN	Gamma-interferon
IL	Interleukin
IV	Intravenous
GTP	Guanosine triphosphate
kDA	Kilodalton
MM	Multiple myeloma
MTD	Maximally tolerated dose
NCI	National Cancer Institute
NF-κB	Nuclear factor kappa B
NSCLC	Non-small cell lung cancer
ORR	Overall response rate
PI	Proteasome inhibitor
RP	Regulatory particle
RCC	Renal cell carcinoma
TNF-α	Tumor necrosis factor-α
Ub	Ubiquitin
UPS	Ubiquitin-proteasome system
UPR	Unfolded protein response
US	United States
VEGFR	Vascular endothelial growth factor receptor

9.1 The Ubiquitin-Proteasome System

Living organisms contain thousands of protein-encoding genes and a far greater number of proteins are encoded by these genes. Innumerable studies over the past century have been devoted to analyzing protein synthesis, but the reverse process of protein degradation for many decades long remained outside the scope of focused attention. In the 1930s, pioneering studies by Schoenheimer described the dynamic turnover of cellular proteins [1]. In the 1950s, it was then shown that protein half-lives required energy utilization and that different enzymes in eukaryotic cells have widely varying half-lives which made it evident that protein degradation was a highly selective process [2]. Up until that time, the lysosome was considered to be the sole site of protein degradation, but it was clear that the activity of lysosomal proteases was not selective [3]. A biochemical reductionist approach led to the discovery of a small (8.5 kDa) protein (Ub) that exists ubiquitously in eukaryotes [4]. Ub performs its myriad functions through conjugation to a large range of targets through a sequential process in three steps: E1-mediated Ub activation, transfer of Ub from the E1 to an E2 Ub-conjugating enzyme (mammalian genomes contain ~40 E2s) and formation of an isopeptide bond between a lysine residue of the target and the C-terminal glycine of the Ub moiety. E3 Ub-protein ligases function as the substrate recognition modules of the UPS to promote interaction with the E2 [5]. The structure responsible for the destruction of Ub-protein conjugates was identified as a labile 26S ATP-dependent complex that utilizes the 20S proteasome as its catalytic core particle (CP) [6, 7] capped at either end by 19S regulatory particles (RP) that provide substrate recognition, deubiquitinating, and ATP-hydrolyzing functions. Subsequently, the immunoproteasome was described and it was demonstrated that gamma-interferon (γ-IFN) replacement of constitutive proteasome subunits modulated individual catalytic activities [8, 9]. Protein degradation is a highly complex, temporally controlled, tightly regulated process that plays a critical role in numerous cellular pathways in both normal and transformed cells [10]. It is now realized that in eukaryotic cells, the degradation of most intracellular proteins is fulfilled by proteasomes. In 2004, the importance of the UPS resulted in awarding of the Nobel Prize in Chemistry jointly to Aaron Ciechanover, Avram Hershko, and Irwin Rose "for the discovery of Ub-mediated protein degradation" [10].

9.2 Proteasome Inhibitors for the Treatment of Solid Tumors

The field of oncology and cancer drug discovery has placed a significant emphasis on the identification and validation of novel molecular targets specific to tumor cells. The UPS consists of separate, linked reactions, e.g., substrate ubiquitination, proteasomal assembly, substrate cleavage, and deubiquitination, to provide a multitude of such targets for therapeutic intervention. The first component in the UPS to be targeted therapeutically is the proteasome itself. In the United States, Federal Drug Administration (FDA) approval of the PI bortezomib (Velcade, Millennium-Takeda Oncology Co., Cambridge, MA) represented a significant milestone as the first PI investigated in human clinical trials and eventually implemented for the treatment of a human malignancy [11, 12]. Bortezomib is a highly selective, reversible PI, which has demonstrated substantial benefit alone or as part of combinations that induce chemo- or radiosensitization [11]. While bortezomib is the first PI to change the natural history of a specific hematologic malignancy, preclinical studies and clinical efficacy in the treatment of the majority solid tumors have been less effective. Bortezomib is a synthetic, dipeptidyl boronate that induces apoptosis in tumor cells quite possibly through inhibiting the degradation of key regulatory and pro-apoptotic proteins. As a potent small molecule that binds the proteasome β5 subunit and hence predominantly inhibits the chymotryptic-like (Ct-L) activity of both the constitutive and immunoproteasome. The antiproliferative effect of bortezomib has been demonstrated in numerous cell lines and xenograft models of lung, breast, prostate, pancreatic, head and neck, and colon cancers and melanoma [11–15]. Numerous mechanisms of action have been proposed to explain the mechanism of selective cytotoxicity.

Newer PIs offer several potential advantages such as increased target specificity, improved safety, better tolerability, and the capacity to overcome bortezomib resistance (Table 9.1). Next generation PIs in clinical development include carfilzomib [16], ONX-0912 [17] (Onyx Pharmaceuticals, San Francisco, CA), MLN9708 [18] (Millennium-Takeda Oncology), Marizomib [19] (NPI-0052, salinosporamide A, Nereus Pharmaceuticals, San Diego, CA), and CEP-18870 [20] (Cephalon, Frazer, PA). Next to carfilzomib, the second most advanced of these PIs is MLN9708 which is a reversible, peptide boronic analog of bortezomib. MLN9708 is an orally bioavailable and is immediately hydrolyzed to its active form, MLN2238, when exposed to aqueous solutions to bind preferentially to the β5

Table 9.1 Agents to target the proteolytic activities within the proteasome complex

Inhibitor	Structural class	Type of inhibitor	Activity inhibited	Development stage	Administration
Bortezomib (Millennium)	Peptide-boronic acid	R	Ct-L Immuno	FDA-approved	IV
Carfilzomib (Onyx)	Tetrapeptide epoxyketone	I	Ct-L	FDA-approved	IV
MLN9708 (Millennium	Peptide boronic acid	R	Ct-L	Phase I	IV/ po
Marizomib (Nereus)	β-lactone-γ-lactam	I	Ct-L, tryptic, caspase-like	Phase Ib	IV
ONX-0912 (Onyx)	Peptide epoxyketone	R	Ct-L	Phase I	IV/ po
Cep-18870 (Cephalon)	Peptide-boronic acid	R	Ct-L	Phase I–III	IV/po

R reversible, *I* irreversible, *Ct-L* chymotryptic-like, *Immuno* immunoproteasome, *IV* intravenous, *po* oral active site. The dissociation half-life of MLN9708 binding to the proteasome is approximately six times shorter than that of bortezomib. Inhibition of proteasome activity and the pharmacodynamic response of the active form (MLN2238) were superior to that of bortezomib in mice bearing human lymphoma (WSU-DLCL2) or human prostate (CWR22) tumor xenografts [21]. The differences improved antitumor activity, particularly in the CWR22 xenografts where MLN2238 demonstrated greater efficacy.

The boronic acid PIs MLN9708 and CEP-18770 are reversible inhibitors of the proteasome ChT-L activity that exhibit inhibitory activity comparable to bortezomib [20]. Carfilzomib is a tetrapeptide that bears an epoxyketone moiety and irreversibly inhibits the Ct-L activity to generate sustained proteasome inhibition [21–28]. Carfilzomib inhibits proliferation and induces apoptosis in bortezomib-resistant MM cell lines and in primary MM cells from patients with clinically established resistance to bortezomib and other conventional agents. ONX-0912 (formerly PR-047, Onyx) is an orally bioavailable analog of carfilzomib investigated in phase I clinical trials with advanced refractory or recurrent solid tumors. Similar to carfilzomib, ONX 0912 is an irreversible inhibitor of the proteasome β5 subunit and induces apoptosis in cells resistant to bortezomib in vitro. In xenograft models, ONX-0912 reduced tumor growth and prolonged survival and elicited a response comparable to that seen with carfilzomib and in rodents and dogs repeated dosing was well tolerated. Although ONX-0912 is based on the same chemistry as carfilzomib, it is designed to provide prolonged proteasome inhibition and the convenience of an oral therapy. ONX-0912 is currently in phase I clinical development in a solid tumor study in the United States. Early data have shown that two-thirds of patients at the 90 mg dose or above achieved a level of proteasome inhibition comparable to what has been observed with carfilzomib. ONX-0914 is an immunoproteasome inhibitor with potential applications in oncology and in autoimmune disease therapy. An immunoproteasome-specific inhibitor may have the potential to selectively target proteasome function in immune cells while exhibiting minimal effects on the proteasome in other tissues and with minimal cross-reactivity for the constitutive proteasome [29]. Recent evidence suggests that the immunoproteasome regulates the production of several inflammatory cytokines, including tumor necrosis factor-α (TNF-α), interleukin-6 (IL-6), IL-17, and IL-23. In models of rheumatoid arthritis and lupus, ONX-0914 blocked progression of disease at well-tolerated doses.

Marizomib (NPI-0052) is a natural β-lactone compound derived from the marine bacterium *Salinospora tropica* [31, 32] and similar to carfilzomib, it is an irreversible inhibitor of the β5 subunit. However, unlike carfilzomib, which preferentially inhibits the Ct-L, and bortezomib, which inhibits the Ct-L and caspase-like activities, Marizomib inhibits the three predominant catalytic activities (Ct-L, tryptic-like and caspase-like) which may yield a long-term benefit to preclude resistance. Preclinical research suggests an improved therapeutic ratio and significant activity in hematologic and solid tumor models through either oral or intravenous (IV) administration. Toxicities of Marizomib are comparable to those of bortezomib except for lack of peripheral neuropathy.

9.3 Preclinical Studies to Demonstrate the Efficacy of Proteasome Inhibitors in Solid Tumor Cells

A number of exploratory preclinical and translational studies have investigated the potential benefit of PI for treatment of solid tumors. These studies have provided a sound rationale to advance bortezomib into trials as monotherapy or in combination with chemotherapy, radiation, immunotherapy, or other novel agents [30–38]. As monotherapy, bortezomib has demonstrated poor responses in both phase I and II trials as assessed in a broad number of solid tumors. Phase I studies of bortezomib-based combination regimens provided only a slight improvement in responses, particularly in combination with traditional chemotherapeutic agents such as CPT-11, gemcitabine, docetaxel, and 5-FU. However, they provided the basis for more refined phase II studies. At the maximal tolerated doses observed, toxicities were mild and easily manageable. Phase II clinical trials were performed in focused solid tumor types, e.g., colon, breast, neuroendocrine, renal, melanoma, gastric, and prostate cancers and sarcomas.

In hepatocellular carcinoma cells, phospho-AKT downregulation was a determinant of PI sensitivity and AKT signaling was targeted to overcome resistance. In medullary and anaplastic thyroid carcinoma cells, drug sensitivity was partially decreased by Bcl-2 overexpression or IGF-I treatment. The PI-induced activation of essential cellular pathways, e.g., AKT, MAPK, p53, c-Jun, and destabilization of NF-κB, has been implicated in dictating response in solid tumors. Bortezomib-induced G_2M arrest mediated through inhibition of cell-cycle regulators turnover has been demonstrated as well, mediated by the induction of p21/cip/waf-1 in either p53-dependent or independent mechanisms. PI induction of a terminal unfolded protein response (UPR) and endoplasmic reticulum (ER) stress was shown to correlate with the accumulation of misfolded proteins and apoptosis while combination of PIs and ER-stress-inducing agents increased cytotoxicity in glioblastoma and metastatic melanoma [39–41]. Importantly, bortezomib was generally well tolerated and did not appear to produce additive toxicities when combined with other therapies in the dosing regimens used in these preclinical in vivo studies. Marizomib has also been found to inhibit brain proteasome activity in a mouse model, to suggest use in the treatment of central nervous system tumors. CEP-18770 is an orally active peptide boronic acid PI that reversibly inhibits the CT-L activity of the proteasome. Antitumor activity, survival benefit, and complete tumor regressions have been demonstrated in myeloma xenograft models using CEP-18770. CEP-18770 also has shown a more favorable cytotoxicity profile toward human bone marrow progenitors and bone marrow-derived stromal cells when compared with bortezomib [28].

9.4 Clinical Trials of Proteasome Inhibitors for Solid Tumors

There is tremendous interest in expanding the use of PI for cancer treatment beyond hematological malignancies (Tables 9.2, and 9.3) [42–45]. Successful application of PIs for certain types of B-cell lymphomas has shown improved response rates.

Table 9.2 Completed trials to assess the efficacy of proteasome inhibitors as monotherapy or in combination to treat solid tumors

Solid tumor	Proteasome inhibitor	Dosing schedule	PI treatment regimen	Outcome
Metastatic breast cancer	Bortezomib	1.5 mg/m^2 administered biweekly	Monotherapy	1 SD,11 PD
NSCLC	Bortezomib	1.3 mg/m^2/day on days 1, 4, 8, and 11	Monotherapy	NR in all 14 patients
Advanced solid tumors	Bortezomib	Varied	PI + paclitaxel and carboplatin	24 % PR in group A,4 % PR in group B
Advanced solid tumors	Bortezomib	Bortezomib (1.0, 1.3, or 1.5 mg/m^2	PI + irinotecan (from 50–125 mg/m^2)	NR
Advanced solid tumors	Bortezomib	Bortezomib 1.0–1.5 mg/m^2	PI + gemcitabine 500–1,000 mg/m^2	1/31 PR, 7 /31SD
Advanced solid tumors	Bortezomib	Dose escalation (7 levels)	PI + sunitinib	4/33 PR,6/33 SD
Advanced solid tumors	Bortezomib	0.9–1.5 mg/m^2	PI + doxorubicin 30 mg/m^2	1/37 nCR,2/37 PR,4/37 SD
Advanced solid tumors	Bortezomib	Dose-escalation study	PI + tanespimycin	1/9 SD
NSCLC	Bortezomib	1.5 mg/m^2) twice a week	Monotherapy	NR
Unresectable solid tumors	Bortezomib	Dose-escalation study	PI + sorafenib	1/14 PR,5 /14SD, 10 PD
Metastatic breast cancer	Bortezomib	1.3 mg/m^2	PI + doxorubicin 30 mg/m^2	1/12 PR,3/12 SD
Metastatic gastric/ gastroesophageal adenocarcinoma	Bortezomib	1.3 mg/m^2	Monotherapy	NR
Previously treated urothelial tract carcinoma	Bortezomib	1.3 mg/m^2	Monotherapy	NR
Metastatic breast cancer	Bortezomib	1–1.3 mg/m^2	PI + capecitabine, 1,500–2,500 mg/m^2	15 % PR,40%SD at MTD
Malignant high grade glioma	Bortezomib	Dose escalation	None	2/66 PR
Advanced solid tumors	Bortezomib	Dose escalation	PI + temozolomide	7/12 SD, 4 /12PD
Advanced solid tumors[a]	MLN9708	–	Monotherapy	26/75 SD,PR in H&N Cohort

[a]Ongoing

Table 9.3 Ongoing trials to assess the efficacy of proteasome inhibitors as monotherapy or in combination to treat solid tumors

Proteasome Inhibitor	Treatment regimen	Tumor type	Phase	Objective
MLN9708	Monotherapy	Advanced non-hematological malignancies	1	To determine safety, MTD and inform phase 2 dose
Oprozomib	Monotherapy	Recurrent or refractory solid tumors	1	
MLN9708	Monotherapy	Advanced solid and hematological malignancies	1, 2-part	Pharmacokinetics of MLN9708 in varying degree of liver dysfunction
Bortezomib	Lapatinib	Advanced solid tumors	1	To test the safety and efficacy of the combination of lapatinib and bortezomib
Bortezomib	Monotherapy	Refractory solid tumors in pediatric patients	1	To determine MTD, 20S proteasome inhibition and progression free survival

For example, the phase II VERTICAL trial studied a combination of bortezomib, bendamustine, and rituximab in patients with relapsed or refractory follicular lymphoma and proved to be highly active (ORR of 88 % and complete response (CR) of 53 %) [46]. A rapidly expanding number of clinical trials have evaluated bortezomib and other PIs either as monotherapy or in combinations to treat patients with solid tumors. Bortezomib was used as monotherapy to treat chemotherapy-naïve patients diagnosed with advanced stage non-small cell lung cancer (NSCLC). The trial was terminated in the first stage due to lack of response in all patients [47]. Separately, bortezomib as monotherapy was also inactive in patients with unresectable or metastatic gastric and gastroesophageal junction adenocarcinoma [48].

Bortezomib was combined with paclitaxel and carboplatin as a first-line regimen in the treatment of patients with metastatic esophageal, gastric, and gastroesophageal cancer and was a disappointment [49]. A phase I/II trial combined Vandetanib (Caprelsa, AstraZeneca USA, Wilmington, DE) with bortezomib in adult patients diagnosed with solid tumors with a focus on hereditary or sporadic, locally advanced, or metastatic medullary thyroid cancers [50]. Vandetanib potently inhibits vascular endothelial growth factor receptor-2 (VEGFR-2), and shows additional inhibitory activity against the rearranged during transfection receptor, Flt-4, and EGF receptor tyrosine kinases [51]. Bortezomib in combination with celecoxib in patients with advanced solid tumors was also studied in a phase I trial and was well tolerated, without dose limiting toxicities (DLT) observed [52]. In patients with metastatic renal cell carcinoma (RCC), the results suggested that bortezomib has an antitumor effect in individual patients with metastatic RCC but the small proportion of patients who did achieve a partial response did not support routine use in metastatic RCC [53, 54].

Lung cancer continues to be the leading cause of cancer-related deaths in the United States, with approximately 160,000 estimated deaths per year [55]. More effective drugs such as bortezomib have been used and based upon some encouraging single-agent activity, bortezomib was combined with other agents in phase I studies to demonstrate significant activity in pretreated patients as a single agent and greater activity in combination with docetaxel [56–58]. Given that the duration of proteasome inhibition is 48–72 h, all clinical studies have used a regimen of bortezomib administered on days 1, 4, 8, and 11. A phase I trial tested a schedule of twice-weekly drug administration for 4 weeks followed by 2 weeks of rest [59]. Toxicities included thrombocytopenia and nonmyeloid toxicities, such as anorexia, fatigue, electrolyte disturbances, and nausea. Another phase I study, conducted in a variety of solid tumors, administered bortezomib on days 1, 4, 8, and 11 of a 21-day cycle [60]. Forty-three patients were treated on this schedule. The DLTs were diarrhea and sensory neuropathy. No hematologic toxicities were observed. One major response was seen in an NSCLC patient. In phase II studies, minimally pretreated (≤1 prior chemotherapy regimens) 23 NSCLC patients were treated with single-agent bortezomib at doses of 1.3–1.5 mg/m^2 in thrice-weekly cycles [61]. One patient experienced a partial response and nine others had stable disease. The duration of response was >4 cycles in 5 patients. Grade 3 toxicities included nausea (3 patients), sensory neuropathy (1 patient), constipation (2 patients), rash (1 patient), and thrombocytopenia (2 patients). Effects on NF-κB reached a maximum 4 h after drug administration, with recovery beginning in 24 h to demonstrate a measurable effect on the biologic target. A recently completed randomized phase II study compared a 1.5-mg/m^2 bortezomib dose with the combination of 1.3 mg/m^2 of bortezomib and 75 mg/m^2 of docetaxel in pretreated patients with NSCLC [62]. Docetaxel was administered on day 1 of a 21-day cycle. Preliminary results indicate that adverse events, including nausea (59 % versus 35 %), fatigue (38 % versus 48 %), diarrhea (38 % versus 29 %), and neutropenia (55 % versus 3 %), respectively, were more common in the combination arm than in the single-agent bortezomib arm. An interim analysis revealed partial response rates of 10.3 % in the bortezomib arm and 16 % in the combination arm.

The clinical observation of intrinsic or acquired resistance to bortezomib; the occurrence of severe and cumulative toxicities, namely painful peripheral neuropathy and fatigue; its IV administration; and the lack of efficacy for solid tumors all prompted the development of second-generation PIs. Phase I studies with MLN9708, alone or in combination, are ongoing in patients with newly diagnosed and refractory MM, lymphomas, and non-hematologic malignancies. In phase I studies, carfilzomib was well tolerated when administered in highly intensive daily dosage regimens to suggest that proteasome inhibition sustained for extended periods was tolerable [63–66]. The safety, pharmacokinetics, and pharmacodynamics of CEP-18770 were investigated after IV administration on days 1, 4, 8, and 11 of every 21-day cycle in patients with MM and solid tumors [67]. CEP-18770 exhibited a favorable safety profile with a lack of toxicity and linear plasma PK to indicate future potential. A phase Ib trial evaluated safety and tolerability of single-agent carfilzomib in relapsed solid tumors, relapsed and/or refractory MM, and refractory lymphoma, while the phase II evaluated the overall response rate after four cycles of carfilzomib in relapsed solid tumors in heavily pretreated patients. The incidence of newly emergent peripheral neuropathy was low despite high rates at baseline in heavily pretreated patients. Worsening neuropathy during treatment with carfilzomib is uncommon to suggest that carfilzomib may be effective for those who have neuropathy due to prior treatment.

A recent phase I study undertaken to define toxicity and the maximum tolerated doses (MTD) of the combination of sorafenib and bortezomib in patients with advanced solid tumors has demonstrated the combination was tolerated well [68]. The combination shows preliminary signs of efficacy, supporting phase 2 studies. A phase I study of the HER1, HER2 dual kinase inhibitor, and lapatinib in combination with bortezomib in patients with advanced malignancies is ongoing [69]. Preclinical cell line and animal studies indicate that combination of these agents was much more effective than administration of either drug alone. Jones et al. demonstrated in their study using mice that bortezomib effectively suppresses breast cancer tumor growth within bone and stimulates new bone formation in the presence of metastatic disease. Antitumor growth effects by bortezomib also occurs in the bone microenvironment where the cycle of tumor growth and osteolytic disease is activated in response to breast cancer cells [69]. Another phase 1 study is being conducted by the National Cancer Institute (NCI) to demonstrate MTD and 20S proteasome inhibition. Patients receive bortezomib IV on days 1, 4, 8, and 11. It is apparent that more effort is required, both in preclinical and clinic studies, to better define the role of PI in the treatment of solid tumors. The NCI clinical trials database includes ~200 currently active trials listed studying bortezomib's potential in the treatment of these various cancer types, although delineating the mechanism by which bortezomib fails in these cases may be the first critical step in improving its efficacy.

9.5 Targeting Non-proteolytic Activities Associated with Proteasome Complex

The clinical development of PIs suggests that targeting other components within the UPS is a useful strategy for the treatment of malignancies (Table 9.4). Substrate recognition by the proteasome is mediated through the multi-Ub chain followed by ATP-dependent unfolding and translocation of the substrate from the RP into the proteolytic chamber of the CP to facilitate degradation [70]. Substrate-bound Ub chains are not delivered directly to the proteolytic active sites but rather recycled as

Table 9.4 Non-proteolytic targets associated with the proteasome complex

Rpn11	19S component that contains an essential JAMM metal-binding motif
Blm10	Proposed role in proteasome maturation
Ecm29	Tethers the 19S RP and 20S CP to unite the 26S proteasome complex
Hul5	Ub-protein ligase
Ubp6	Deubiquitinating enzyme
Rpt2	19S component regulates access to the 20S proteasome core and proteolytic chamber

intact free Ub or Ub chains [71]. Substrate deubiquitination is mediated by three distinct enzymes associated with the RP: RPN11, UCH37, and USP14 [72–74]. RPN11 cleaves at the base of the Ub chain where it is linked to the substrate, whereas UCH37 and USP14 mediate stepwise removal of Ub from the substrate by disassembling the chain from its distal tip. USP14 can inhibit the degradation of Ub-protein conjugates both in vitro and in vivo. A catalytically inactive variant of USP14 was shown to reduce inhibitory activity and to indicate such inhibition was mediated by trimming of the Ub chain on the substrate. A high-throughput screen identified a selective small-molecule inhibitor of human USP14 deubiquitinating activity and treatment of cultured cells with this compound enhanced degradation of several proteasome substrates. Another small molecule, b-AP15, is a newly identified PI that abrogates the deubiquitinating activity of the 19S RP [74]. b-AP15 inhibited the activity of two 19S RP deubiquitinases, UCHL5 and USP14, to result in the accumulation of polyubiquitin and was shown to inhibit tumor progression in in vivo solid tumor models. Other novel activities associated with the proteasome but not directly involved in substrate hydrolysis are Blm10 which functions in maturation of the multi-subunit 26S proteasome and Ecm29 which tethers the RP to the CP [75–78]. The protein ligase Hul5 and Rad23 each deliver Ub conjugates to the proteasome to suggest that substrate delivery may be targeted as well.

9.6 Concluding Remarks

The precise molecular events that underlie the cellular response to proteasome inhibitors remain to be clearly elucidated in solid tumor models. Evidence suggests that the ability of a cell to manage the amount of proteotoxic stress following proteasome inhibition dictates or contributes to survival. Mammalian cells initiate and retain tight control of protein synthesis during stress conditions. Biologically, it is reasonable to reduce protein synthesis during cell stress to prevent the accumulation of translational mistakes. The primary mechanism used to control translation rates involves inhibitory phosphorylation of the eIF2 translation initiation factor at the Ser51 residue of its α subunit [79]. In its active, unphosphorylated form, eIF2 bound with GTP and the Met-tRNAi assembles with eIF1, eIF1A, eIF3, eIF4F, and eIF5 to form the 43S pre-initiation complex. The complex scans the 5′ cap of the mRNA being translated, and once the start codon is recognized, the eIF2-bound GTP is hydrolyzed to GDP and the initiator Met-tRNA binds to the 40S ribosome to provide the initial amino acid for the polypeptide [79, 80]. Inactivated eIF2-GDP is recycled back to its active GTP-bound form by eIF2B, a guanine nucleotide exchange factor. Upon proteotoxic stress, the α subunit of eIF2 is phosphorylated and directly binds to and inhibits the nucleotide exchange capacity eIF2B, thus significantly reducing decreasing eIF2-GTP levels and reducing translation rates. Recent studies have suggested that the ability of cancer cells to induce eIF2α phosphorylation upon stress promotes survival. A lack of inducible eIF2α-P led to the excessive accumulation of aggregated proteins, reactive oxygen species, and ultimately cell death [81–83].

Remarkable progress has been made in understanding the basic biology of cellular mechanisms to target and degrade intracellular proteins. However, much of the complexity within the Ub system remains to be unraveled, especially defining the alterations in the pathway that play a primary role in many pathological states, such as solid tumors. Similar to the UPS, cancer is likewise, a complex system that has acquired the ability to maintain stable functioning despite perturbations and poses a formidable hurdle in cancer therapeutics. Since complex systems are maintained through invulnerability to both internal and external stresses and tumor robustness is achieved through functional redundancy and multilayered feedback control systems, targeting the unique effectors within the UPS may eventually yield the most specific and effective agents that provide a durable survival benefit in the treatment of solid tumors.

Disclosures The authors disclose no conflicts of interest

References

1. Schoenheimer R (1942) The dynamic state of body constituents. Harvard University Press, Cambridge
2. Simpson MV (1953) The release of labeled amino acids from proteins in liver slices. J Biol Chem 201:143–54
3. De Duve C, Gianetto R, Appelmans F, Wattiaux R (1953) Enzymic content of the mitochondria fraction. Nature 172:1143–44
4. Ciechanover A, Hod Y, Hershko A (1978) A heat-stable polypeptide component of an ATP-dependent proteolytic system from reticulocytes. Biochem Biophys Res Commun 81:1100–05
5. Ciechanover A (2005) From the lysosome to ubiquitin and the proteasome. Nat Rev Mol Cell Biol 6:79–86
6. Eytan E, Ganoth D, Armon T, Hershko A (1989) ATP-dependent incorporation of 20S protease into the 26S complex that degrades proteins conjugated to ubiquitin. Proc Natl Acad Sci U S A 86:7751–55
7. Driscoll J, Goldberg AL (1990) The proteasome (multicatalytic protease) is a component of the 1500-kDa proteolytic complex which degrades ubiquitin-conjugated proteins. J Biol Chem 265:4789–92
8. Brown MG, Driscoll J, Monaco JJ (1991) Structural and serological similarity of MHC-linked LMP and proteasome (multicatalytic proteinase) complexes. Nature 353:355–7
9. Driscoll J, Brown MG, Finley D, Monaco JJ (1993) *MHC*-linked *LMP* gene products specifically alter peptidase activities of the proteasome. Nature 365:262–4
10. Ciechanover A, Hershko A, Rose I. (2004) http://www.nobelprize.org/nobel_prizes/chemistry/laureates/2004
11. Chen D, Dou QP (2010) The ubiquitin-proteasome system as a prospective molecular target for cancer treatment and prevention. Curr Protein Pept Sci 11(6):459–70
12. Orlowski RZ, Kuhn DJ (2008) Proteasome inhibitors in cancer therapy: lessons from the first decade. Clin Cancer Res 1649–57
13. Nawrocki ST, Bruns CJ, Harbison MT et al (2002) Effects of the proteasome inhibitor PS-341 on apoptosis and angiogenesis in orthotopic human pancreatic tumor xenografts. Mol Cancer Ther 1:1243–53
14. Williams S, Pettaway C, Song R (2003) Differential effects of the proteasome inhibitor bortezomib on apoptosis and angiogenesis in human prostate tumor xenografts. Mol Cancer Ther 2:835–43

15. Hideshima T, Richardson P, Chauhan D et al (2006) The proteasome inhibitor PS-341 inhibits growth, induces apoptosis, and overcomes drug resistance in human multiple myeloma cells. Cancer Res 61:3071–6
16. Kupperman E, et al. Cancer Res. Phase II results of Study PX-171-007: a phase Ib/II study of carfilzomib (CFZ), a selective proteasome inhibitor, in patients with selected advanced metastatic solid tumors. ASCO. 2009; Abstract 3515
17. Development: ONX 0914 (PR-957). www.onyx-pharm.com/view.cfm/679/ONX-0914
18. Rodler ET, Infante JR, Siu LL. First-in-human, phase I dose-escalation study of investigational drug MLN9708, a second-generation proteasome inhibitor, in advanced nonhematologic malignancies. J Clin Oncol 2010;28:15s (suppl; abstr 3071)
19. Groll M, Huber R, Potts BC (2006) Crystal structures of salinosporamide A (NPI-0052) and B (NPI-0047) in complex with the 20S proteasome reveal important consequences of β-lactone ring opening and a mechanism for irreversible binding. J Am Chem Soc 128:5136–41
20. Piva R, Ruggeri B, Williams M et al (2008) CEP-18770: a novel, orally active proteasome inhibitor with a tumor-selective pharmacologic profile competitive with bortezomib. Blood 111(5):2765–75
21. Dick LR, Fleming PE (2010) Building on bortezomib: second-generation proteasome inhibitors as anti-cancer therapy. Drug Discov Today 15:243–9
22. ClinicalTrials.gov. NCT00531284—Phase 1b/2 Study of Carfilzomib in relapsed solid tumors and multiple myeloma
23. Demo SD, Kirk CJ, Aujay MA et al (2007) Antitumor activity of PR-171, a novel irreversible inhibitor of the proteasome. Cancer Res 67(13):6383–91
24. Min CK, Lee SE, Yahng SA et al (2013) The impact of novel therapeutic agents before and after frontline autologous stem cell transplantation in patients with multiple myeloma. Blood Res 48(3):198–205
25. Yaqub S, Ballester G, Ballester O (2013) Frontline Therapy for multiple myeloma: a concise review of the evidence based on randomized clinical trials. Cancer Invest 31(8):529–537
26. De la Puente P, Azab AK (2013) Contemporary drug therapies for multiple myeloma. Drugs Today (Barc) 49(9):563–73
27. Parlati F, Lee SJ, Aujay M et al (2009) Carfilzomib can induce tumor cell death through selective inhibition of the chymotrypsin-like activity of the proteasome. Blood 114:3439–3447
28. Chauhan D, Catley L, Li G et al (2005) A novel orally active proteasome inhibitor induces apoptosis in multiple myeloma cells with mechanisms distinct from Bortezomib. Cancer Cell 8:407–19
29. Huber EM, Basler M, Schwab R, Heinemeyer W, Kirk CJ, Groettrup M, Groll M (2012) Immuno- and constitutive proteasome crystal structures reveal differences in substrate and inhibitor specificity. Cell 148:727–738
30. Korteum KM, Stewart AK (2013) Carfilzomib. Blood 121:893–7
31. Potts BC, Albitar MX, Anderson KC et al (2011) Marizomib, a proteasome inhibitor for all seasons: preclinical profile and a framework for clinical trials. Curr Cancer Drug Targets 11(3):254–284
32. Feling RH, Buchanan GO, Mincer TJ et al (2003) A highly cytotoxic proteasome inhibitor from a novel microbial source, a marine bacterium of the new genus Salinospora. Angew Chem Int Ed Engl 42(3):355–7
33. Chen KF, Yeh PY, Hsu C et al (2009) Bortezomib overcomes tumor necrosis factor-related apoptosis-inducing ligand resistance in hepatocellular carcinoma cells in part through the inhibition of the phosphatidylinositol 3-kinase/Akt pathway. J Biol Chem 284:11121–33
34. Mitsiades CS, McMillin D, Kotoula V (2006) Antitumor effects of the proteasome inhibitor bortezomib in medullary and anaplastic thyroid carcinoma cells in vitro. J Clin Endocrinol Metab 91:4013–21
35. Lioni M, Noma K, Snyder A et al (2008) Bortezomib induces apoptosis in esophageal squamous cell carcinoma cells through activation of the p38 mitogen-activated protein kinase pathway. Mol Cancer Ther 7(9):2866–75
36. Ooi MG, Hayden PJ, Kotoula V et al (2009) Interactions of the Hdm2/p53 and proteasome pathways may enhance the antitumor activity of bortezomib. Clin Cancer Res 15:7153–60

37. Yu C, Friday BB, Lai JP et al (2006) Cytotoxic synergy between the multikinase inhibitor sorafenib and the proteasome inhibitor bortezomib in vitro: induction of apoptosis through Akt and c-Jun NH2-terminal kinase pathways. Mol Cancer Ther 5:2378–87
38. Sunwoo JB, Chen Z, Dong G et al (2008) Novel proteasome inhibitor PS-341 inhibits activation of nuclear factor-kappa B, cell survival, tumor growth, and angiogenesis in squamous cell carcinoma. Clin Cancer Res 7:1419–28
39. Mitsiades N, Mitsiades CS, Poulaki V et al (2002) Molecular sequelae of proteasome inhibition in human multiple myeloma cells. Proc Natl Acad Sci U S A 99:14374–9
40. Canfield SE, Zhu K, Williams SA (2006) Bortezomib inhibits docetaxel-induced apoptosis via a p21-dependent mechanism in human prostate cancer cells. Mol Cancer Ther 5:2043–50
41. Wu J, Kaufman RJ (2006) From acute ER stress to physiological roles of the unfolded protein response. Cell Death Differ 13:374–84
42. Kardosh A et al (2008) Aggravated endoplasmic reticulum stress as a basis for enhanced glioblastoma cell killing by bortezomib in combination with celecoxib or its non-coxib analogue, 2,5-dimethyl-celecoxib. Cancer Res 68:843–51
43. Hill DS, Martin S, Armstrong JL (2009) Combining the endoplasmic reticulum stress-inducing agents bortezomib and fenretinide as a novel therapeutic strategy for metastatic melanoma. Clin Cancer Res 15:1192–8
44. Williamson MJ, Silva MD, Terkelsen J (2009) The relationship among tumor architecture, pharmacokinetics, pharmacodynamics, and efficacy of bortezomib in mouse xenograft models. Mol Cancer Ther 8:3234–43
45. Buac D, Shen M, Schmitt S et al (2013) From bortezomib to other inhibitors of the proteasome and beyond. Curr Pharm Des 19(22):4025–4038
46. Caravita T, De Fabritiis P, Palumbo A (2006) Bortezomib: efficacy comparisons in solid tumors and hematologic malignancies. Nat Clin Pract Oncol 3:374–87
47. Wright JJ (2010) Combination therapy of bortezomib with novel targeted agents: an emerging treatment strategy. Clin Cancer Res 16(16):4094–04
48. Milano A, Perri F, Caponigro F (2009) The ubiquitin-proteasome system as a molecular target in solid tumors: an update on bortezomib. Oncotargets Ther 2:171–8
49. Fowler N, Kahl BS, Lee P et al (2011) Bortezomib, bendamustine, and rituximab in patients with relapsed or refractory follicular lymphoma: the phase II VERTICAL study. J Clin Oncol 29(25):3389–95
50. Li TH, Ho L, Piperdi B et al (2010) Phase II study of the proteasome inhibitor bortezomib (PS-341, Velcade) in chemotherapy-naive patients with advanced stage non-small cell lung cancer (NSCLC)Lung. Cancer 68(1):89–93
51. Shah MA, Power DG, Kindler HL et al (2011) A multicenter, phase II study of Bortezomib (PS-341) in patients with unresectable or metastatic gastric and gastroesophageal junction adenocarcinoma. Invest New Drugs 29(6):1475–81
52. Jatoi A, Dakhil SR, Foster NR et al (2008) Bortezomib, paclitaxel, and carboplatin as a first-line regimen for patients with metastatic esophageal, gastric, and gastroesophageal cancer - Phase II Results from the North Central Cancer Treatment Group (N044B). J Thorac Oncol 3(5):516–20
53. ClinicalTrials.gov. http://clinicaltrials.gov/show/NCT00923247
54. Carlomagno F, Vitagliano D, Guida T et al (2002) ZD6474, an orally available inhibitor of KDR tyrosine kinase activity, efficiently blocks oncogenic RET kinases. Cancer Res 62:7284–90
55. Dubrey S, Schiller JH (2005) Three emerging new drugs for NSCLC: pemetrexed, bortezomib and cetuximab. Oncologist 10(4):282–291
56. Hayslip J, Chaudhary U, Green M, Meyer M, Dunder S, Sherman C et al (2007) Bortezomib in combination with celecoxib in patients with advanced solid tumors: a phase I trial. BMC Cancer 7:221
57. Kondagunta GV, Drucker B, Schwartz L et al (2004) Phase II trial of bortezomib for patients with advanced renal cell carcinoma. J Clin Oncol 22:3720–5

58. Davies AM, Lara PN, Lau DH et al (2004) The proteasome inhibitor, bortezomib, in combination with gemcitabine (Gem) and carboplatin (Carbo) in advanced non-small cell lung cancer (NSCLC): final results of a phase I California Cancer Consortium study. Proc Am Soc Clin Oncol 23:639a
59. Ryan DP, O'Neil B, Lima CR et al (2003) Phase I dose-escalation study of the proteasome inhibitor, bortezomib, plus irinotecan in patients with advanced solid tumors. Proc Am Soc Clin Oncol 22:228a
60. Erlichman C, Adjei AA, Thomas JPT et al (2001) A phase I trial of the proteasome inhibitor PS-341 in patients with advanced cancer. Proc Am Soc Clin Oncol 20:85a
61. Aghajanian C, Soignet S, Dizon D et al (2001) A phase I trial of the novel proteasome inhibitor PS341 in advanced solid tumor malignancies. Proc Am Soc Clin Oncol 20:85a
62. Fanucchi MP, Belt RJ, Fossella FV et al (2004) Phase (ph) 2 study of bortezomib ± docetaxel in previously treated patients (pts) with advanced non-small cell lung cancer (NSCLC): preliminary results. Proc Am Soc Clin Oncol 23:640a
63. Stevenson JP, Nho CW, Johnson SW et al (2004) Effects of bortezomib (PS-341) on NF-κB activation in peripheral blood mononuclear cells (PBMCs) of advanced non-small cell lung cancer (NSCLC) patients: a phase II/pharmacodynamic trial. Proc Am Soc Clin Oncol 23:649a
64. Rosen PJ, Gordon M, Lee PN. Phase II results of study PX-171-007: a phase Ib/II study of carfilzomib (CFZ), a selective proteasome inhibitor, in patients with selected advanced metastatic solid tumors. J Clin Oncol 2009;27:15s (suppl; abstr 3515)
65. Papadopoulos KP, Mendelson DS, Tolcher AW. A phase I, open-label, dose-escalation study of the novel oral proteasome inhibitor (PI) ONX 0912 in patients with advanced refractory or recurrent solid tumors, J Clin Oncol 2011;29: (suppl; abstr 3075)
66. Muchamuel T, Basler M, Aujay MA, Groettrup M (2009) A selective inhibitor of the immunoproteasome subunit LMP7 blocks cytokine production and attenuates progression of experimental arthritis. Nat Med 15(7):781–7
67. Kumar SK, Jett J, Marks R, Richardson R, Quevedo F, Moynihan T, Croghan G, Adjei AA (2013) Phase 1 study of sorafenib in combination with bortezomib in patients with advanced malignancies. Invest New Drugs 31(5):1201–6
68. Gallerani E, Zucchetti M, Brunelli D et al (2013) A first in human phase I study of the proteasome inhibitor CEP-18770 in patients with advanced solid tumours and multiple myeloma. Eur J Cancer 49(2):290–6
69. Jones MD, Liu JC, Barthel TK, Hussain S, Lian JB (2010) A proteasome inhibitor, bortezomib, inhibits breast cancer growth and reduces osteolysis by downregulating metastatic genes. Clin Cancer Res 16(20):4978–4989
70. Finley D (2009) Recognition and processing of ubiquitin-protein conjugates by the proteasome. Annu Rev Biochem 78:477–513
71. Husnjak K, Elsasser S, Zhang N, Chen X, Randles L, Shi Y et al (2008) Proteasome subunit Rpn13 is a novel ubiquitin receptor. Nature 453:481–8
72. Lee BH, Lee MJ, Park S, Oh DC, Elsasser S, Chen PC et al (2010) Enhancement of proteasome activity by a small-molecule inhibitor of USP14. Nature 467:179–84
73. Lee MJ, Lee BH, Hanna J, King RW, Finley D (2011) Trimming of ubiquitin chains by proteasome-associated deubiquitinating enzymes. Mol Cell Proteomics 10:R110.003871
74. D'Arcy P, Brnjic S, Olofsson MH et al (2011) Inhibition of proteasome deubiquitinating activity as a new cancer therapy. Nat. Med, Epub
75. Fehlker M, Wendler P, Lehmann A, Enenkel C (2004) Blm3 is part of nascent proteasomes and is involved in a late stage of nuclear proteasome assembly. EMBO Rep 4:959–63
76. Leggett DS, Hanna J, Borodovsky A et al (2002) Multiple associated proteins regulate proteasome structure and function. Mol Cell 10:495–507
77. Crosas B, Hanna J, Kirkpatrick DS et al (2006) Ubiquitin chains are remodeled at the proteasome by opposing ubiquitin ligase and deubiquitinating activities. Cell 127:1401–13
78. Ortolan TG, Tongaonkar P, Lambertson D et al (2000) The Rad23 DNA repair protein is a negative regulator of substrate-linked multi-ubiquitin chain assembly. Nat Cell Biol 2:601–8

79. Baird TD, Wek RC (2012) Eukaryotic initiation factor 2 phosphorylation and translational control in metabolism. Adv Nutr 3:307–321
80. Harding HP, Calfon M, Urano F, Novoa I, Ron D (2002) Transcriptional and translational control in the mammalian unfolded protein response. Annu Rev Cell Dev Biol 18:575–599
81. Zhu K, Dunner K Jr, McConkey DJ (2010) Proteasome inhibitors activate autophagy as a cytoprotective response in human prostate cancer cells. Oncogene 29:451–462
82. Trinh MA, Kaphzan H, Wek RC, Pierre P, Cavener DR, Klann E (2012) Brain-specific disruption of the eIF2T kinase PERK decreases ATF4 expression and impairs behavioral flexibility. Cell Rep 1:676–678
83. Hetz C, Chevet E, Harding HP (2013) Targeting the unfolded protein response in disease. Nat Rev Drug Discov 12:703–719

Chapter 10
Oxidative Stress and the Proteasome: Mechanisms and Therapeutic Relevance

Christa Manton and Joya Chandra

Abstract The proteasome is a key mediator of the oxidative environment in cells. Reactive oxygen species (ROS) are produced by normal cellular metabolic processes, and the proteasome can mediate ROS levels by degrading proteins that generate ROS and by controlling antioxidant turnover, as well as by clearing oxidatively damaged proteins from cells. The proteasome itself is also regulated by ROS, with certain subunits being susceptible to oxidative modification and damage, while other subunits are transcriptionally up-regulated as part of the antioxidant response. Proteasome inhibition has been shown to increase ROS in many cellular contexts, and this increase in ROS is often integral to cell death induction. Cells that have elevated basal levels of antioxidants, or that can mount a quick antioxidant response that often includes increasing proteasome subunit levels, can neutralize ROS and escape proteasome inhibitor-induced death. Many current studies are focused on overcoming this resistance by combining proteasome inhibitors with other ROS-generating agents, such as histone deacetylase inhibitors and certain kinase inhibitors, which can cause synergistic ROS induction and death.

Keywords Oxidative stress • Antioxidant • Proteasome • Bortezomib resistance • Nrf2 • Combination therapy

Abbreviations

AML	Acute myeloid leukemia
ARE	Antioxidant responsive element
ASK1	Apoptosis signal-related kinase 1
(-)-EGCG	(-)-Epigallocatechin gallate
GSH	Glutathione
GSSG	Glutathione disulfide

C. Manton • J. Chandra, Ph.D. (✉)
Department of Pediatrics Research, The University of Texas MD Anderson Cancer Center, 515 Holcombe Boulevard, Unit 0853, Houston, TX 77030, USA
e-mail: jchandra@mdanderson.org

Q.P. Dou (ed.), *Resistance to Proteasome Inhibitors in Cancer*, Resistance to Targeted Anti-Cancer Therapeutics, DOI 10.1007/978-3-319-06752-0_10

F_1	Ferritin
H_2O_2	Hydrogen peroxide
HDACi	Histone deacetylase inhibitor
HO^-	Hydroxyl radical
HO-1	Heme oxygenase-1
IκBα	NF-κB inhibitor α
IRE	Iron responsive element
IRP2	Iron regulatory protein 2
MEFs	Mouse embryonic fibroblasts
mTOR	Mammalian target of rapamycin
mTORC1	Mammalian target of rapamycin complex 1
NAC	*N*-acetyl cysteine
NF-κB	Nuclear factor-κB
Nox	NADPH oxidase
Nrf2	Nuclear factor-like 2
O_2^-	Superoxide
ROS	Reactive oxygen species
SOD	Superoxide dismutase
SOD2	Superoxide dismutase 2
TNF-α	Tumor necrosis factor-α
Trx	Thioredoxin

10.1 Introduction

Regulation of the cellular redox environment is one of the many functions of the proteasome. As the major guardian of cellular protein quality control, the proteasome plays a significant role in the cellular response to oxidative stress. In fact, the proteasome is key to multiple aspects of how cells are affected by and cope with increased oxidative stress. Turnover of proteins that contribute to generation of free radicals and turnover of antioxidant proteins are amongst the tasks conducted by the proteasome; therefore, degradation of these specific substrates can influence oxidative stress. In addition to regulating the redox environment, a primary function of the proteasome is dealing with the consequences of oxidative stress since oxidatively damaged proteins constitute a large portion of proteasomal substrates. Furthermore, the proteasome itself is susceptible to oxidative modifications and regulation since some proteasome components can be oxidized, while others are transcriptionally up-regulated in response to oxidative stress.

Given how integral the proteasome is in oxidative processes, it is logical that proteasome inhibition by bortezomib would alter the cellular oxidative environment in key ways that could be important for drug activity. For example, inhibition of the proteasome causes accumulation of reactive oxygen species (ROS)-generating proteins as well as the antioxidants that are classical proteasome substrates. This disrupts the redox balance in cells. At the same time, proteasome inhibition can

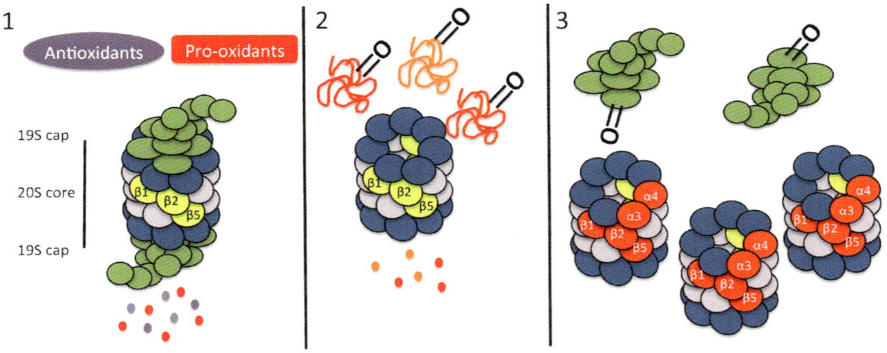

Fig. 10.1 The proteasome is involved in oxidative balance at multiple points. (*1*) The proteasome degrades many targets involved in redox balance, including antioxidants and ROS generating proteins. (*2*) The proteasome clears oxidized proteins from cells, preventing their toxic accumulation. (*3*) The proteasome is itself modified by oxidative stress, with cap components being oxidized, while other components are transcriptionally up-regulated (in *red*)

prevent degradation of oxidized proteins, causing their toxic accumulation within cells. Also, inhibition of proteasome catalytic activity by bortezomib may combine with ROS-induced damage to proteasome subunits to cause a further decrease in proteasome function. Additionally, ROS-induced transcriptional increases in proteasome subunits may be countered by the presence of bortezomib, which can prevent these newly produced subunits from functioning.

In a broad picture of cellular redox regulation, the proteasome appears at pivotal points as it functions to degrade oxidized proteins and key substrates that affect oxidative balance, and as it is modified and transcriptionally altered in response to ROS (Fig. 10.1). All of these roles can contribute to sensitivity to proteasome inhibitors by tipping the oxidative balance toward increased ROS and cellular damage that leads to cell death. Alternatively, some cells can circumvent the toxic effects of proteasome inhibitor-induced oxidative stress, leading to resistance to inhibitors such as bortezomib. This chapter will give examples of how the proteasome is a key regulator of the oxidative environment, and explore how alterations in cellular redox components can contribute to bortezomib resistance.

10.2 Proteasomal Regulation of Reactive Oxygen Species Formation

Oxidative stress refers to an imbalance in the ratio of pro- and antioxidants. Pro-oxidants arise from endogenous sources and include breakdown products of molecular oxygen that are natural by-products of respiration. The term ROS collectively describes derivatives of molecular oxygen that interact with biomolecules.

Types of ROS include superoxides (O_2^-), hydrogen peroxide (H_2O_2), and the hydroxyl radical (HO^-). ROS are produced as a natural part of cellular processes. Mitochondrial respiration is the root source of an estimated 90 % of intracellular ROS [1]. Molecular oxygen takes on electrons produced by complexes I and II in the mitochondrial electron transport chain, producing superoxide. Other ROS are then produced as superoxide is converted to hydrogen peroxide by superoxide dismutase (SOD). Hydrogen peroxide can be inactivated by several cellular antioxidants including thioredoxin-dependent peroxidases (peroxiredoxins) or glutathione peroxidases. Notably, if transition metals are present, they are capable of transferring electrons to hydrogen peroxide (the Fenton reaction) to produce the highly reactive hydroxyl radical. Despite its very short half-life, the hydroxyl radical is extremely toxic to cells. While all ROS are capable of causing cellular damage to DNA, lipids, and proteins, the hydroxyl radical is particularly damaging because it is the most reactive form of ROS.

The proteasome is a gatekeeper for this initial ROS formation through its ability to regulate the enzymes that inactivate ROS as well as proteins that regulate the intracellular iron pool. Several antioxidant proteins are elevated following proteasome inhibition, including SOD and catalase [2, 3]. More detailed studies have determined that several ROS eliminating enzymes, such as catalase and peroxiredoxin III, undergo ubiquitin-dependent proteasomal degradation [4, 5].

The proteasome also controls levels of ferritin, an intracellular iron storage protein that stores iron in an inactive state, preventing it from participating in reactions such as the Fenton reaction to form the damaging hydroxyl radical. Ferritin is a proteasome substrate, and has been shown to be degraded if oxidatively damaged [6]. Ferritin was also degraded by the proteasome after tumor necrosis factor treatment in a prostate cancer cell line. This degradation of ferritin increased the amount of reactive iron in cells, which could facilitate ROS formation [7].

Another element of proteasome control of the iron pool involves iron regulatory protein 2 (IRP2), an iron-sensing protein that binds to iron responsive elements (IREs) in RNA to regulate iron metabolism. IRP2 is oxidized and ubiquitinated, followed by proteasomal degradation, in iron replete cells [8–10]. Mice lacking IRP2 were found to accumulate iron in neurons and oligodendrocytes, and showed characteristics of neurodegenerative disease [11]. Control of ferritin and IRP2 protein levels makes the proteasome a key player in the regulation of cellular free iron levels and, by extension, ROS formation by the Fenton reaction.

An additional layer of control of the iron pool is through up-regulation of the ferritin heavy chain by nuclear factor-κB (NF-κB) [12]. NF-κB suppresses tumor necrosis factor-α (TNF-α)-induced ROS accumulation, abrogating TNF-α initiated cell death [13]. This occurs through transcriptional up-regulation of the ferritin heavy chain by NF-κB, which then sequesters iron and prevents ROS production (Fig. 10.2) [12]. This pathway is also controlled by the proteasome, because NF-κB inhibitor alpha (IκBα) is a key proteasome substrate that must be degraded to allow for NF-κB stabilization and ROS suppression [14]. Proteasome inhibition leads to IκBα stabilization and NF-κB inhibition, which can lead to increased ROS after certain stimuli due to failure to induce the ferritin heavy chain [12, 14, 15]. NF-κB also increases transcription of other target genes that attenuate oxidative stress, such

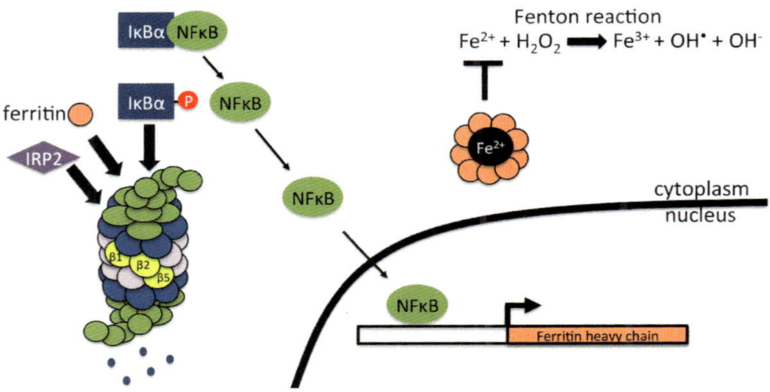

Fig. 10.2 Proteasome regulation of NF-κB lowers free iron, and therefore ROS generation. Degradation of the IκBα by the proteasome leads to NF-κB activation. NF-κB transcriptionally up-regulates ferritin heavy chain, which sequesters iron in cells [12, 14]. Lower levels of available iron can lead to less hydroxyl radical generation by the Fenton reaction. The proteasome also regulates iron levels by degrading its substrates ferritin and IRP2 [6, 8–10]

as Cu/Zn SOD [12, 16]. NF-κB is up-regulated in response to oxidative stress, though this regulation appears to be dependent on the cell type [17–19]. The ability of proteasome inhibitors to stabilize IκBα, and thereby cause NF-κB suppression, has been listed as a key way these inhibitors cause cell death [20, 21]. This pathway is of additional interest due to the fact that several types of chemotherapy and radiation cause an increase in NF-κB, which is suppressed by the addition of a proteasome inhibitor, leading to sensitization of cancer cells to these treatments [21–23]. Suppression of NF-κB activity by proteasome inhibitors is one way in which these drugs may prevent an antioxidant response by reducing levels of genes such as ferritin and Cu/Zn SOD.

Other cellular sources of ROS besides the mitochondria include dehydrogenases located in the mitochondrial membrane as well as cellular oxidases such as NADPH oxidase (Nox) complexes [24, 25]. Rac1, a small G protein that induces Nox activation, is a proteasome substrate, as is the Nox component p22phox. Degradation of either of these proteins reduces Nox activity and, therefore, lowers superoxide production [26, 27]. Though these are minor sources of ROS compared to the mitochondria, they are notable because even a small increase in cellular ROS can lead to formation of highly reactive hydroxyl radicals and therefore damage.

10.3 Proteasome Degradation of Oxidized Proteins

ROS can oxidatively damage proteins, which must then be turned over within cells; this is a major housekeeping function of the proteasome. Tracking of protein carbonyl groups, which indicate oxidative damage, in fibroblasts exposed to hydrogen peroxide revealed that cells were able to turn over these damaged proteins.

However, this ability was blocked by the proteasome inhibitor lactacystin, indicating that the proteasome is key to degradation of oxidized proteins [28]. Further studies showed that low levels of oxidation can increase susceptibility of proteins to proteasome degradation [29, 30]. Oxidation likely does this through an increase in surface hydrophobicity of the proteins, as well as a loss of secondary protein structure [29, 31–33]. Specific examination of calmodulin that was oxidized by exposure to hydrogen peroxide showed that there was a clear correlation between a loss of secondary protein structure caused by oxidation and increased proteasome degradation [29].

Oxidation status of a protein substrate can influence the specific recognition and degradation process by the proteasome. The proteasome consists of a barrel-shaped, 20S core component that contains the catalytic activities involved in protein breakdown. This core can be attached to several different regulatory subunits that are interchangeable, with the standard regulatory component being the 19S cap. Alteration of protein properties by oxidation may make them more susceptible to degradation by the 20S catalytic core of the proteasome without a need for the 19S cap subunits. 19S caps are important for recognizing ubiquitinated proteins and unwinding them so they can be fed into the 20S core. However, proteins that have a loss of secondary structure and a gain of surface hydrophobic regions would not need to be unwound further to be degraded by the 20S core. Indeed, studies indicate that the proteasome can often degrade oxidized proteins in a ubiquitin and ATP-independent manner, indicating a large role for the 20S core, but not the 19S caps, in degradation of oxidized proteins [31, 33–35]. Cells that have impaired ubiquitin conjugating ability and, therefore, a decrease in protein ubiquitination were still able to degrade oxidized proteins at nearly normal rates [33].

Regardless of the pathway for how proteins are oxidized, if these damaged proteins are allowed to accumulate, they can form aggresomes; large structures of cross-linked proteins. The proteasome is largely responsible for clearing oxidized proteins, preventing aggregate formation (Fig. 10.3) [36, 37]. There is evidence that aggresomes can be degraded by either the proteasome or autophagy. It seems likely that, in some circumstances, autophagy can be up-regulated as a cytoprotective response following proteasome inhibition to clear the resulting protein aggregates. While inhibition of either the proteasome or autophagy alone does not cause a strong increase in aggresomes, dual inhibition of both pathways leads to aggresome formation [38]. Aggresome formation can be toxic to cells, and is associated with several neurodegenerative diseases as well as aging [30]. Dual inhibition of the proteasome and autophagy not only led to a visible increase in aggregates but also caused a significant increase in cell death [38].

Failure of proteasomes to clear these aggresomes may lead to a positive feedback loop whereby aggresomes cause further inhibition of the ubiquitin proteasome system. A study was conducted of two proteins prone to aggregation, a fragment of the huntingtin protein and the cystic fibrosis transmembrane conductance regulator. When these proteins were expressed, they formed aggregates and also caused accumulation of a GFP-tagged degron that was normally degraded by the proteasome. This suggests that the aggregates themselves somehow decrease proteasome-mediated protein degradation [39].

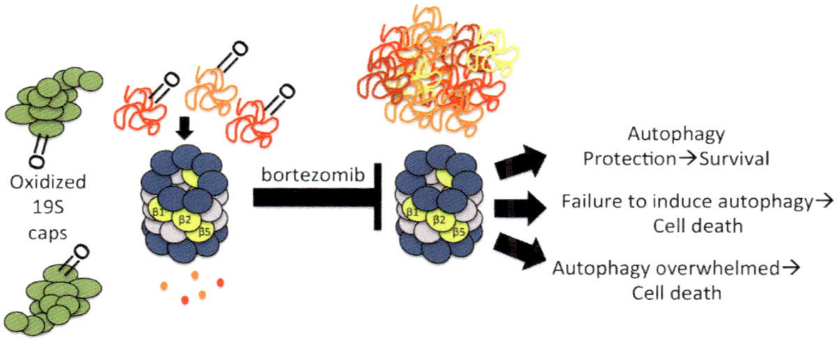

Fig. 10.3 Degradation of oxidized proteins by the proteasome. Oxidized proteins can be degraded by the proteasome, perhaps more by 20S cores than by intact 26S complexes, as subunits in 19S caps tend to be sensitive to oxidation themselves [31, 33–35]. If the proteasome is inhibited, as by bortezomib, oxidized proteins accumulate and form cross-linked structures termed aggresomes that can be toxic to cells [36, 37]. In some cases, up-regulation of autophagy may facilitate degradation of oxidized proteins and lead to cell survival. However, in some cases autophagy is not induced, or autophagy is unable to cope with the increased protein load and is overwhelmed, leading to cell death

10.4 Regulation of the Proteasome by Antioxidant Status

In addition to participating in the generation of ROS, the proteasome itself can be modified by redox status. The proteasome consists of a barrel-shaped 20S catalytic core that includes four heptameric rings. Beta subunits make up the two inner rings and contain the catalytic sites of the proteasome, while the alpha subunits that form the two outer rings have a role in regulating access to the catalytic sites. Multiple regulator complexes can bind to the 20S core. The standard proteasome, or 26S proteasome, occurs when the 19S cap complexes bind to the 20S core. These complexes recognize ubiquitinated substrates and begin unfolding them so they can be fed into the core of the proteasome. The 19S complex is just one type of cap, however, and other regulators such as PA28α/β or PA28γ can also bind to the 20S core. In addition to alternative cap complexes, there is also a different set of catalytic subunits, known as immunoproteasome (i-proteasome) subunits, that are inducible and can replace the standard catalytic subunits. The ways in which these various proteasome components are affected by changes in the oxidative environment reveals important information about how proteasome function is impacted by oxidative stress.

An oxidative cellular environment can directly impact proteasome function via posttranslational modifications of subunits. Also, specific oxidative stimuli have been found to transcriptionally up-regulate expression of other subunits through stimulation of specific transcription factors.

10.5 Oxidative Modification of Proteasome Subunits

Supporting the importance of the 20S core over the 19S caps in the degradation of oxidized proteins, studies show that ATPase subunits within the 19S caps are vulnerable to oxidative damage [34, 35]. ROS-induced decreases in the catalytic activity of the proteasome have also been noted [35, 40–42]. A comparison of the 26S and 20S proteasomes found that 26S complexes were more sensitive to oxidative inactivation than 20S complexes, further supporting a role for the 20S proteasome or alternative proteasome forms in degradation of oxidized proteins [35, 43]. Heat shock proteins, specifically hsp90 and HDJ40 (an hsp40 family member), were found to protect the proteasome from oxidative damage [40–42].

Alternative forms of the proteasome may also contribute to degradation of oxidized proteins. In particular, the immunoproteasome, which consists of the alternative catalytic subunits LMP2, LMP7, and MECL-1, has been postulated to help in this capacity. LMP2 and LMP7 protein levels increase following hydrogen peroxide treatment [43]. Also, interferon-γ induces expression of immunoproteasome subunits, and also increases oxidative stress by an increase in nitric oxide synthase [44]. The immunoproteasome was found to be key to degrading the oxidized proteins that resulted from this increased stress [45].

10.6 Regulation of the Proteasome by the Antioxidant Response

The need to quickly neutralize ROS and repair oxidative damage is evidenced by the robust antioxidant defense system in cells. Central to the antioxidant system is glutathione (GSH), which acts as a reducing agent to maintain a proper redox environment. The balance between reduced GSH and its oxidized form, glutathione disulfide (GSSG), is tightly controlled by the enzyme glutathione reductase, which functions to ensure the majority of glutathione is in the reduced form [46, 47]. In addition to the GSH regulatory network of enzymes, the antioxidant thioredoxin (Trx), its isoforms, and reductase family members complement the function of GSH in maintaining a reduced cellular environment.

Pools of proteins such as GSH and Trx are maintained in a reduced state, allowing for quick neutralization of ROS and repair of oxidative damage in cells. However, in some cases this defense system can be overwhelmed. This usually occurs due to a toxic insult to cells, which includes certain chemotherapy drugs and radiation. When the production of ROS and resulting damage outweighs the ability of the antioxidants to protect cells, this is called oxidative stress. The result of oxidative stress in cells is complex and highly dependent on the levels of pro- and antioxidants in various cell types. Furthermore, cell fates as diverse as life versus death are promoted by ROS, the molecular details of which are only now being fully understood.

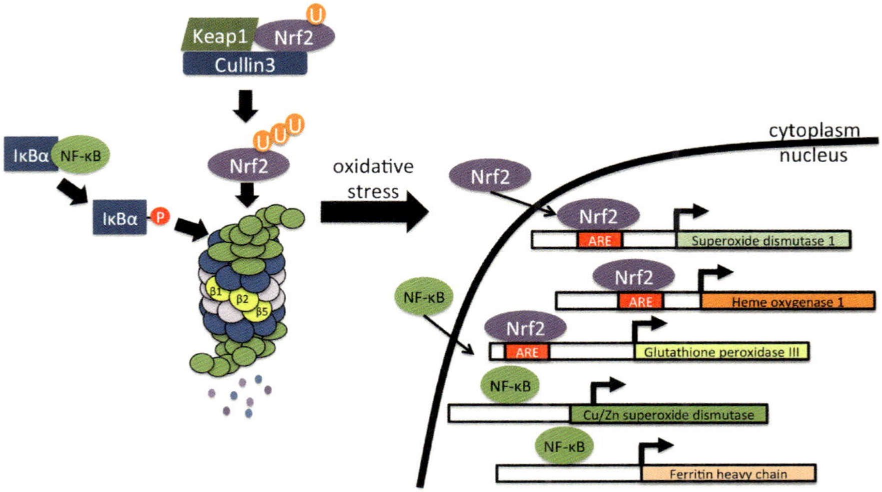

Fig. 10.4 Proteasome modulation of the antioxidant response through Nrf2 and NF-κB. In the absence of oxidative stress, Nrf2 is bound to Keap1, and is sent to the proteasome to be degraded. The proteasome also degrades IκBα, an inhibitor of NF-κB. Under conditions of oxidative stress, both NF-κB and Nrf2 activity is increased, leading to translocation of these transcription factors to the nucleus. Nrf2 binds to antioxidant response elements (AREs) to transcriptionally up-regulate genes to attenuate oxidative damage, while NF-κB also up-regulates genes involved in the antioxidant response [12, 16, 46, 52]

Cells must quickly up-regulate antioxidant genes in response to oxidative stress. One of the main mechanisms by which this is accomplished is through translocation of the transcription factor nuclear factor-like 2 (Nrf2) to the nucleus, where it binds to antioxidant responsive elements (AREs) in the promoters of genes that are involved in helping cells combat increased ROS levels (Fig. 10.4). When ROS levels are low, Nrf2 is sequestered in the cytoplasm bound to Keap1, which also interacts with the E3 ligase Cullin3 to send Nrf2 for proteasomal degradation [48–51]. Elevated ROS levels cause dissociation of Nrf2 from Keap1, allowing it to enter the nucleus and bind its target genes [46, 52].

A key target of Nrf2 is the proteasome catalytic subunit PSMB5, which has 2 tandem AREs in its promoter [48, 52]. This confirms the importance of the proteasome in the antioxidant response system as a key line of defense in protecting cells from oxidative damage. AREs have also been identified in the promoters of several other 20S catalytic core components, as well as in one of the immunoproteasome catalytic subunits (Fig. 10.5) [52]. Additionally, the proteasome regulator PA28α/β is induced by oxidative stress in an Nrf2-dependent manner [52].

In mouse embryonic fibroblasts (MEFs), hydrogen peroxide induced an increase in proteasome activity, which was blocked by silencing of Nrf2. The importance of the proteasome in adaptation to oxidative stress was also shown in a system in which MEFs were pretreated with a low dose (1 μM) of hydrogen peroxide, which

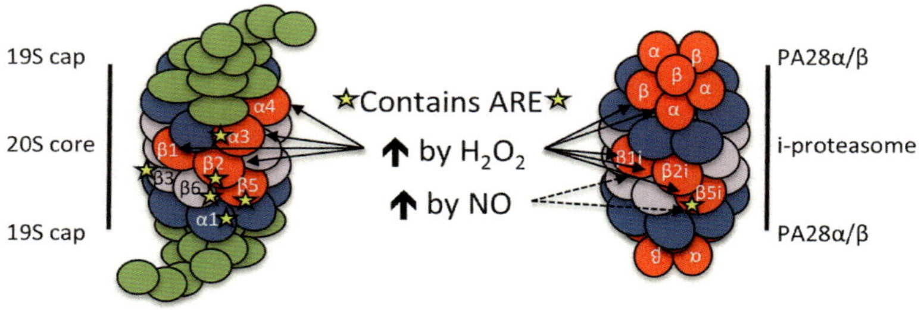

Fig. 10.5 Proteasome subunits regulated by oxidative stress. Many proteasome subunits, such as α3, α4, β1, β2, β5, β1i, β2i, β5i, and the PA28α/β regulatory subunits, have been shown to be up-regulated in response to various oxidative stress stimuli. These subunits are shown in *red*. The *starred* subunits, α1, α3, β2, β3, β5, β6, and β5i, have been reported to contain AREs in their promoters [48, 52]

causes gene expression changes that allow cells to adapt to survive a higher dose (1 mM). However, when either the 20S proteasome subunit PSMB1 or the immunoproteasome subunit LMP2 were silenced, it prevented this adaptation from occurring, as evidenced by lower cell counts after the higher dose, thereby tying expression of these two subunits (one from the classical proteasome and one from the immunoproteasome) to protection from ROS-induced cell death [52].

Other immunoproteasome subunits are also up-regulated after oxidative stress in a manner that appears to be independent of Nrf2, indicating that there are yet other mechanisms at play in proteasome regulation in response to oxidative stress [52]. When put together, current evidence strongly supports a key role for the proteasome as a regulator of the antioxidant response system.

10.7 Effect of Proteasome Inhibition on ROS

Proteasome inhibition by bortezomib has been shown to increase levels of cellular ROS in many cancer types, including the two cancers for which bortezomib is FDA-approved: multiple myeloma [53] and mantle cell lymphoma [54]. Proteasome inhibitors also induce ROS in some solid tumors, including lung cancer [55], colon cancer [56], endometrial cancer [57], and head and neck squamous cell carcinoma [58]. These ROS increases have two main functions: induction of cell death, primarily apoptosis, in response to higher levels and changes in cellular growth signaling upon exposure to lower levels of ROS.

10.8 ROS and Cell Death

The role of ROS in proteasome inhibitor-induced cell death is well documented. Key studies show that ROS generation occurs upstream of apoptosis activation. In mantle cell lymphoma, a pan-caspase inhibitor was capable of blocking apoptosis, but not ROS generation. However, treatment with the antioxidants glutathione-reduced ethyl ester or *N*-acetyl cysteine (NAC) prevented both ROS formation and apoptosis in cells treated with bortezomib [54].

Other studies have questioned these findings, with one report showing that NAC and glutathione did not protect two lung cancer cell lines from bortezomib-induced death [59]. One explanation for this is a cell specific effect, where some cells are more susceptible to ROS increases than others, perhaps due to intrinsic differences in antioxidant systems or relative levels of pro- versus anti-apoptotic Bcl-2 family members that regulate mitochondrial membrane permeability.

In systems where proteasome inhibitors do induce ROS, there is evidence that it is integral to the mechanism of cell death. Multiple studies show that treatment with antioxidants blunts the effect of bortezomib, while combinations that lead to further increases in ROS cause synergistic cell death with bortezomib [53, 56, 57]. In lung cancer cells, the superoxide scavenger Tiron protected against bortezomib-induced increases in ROS and ultimately PARP cleavage and cell death [55].

Mitochondrial dysfunction is key to the production of ROS after bortezomib treatment. Inhibitors of the mitochondrial electron transport chain complexes I and II prevented ROS increases after bortezomib treatment as well as the loss of mitochondrial membrane potential and cytochrome C release that usually follows bortezomib treatment [55]. This brings to light an important mechanism by which bortezomib induces ROS-dependent apoptosis through mitochondrial dysfunction leading to activation of the intrinsic pathway of apoptosis.

This happens in two main steps. First, cardiolipin, which binds cytochrome C inside the mitochondria, can be oxidized facilitating cytochrome C release from mitochondria [60]. Secondly, oxidative stress triggers the mitochondrial permeability transition, which allows release of multiple pro-apoptotic mitochondrial proteins, including cytochrome C, into the cytoplasm [61]. Cytochrome C then goes on to form the apoptosome together with Apaf-1, leading to caspase 9 activation and apoptosis [62].

Other forms of cell death that are regulated by ROS likely play roles in proteasome inhibitor-mediated cell death. Proteasome inhibition can induce autophagy as a cytoprotective mechanism to degrade proteins and rescue cells from nutrient starvation [38]. However, autophagy can pass a tipping point and also lead to cell death. A primary regulator of autophagy, mammalian target of rapamycin (mTOR), which inhibits autophagy induction, can be inhibited by oxidative modification, likely leading to autophagy induction in the presence of oxidative stress [63, 64]. Supporting this, inhibition of mitochondrial electron transport chain complexes I or II in transformed cells induces ROS and also induces autophagy and cell death. Mitigation of ROS levels by the ROS scavenger Tiron or by overexpression of superoxide dismutase 2 (SOD2) blunts autophagy induction and also reduces cell death [65]. This indicates an important ROS-regulated role of autophagy, though the exact balance of factors that lead to cytoprotective autophagy versus lethal autophagy is likely cell context specific.

Another cell death pathway with implicated ROS involvement is programmed necrosis, referred to as necroptosis. The necroptosis pathway involves death dependent on RIP1 kinase and is characterized by rapid loss of mitochondrial membrane potential and ROS accumulation [66, 67]. Interestingly, NF-κB protects cells from necroptosis, possibly in a role that involves ROS attenuation as described earlier in this chapter [68]. Since proteasome inhibitors prevent NF-κB activation, it is likely that they also facilitate necroptosis in response to stress that activates RIP1 kinase.

10.9 ROS Effects on Cell Signaling

While the role of ROS in apoptosis is more clearly defined, recent research is pointing to an important role of ROS in promoting cellular signaling. A key difference between these two outcomes appears to be dose, with higher levels of ROS leading to cell death and lower levels of ROS effecting signaling pathways. In particular, oxidative modification of several key proteins has been shown to regulate their function. Since the proteasome is a key mediator of the oxidative environment, the function of the proteasome is likely linked to the regulation of these pathways. Several of the targets identified so far are part of pathways that are frequently deregulated in cancer.

For example, multiple protein tyrosine phosphatases are inactivated by oxidation [69–72]. This corresponds with the observation of increased receptor tyrosine kinase phosphorylation after ROS exposure [73]. This inactivation of phosphatases could allow for unchecked activity of many kinases that signal for cell growth and proliferation.

One notable phosphatase that is inactive after oxidation is the tumor suppressor PTEN [74–77]. PTEN mutations are frequently reported in cancer, and oxidation provides a mutation-independent way for cells to gain sustained activation of PI3K/Akt growth signaling.

Other proteins are regulated by their interaction with redox-sensitive proteins. The reduced form of the antioxidant Trx interacts with apoptosis signal-related kinase 1 (ASK1), a member of the mitogen-activated protein kinase signaling pathway, preventing its activation [78]. When Trx becomes oxidized, it dissociates from ASK1, allowing it to activate downstream pathways including JNK/p38 and apoptosis [79]. ASK1 has also been shown to have a role in other cellular processes such as differentiation [80]. The ASK1 model demonstrates that effects on signaling by proteasome inhibitor-induced ROS can converge with cell death pathways, but other nontoxic cellular end points can also be achieved.

10.10 Bortezomib Resistance and Oxidative Stress

Despite initial success of bortezomib for cancer therapy, a few mechanisms of resistance have come to light. Some cell types may be intrinsically resistant to proteasome inhibition due to factors such as increased basal levels of antioxidant response factors [81]. Cells may also acquire resistance to bortezomib treatment. The proteasome itself is often changed in response to proteasome inhibitor treatment, with increased proteasome subunit expression and point mutations to the catalytic subunit β5 being associated with resistance [82–85]. Sometimes this resistance is bortezomib-specific, which is apparent when some bortezomib resistant cells are still sensitive to other unique proteasome inhibitors, such as the second-generation proteasome inhibitors marizomib and carfilzomib [86, 87]. Targeting different proteasome components, such as the immunoproteasome (which is now possible through compounds poised for clinical trials), can also overcome resistance in some cell types [88].

Proteasome inhibition also up-regulates many genes that have the potential to lead to resistance. For example, REDD1, a negative regulator of the mammalian target of rapamycin complex 1 (mTORC1), is up-regulated following bortezomib and dexamethasone combination treatment in myeloma cells. Knockdown of REDD1 increases bortezomib sensitivity [89]. Since mTOR has an important role in autophagy suppression, this could be a mechanism by which proteasome inhibition triggers a protective autophagy response. Knockdown of REDD1 would then abrogate that response.

The dependence of proteasome inhibitors on ROS for cell death may also meet resistance in cells. This can occur by up-regulation of antioxidants, an intrinsically higher level of antioxidant response, or up-regulation of the proteasome itself by oxidative stress (Fig. 10.6).

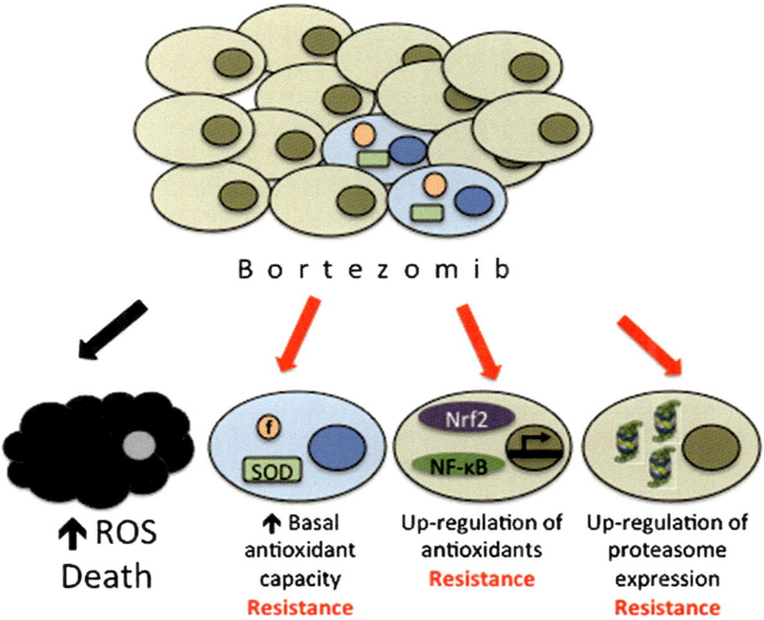

Fig. 10.6 Mechanisms of bortezomib resistance mediated by the antioxidant response. When treated with bortezomib, increased ROS levels in many cancer cells cause death. However, some cells are resistant to bortezomib through (1) higher basal antioxidant capacity, (2) their ability to up-regulate antioxidants, or (3) their capacity to up-regulate the proteasome itself

10.11 Resistance to Proteasome Inhibitors Through Antioxidant Up-regulation

Proteasome inhibition prevents degradation of Nrf2, which can then induce an antioxidant response may sufficiently neutralize ROS to prevent cell death [51]. In a study that examined gene expression changes following treatment of HUVEC cells with toxic versus nontoxic doses of the proteasome inhibitor MG132, researchers found that the nontoxic doses specifically up-regulated a range of antioxidant genes including SOD, *heme oxygenase-1* (*HO-1*), *glutathione peroxidase-3*, *and multiple glutathione S-transferases* [90]. The implication of this study is that the up-regulation of these antioxidants following lower levels of proteasome inhibition may have prevented the proteasome inhibitor from achieving a toxic effect. Due to the complexity of clinical situations, it is logical that this same situation may occur in patients where some cancer cells do not reach the threshold dose needed for toxicity, and instead manage to escape death due to an increased antioxidant response.

Another study showed up-regulation of antioxidant proteins such as SOD and HO-1 after treatment with the proteasome inhibitor MG132. Following this up-regulation, cardiomyocytes were protected from hydrogen peroxide-induced death. Cardiomyocytes lacking Nrf2 were unable to induce these antioxidants, and MG132 pretreatment no longer protected the cells from hydrogen peroxide [91]. This indicates that a certain, sublethal degree of proteasome inhibition can trigger an antioxidant response, making the cells more capable of dealing with future ROS increases, such as that induced by a second dose of proteasome inhibitor. This study emphasizes the impact that an Nrf2-dependent antioxidant response may have, both in protection of normal cells from proteasome inhibitor treatment and possibly in protection of cancer cells. Proteasome inhibitor-induced ROS increases may be a main cause of resulting cell death, but at the same time cells can counter this increased ROS with an antioxidant response. If the proteasome inhibitor is unable to cause a strong enough increase in ROS, or if cells are capable of a robust antioxidant response, cellular antioxidant defenses can protect the cells from death.

10.12 Antioxidant Capacity and Resistance to Bortezomib

As was briefly mentioned earlier, it appears that bortezomib-induced ROS increases may be cell specific. One factor that can make a certain cell line sensitive while another is more resistant to bortezomib is the cellular capacity to quickly neutralize ROS produced by the treatment. In fact, Nrf2 (previously mentioned as a key transcriptional inducer of the antioxidant response) has been found to be basally elevated in some types of cancer [81, 92]. In one study, acute myeloid leukemia (AML) cell lines were found to be more resistant to bortezomib than normal myeloid cells. Investigation of this difference led to the revelation that the resistant cells had higher basal levels of nuclear Nrf2. After bortezomib treatment, the AML cells quickly translocated the antioxidant transcriptional repressor Bach1 to the cytoplasm, and the already-present levels of Nrf2 were able to lead to a quick antioxidant response and detoxify the ROS in cells [81]. Knockdown of Nrf2 sensitized the AML cells to bortezomib treatment. This suggests that a high basal level of antioxidant response pathway components can, in some cases, predict resistance to bortezomib.

Another study in mantle cell lymphoma described the somewhat counterintuitive result that cell lines that had a great increase in oxidative stress responsive genes after bortezomib treatment were actually the most sensitive lines when cell death was measured. Further investigation of this phenomenon revealed that though bortezomib-resistant cells did not have large increases in these oxidant responsive genes, they did have higher baseline levels of antioxidant gene expression prior to treatment [93]. All together, these findings suggest that cells can induce an antioxidant response to bortezomib, but that it may be a case of "too little too late" unless elevated basal levels of proteins such as Nrf2 are already in place to allow for an extraordinarily quick antioxidant response.

Increased Nrf2 is just one of several ways the antioxidant system can be deregulated in cancer. Many cancers also overexpress Bcl-2, which has been shown to increase cellular GSH levels [94, 95]. High Bcl-2 levels are associated with resistance to radiation-induced apoptosis, and depletion of cellular thiols (including GSH) sensitized cells to the radiation [96]. This demonstrates another way in which elevation of antioxidants can cause resistance to therapy that induces ROS as part of its mechanism.

10.13 Resistance by Antioxidant Response Up-regulation of the Proteasome

Increased proteasome subunit expression following proteasome inhibitor treatment is a frequently cited mechanism of resistance [85, 93]. The level of proteasome expression has been tightly correlated with sensitivity to proteasome inhibitors. One study found an inverse correlation between proteasome activity and proteasome inhibitor sensitivity in multiple myeloma cells. In other words, cells with the lowest level of proteasome activity were generally most sensitive to proteasome inhibitors [97]. This supports the idea that any increase in proteasome protein levels could make cells more resistant to proteasome inhibitors.

In another model of bortezomib resistance, THP1 monocytic/macrophage cells were grown in the presence of increasing concentrations of bortezomib to develop a resistant line. The study found that levels of the proteasome subunit β5 were increased up to 60-fold in resistant cells versus the normal cells [85].

As briefly outlined previously, several proteasome subunits, such as the β5 catalytic subunit, contain AREs in their promoters. This allows them to be up-regulated as part of the antioxidant response by Nrf2 binding to their promoters. Abrogating this increased expression, perhaps by inhibiting Nrf2 function, could prove beneficial to proteasome inhibitor therapy.

10.14 Overcoming Resistance: Combinations That Amplify ROS

Bortezomib-induced increases in ROS have been shown to be capable of causing cell death. In some cases, however, an antioxidant response can attenuate the ability of bortezomib to achieve the level of ROS necessary to push cancer cells over the edge into cell death. Several other therapeutic agents, many of which are already utilized clinically, have also been shown to increase ROS. Studies are now finding that combining bortezomib with another agent that also amplifies ROS can lead to a synergistic effect on cell death and more promising clinical outcomes (Fig. 10.7). Specifically, combinations with histone deacetylase inhibitors (HDACi) and kinase inhibitors such as adaphostin have been successful and are now being tested in the clinic.

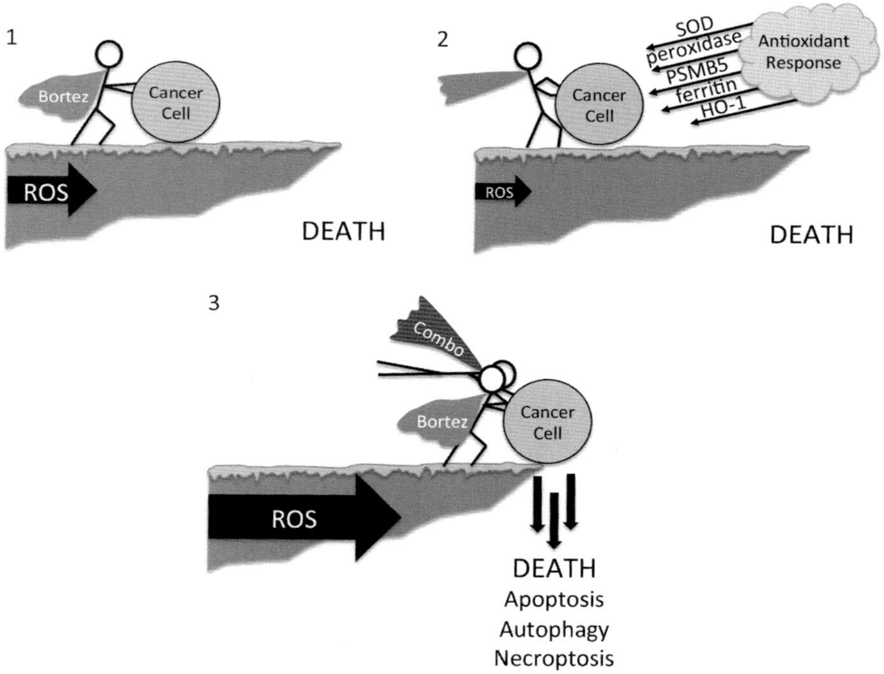

Fig. 10.7 Combination therapy overcomes resistance due to the antioxidant response. (*1*) Bortezomib increases ROS in cancer cells, pushing them toward the "cliff" of cell death. (*2*) Up-regulation of antioxidants can eliminate ROS, reducing the ability of bortezomib to cause death. (*3*) Combination treatments amplify ROS too much for an antioxidant response, pushing cells off the "cliff" of death. Modes of cell death induced by combinations include apoptosis, autophagy, and potentially necroptosis

10.15 Overcoming Resistance: Combination with Histone Deacetylase Inhibitors

HDACi are a class of agents that have been developed to impact epigenetic alterations that occur in cancer cells. HDACi cause an overall increase in acetylation of both histone and nonhistone proteins. Several HDACi have been developed and are in differing stages of clinical development, with the HDACi vorinostat being FDA-approved for the treatment of cutaneous T-cell lymphoma [98].

Several in vitro studies have shown a synergistic effect of the combination of proteasome inhibitors plus HDACi on both ROS production and cell death in several cancer cell types including multiple myeloma [53, 99], acute lymphoblastic leukemia [100], Bcr/Abl+ leukemia [101], and mantle cell lymphoma [102]. In these studies, the synergistic effect was blocked by treatment with NAC [99–102]. The combination of bortezomib and vorinostat also reduced tumor size in a mouse xenograft model of multiple myeloma [103]. The cell death in these studies was marked by increased cleavage of multiple caspases and PARP cleavage, as well as mitochondrial dysfunction [53, 99–102].

Because of these promising results, the combination of bortezomib plus vorinostat has been utilized in multiple clinical trials. Completed trials of this combination in multiple myeloma have been especially promising, and are now in a phase III investigation [104]. The combination also entered into phase II clinical trials for the treatment of several other types of cancer, including AML, mantle cell lymphoma, diffuse large B-cell lymphoma, soft tissue sarcoma, glioblastoma, non-small cell lung cancer, and acute lymphoblastic leukemia (clinicaltrials.gov). Panobinostat, another HDACi that has been shown to be more potent than vorinostat in many cases, is also in clinical trials in combination with bortezomib for multiple myeloma treatment [105, 106] (clinicaltrials.gov).

10.16 Overcoming Resistance: Combination with Kinase Inhibitors

The combination of proteasome inhibitors with kinase inhibitors that are already in clinical development has been quite promising. Sorafenib, a multikinase inhibitor that mainly targets the Raf family, causes synergistic cell death in combination with bortezomib in a broad variety of cancer cell types [107]. ROS may play a role, as other studies have indicated that sorafenib acts in a ROS-dependent manner to cause cell death in hepatocellular carcinoma [108].

Another combination under study is bortezomib with herceptin, an inhibitor of the Her2 receptor tyrosine kinase that has been quite effective in Her2+ breast cancer. Low doses of bortezomib augment the effect of herceptin in Her2+ breast cancer cells, allowing lower doses to be used to achieve a potent anticancer effect in cell lines [109]. Notably, herceptin has also been shown to increase levels of ROS in some cell types [110]. Though the increased ROS effects caused by herceptin can cause cardiotoxicity, refinement of dosing and combination therapy may allow clinicians to maximize the antitumor effect while minimizing negative side effects.

ROS also plays a role in the combination of proteasome inhibition plus the tyrosine kinase inhibitor adaphostin. Though it was originally developed as a Bcr/Abl inhibitor, adaphostin has been shown to have antitumor effects in lines that are not Bcr/Abl+, indicating that it has broader activity [111]. In fact, adaphostin has been shown to increase levels of ROS in leukemia cells and cause cell death. The ROS were tightly linked to the cell death as NAC attenuated the death, while buthionine sulfoximine, which inhibits GSH synthesis, increased the effect [112].

A preliminary study of the combination of adaphostin with the proteasome inhibitor MG-132 in leukemia cell lines and patient samples showed promising increased effects on ROS levels, cytochrome C release from the mitochondria, caspase activation, and ultimately cell death [113].

10.17 Conclusions

The balance of oxidants and antioxidants in cells helps to determine what proteasome subunits are produced and active within cells through both transcriptional and posttranslational controls. The proteasome is then able to regulate redox balance in cells through degradation of oxidized proteins as well as key substrates such as antioxidants, iron regulatory proteins, and autophagy regulators.

This complex relationship leads to a disruption of balance following proteasome inhibition, and increased levels of ROS are seen in many types of cells treated with bortezomib. This increase in ROS has been implicated in the ability of proteasome inhibitors to cause cell death, and attenuation of ROS with agents such as NAC often protects cancer cells from bortezomib-induced cell death.

There are also dietary antioxidants that have been shown to antagonize bortezomib. Vitamin C and (-)-epigallocatechin gallate (EGCG), a component of green tea, have both been shown to impede boronic acid inhibitors, including bortezomib, through a direct interaction that diminishes the proteasome inhibitor's ability to cause reduced proteasome activity [59, 114–116]. Though these agents act by directly inactivating bortezomib, not necessarily through their antioxidant functions, this does highlight an important consideration when developing a strategy that optimizes the efficacy of bortezomib. In one mouse study, researchers showed that normal dietary consumption of Vitamin C and EGCG was not sufficient to blunt the antiprostate cancer effect of bortezomib [117]. There is an additional layer to this story, as EGCG is one of several plant polyphenols, including such compounds as genistein, curcumin, and tannic acid, that can actually cause proteasome inhibition [118]. The proteasome inhibitory activity of these agents has been shown to act as a sensitizer to overcome resistance to chemotherapy in a variety of tumor types. Additional careful studies that examine the effect of these agents on bortezomib and proteasome activity in human patients are necessary to determine the clinically relevant effects of these interactions between dietary antioxidants, the proteasome, and therapeutics.

Cancer cells can also combat proteasome inhibitor-mediated cell death through several mechanisms, including having increased basal antioxidant levels, as well as inducing an antioxidant response, including production of more proteasome subunits, upon oxidative stress stimulation. This may be one explanation for why bortezomib is sometimes not very effective as a single agent, particularly in solid tumors [119–121]. In particular, a study of advanced renal cell carcinoma found that a subset of patients did seem to have a response, and highlighted the need for molecular profiling to preselect a patient population most likely to respond [121]. Future studies will likely determine whether examination of components of oxidative stress pathways could be part of the solution for predicting patient response. In addition to aiding in the selection of patient populations, the realization that cancer cells can avoid cell death by regulating the redox state has led to several new strategies that involve drug combinations that further amplify ROS levels, leading to a synergistic increase in cell death.

This is the first step toward utilizing our knowledge of oxidative stress for the more effective treatment of cancer. This information could be put to other uses as well. For example, patient sensitivity to an agent such as bortezomib could be predicted by screening patient basal antioxidant capacity by looking at levels of Nrf2. This would allow for selection of patients who would most benefit from bortezomib treatment.

There are other applications for this information, as well. For instance, drugs that more specifically target antioxidant response components could be used to amplify the effects of bortezomib. Additionally, information about how the antioxidant response can lead to up-regulation of specific proteasome subunits gives information about how repeated doses with bortezomib, or perhaps co-treatment with inhibitors that target up-regulated i-proteasome subunits, can lead to a more sustained inhibition of the proteasome and more effective therapy. Current efforts to alter the redox status of cells through combination therapies have been quite promising, warranting further examination into how the oxidative environment can amplify or blunt bortezomib therapeutic effectiveness.

References

1. Balaban RS, Nemoto S, Finkel T (2005) Mitochondria, oxidants, and aging. Cell 120(4): 483–495
2. Lee MH, Hyun DH, Jenner P, Halliwell B (2001) Effect of proteasome inhibition on cellular oxidative damage, antioxidant defences and nitric oxide production. J Neurochem 78(1):32–41
3. Leak RK, Zigmond MJ, Liou AKF (2008) Adaptation to chronic MG132 reduces oxidative toxicity by a CuZnSOD-dependent mechanism. J Neurochem 106(2):860–874
4. Li X, Lu D, He F, Zhou H, Liu Q, Wang Y, Shao C, Gong Y (2011) Cullin 4B protein ubiquitin ligase targets peroxiredoxin III for degradation. J Biol Chem 286(37):32344–32354
5. Rhee SG, Yang K-S, Kang SW, Woo HA, Chang T-S (2005) Controlled elimination of intracellular H_2O_2: regulation of peroxiredoxin, catalase, and glutathione peroxidase via post-translational modification. Antioxid Redox Signal 7(5–6):619–626
6. Rudeck M, Volk T, Sitte N, Grune T (2000) Ferritin oxidation in vitro: implication of iron release and degradation by the 20S proteasome. IUBMB Life 49(5):451–456

7. Antosiewicz J, Ziolkowski W, Kaczor JJ, Herman-Antosiewicz A (2007) Tumor necrosis factor-α-induced reactive oxygen species formation is mediated by JNK1-dependent ferritin degradation and elevation of labile iron pool. Free Radic Biol Med 43(2):265–270
8. Iwai K, Klausner RD, Rouault TA (1995) Requirements for iron-regulated degradation of the RNA binding protein, iron regulatory protein 2. EMBO J 14(21):5350–5357
9. Iwai K, Drake SK, Wehr NB, Weissman AM, LaVaute T, Minato N, Klausner RD, Levine RL, Rouault TA (1998) Iron-dependent oxidation, ubiquitination, and degradation of iron regulatory protein 2: implications for degradation of oxidized proteins. Proc Natl Acad Sci U S A 95(9):4924–4928
10. Guo B, Phillips JD, Yu Y, Leibold EA (1995) Iron regulates the intracellular degradation of iron regulatory protein 2 by the proteasome. J Biol Chem 270(37):21645–21651
11. LaVaute T, Smith S, Cooperman S, Iwai K, Land W, Meyron-Holtz E, Drake SK, Miller G, Abu-Asab M, Tsokos M (2001) Targeted deletion of the gene encoding iron regulatory protein-2 causes misregulation of iron metabolism and neurodegenerative disease in mice. Nat Genet 27(2):209–214
12. Pham CG, Bubici C, Zazzeroni F, Papa S, Jones J, Alvarez K, Jayawardena S, De Smaele E, Cong R, Beaumont C, Torti FM, Torti SV, Franzoso G (2004) Ferritin heavy chain upregulation by NF-kappaB inhibits TNFalpha-induced apoptosis by suppressing reactive oxygen species. Cell 119(4):529–542
13. Sakon S, Xue X, Takekawa M, Sasazuki T, Okazaki T, Kojima Y, Piao J-H, Yagita H, Okumura K, Doi T, Nakano H (2003) NF-kappaB inhibits TNF-induced accumulation of ROS that mediate prolonged MAPK activation and necrotic cell death. EMBO J 22(15): 3898–3909
14. Palombella VJ, Rando OJ, Goldberg AL, Maniatis T (1994) The ubiquitin-proteasome pathway is required for processing the NF-kappa B1 precursor protein and the activation of NF-kappa B. Cell 78(5):773–785
15. Sunwoo JB, Chen Z, Dong G, Yeh N, Crowl BC, Sausville E, Adams J, Elliott P, Van Waes C (2001) Novel proteasome inhibitor PS-341 inhibits activation of nuclear factor-kappa B, cell survival, tumor growth, and angiogenesis in squamous cell carcinoma. Clin Cancer Res 7(5):1419–1428
16. Rojo AI, Salinas M, Martín D, Perona R, Cuadrado A (2004) Regulation of Cu/Zn-superoxide dismutase expression via the phosphatidylinositol 3 kinase/Akt pathway and nuclear factor-kappaB. J Neurosci 24(33):7324–7334
17. Sen CK, Packer L (1996) Antioxidant and redox regulation of gene transcription. FASEB J 10(7):709–720
18. Schreck R, Rieber P, Baeuerle PA (1991) Reactive oxygen intermediates as apparently widely used messengers in the activation of the NF-kappa B transcription factor and HIV-1. EMBO J 10(8):2247
19. Li N, Karin M (1999) Is NF-kappaB the sensor of oxidative stress? FASEB J 13(10): 1137–1143
20. Traenckner EB, Wilk S, Baeuerle PA (1994) A proteasome inhibitor prevents activation of NF-kappa B and stabilizes a newly phosphorylated form of I kappa B-alpha that is still bound to NF-kappa B. EMBO J 13(22):5433
21. McConkey DJ, Zhu K (2008) Mechanisms of proteasome inhibitor action and resistance in cancer. Drug Resist Updat 11(4):164–179
22. Cusack JC, Liu R, Houston M, Abendroth K, Elliott PJ, Adams J, Baldwin AS (2001) Enhanced chemosensitivity to CPT-11 with proteasome inhibitor PS-341: implications for systemic nuclear factor-κB inhibition. Cancer Res 61(9):3535–3540
23. Russo SM, Tepper JE, Baldwin AS, Liu R, Adams J, Elliott P, Cusack JC (2001) Enhancement of radiosensitivity by proteasome inhibition: implications for a role of NF-kappaB. Int J Radiat Oncol Biol Phys 50(1):183–193
24. Turrens JF (2003) Mitochondrial formation of reactive oxygen species. J Physiol 552(2): 335–344
25. Goetz ME, Luch A (2008) Reactive species: a cell damaging rout assisting to chemical carcinogens. Cancer Lett 266(1):73–83

26. Kovacic HN, Irani K, Goldschmidt-Clermont PJ (2001) Redox regulation of human Rac1 stability by the proteasome in human aortic endothelial cells. J Biol Chem 276(49): 45856–45861
27. Landry WD, Woolley JF, Cotter TG (2013) Imatinib and Nilotinib inhibit Bcr–Abl-induced ROS through targeted degradation of the NADPH oxidase subunit p22phox. Leuk Res 37(2):183–189
28. Sitte N, Merker K, Grune T (1998) Proteasome-dependent degradation of oxidized proteins in MRC-5 fibroblasts. FEBS Lett 440(3):399–402
29. Ferrington DA, Sun H, Murray KK, Costa J, Williams TD, Bigelow DJ, Squier TC (2001) Selective degradation of oxidized calmodulin by the 20 S proteasome. J Biol Chem 276(2):937–943
30. Grune T, Jung T, Merker K, Davies KJA (2004) Decreased proteolysis caused by protein aggregates, inclusion bodies, plaques, lipofuscin, ceroid, and 'aggresomes' during oxidative stress, aging, and disease. Int J Biochem Cell Biol 36(12):2519–2530
31. Shringarpure R, Grune T, Davies K (2001) Protein oxidation and 20S proteasome-dependent proteolysis in mammalian cells. Cell Mol Life Sci 58(10):1442–1450
32. Pacifici RE, Kono Y, Davies KJ (1993) Hydrophobicity as the signal for selective degradation of hydroxyl radical-modified hemoglobin by the multicatalytic proteinase complex, proteasome. J Biol Chem 268(21):15405–15411
33. Shringarpure R, Grune T, Mehlhase J, Davies KJA (2003) Ubiquitin conjugation is not required for the degradation of oxidized proteins by proteasome. J Biol Chem 278(1): 311–318
34. Ishii T, Sakurai T, Usami H, Uchida K (2005) Oxidative modification of proteasome: identification of an oxidation-sensitive subunit in 26 S proteasome. Biochemistry 44(42): 13893–13901
35. Reinheckel T, Sitte N, Ullrich O, Kuckelkorn U, Davies KJ, Grune T (1998) Comparative resistance of the 20S and 26S proteasome to oxidative stress. Biochem J 335(Pt 3):637–642
36. Grune T, Reinheckel T, Davies KJ (1996) Degradation of oxidized proteins in K562 human hematopoietic cells by proteasome. J Biol Chem 271(26):15504–15509
37. Davies KJ (2001) Degradation of oxidized proteins by the 20S proteasome. Biochimie 83(3):301–310
38. Zhu K, Dunner K, McConkey DJ (2009) Proteasome inhibitors activate autophagy as a cytoprotective response in human prostate cancer cells. Oncogene 29(3):451–462
39. Bence NF, Sampat RM, Kopito RR (2001) Impairment of the ubiquitin-proteasome system by protein aggregation. Science 292(5521):1552–1555
40. Conconi M, Friguet B (1997) Proteasome inactivation upon aging and on oxidation-effect of HSP 90. Mol Biol Rep 24(1–2):45–50
41. Conconi M, Petropoulos I, Emod I, Turlin E, Biville F, Friguet B (1998) Protection from oxidative inactivation of the 20S proteasome by heat-shock protein 90. Biochem J 333(Pt 2): 407–415
42. Ding Q, Keller JN (2001) Proteasome inhibition in oxidative stress neurotoxicity: implications for heat shock proteins. J Neurochem 77(4):1010–1017
43. Ding Q, Reinacker K, Dimayuga E, Nukala V, Drake J, Butterfield DA, Dunn JC, Martin S, Bruce-Keller AJ, Keller JN (2003) Role of the proteasome in protein oxidation and neural viability following low-level oxidative stress. FEBS Lett 546(2–3):228–232
44. Stuehr DJ, Marletta MA (1987) Induction of nitrite/nitrate synthesis in murine macrophages by BCG infection, lymphokines, or interferon-gamma. J Immunol 139(2):518–525
45. Seifert U, Bialy LP, Ebstein F, Bech-Otschir D, Voigt A, Schröter F, Prozorovski T, Lange N, Steffen J, Rieger M, Kuckelkorn U, Aktas O, Kloetzel P-M, Krüger E (2010) Immunoproteasomes preserve protein homeostasis upon interferon-induced oxidative stress. Cell 142(4):613–624
46. Dinkova-Kostova AT, Holtzclaw WD, Cole RN, Itoh K, Wakabayashi N, Katoh Y, Yamamoto M, Talalay P (2002) Direct evidence that sulfhydryl groups of Keap1 are the sensors regulating induction of phase 2 enzymes that protect against carcinogens and oxidants. Proc Natl Acad Sci U S A 99(18):11908–11913

47. Townsend DM, Tew KD, Tapiero H (2003) The importance of glutathione in human disease. Biomed Pharmacother 57(3–4):145–155
48. Kwak M-K, Wakabayashi N, Greenlaw JL, Yamamoto M, Kensler TW (2003) Antioxidants enhance mammalian proteasome expression through the Keap1-Nrf2 signaling pathway. Mol Cell Biol 23(23):8786–8794
49. Furukawa M, Xiong Y (2005) BTB protein Keap1 targets antioxidant transcription factor Nrf2 for ubiquitination by the Cullin 3-Roc1 ligase. Mol Cell Biol 25(1):162–171
50. Itoh K, Chiba T, Takahashi S, Ishii T, Igarashi K, Katoh Y, Oyake T, Hayashi N, Satoh K, Hatayama I, Yamamoto M, Nabeshima Y (1997) An Nrf2/small Maf heterodimer mediates the induction of phase II detoxifying enzyme genes through antioxidant response elements. Biochem Biophys Res Commun 236(2):313–322
51. Kobayashi A, Kang M-I, Okawa H, Ohtsuji M, Zenke Y, Chiba T, Igarashi K, Yamamoto M (2004) Oxidative stress sensor Keap1 functions as an adaptor for Cul3-based E3 ligase to regulate proteasomal degradation of Nrf2. Mol Cell Biol 24(16):7130–7139
52. Pickering AM, Linder RA, Zhang H, Forman HJ, Davies KJA (2012) Nrf2-dependent induction of proteasome and Pa28αβ regulator are required for adaptation to oxidative stress. J Biol Chem 287(13):10021–10031
53. Pei X-Y, Dai Y, Grant S (2004) Synergistic induction of oxidative injury and apoptosis in human multiple myeloma cells by the proteasome inhibitor bortezomib and histone deacetylase inhibitors. Clin Cancer Res 10(11):3839–3852
54. Perez-Galan P (2006) The proteasome inhibitor bortezomib induces apoptosis in mantle-cell lymphoma through generation of ROS and Noxa activation independent of p53 status. Blood 107(1):257–264
55. Ling Y-H, Liebes L, Zou Y, Perez-Soler R (2003) Reactive oxygen species generation and mitochondrial dysfunction in the apoptotic response to Bortezomib, a novel proteasome inhibitor, in human H460 non-small cell lung cancer cells. J Biol Chem 278(36): 33714–33723
56. Minami T, Adachi M, Kawamura R, Zhang Y, Shinomura Y, Imai K (2005) Sulindac enhances the proteasome inhibitor bortezomib-mediated oxidative stress and anticancer activity. Clin Cancer Res 11(14):5248–5256
57. Llobet D, Eritja N, Encinas M, Sorolla A, Yeramian A, Schoenenberger JA, Llombart-Cussac A, Marti RM, Matias-Guiu X, Dolcet X (2008) Antioxidants block proteasome inhibitor function in endometrial carcinoma cells. Anticancer Drugs 19(2):115–124
58. Fribley A, Zeng Q, Wang C-Y (2004) Proteasome inhibitor PS-341 induces apoptosis through induction of endoplasmic reticulum stress-reactive oxygen species in head and neck squamous cell carcinoma cells. Mol Cell Biol 24(22):9695–9704
59. Zou W, Yue P, Lin N, He M, Zhou Z, Lonial S, Khuri FR, Wang B, Sun S-Y (2006) Vitamin C inactivates the proteasome inhibitor PS-341 in human cancer cells. Clin Cancer Res 12(1):273–280
60. Shidoji Y, Hayashi K, Komura S, Ohishi N, Yagi K (1999) Loss of molecular interaction between cytochrome c and cardiolipin due to lipid peroxidation. Biochem Biophys Res Commun 264(2):343–347
61. Kowaltowski AJ, Castilho RF, Vercesi AE (2001) Mitochondrial permeability transition and oxidative stress. FEBS Lett 495(1):12–15
62. Li P, Nijhawan D, Budihardjo I, Srinivasula SM, Ahmad M, Alnemri ES, Wang X (1997) Cytochrome c and dATP-dependent formation of Apaf-1/caspase-9 complex initiates an apoptotic protease cascade. Cell 91(4):479–489
63. Dames SA, Mulet JM, Rathgeb-Szabo K, Hall MN, Grzesiek S (2005) The solution structure of the FATC domain of the protein kinase target of rapamycin suggests a role for redox-dependent structural and cellular stability. J Biol Chem 280(21):20558–20564
64. Lee J, Giordano S, Zhang J (2012) Autophagy, mitochondria and oxidative stress: cross-talk and redox signalling. Biochem J 441(2):523–540
65. Chen Y, McMillan-Ward E, Kong J, Israels SJ, Gibson SB (2007) Mitochondrial electron-transport-chain inhibitors of complexes I and II induce autophagic cell death mediated by reactive oxygen species. J Cell Sci 120(23):4155–4166

66. Hitomi J, Christofferson DE, Ng A, Yao J, Degterev A, Xavier RJ, Yuan J (2008) Identification of a molecular signaling network that regulates a cellular necrotic cell death pathway. Cell 135(7):1311–1323
67. Galluzzi L, Kroemer G (2008) Necroptosis: a specialized pathway of programmed necrosis. Cell 135(7):1161–1163
68. Thapa RJ, Basagoudanavar SH, Nogusa S, Irrinki K, Mallilankaraman K, Slifker MJ, Beg AA, Madesh M, Balachandran S (2011) NF-kappaB protects cells from gamma interferon-induced RIP1-dependent necroptosis. Mol Cell Biol 31(14):2934–2946
69. Meng T-C, Fukada T, Tonks NK (2002) Reversible oxidation and inactivation of protein tyrosine phosphatases in vivo. Mol Cell 9(2):387–399
70. Denu JM, Tanner KG (1998) Specific and reversible inactivation of protein tyrosine phosphatases by hydrogen peroxide: evidence for a sulfenic acid intermediate and implications for redox regulation. Biochemistry 37(16):5633–5642
71. Salmeen A, Andersen JN, Myers MP, Meng T-C, Hinks JA, Tonks NK, Barford D (2003) Redox regulation of protein tyrosine phosphatase 1B involves a sulphenyl-amide intermediate. Nature 423(6941):769–773
72. Weibrecht I, Böhmer S-A, Dagnell M, Kappert K, Östman A, Böhmer F-D (2007) Oxidation sensitivity of the catalytic cysteine of the protein-tyrosine phosphatases SHP-1 and SHP-2. Free Radic Biol Med 43(1):100–110
73. Brumell JH, Burkhardt AL, Bolen JB, Grinstein S (1996) Endogenous reactive oxygen intermediates activate tyrosine kinases in human neutrophils. J Biol Chem 271(3):1455–1461
74. Kwon J, Lee S-R, Yang K-S, Ahn Y, Kim YJ, Stadtman ER, Rhee SG (2004) Reversible oxidation and inactivation of the tumor suppressor PTEN in cells stimulated with peptide growth factors. Proc Natl Acad Sci U S A 101(47):16419–16424
75. Lim S, Clément M-V (2007) Phosphorylation of the survival kinase Akt by superoxide is dependent on an ascorbate-reversible oxidation of PTEN. Free Radic Biol Med 42(8): 1178–1192
76. Covey TM, Edes K, Fitzpatrick FA (2007) Akt activation by arachidonic acid metabolism occurs via oxidation and inactivation of PTEN tumor suppressor. Oncogene 26(39): 5784–5792
77. Lee SR (2002) Reversible Inactivation of the Tumor Suppressor PTEN by H_2O_2. J Biol Chem 277(23):20336–20342
78. Saitoh M, Nishitoh H, Fujii M, Takeda K, Tobiume K, Sawada Y, Kawabata M, Miyazono K, Ichijo H (1998) Mammalian thioredoxin is a direct inhibitor of apoptosis signal-regulating kinase (ASK) 1. EMBO J 17(9):2596–2606
79. Tobiume K, Matsuzawa A, Takahashi T, Nishitoh H, Morita K, Takeda K, Minowa O, Miyazono K, Noda T, Ichijo H (2001) ASK1 is required for sustained activations of JNK/p38 MAP kinases and apoptosis. EMBO Rep 2(3):222–228
80. Choi TG, Lee J, Ha J, Kim SS (2011) Apoptosis signal-regulating kinase 1 is an intracellular inducer of p38 MAPK-mediated myogenic signalling in cardiac myoblasts. Biochem Biophys Acta 1813(8):1412–1421
81. Rushworth SA, Bowles KM, MacEwan DJ (2011) High basal nuclear levels of Nrf2 in acute myeloid leukemia reduces sensitivity to proteasome inhibitors. Cancer Res 71(5): 1999–2009
82. Fuchs D, Berges C, Opelz G, Daniel V, Naujokat C (2008) Increased expression and altered subunit composition of proteasomes induced by continuous proteasome inhibition establish apoptosis resistance and hyperproliferation of Burkitt lymphoma cells. J Cell Biochem 103(1):270–283
83. Busse A, Kraus M, Na I-K, Rietz A, Scheibenbogen C, Driessen C, Blau IW, Thiel E, Keilholz U (2008) Sensitivity of tumor cells to proteasome inhibitors is associated with expression levels and composition of proteasome subunits. Cancer 112(3):659–670
84. Lü S, Yang J, Song X, Gong S, Zhou H, Guo L, Song N, Bao X, Chen P, Wang J (2008) Point mutation of the proteasome beta5 subunit gene is an important mechanism of bortezomib resistance in bortezomib-selected variants of Jurkat T cell lymphoblastic lymphoma/leukemia line. J Pharmacol Exp Ther 326(2):423–431

85. Oerlemans R, Franke NE, Assaraf YG, Cloos J, van Zantwijk I, Berkers CR, Scheffer GL, Debipersad K, Vojtekova K, Lemos C, van der Heijden JW, Ylstra B, Peters GJ, Kaspers GL, Dijkmans BAC, Scheper RJ, Jansen G (2008) Molecular basis of bortezomib resistance: proteasome subunit beta5 (PSMB5) gene mutation and overexpression of PSMB5 protein. Blood 112(6):2489–2499
86. Chauhan D, Catley L, Li G, Podar K, Hideshima T, Velankar M, Mitsiades C, Mitsiades N, Yasui H, Letai A, Ovaa H, Berkers C, Nicholson B, Chao T-H, Neuteboom STC, Richardson P, Palladino MA, Anderson KC (2005) A novel orally active proteasome inhibitor induces apoptosis in multiple myeloma cells with mechanisms distinct from Bortezomib. Cancer Cell 8(5):407–419
87. Kuhn DJ, Chen Q, Voorhees PM, Strader JS, Shenk KD, Sun CM, Demo SD, Bennett MK, Van Leeuwen FW, Chanan-Khan AA (2007) Potent activity of carfilzomib, a novel, irreversible inhibitor of the ubiquitin-proteasome pathway, against preclinical models of multiple myeloma. Blood 110(9):3281–3290
88. Kuhn DJ, Hunsucker SA, Chen Q, Voorhees PM, Orlowski M, Orlowski RZ (2009) Targeted inhibition of the immunoproteasome is a potent strategy against models of multiple myeloma that overcomes resistance to conventional drugs and nonspecific proteasome inhibitors. Blood 113(19):4667–4676
89. Decaux O, Clément M, Magrangeas F, Gouraud W, Charbonnel C, Campion L, Loiseau HA, Minvielle S (2010) Inhibition of mTORC1 activity by REDD1 induction in myeloma cells resistant to bortezomib cytotoxicity. Cancer Sci 101(4):889–897
90. Meiners S, Ludwig A, Lorenz M, Dreger H, Baumann G, Stangl V, Stangl K (2006) Nontoxic proteasome inhibition activates a protective antioxidant defense response in endothelial cells. Free Radic Biol Med 40(12):2232–2241
91. Dreger H, Westphal K, Weller A, Baumann G, Stangl V, Meiners S, Stangl K (2009) Nrf2-dependent upregulation of antioxidative enzymes: a novel pathway for proteasome inhibitor-mediated cardioprotection. Cardiovasc Res 83(2):354–361
92. Ohta T, Iijima K, Miyamoto M, Nakahara I, Tanaka H, Ohtsuji M, Suzuki T, Kobayashi A, Yokota J, Sakiyama T, Shibata T, Yamamoto M, Hirohashi S (2008) Loss of Keap1 function activates Nrf2 and provides advantages for lung cancer cell growth. Cancer Res 68(5): 1303–1309
93. Weniger MA, Rizzatti EG, Pérez-Galán P, Liu D, Wang Q, Munson PJ, Raghavachari N, White T, Tweito MM, Dunleavy K, Ye Y, Wilson WH, Wiestner A (2011) Treatment-induced oxidative stress and cellular antioxidant capacity determine response to bortezomib in mantle cell lymphoma. Clin Cancer Res 17(15):5101–5112
94. Meredith MJ, Cusick CL, Soltaninassab S, Sekhar KS, Lu S, Freeman ML (1998) Expression of Bcl-2 increases intracellular glutathione by inhibiting methionine-dependent GSH efflux. Biochem Biophys Res Commun 248(3):458–463
95. Hockenbery DM, Oltvai ZN, Yin X-M, Milliman CL, Korsmeyer SJ (1993) Bcl-2 functions in an antioxidant pathway to prevent apoptosis. Cell 75(2):241–251
96. Mirkovic N, Voehringer DW, Story MD, McConkey DJ, McDonnell TJ, Meyn RE (1997) Resistance to radiation-induced apoptosis in Bcl-2-expressing cells is reversed by depleting cellular thiols. Oncogene 15(12):1461–1470
97. Bianchi G, Oliva L, Cascio P, Pengo N, Fontana F, Cerruti F, Orsi A, Pasqualetto E, Mezghrani A, Calbi V, Palladini G, Giuliani N, Anderson KC, Sitia R, Cenci S (2009) The proteasome load versus capacity balance determines apoptotic sensitivity of multiple myeloma cells to proteasome inhibition. Blood 113(13):3040–3049
98. Mann BS, Johnson JR, He K, Sridhara R, Abraham S, Booth BP, Verbois L, Morse DE, Jee JM, Pope S, Harapanhalli RS, Dagher R, Farrell A, Justice R, Pazdur R (2007) Vorinostat for treatment of cutaneous manifestations of advanced primary cutaneous T-cell lymphoma. Clin Cancer Res 13(8):2318–2322
99. Feng R, Oton A, Mapara MY, Anderson G, Belani C, Lentzsch S (2007) The histone deacetylase inhibitor, PXD101, potentiates bortezomib-induced anti-multiple myeloma effect by induction of oxidative stress and DNA damage. Br J Haematol 139(3):385–397

100. Miller CP, Ban K, Dujka ME, McConkey DJ, Munsell M, Palladino M, Chandra J (2007) NPI-0052, a novel proteasome inhibitor, induces caspase-8 and ROS-dependent apoptosis alone and in combination with HDAC inhibitors in leukemia cells. Blood 110(1):267–277
101. Yu C (2003) The proteasome inhibitor bortezomib interacts synergistically with histone deacetylase inhibitors to induce apoptosis in Bcr/Abl + cells sensitive and resistant to STI571. Blood 102(10):3765–3774
102. Heider U, Metzler IV, Kaiser M, Rosche M, Sterz J, Rötzer S, Rademacher J, Jakob C, Fleissner C, Kuckelkorn U, Kloetzel P-M, Sezer O (2007) Synergistic interaction of the histone deacetylase inhibitor SAHA with the proteasome inhibitor bortezomib in mantle cell lymphoma. Eur J Haematol 80(2):133–142
103. Campbell RA, Sanchez E, Steinberg J, Shalitin D, Li Z-W, Chen H, Berenson JR (2010) Vorinostat enhances the antimyeloma effects of melphalan and bortezomib. Eur J Haematol 84(3):201–211
104. Badros A, Burger AM, Philip S, Niesvizky R, Kolla SS, Goloubeva O, Harris C, Zwiebel J, Wright JJ, Espinoza-Delgado I, Baer MR, Holleran JL, Egorin MJ, Grant S (2009) Phase I study of vorinostat in combination with bortezomib for relapsed and refractory multiple myeloma. Clin Cancer Res 15(16):5250–5257
105. Maiso P, Carvajal-Vergara X, Ocio EM, López-Pérez R, Mateo G, Gutiérrez N, Atadja P, Pandiella A, San Miguel JF (2006) The histone deacetylase inhibitor LBH589 is a potent antimyeloma agent that overcomes drug resistance. Cancer Res 66(11):5781–5789
106. Ocio EM, Vilanova D, Atadja P, Maiso P, Crusoe E, Fernandez-Lazaro D, Garayoa M, San-Segundo L, Hernandez-Iglesias T, de Alava E, Shao W, Yao YM, Pandiella A, San-Miguel JF (2010) In vitro and in vivo rationale for the triple combination of panobinostat (LBH589) and dexamethasone with either bortezomib or lenalidomide in multiple myeloma. Haematologica 95(5):794–803
107. Yu C, Friday BB, Lai J-P, Yang L, Sarkaria J, Kay NE, Carter CA, Roberts LR, Kaufmann SH, Adjei AA (2006) Cytotoxic synergy between the multikinase inhibitor sorafenib and the proteasome inhibitor bortezomib in vitro: induction of apoptosis through Akt and c-Jun NH2-terminal kinase pathways. Mol Cancer Ther 5(9):2378–2387
108. Chiou J-F, Tai C-J, Wang Y-H, Liu T-Z, Jen Y-M, Shiau C-Y (2009) Sorafenib induces preferential apoptotic killing of a drug- and radio-resistant Hep G2 cells through a mitochondria-dependent oxidative stress mechanism. Cancer Biol Ther 8(20):1904–1913
109. Cardoso F, Durbecq V, Laes JF, Badran B, Lagneaux L, Bex F, Desmedt C, Willard-Gallo K, Ross JS, Burny A, Piccart M, Sotiriou C (2006) Bortezomib (PS-341, Velcade) increases the efficacy of trastuzumab (Herceptin) in HER-2-positive breast cancer cells in a synergistic manner. Mol Cancer Ther 5(12):3042–3051
110. Gordon LI, Burke MA, Singh ATK, Prachand S, Lieberman ED, Sun L, Naik TJ, Prasad SVN, Ardehali H (2008) Blockade of the erbB2 receptor induces cardiomyocyte death through mitochondrial and reactive oxygen species-dependent pathways. J Biol Chem 284(4):2080–2087
111. Avramis IA, Christodoulopoulos G, Suzuki A, Laug WE, Gonzalez-Gomez I, McNamara G, Sausville EA, Avramis VI (2002) In vitro and in vivo evaluations of the tyrosine kinase inhibitor NSC 680410 against human leukemia and glioblastoma cell lines. Cancer Chemother Pharmacol 50(6):479–489
112. Chandra J (2003) Involvement of reactive oxygen species in adaphostin-induced cytotoxicity in human leukemia cells. Blood 102(13):4512–4519
113. Dasmahapatra G (2006) The tyrphostin adaphostin interacts synergistically with proteasome inhibitors to induce apoptosis in human leukemia cells through a reactive oxygen species (ROS)-dependent mechanism. Blood 107(1):232–240
114. Perrone G, Hideshima T, Ikeda H, Okawa Y, Calabrese E, Gorgun G, Santo L, Cirstea D, Raje N, Chauhan D (2009) Ascorbic acid inhibits antitumor activity of bortezomib in vivo. Leukemia 23(9):1679–1686
115. Golden EB, Lam PY, Kardosh A, Gaffney KJ, Cadenas E, Louie SG, Petasis NA, Chen TC, Schonthal AH (2009) Green tea polyphenols block the anticancer effects of bortezomib and other boronic acid-based proteasome inhibitors. Blood 113(23):5927–5937

116. Shah JJ, Kuhn DJ, Orlowski RZ (2009) Bortezomib and EGCG: no green tea for you? Blood 113(23):5695–5696
117. Bannerman B, Xu L, Jones M, Tsu C, Yu J, Hales P, Monbaliu J, Fleming P, Dick L, Manfredi M, Claiborne C, Bolen J, Kupperman E, Berger A (2011) Preclinical evaluation of the antitumor activity of bortezomib in combination with vitamin C or with epigallocatechin gallate, a component of green tea. Cancer Chemother Pharmacol 68(5):1145–1154
118. Shen M, Chan TH, Dou QP (2012) Targeting tumor ubiquitin-proteasome pathway with polyphenols for chemosensitization. Anticancer Agents Med Chem 12(8):891–901
119. Engel RH, Brown JA, Von Roenn JH, O'Regan RM, Bergan R, Badve S, Rademaker A, Gradishar WJ (2007) A phase II study of single agent bortezomib in patients with metastatic breast cancer: a single institution experience. Cancer Invest 25(8):733–737
120. Shah MH, Young D, Kindler HL, Webb I, Kleiber B, Wright J, Grever M (2004) Phase II study of the proteasome inhibitor bortezomib (PS-341) in patients with metastatic neuroendocrine tumors. Clin Cancer Res 10(18):6111–6118
121. Kondagunta GV, Drucker B, Schwartz L, Bacik J, Marion S, Russo P, Mazumdar M, Motzer RJ (2004) Phase II trial of bortezomib for patients with advanced renal cell carcinoma. J Clin Oncol 22(18):3720–3725

Chapter 11
Proteotoxic Stress and Proteasome Inhibitor Efficacy and Resistance

David McConkey

Abstract Proteasome inhibitors have established themselves as the frontline therapy for multiple myeloma (MM) and they are displaying strong clinical activity in a variety of other hematological cancers. However, as is observed with other targeted agents, resistance to proteasome inhibitor therapy is emerging as a major clinical challenge. Accumulating evidence has implicated proteotoxicity in the cytotoxic mechanisms of proteasome inhibitors in cancer cells, and it is therefore not surprising that key resistance mechanisms involve inducible, physiological cytoprotective responses to proteotoxicity. Here I will discuss our current understanding of the role of proteotoxicity in the antitumor activities of proteasome inhibitors and the evidence that induced cytoprotective mechanisms could play important roles in mediating resistance.

Keywords Proteotoxicity • Integrated stress response • Translation • eIF2-alpha

Abbreviations

ATF	Activating transcription factor
ATG	Autophagy-related gene
CHOP	C/EBP-homologous protein
ER	Endoplasmic reticulum
GADD	Growth arrest and DNA damage-induced
GCN2	General control nonderepressible 2 kinase
Grp	Glucose-regulated protein
HDAC	Histone deacetylase
HRI	Heme-regulated inhibitor
HSP	Heat shock protein

D. McConkey (✉)
Departments of Urology and Cancer Biology, U.T. M.D. Anderson Cancer Center, Houston, TX 77030, USA
e-mail: dmcconke@mdanderson.org

Q.P. Dou (ed.), *Resistance to Proteasome Inhibitors in Cancer*, Resistance to Targeted Anti-Cancer Therapeutics, DOI 10.1007/978-3-319-06752-0_11

ISR	Integrated stress response
IκBα	Inhibitor of nuclear factor kappa B, alpha isoform
LC3	Microtubule-associated protein light chain 3
MEF	Mouse embryonic fibroblast
MM	Multiple myeloma
NF-κB	Nuclear factor kappa B
PERK	Pancreatic ER kinase
PKR	Protein kinase R
ROS	Reactive oxygen species
UPR	Unfolded protein response
XBP-1	X-box binding protein-1

11.1 Introduction

Julian Adams and his colleagues at ProScript, Inc. developed the peptide boronate inhibitor of the proteasome known as PS-341 as a first-in-class cancer therapeutic in the late 1990s [1]. The drug attracted immediate attention because of its uniquely strong activity in the NCI's panel of 60 cell lines (the "NCI-60"), where it produced broad tumor cell growth inhibition at low nanomolar concentrations [1]. These effects were initially attributed to PS-341's ability to cause stabilization of specific proteins involved in the control of tumor cell proliferation and survival, including NF-κB's physiological inhibitor (IκBα) [2] and cell cycle inhibitors like p21 and p53 [3]. Investigators also noted that PS-341 blocked tumor production of vascular endothelial growth factor (VEGF) in vitro and strongly inhibited angiogenesis in vivo [4–7], suggesting that its indirect effects on the tumor-associated stroma might also contribute to growth inhibition.

However, these preclinical studies did not really predict the strong and unique clinical activity of PS-341 (now known as bortezomib or Velcade) in patients with multiple myeloma (MM). ProScript initiated a number of Phase I clinical trials in patients with solid and hematologic tumors, using a novel pharmacodynamic bioassay [1] to closely monitor 20S proteasome inhibition in the peripheral blood during dose escalation because preclinical studies in rodents and primates indicated that doses that produced greater than 80 % inhibition produced acute toxicity [8]. The early Phase I results indicated that PS-341 had modest single-agent activity in multiple solid and hematologic tumors, but it produced striking clinical responses in refractory MM [9], results that were confirmed in a subsequent Phase II clinical trial [10]. Bortezomib received FDA approval for the treatment of MM in 2003 [11, 12], and its success prompted other companies to enter the field [13, 14]. The next-generation proteasome inhibitor carfilzomib also recently received FDA approval for the treatment of MM [15, 16], and the development of several other, structurally distinct inhibitors is well underway.

What is it about the biology of MM that makes it so uniquely sensitive to proteasome inhibitors? Early work established that NF-κB inhibition did not account for

PS-341's cytotoxic effects [2]. Rather, the potent effects of proteasome inhibitors in MM cells appear to be related to proteotoxicity, and more specifically to the importance of proteasome-mediated degradation of misfolded and/or aggregated proteins that can accumulate rapidly within the endoplasmic reticulum (ER) of highly active secretory cells [17]. Therefore, the extremely high production of monoclonal immunoglobulin in MM cells causes them to be exquisitely sensitive to proteasome inhibitor-induced ER stress [18]—proteasome inhibitor sensitivity correlates with cellular immunoglobulin production [18, 19], and enforced immunoglobulin expression also promoted proteasome inhibitor-induced cell death [20].

11.2 Proteasome Inhibitors and the Integrated Stress Response

The integrated stress response (ISR) is an adaptive response that enables normal cells to survive ER stress and other examples of proteotoxicity. Exposure to a variety of endogenous stimuli, including oxidative stress, heat shock, heavy metals, and viruses, can cause protein denaturation and exposure of normally buried hydrophobic regions that are prone to aggregation [21–25]. These aggregation-prone proteins rapidly attract members of the HSP70 family of protein chaperones away from their constitutive binding partners, which result simultaneously in chaperone-mediated aggregate recognition by ubiquitin ligases and activation of a family of four related serine/threonine protein kinases (PERK, GCN2, HRI, and PKR) that activate a cytoprotective pathway known as the ISR (Fig. 11.1) [26]. The best-studied downstream consequence of ISR kinase activation is phosphorylation of the translation initiation factor, eIF2α, on serine 51 (S52 in mice) [27–30]. Phosphorylation of eIF2α inhibits the translation of most mRNAs (including the essential cell cycle regulator cyclin D) while enhancing the expression of a discrete set of proteins that attenuate proteotoxic stress [26]. Central to these effects are the transcription factors, ATF-4 and GADD153/CHOP, which induce the expression of cytoprotective factors and a protein phosphatase (GADD34) that dephosphorylates eIF2α and restores translation once proteotoxic protein aggregates have been cleared. The rapid downregulation of protein synthesis that is caused by eIF2α phosphorylation provides immediate cytoprotective benefit by preventing new misfolded proteins from being formed. Because proliferating cells tend to be intrinsically more sensitive to apoptosis than are quiescent cells [31, 32], the cell cycle arrest that is caused by eIF2α phosphorylation also produces cytoprotective effects.

Phosphorylation of eIF2α also enhances cell survival by stimulating autophagy [33, 34]. Although the precise molecular mechanisms involved in this coupling are still not completely clear, eIF2α phosphorylation causes increased expression of the central autophagy genes *LC3*, *ATG5*, and *ATG7* via *ATF4* and *CHOP* [33, 35]. Autophagy provides another route for protein aggregate disposal. Because the proteasome cannot degrade large protein aggregates without unwinding them first, autophagy complements the proteasome within the ISR.

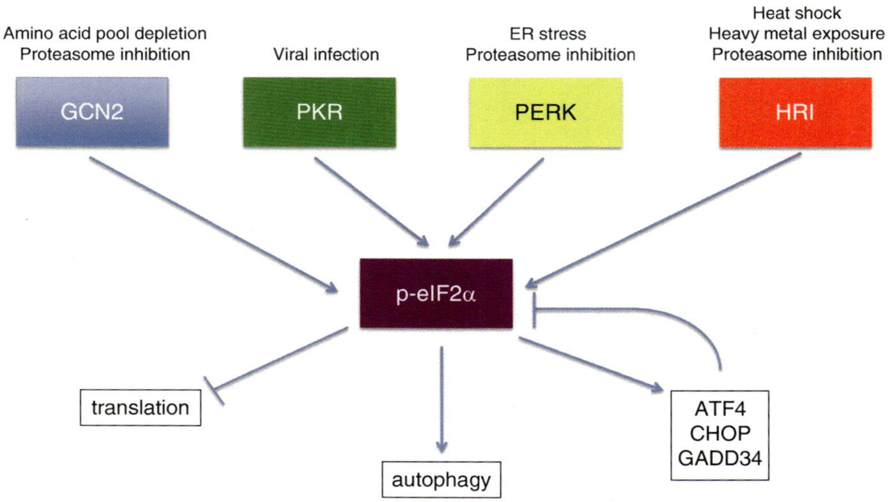

Fig. 11.1 Kinase control of the integrated stress response (ISR). Upstream signals leading to activation of one or more of the 4 eIF2α kinases coordinate multiple cytoprotective responses in cells experiencing proteotoxic stress. Phosphorylation of eIF2α results in suppression of translation, upregulation of autophagy, and downregulation of cyclin D, leading to cell cycle arrest. Persistent activation of the ISR subsequently leads to CHOP-mediated upregulation of GADD34, which dephosphorylates eIF2α and terminates the response. Therefore, if GADD34 is strongly induced before proteotoxic stress is resolved, it exacerbates the stress and promotes cell death. This probably explains how the ISR can be sequentially involved in inhibiting or promoting cell death

11.3 Proteasome Inhibitor-Induced Cell Death

11.3.1 Role of the ISR: Cytoprotective or Cytotoxic?

Although the cytotoxic effects of proteasome inhibition clearly involve misfolded protein accumulation, the precise mechanisms that mediate cell killing are still being elucidated. One possibility is that cell death is caused by some of the same ISR-dependent mechanisms that mediate the early cytoprotective response. Early work established that proteasome inhibitors cause changes consistent with ER stress in MM cells and some other cancer cell lines, including activation of the ER-localized ISR kinase, PERK, eIF2α phosphorylation, and activation of ATF4 and CHOP, leading to induction of the ER chaperone and HSP70 family member, Grp78/BIP in MM cells, and mechanistic studies demonstrated that eIF2α phosphorylation and CHOP induction promoted cell death, consistent with the conclusion that bortezomib causes a "terminal unfolded protein response" (UPR) [18, 19, 36, 37]. However, RNAi-mediated knockdown of the eIF2α kinases or CHOP greatly potentiated cell death in human pancreatic cancer cells (M. White et al., manuscript under revision), which is more consistent with their known cytoprotective effects within the context of the ISR that were discussed above. Although the molecular mechanisms that dictate whether the UPR promotes cell death or survival are likely to be highly complex and cell type dependent, exposing cancer cells to cycloheximide (a chemical protein synthesis inhibitor) consistently mimics the effects of eIF2α phosphorylation to block protein synthesis and protect cancer cells from proteasome inhibitor-induced cell death [38]. Therefore, the CHOP-mediated induction of GADD34 that occurs after ISR kinase-induced eIF2α phosphorylation has produced its cytoprotective effects could provide an explanation [39]. GADD34 dephosphorylates eIF2α, resulting in restoration of protein translation and cell cycle progression. In the face of ongoing proteasome inhibition, these effects will greatly exacerbate proteotoxic stress and intrinsic apoptosis susceptibility.

11.3.2 Role of ER Versus Cytosolic Stress

The precise nature of the stress induced by proteasome inhibition also appears to be cell type dependent. In highly secretory cells like MM, it makes sense that ER stress would play a major role, but in many other cancers derived from endocrine (prostate) or exocrine (pancreatic) tissues, the secretory machinery may be drastically downregulated as a consequence of cancer-associated dedifferentiation. On the other hand, global rates of translation are markedly elevated in cancer cells to offset the need for protein synthesis in proliferation and tumor cell metabolism. We directly compared the effects of bortezomib on activation of each of the eIF2α kinases in human pancreatic cancer cells and discovered that HRI (not PERK) was most strongly activated (M. White et al., manuscript under revision). Consistent with these observations, proteasome inhibitors caused much stronger induction of the cytosolic chaperone, HSP72 (the inducible HSP70 isoform), than they did induction of the ER chaperone Grp78, and knockdown of HRI (not PERK) had the strongest effects on proteasome inhibitor-induced cell death. Therefore, in pancreatic cancer cells the effects of proteasome inhibitors may more closely resemble the changes induced by heat shock or heavy metals that are primarily localized to the cytosol rather than the ER, and similar results were obtained by another group using mouse embryonic fibroblasts (MEFS) [40]. Nevertheless, still other studies have implicated the amino acid pool-controlled ISR kinase, GCN2, in proteasome inhibitor-induced eIF2α phosphorylation in MEFs and several other cell types [36, 37]. The authors concluded that GCN2 activation was caused by amino acid pool depletion and was rescued by exogenous amino acids [37]. It is not clear why two groups working with the same cells (MEFs) advanced two different conclusions about which ISR kinase was most relevant to the effects of proteasome inhibitors.

11.3.3 Role of Protein Aggregates: Cytoprotective or Cytotoxic?

There is a close correlation between the sensitivity of cancer cells to proteasome inhibitors and their tendency to form protein aggregates [41–43]. These aggregates tend to coalesce into discrete perinuclear structures that are termed "aggresomes" [44].

Aggresome formation is dependent on the activities of histone deacetylases, and in particular HDAC6 [45]. Aggresomes may represent an intermediate step in the shuttling of protein aggregates to lysosomes during autophagy-mediated degradation. Therefore, chemical HDAC inhibitors or HDAC6 knockdown prevents proteasome inhibitor-induced aggresome formation and promotes cell death [42, 43, 45]. These data suggest that it is not the presence of protein aggregates per se that causes cytotoxicity, but rather the nature of the protein aggregates and whether or not they are bound by chaperones and/or compartmentalized to aggresomes.

11.3.4 Role of Reactive Oxygen Species

If misfolded proteins are toxic, what are the biochemical mechanisms underlying their cytotoxicity? The most consistent downstream mechanism is reactive oxygen species (ROS) production [46–50]. All of the chemical proteasome inhibitors analyzed to date cause early increases in ROS production, and radical scavenging agents (particularly the thiol antioxidant *N*-acetylcysteine) block proteasome inhibitor-induced cell death [46–50]. The origin of these free radicals appears to be the mitochondria, but precisely how protein aggregates trigger mitochondrial ROS production is not yet known.

11.3.5 Downstream Caspase Activation

Proteasome inhibitors can trigger either apoptosis or necrosis in human cancer cells [33, 51], and caspase activation is required only for the former [33]. In addition, precisely which caspase(s) initiates proteasome inhibitor-induced apoptosis appears to vary among cell lines and proteasome inhibitors. One study concluded that the ER-localized caspase-4 was required for bortezomib-induced apoptosis in human pancreatic cancer cells [38], but another study concluded that caspase-4 was not necessary for proteasome inhibitor-induced apoptosis in MM cells [18], and other studies implicated caspases-2 [52, 53], -8 [14], and -9 [14] as the relevant initiator caspases in different cell lines exposed to different inhibitors. Because a distinct adaptor protein controls the activation of each initiator caspase, the upstream signals that lead to their activation are also distinct. Identifying the nature of these signals will require further investigation.

11.3.6 Amino Acid Pool Depletion

Exciting recent results indicate that the constitutive protein "recycling" that is mediated by the proteasome is important for maintaining intracellular amino acid pool levels. According to this model, proteasome inhibition depletes intracellular amino acid pool levels, resulting in GCN2 activation, eIF2α phosphorylation, ATF4 and CHOP induction, and autophagy [37]. Although translational arrest mitigated proteotoxicity and autophagy staved off complete amino acid pool depletion, ultimately cells succumbed via CHOP-mediated cell death [37]. Again, we failed to observe a significant role for GCN2 in proteasome inhibitor-induced cell death in human pancreatic cancer cells (M. White, manuscript under revision). Therefore, the metabolic and molecular determinants of susceptibility to this mechanism await further characterization.

11.4 Determinants of Proteasome Inhibitor Sensitivity

If proteasome inhibitors kill cancer cells via proteotoxicity, then molecular features that enhance proteotoxicity should be associated with drug sensitivity. The argument that high-level immunoglobulin secretion underlies the relative sensitivity of MM cells has been outlined above, but there are other cancer-specific features that also appear to be involved. Overall, these mechanisms tend to be associated with increased translation and/or resistance to eIF2α-mediated translational arrest. These mechanisms could determine the "therapeutic window" that allows proteasome inhibitors to kill certain cancer cells at doses that do not cause excessive toxicity to normal tissues.

11.4.1 Abnormal Control of Translation

Mutations and DNA copy number alterations that cause abnormal activation of the PI-3 kinase/AKT/mTOR pathway are among the most common molecular abnormalities in human cancer. The increased translation caused by these alterations probably increases cellular dependence on protein quality control mechanisms and therefore renders cancer cells vulnerable to proteasome inhibition. Similarly, Myc overexpression dramatically increases baseline rates of translation and intrinsic apoptosis [32] and proteasome inhibitor sensitivity [41]. Normal cells tend to be resistant to proteasome inhibitor-induced aggresome formation, a phenotype that is linked to lower baseline translation [42]. Therefore, proliferation markers and mutations that upregulate protein synthesis may prove to be informative predictive biomarkers of proteasome inhibitor clinical activity.

11.4.2 Defective Chaperone Induction

Members of the HSP70 family of protein chaperones play central roles in the response to proteotoxic stress. We recently uncovered a potential contribution of defective HSP72 induction in the responses of human bladder cancer cells to proteasome inhibitor-induced apoptosis [51]. We used whole genome mRNA expression profiling to compare the proteasome inhibitor-induced changes in gene expression in cells that were sensitive or resistant to bortezomib. The results revealed that HSP72 induction was defective in the sensitive cells due to hypermethylation of the HSP72 promoter, and analysis of additional cell lines and primary human tumors identified HSP72 methylation in 40–50 % of cases. HSP72 knockdown increased bortezomib sensitivity in the drug-resistant cells that were linked to lysosomal destabilization [51]. Therefore, HSP72 methylation could serve as a predictive biomarker for bortezomib sensitivity in bladder cancers and other cancers that display this phenotype.

11.4.3 Constitutive eIF2α Phosphorylation

We have found that many solid tumor cell lines display high eIF2α phosphorylation at baseline [26, 33]. In these cells, diverse stimuli that activate the eIF2α protein kinases (including proteasome inhibitors) fail to cause further increases in eIF2α phosphorylation. As a consequence, protein synthesis continues unabated and the cells rapidly accumulate protein aggregates and die. The precise mechanisms leading to this elevated basal eIF2α phosphorylation are still under investigation, but it appears that GCN2 is involved (M. White, manuscript under revision), suggesting the involvement of metabolic stress. It is possible that this basal stress involves some of the same mechanisms (AKT pathway, Myc) that cause deregulated protein synthesis overall.

11.4.4 High Basal ROS Production

Recent studies have demonstrated that cancers have elevated baseline ROS levels, rendering them vulnerable to oxidative stress. As introduced above, oxidative stress also damages proteins and can lead to the accumulation of damaged and misfolded proteins. Elevated ROS levels have also been implicated in mitochondrial injury, which causes pressure on mitochondrial quality control mechanisms involving autophagy (termed "mitophagy"). Therefore, the high basal ROS levels observed in cancer cells place pressures on protein quality control mechanisms and probably contribute to cancer cell susceptibility to proteasome inhibitors. Whether basal ROS levels can be used as a predictive biomarker (e.g., in MM) remains to be determined.

11.5 Determinants of Proteasome Inhibitor Resistance

The recent insights into the cytotoxic mechanisms underlying the tumor growth inhibitory effects of proteasome inhibitors allow for predictions to be made about relevant mechanisms of resistance (Fig. 11.2). Unfortunately, most of the direct evidence that is available comes from studies in human cell lines and other

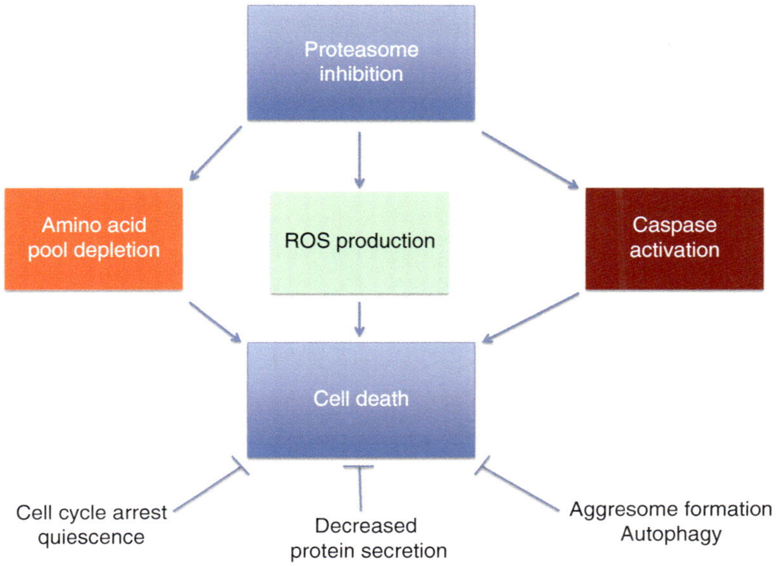

Fig. 11.2 Proteasome inhibitor resistance mechanisms. The cytoprotective effects of the ISR and selection processes probably contribute to de novo and acquired resistance to proteasome inhibitors in cancer. Among the induced mechanisms, growth arrest, translational suppression, and aggresome-mediated protein aggregate clearance via autophagy appear to play particularly important roles. In addition, recent work indicates that proteasome inhibitors select for drug-resistant progenitors characterized by reduced immunoglobulin production. Clinically available HDAC and autophagy inhibitors may represent immediate strategies to overcome some of these resistance mechanisms to enhance therapeutic efficacy

preclinical models rather than refractory tumors from patients. However, the limited data that are available from refractory MM patients support the involvement of the pathways as introduced in Fig. 11.2.

11.5.1 *Quiescence*

As introduced earlier, bortezomib first attracted attention because of its unique potency in the NCI-60 panel of cell lines [1]. Subsequent studies have confirmed that proteasome inhibitors produce strong growth inhibitory effects in MTT assays and other high throughput screens, but the bulk of this activity (especially in solid tumor cell lines) involves cell cycle arrest rather than cell death. This growth arrest is mediated via multiple mechanisms including direct stabilization and accumulation of cell cycle inhibitors (p21, p27) [54–56] as well as phosphorylation of eIF2α and subsequent downregulation of cyclin D [57]. Therefore, most cells are sensitive to these effects, and cell cycle arrest probably generally limits the cytotoxic effects of proteasome inhibitors, and it can lead to interference with conventional chemotherapy if proper scheduling is not employed [54]. One means of bypassing this resistance is to combine proteasome inhibitors with agents like TNF-related apoptosis-inducing ligand (TRAIL) whose effects are not as sensitive to cancer cell proliferation status [58].

11.5.2 Aggresome Formation

As introduced above, the misfolded proteins that accumulate in response to proteasome inhibition are directed to aggresomes for disposal in lysosomes, and this process appears to protect cells from death. Therefore, agents that disrupt aggresome formation will promote proteasome inhibitor-induced cell death. Pan-specific HDAC inhibitors are potent inhibitors of aggresome formation, and they synergize with proteasome inhibitors to induce cancer cell death [42, 43, 47, 48, 59–61]. Several academic groups and companies have developed HDAC6-selective inhibitors, and they also prevent aggresome formation and promote cell death. Early data from clinical trials employing combinations of proteasome and pan HDAC inhibitors have yielded some encouraging results [62]. Likewise, promising clinical activity has been observed in a clinical trial employing the HDAC6-selective inhibitor ACY-1215 (Acetylon, Inc) plus bortezomib in patients with refractory MM (ASH, 2013).

11.5.3 Autophagy

The protein aggregates that are formed in response to proteasome inhibition are redirected to lysosomes for degradation [63]. As discussed above, this process is coordinated by eIF2α phosphorylation and results in a reduction of cytotoxic stress [26, 63]. Therefore, combined inhibition of the proteasome and autophagy results in additive or synergistic cell killing [33, 64]. Importantly, although combinations of proteasome and autophagy inhibitors induce apoptosis, apoptosis is not required for cell death [33]. Combination therapy with bortezomib plus hydroxychloroquine (an antimalarial autophagy inhibitor) was well tolerated and led to growth inhibition in xenografts in vivo [65]. Given that HDAC inhibitors are also thought to disrupt autophagy-mediated aggregate clearance, it will be interesting to determine whether HDAC or autophagy inhibitors produce stronger tumor growth inhibitory effects in head-to-head evaluations.

11.5.4 Decreased ER Stress

As discussed above, proteasome inhibitor sensitivity correlated with baseline immunoglobulin production in MM cell lines, whereas enforced overexpression of immunoglobulin promoted cell death [18, 19]. An elegant recent study illustrated the importance of reduced immunoglobulin production in MM resistance to proteasome inhibitors and identified a novel molecular mechanism that mediated these effects [66]. Knockdown of Xbp-1s, a transcription factor that serves as a central component of one of the 3 arms of the unfolded protein response, produced proteasome inhibitor resistance in MM cells. The effects were not associated with effects of Xbp-1s on ER stress but rather to its role in promoting immunoglobulin production during B cell differentiation. Importantly, proteasome inhibitor-resistant Xbp-1s-B cell progenitors in MM patients who developed resistance to proteasome inhibitors. The authors failed to observe a variety of other candidate resistance mechanisms that had been identified in preclinical studies, underscoring the importance of studying acquired resistance within the context of carefully designed clinical trials.

11.6 Summary and Future Directions

Proteasome inhibitors rank among the most successful targeted agents developed to date, and they have completely changed the natural history of disease progression in patients with multiple myeloma. The molecular mechanisms underlying their actions are becoming clearer, and with this information new predictions can be made about strategies that could synergize with proteasome inhibitors to promote cell death. Although strategies to target HDACs and autophagy are already clinically available, it will be much more challenging to develop strategies to target proteasome inhibitor-induced cell cycle arrest, which may be the most common de novo and acquired proteasome inhibitor resistance mechanism in cancer. Likewise, it may be necessary to develop a completely different approach to target the Xbp-1s-progenitor population that emerges in proteasome inhibitor-refractory MM and possibly mantle cell lymphomas.

Another challenge for the future will be to develop active proteasome inhibitor-based combinations for solid tumor therapy. This effort will hopefully be informed by the large-scale genomic efforts that are being led by The Cancer Genome Atlas and other private groups. We recently completed a clinical trial with bortezomib plus gemcitabine and doxorubicin in patients with refractory, metastatic bladder cancer and observed objective clinical responses in over half of the patients. To our knowledge, this is the first active proteasome inhibitor-based clinical trial in any solid tumor, and we are initiating genomic studies to characterize the molecular profiles of drug sensitivity and resistance in depth. We are also planning a follow-up to this trial, this time employing the next-generation proteasome inhibitor ixazomib [67].

References

1. Adams J, Palombella VJ, Sausville EA, Johnson J, Destree A, Lazarus DD et al (1999) Proteasome inhibitors: a novel class of potent and effective antitumor agents. Cancer Res 59(11):2615–2622, Epub 1999/06/11
2. Hideshima T, Chauhan D, Richardson P, Mitsiades C, Mitsiades N, Hayashi T et al (2002) NF-kappa B as a therapeutic target in multiple myeloma. J Biol Chem 277(19):16639–16647, Epub 2002/03/02

3. Williams SA, McConkey DJ (2003) The proteasome inhibitor bortezomib stabilizes a novel active form of p53 in human LNCaP-Pro5 prostate cancer cells. Cancer Res 63(21): 7338–7344, Epub 2003/11/13
4. Sunwoo JB, Chen Z, Dong G, Yeh N, Crowl Bancroft C, Sausville E et al (2001) Novel proteasome inhibitor PS-341 inhibits activation of nuclear factor-kappa B, cell survival, tumor growth, and angiogenesis in squamous cell carcinoma. Clin Cancer Res 7(5):1419–28, Epub 2001/05/15
5. Nawrocki ST, Bruns CJ, Harbison MT, Bold RJ, Gotsch BS, Abbruzzese JL et al (2002) Effects of the proteasome inhibitor PS-341 on apoptosis and angiogenesis in orthotopic human pancreatic tumor xenografts. Mol Cancer Ther 1(14):1243–1253, Epub 2003/01/09
6. Zhu K, Chan W, Heymach J, Wilkinson M, McConkey DJ (2009) Control of HIF-1alpha expression by eIF2 alpha phosphorylation-mediated translational repression. Cancer Res 69(5):1836–1843, Epub 2009/02/27
7. Williams S, Pettaway C, Song R, Papandreou C, Logothetis C, McConkey DJ (2003) Differential effects of the proteasome inhibitor bortezomib on apoptosis and angiogenesis in human prostate tumor xenografts. Mol Cancer Ther 2(9):835–843, Epub 2003/10/14
8. Adams J (2004) The development of proteasome inhibitors as anticancer drugs. Cancer Cell 5(5):417–421, Epub 2004/05/18
9. Orlowski RZ, Stinchcombe TE, Mitchell BS, Shea TC, Baldwin AS, Stahl S et al (2002) Phase I trial of the proteasome inhibitor PS-341 in patients with refractory hematologic malignancies. J Clin Oncol 20(22):4420–4427, Epub 2002/11/15
10. Richardson PG, Barlogie B, Berenson J, Singhal S, Jagannath S, Irwin D et al (2003) A phase 2 study of bortezomib in relapsed, refractory myeloma. N Engl J Med 348(26):2609–2617, Epub 2003/06/27
11. Twombly R (2003) First proteasome inhibitor approved for multiple myeloma. J Natl Cancer Inst 95(12):845, Epub 2003/06/19
12. Kane RC, Bross PF, Farrell AT, Pazdur R (2003) Velcade: U.S. FDA approval for the treatment of multiple myeloma progressing on prior therapy. Oncologist 8(6):508–513
13. Kuhn DJ, Chen Q, Voorhees PM, Strader JS, Shenk KD, Sun CM et al (2007) Potent activity of carfilzomib, a novel, irreversible inhibitor of the ubiquitin-proteasome pathway, against preclinical models of multiple myeloma. Blood 110(9):3281–3290, Epub 2007/06/27
14. Chauhan D, Catley L, Li G, Podar K, Hideshima T, Velankar M et al (2005) A novel orally active proteasome inhibitor induces apoptosis in multiple myeloma cells with mechanisms distinct from Bortezomib. Cancer Cell 8(5):407–419, Epub 2005/11/16
15. Katsnelson A (2012) Next-generation proteasome inhibitor approved in multiple myeloma. Nat Biotechnol 30(11):1011–1012, Epub 2012/11/10
16. Herndon TM, Deisseroth A, Kaminskas E, Kane RC, Koti KM, Rothmann MD et al (2013) U.S. Food and Drug Administration approval: carfilzomib for the treatment of multiple myeloma. Clin Cancer Res 19(17):4559–4563
17. Smith MH, Ploegh HL, Weissman JS (2011) Road to ruin: targeting proteins for degradation in the endoplasmic reticulum. Science 334(6059):1086–1090, Epub 2011/11/26
18. Obeng EA, Carlson LM, Gutman DM, Harrington WJ Jr, Lee KP, Boise LH (2006) Proteasome inhibitors induce a terminal unfolded protein response in multiple myeloma cells. Blood 107(12):4907–4916, Epub 2006/03/02
19. Schewe DM, Aguirre-Ghiso JA (2009) Inhibition of eIF2alpha dephosphorylation maximizes bortezomib efficiency and eliminates quiescent multiple myeloma cells surviving proteasome inhibitor therapy. Cancer Res 69(4):1545–1552, Epub 2009/02/05
20. Meister S, Schubert U, Neubert K, Herrmann K, Burger R, Gramatzki M et al (2007) Extensive immunoglobulin production sensitizes myeloma cells for proteasome inhibition. Cancer Res 67(4):1783–1792, Epub 2007/02/20
21. Hightower LE (1991) Heat shock, stress proteins, chaperones, and proteotoxicity. Cell 66(2):191–197, Epub 1991/07/26
22. Morimoto RI (2011) The heat shock response: systems biology of proteotoxic stress in aging and disease. Cold Spring Harb Symp Quant Biol 76:91–9, Epub 2012/03/01

23. Morimoto RI (1993) Cells in stress: transcriptional activation of heat shock genes. Science 259(5100):1409–1410, Epub 1993/03/05
24. Westerheide SD, Morimoto RI (2005) Heat shock response modulators as therapeutic tools for diseases of protein conformation. J Biol Chem 280(39):33097–33100, Epub 2005/08/04
25. Goldberg AL (2003) Protein degradation and protection against misfolded or damaged proteins. Nature 426(6968):895–899, Epub 2003/12/20
26. McConkey DJ, White M, Yan W (2012) HDAC inhibitor modulation of proteotoxicity as a therapeutic approach in cancer. Adv Cancer Res 116:131–163, Epub 2012/10/24
27. Harding HP, Novoa I, Zhang Y, Zeng H, Wek R, Schapira M et al (2000) Regulated translation initiation controls stress-induced gene expression in mammalian cells. Mol Cell 6(5): 1099–1108, Epub 2000/12/07
28. Harding HP, Zhang Y, Bertolotti A, Zeng H, Ron D (2000) Perk is essential for translational regulation and cell survival during the unfolded protein response. Mol Cell 5(5):897–904, Epub 2000/07/06
29. Harding HP, Zhang Y, Ron D (1999) Protein translation and folding are coupled by an endoplasmic-reticulum-resident kinase. Nature 397(6716):271–274, Epub 1999/02/04
30. Shi Y, Vattem KM, Sood R, An J, Liang J, Stramm L et al (1998) Identification and characterization of pancreatic eukaryotic initiation factor 2 alpha-subunit kinase, PEK, involved in translational control. Mol Cell Biol 18(12):7499–7509, Epub 1998/11/20
31. Evan G, Harrington E, Fanidi A, Land H, Amati B, Bennett M (1994) Integrated control of cell proliferation and cell death by the c-myc oncogene. Philos Trans R Soc Lond B Biol Sci 345(1313):269–275, Epub 1994/08/30
32. Harrington EA, Fanidi A, Evan GI (1994) Oncogenes and cell death. Curr Opin Genet Dev 4(1):120–129, Epub 1994/02/01
33. Zhu K, Dunner K Jr, McConkey DJ (2010) Proteasome inhibitors activate autophagy as a cytoprotective response in human prostate cancer cells. Oncogene 29(3):451–462, Epub 2009/11/03
34. Talloczy Z, Jiang W, Virgin HW 4th, Leib DA, Scheuner D, Kaufman RJ et al (2002) Regulation of starvation- and virus-induced autophagy by the eIF2alpha kinase signaling pathway. Proc Natl Acad Sci U S A 99(1):190–5, Epub 2002/01/05
35. Rouschop KM, van den Beucken T, Dubois L, Niessen H, Bussink J, Savelkouls K et al (2010) The unfolded protein response protects human tumor cells during hypoxia through regulation of the autophagy genes MAP1LC3B and ATG5. J Clin Invest 120(1):127–141, Epub 2009/12/30
36. Jiang HY, Wek RC (2005) Phosphorylation of the alpha-subunit of the eukaryotic initiation factor-2 (eIF2alpha) reduces protein synthesis and enhances apoptosis in response to proteasome inhibition. J Biol Chem 280(14):14189–14202, Epub 2005/02/03
37. Suraweera A, Munch C, Hanssum A, Bertolotti A (2012) Failure of amino acid homeostasis causes cell death following proteasome inhibition. Mol Cell 48(2):242–253, Epub 2012/09/11
38. Nawrocki ST, Carew JS, Dunner K Jr, Boise LH, Chiao PJ, Huang P et al (2005) Bortezomib inhibits PKR-like endoplasmic reticulum (ER) kinase and induces apoptosis via ER stress in human pancreatic cancer cells. Cancer Res 65(24):11510–11519, Epub 2005/12/17
39. Marciniak SJ, Yun CY, Oyadomari S, Novoa I, Zhang Y, Jungreis R et al (2004) CHOP induces death by promoting protein synthesis and oxidation in the stressed endoplasmic reticulum. Genes Dev 18(24):3066–3077, Epub 2004/12/17
40. Yerlikaya A, Kimball SR, Stanley BA (2008) Phosphorylation of eIF2alpha in response to 26S proteasome inhibition is mediated by the haem-regulated inhibitor (HRI) kinase. Biochem J 412(3):579–588, Epub 2008/02/23
41. Nawrocki ST, Carew JS, Maclean KH, Courage JF, Huang P, Houghton JA et al (2008) Myc regulates aggresome formation, the induction of Noxa, and apoptosis in response to the combination of bortezomib and SAHA. Blood 112(7):2917–2926, Epub 2008/07/22
42. Nawrocki ST, Carew JS, Pino MS, Highshaw RA, Andtbacka RH, Dunner K Jr et al (2006) Aggresome disruption: a novel strategy to enhance bortezomib-induced apoptosis in pancreatic cancer cells. Cancer Res 66(7):3773–3781, Epub 2006/04/06

43. Hideshima T, Bradner JE, Wong J, Chauhan D, Richardson P, Schreiber SL et al (2005) Small-molecule inhibition of proteasome and aggresome function induces synergistic antitumor activity in multiple myeloma. Proc Natl Acad Sci U S A 102(24):8567–8572, Epub 2005/06/07
44. Johnston JA, Ward CL, Kopito RR (1998) Aggresomes: a cellular response to misfolded proteins. J Cell Biol 143(7):1883–1898, Epub 1998/12/29
45. Kawaguchi Y, Kovacs JJ, McLaurin A, Vance JM, Ito A, Yao TP (2003) The deacetylase HDAC6 regulates aggresome formation and cell viability in response to misfolded protein stress. Cell 115(6):727–738, Epub 2003/12/17
46. Chandra J (2009) Oxidative stress by targeted agents promotes cytotoxicity in hematologic malignancies. Antioxid Redox Signal 11(5):1123–1137, Epub 2008/11/21
47. Miller CP, Ban K, Dujka ME, McConkey DJ, Munsell M, Palladino M et al (2007) NPI-0052, a novel proteasome inhibitor, induces caspase-8 and ROS-dependent apoptosis alone and in combination with HDAC inhibitors in leukemia cells. Blood 110(1):267–277, Epub 2007/03/16
48. Pei XY, Dai Y, Grant S (2004) Synergistic induction of oxidative injury and apoptosis in human multiple myeloma cells by the proteasome inhibitor bortezomib and histone deacetylase inhibitors. Clin Cancer Res 10(11):3839–3852, Epub 2004/06/03
49. Yu C, Rahmani M, Conrad D, Subler M, Dent P, Grant S (2003) The proteasome inhibitor bortezomib interacts synergistically with histone deacetylase inhibitors to induce apoptosis in Bcr/Abl+ cells sensitive and resistant to STI571. Blood 102(10):3765–3774, Epub 2003/08/02
50. Yu C, Rahmani M, Dent P, Grant S (2004) The hierarchical relationship between MAPK signaling and ROS generation in human leukemia cells undergoing apoptosis in response to the proteasome inhibitor Bortezomib. Exp Cell Res 295(2):555–566, Epub 2004/04/20
51. Qi W, White MC, Choi W, Guo C, Dinney C, McConkey DJ et al (2013) Inhibition of inducible heat shock protein-70 (hsp72) enhances bortezomib-induced cell death in human bladder cancer cells. PLoS One 8(7):e69509, Epub 2013/07/23
52. Sorolla A, Yeramian A, Dolcet X, Perez de Santos AM, Llobet D, Schoenenberger JA et al (2008) Effect of proteasome inhibitors on proliferation and apoptosis of human cutaneous melanoma-derived cell lines. Br J Dermatol 158(3):496–504, Epub 2008/01/22
53. Gu H, Chen X, Gao G, Dong H (2008) Caspase-2 functions upstream of mitochondria in endoplasmic reticulum stress-induced apoptosis by bortezomib in human myeloma cells. Mol Cancer Ther 7(8):2298–2307, Epub 2008/08/30
54. Canfield SE, Zhu K, Williams SA, McConkey DJ (2006) Bortezomib inhibits docetaxel-induced apoptosis via a p21-dependent mechanism in human prostate cancer cells. Mol Cancer Ther 5(8):2043–2050, Epub 2006/08/25
55. Nawrocki ST, Sweeney-Gotsch B, Takamori R, McConkey DJ (2004) The proteasome inhibitor bortezomib enhances the activity of docetaxel in orthotopic human pancreatic tumor xenografts. Mol Cancer Ther 3(1):59–70, Epub 2004/01/30
56. An B, Goldfarb RH, Siman R, Dou QP (1998) Novel dipeptidyl proteasome inhibitors overcome Bcl-2 protective function and selectively accumulate the cyclin-dependent kinase inhibitor p27 and induce apoptosis in transformed, but not normal, human fibroblasts. Cell Death Differ 5(12):1062–1075, Epub 1999/01/23
57. Brewer JW, Diehl JA (2000) PERK mediates cell-cycle exit during the mammalian unfolded protein response. Proc Natl Acad Sci U S A 97(23):12625–12630, Epub 2000/10/18
58. Lashinger LM, Zhu K, Williams SA, Shrader M, Dinney CP, McConkey DJ (2005) Bortezomib abolishes tumor necrosis factor-related apoptosis-inducing ligand resistance via a p21-dependent mechanism in human bladder and prostate cancer cells. Cancer Res 65(11):4902–4908, Epub 2005/06/03
59. Dasmahapatra G, Lembersky D, Son MP, Attkisson E, Dent P, Fisher RI et al (2011) Carfilzomib interacts synergistically with histone deacetylase inhibitors in mantle cell lymphoma cells in vitro and in vivo. Mol Cancer Ther 10(9):1686–1697, Epub 2011/07/14
60. Dasmahapatra G, Lembersky D, Kramer L, Fisher RI, Friedberg J, Dent P et al (2010) The pan-HDAC inhibitor vorinostat potentiates the activity of the proteasome inhibitor carfilzomib in human DLBCL cells in vitro and in vivo. Blood 115(22):4478–4487, Epub 2010/03/18

61. Dai Y, Chen S, Kramer LB, Funk VL, Dent P, Grant S (2008) Interactions between bortezomib and romidepsin and belinostat in chronic lymphocytic leukemia cells. Clin Cancer Res 14(2):549–558, Epub 2008/01/29
62. Millward M, Price T, Townsend A, Sweeney C, Spencer A, Sukumaran S et al (2012) Phase 1 clinical trial of the novel proteasome inhibitor marizomib with the histone deacetylase inhibitor vorinostat in patients with melanoma, pancreatic and lung cancer based on in vitro assessments of the combination. Invest New Drugs 30(6):2303–2317, Epub 2011/11/15
63. Amaravadi RK, Lippincott-Schwartz J, Yin XM, Weiss WA, Takebe N, Timmer W et al (2011) Principles and current strategies for targeting autophagy for cancer treatment. Clin Cancer Res 17(4):654–666, Epub 2011/02/18
64. Ding WX, Ni HM, Gao W, Yoshimori T, Stolz DB, Ron D et al (2007) Linking of autophagy to ubiquitin-proteasome system is important for the regulation of endoplasmic reticulum stress and cell viability. Am J Pathol 171(2):513–524, Epub 2007/07/11
65. Ding WX, Ni HM, Gao W, Chen X, Kang JH, Stolz DB et al (2009) Oncogenic transformation confers a selective susceptibility to the combined suppression of the proteasome and autophagy. Mol Cancer Ther 8(7):2036–2045, Epub 2009/07/09
66. Leung-Hagesteijn C, Erdmann N, Cheung G, Keats JJ, Stewart AK, Reece DE et al (2013) Xbp1s-negative tumor B cells and pre-plasmablasts mediate therapeutic proteasome inhibitor resistance in multiple myeloma. Cancer Cell 24(3):289–304, Epub 2013/09/14
67. Kuhn DJ, Orlowski RZ (2012) The immunoproteasome as a target in hematologic malignancies. Semin Hematol 49(3):258–262, Epub 2012/06/26

Chapter 12
Proteasome Inhibitors Versus E3 Ligase Inhibitors for Cancer Therapy

Michael R. Mattern, Michael J. Eddins, Saket Agarwal, David E. Sterner, Matthew P. Kodrasov, K.G. Suresh Kumar, Jian Wu, and Benjamin Nicholson

Abstract Molecular oncology has the potential to revolutionize cancer treatment owing to its focus on discrete, cancer-selective targets, as evident in the recent success of kinase inhibitors and antibody-based therapies. Because of the heterogeneous nature of cancer, however, not every tumor type can be addressed with an appropriately selective therapy and some respond best to drug combinations that include classical "toxic" agents. The ubiquitin-proteasome pathway, recently harnessed for cancer treatment with the clinical use of "toxic" proteasome inhibitors bortezomib and carfilzomib, affords targets that intuitively are highly selective, exemplified by inhibitors of E3 ligases, the ubiquitin-conjugating enzymes, as well as those that are intuitively nonselective, exemplified by the proteasomal proteases. In the last two decades, anticancer drug development based on these two target classes has proceeded in parallel, with the early results suggesting that the nonselective proteasome is the better target. Lately, however, it has become clear that (1) the "nonselective" proteasome target may be addressed in selective ways and (2) a clearer understanding of the E3 ligase reaction can lead to the design or discovery of efficacious inhibitors. Evidence supporting these notions and implications for cancer treatment going forward will be discussed.

Keywords Proteasome inhibitor • E3 ligase • Drug resistance • Clinical trial • Binding pocket • Cancer pharmacology

M.R. Mattern (✉) • M.J. Eddins • S. Agarwal • D.E. Sterner • M.P. Kodrasov • K.G.S. Kumar
J. Wu • B. Nicholson
Progenra, Inc., 277 Great Valley Parkway, Malvern, PA 19355, USA
e-mail: mattern@progenra.com; eddins@progenra.com; agarwal@progenra.com; sterner@progenra.com; kodrasov@progenra.com; kumar@progenra.com; wu@progenra.com; nicholson@progenra.com

Q.P. Dou (ed.), *Resistance to Proteasome Inhibitors in Cancer*, Resistance to Targeted Anti-Cancer Therapeutics, DOI 10.1007/978-3-319-06752-0_12

Abbreviations

ADME	Absorption distribution, metabolism, excretion
DUB	Deubiquitylating enzyme
ERAD	Endoplasmic reticulum-associated degradation
HDM2	Human variant of MDM2 = murine double minute 2 homologue (an E3 ligase)
IAP	Inhibitor of apoptosis
RING	Really interesting new gene
USP	Ubiquitin-specific protease

12.1 Introduction

Molecularly targeted therapy, according to the National Cancer Institute (National Institutes of Health) dictionary of cancer terms, is a type of medication that blocks the growth of cancer cells by interfering with specific targeted molecules needed for carcinogenesis and tumor growth. In the last two or three decades, this class of therapy has been heralded as the successor to traditional toxicity-based cancer chemotherapy and radiation, directed at all rapidly dividing cells, and it arguably has the potential to deliver anticancer activity with greatly reduced toxicity to the patient. Despite successes with certain kinase inhibitors used against genetically receptive tumors, and with the use of highly specific antibody-based therapies, however, the fact remains that cancer is a heterogeneous collection of hyperproliferative diseases, and oncologists treating patients with available chemical and biological agents have not yet uniformly replaced "toxic" therapies with highly targeted tumor-selective interventions. The lack of a rapid and complete changeover to exclusive use of molecularly targeted therapy is exemplified by the significant component of anticancer drug development currently focused on the ubiquitin-proteasome pathway for cellular protein regulation (Fig. 12.1).

This pathway is now recognized as a useful source of new medicines, following on the success of the proteasome inhibitors bortezomib/Velcade by Takeda/Millennium Pharmaceuticals and more recently, carfilzomib/Kyprolis by Onyx Pharmaceuticals. Inhibition of the proteasome is, in one sense, molecularly targeted therapy, as proteasome inhibitors act on at most three proteolytic enzymes (and perhaps a few additional ancillary enzymes) in the catalytic core of the proteasome. On the other hand, nearly 90 % of the cell's soluble proteins are degraded by the proteasome, suggesting that inhibiting proteasome activity should result in a global (and, perhaps intuitively, devastating) effect on cells. It was difficult early on, in fact, to envision any sort of therapeutic window achievable by administering proteasome inhibitors to patients. Clinical trials with bortezomib (known originally as PS-341), however, would later show that proteasome inhibition was tolerated far better than anticipated ([1]; summarized in [2]). On the other hand, an alternative

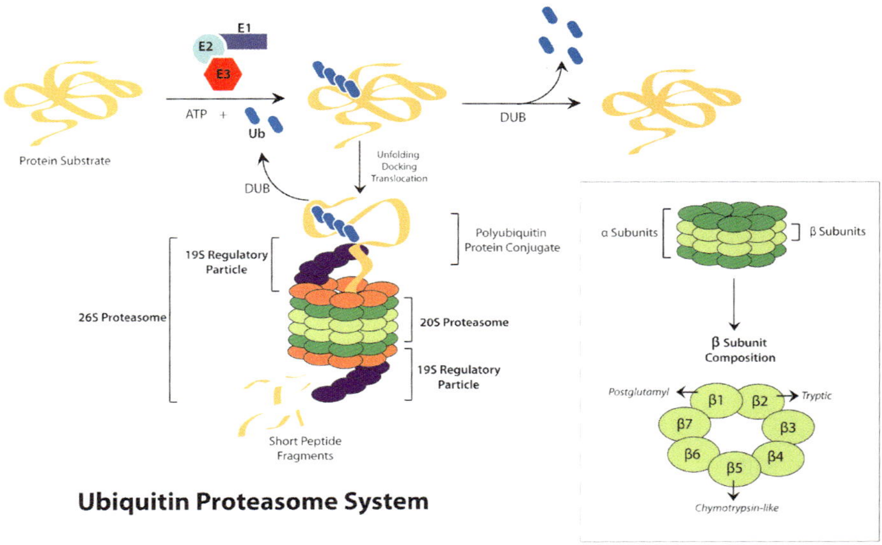

Fig. 12.1 The ubiquitin-proteasome pathway. Targeting of protein substrates by ubiquitin requires the sequential action of three enzymes: ubiquitin is activated by a specific activating enzyme (E1) to yield a ubiquitin-E1-thiolester. Activated ubiquitin is transferred to a carrier protein or "conjugase," E2. Ubiquitin is subsequently transferred by a ligase (E3) and linked by an isopeptide bond to a lysine residue on the substrate protein. After linkage of ubiquitin to the substrate, a polyubiquitin chain is usually formed. Ubiquitinated proteins can be deubiquitinated by specific isopeptidases (DUBs) or can be recognized and processed to short peptide fragments by the 26S proteasome. Proteasomes also contain ubiquitin isopeptidase activity which allows recycling of ubiquitin. Also shown above are the α and β subunits of the 20S proteasome core. β1, β2, and β5 subunits possess trypsin-, chymotrypsin-, and caspase (postglutamyl)-like protease activities, respectively, and are targeted by various clinical and experimental proteasome inhibitors

target class in the pathway, ubiquitin E3 ligases, each of which marks a limited number of substrate proteins for degradation in the proteasome by conjugating them with (poly)ubiquitin chains, were believed to be more promising than the proteasome, as they would spare a small subset of proteins, rather than (at least theoretically) most or all proteins, from degradation (Fig. 12.2). If the proteins spared from degradation by E3 ligase inhibitors happened to be tumor suppressors (e.g., p53), a selective anticancer effect upon treating with appropriate ligase inhibitors was intuitive. Because there are approximately 600 ubiquitin E3 ligases in humans, each with a limited number of substrates and several with biochemical or genetic links to various cancers, it seemed reasonable that at least a few ligases would be ideal anticancer targets. Since these early days of limited expectations for proteasome inhibitors and great hopes for E3 ligase inhibitors, the relatively "unselective" proteasome inhibitors have undergone extensive clinical evaluation, resulting in two approvals so far by the USFDA [3, 4], while their more "selective" counterparts, inhibitors of ubiquitin E3 ligases, have struggled in development by comparison (although several

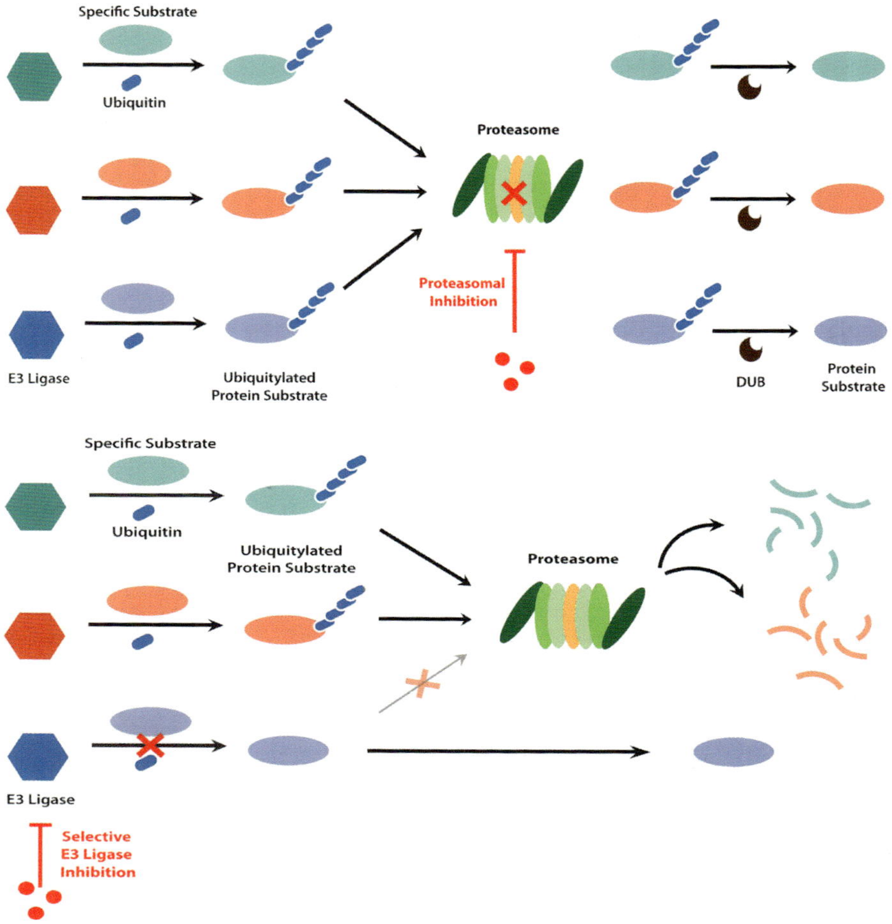

Fig. 12.2 Basis for purported selectivity of inhibition of E3 ligase inhibitors as compared to protease inhibitors. *Top*: Inhibition of proteasome activity and removal of polyubiquitin tags by DUBs regenerates all three ligase-targeted protein substrates, essentially prolonging their cellular half-lives. *Bottom*: Inhibition of one of the three ligases shown spares its substrate from ubiquitination and proteasomal degradation. Degradation of the other substrates is unaffected

new inhibitors are currently in preclinical development or Phase I clinical trials). While FDA approval had been granted to one ligase-targeting drug class (thalidomide and analogues lenalidomide and pomalidomide) as of 2013, its link to the E3 ligase target was established subsequent to the initiation of clinical development of the class [5].

The foregoing describes the current situation, if perhaps in a somewhat simplified manner. In the following, potential reasons for this apparent paradox will be examined and the current state of proteasome inhibitor and ligase-based anticancer drug discovery will be reviewed, leading to projections based on recent developments in these two paths to ubiquitin-based cancer treatment. The developmental strategy for proteasome inhibitors is proceeding in a rather conventional manner, addressing issues of side effects and resistance [3]. On the ligase side, it is acknowledged that the really interesting new gene (RING) E3 ligases (a majority of the identified ligase anticancer targets) are really not enzymes in the classical sense, perhaps precluding the identification of pharmacologically useful molecules in high-throughput screening (or rational design) efforts to discover "catalytic inhibitors" of ubiquitylation, and supporting the continued development of non-catalytic discovery strategies, which has been initiated and has actually led to some promising results.

12.2 Proteasome Inhibitors

12.2.1 The Proteasome

Cellular proteins are degraded by two major types of endoprotease activity, which take place in lysosomes or proteasomes. Proteasomal degradation, occurring in both the cytoplasm and the nucleus of cells, is the major route for hydrolysis of most soluble short-lived regulatory proteins and serves as a mechanism for controlling protein half-lives as well as a means of quality control, the latter by eliminating misfolded proteins [6–8]. The proteasome is a huge cylindrical intracellular structure consisting of a catalytic 20S core (cylinder) and regulatory units (19S) at each end appearing as bases with lids. The 20S core is made from precise structural arrangements of four rings containing seven subunits each (Fig. 12.1). The two outer rings are composed of regulatory subunits called α, which are related to gate opening, and the inner two of β, or catalytic subunits, which include caspase-like (β1 subunit), trypsin-like (β2 subunit), and chymotrypsin-like (β5 subunit) proteolytic activities [9]. The regulatory "lids" detect polyubiquitylated proteins and, in a series of further molecular recognition, deubiquitylation, and unfolding events performed by various constituent proteins facilitate the entry of the "prepared" protein into the 20S core for degradation [6]. A second type of proteasome—the immunoproteasome—has been identified in cells that are exposed to inflammatory cytokines (e.g., TNFα, interferon), are of hematopoietic lineage, or are neoplastic [10]. The immunoproteasome differs from the classical ("constitutive") proteasome in its β catalytic subunits responsible for caspase-, trypsin-, and chymotrypsin-like protease activities, respectively; the corresponding immunoproteasome subunits are named β1i, β2i, and β5i or, alternatively, LMP2, MECL1, and LMP7 [11–13]. Regulatory ends of immunoproteasomes are 11S rather than 19S structures. While both proteasome classes receive polyubiquitylated proteins and degrade these tagged substrates by endoprotease activity, the immunoproteasome is enabled by virtue of its altered β subunit structures to catalyze proteolysis in a specific manner leading to the production of antigenic peptides [12] and perhaps to perform additional directed proteolysis functions [14].

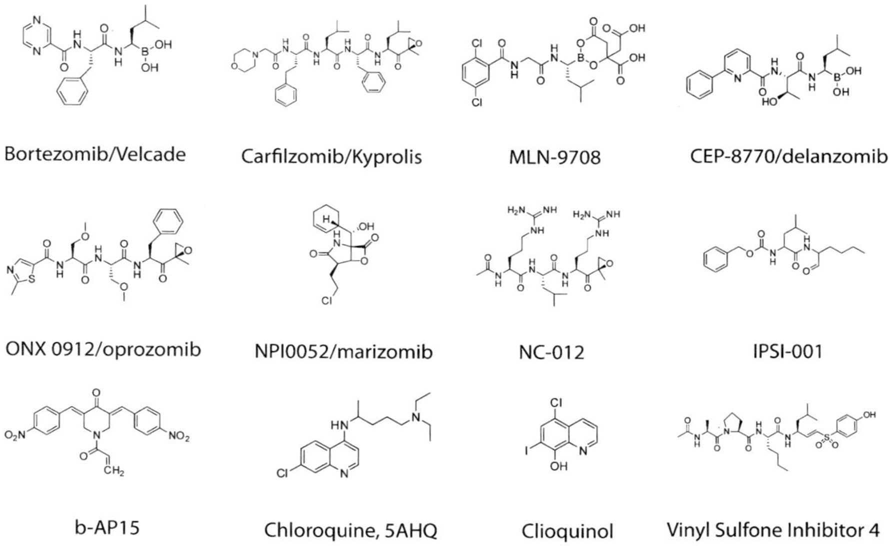

Fig. 12.3 Structures of selected proteasome inhibitors (see text)

12.2.2 Success and Limitations of Proteasome Inhibitors

12.2.2.1 Bortezomib

The first (and until 2012 the only) clinically approved proteasome inhibitor, bortezomib (VELCADE®), a synthetic peptidyl boronate developed by Millennium Pharmaceuticals (Takeda) (Fig. 12.3) [15, 16], was initially approved as an injectable treatment for refractory relapsed multiple myeloma and, shortly afterward, for first-line treatment of multiple myeloma and treatment of relapsed mantle cell lymphoma [4, 17, 18]. Bortezomib binds reversibly to the β5 subunit of the 20S core (Fig. 12.1) and inhibits the threonine protease activity of the chymotrypsin-like subunit, the rate-limiting step of proteolysis, by forming a complex between its boronic acid group and the threonine hydroxyl group at the catalytic site [6, 19]. Bortezomib is active as a single agent or as a component of combination therapy protocols; impressive progression-free survival has been achieved, but despite these therapeutic gains, enabled in part by the use of proteasome inhibitors such as bortezomib and the recently approved carfilzomib (KYPROLIS®) (for relapsed multiple myeloma), multiple myeloma remains incurable [3, 17].

The cellular response to proteasome inhibition, resulting in accumulation of numerous proteins normally destined for removal by degradation in the proteasome, is characterized by both antitumor efficacy and toxicity. Proteasome inhibitors are thus toxic chemotherapy agents, as are most anticancer drugs, including those that are generally considered to be targeted therapeutics. Bortezomib has produced side effects, which differ in nature and intensity among patients. Its two major toxicities are peripheral neuropathy and fatigue, and other toxicities common to anticancer chemotherapeutic agents have been reported, in addition to bone and muscle pain [17]. The therapeutic window for the first proteasome inhibitors is not huge, as dose-limiting toxicities are evident just above the treatment dose, and therapeutic strategies for second-generation proteasome inhibitors are aimed at increasing it.

12.2.2.2 Proteasome Inhibitors Kill Cancer Cells Selectively

The anticancer mechanism of proteasome inhibitors is multifactorial, since the cellular levels of a considerable number of proteins are altered by blocking proteasomal degradation (reviewed in [20]). Some, but likely not all, of the relevant molecular mechanisms have been described. Many currently used anticancer drugs attack oncogenic targets that either stimulate growth/cell cycling or block apoptosis. It was established early on that proteasomal activity is necessary for both processing of the precursor of the pro-survival (antiapoptotic) protein NFκB and activation of NFκB [21]. Thus, treatment with proteasome inhibitors should induce or augment apoptosis. Results similar to those of Hideshima et al., who found an approximately three log difference between tumor-derived cells and normal plasma cells in their sensitivity to bortezomib-induced apoptosis [22], made proteasome inhibitors clinically attractive. Several elements of the antitumor mechanism of proteasome inhibitors have been studied, and many of these are related to either extrinsic (mediated by death receptors) or intrinsic (mitochondria-dependent) apoptotic pathways.

As an example of extrinsic pathways, bortezomib, in appropriate experimental therapeutic combinations, has been shown to facilitate FADD-induced activation of caspase 8, thereby sensitizing tumor cells to extrinsic apoptosis [23, 24]. Some of the earliest in vitro experiments performed with bortezomib demonstrated that the proteasome inhibitor also affects the intrinsic mitochondrial Bcl-2 pathway in a manner that results in the activation of caspase 9 [25, 26]. More recently, additional molecular mechanisms have been identified whereby proteasome inhibitor treatment augments apoptosis, e.g., via the apoptosis-inducing tumor suppressor p53 and its activated gene products such as p21; as is usual in cancer biology, however, there are still areas of uncertainty regarding mechanism and some contradictory literature reports [2, 6, 27]. Nevertheless, with respect to p53 wild-type tumors it is clear that sparing p53 from degradation in the proteasome would be expected to contribute to the net increase in apoptosis seen after bortezomib treatment. Because of the multiple proapoptotic (or anti-antiapoptotic) effects demonstrated by proteasome inhibitors, bortezomib has been used clinically in combination with agents that induce apoptosis [3].

12.2.2.3 Proteasome Inhibitors and Autophagy

Cells undergoing stress are also subject to autophagy, an alternative to the ubiquitin-proteasome pathway for effecting degradation, wherein they sequester large parts of their cytoplasm in vacuoles (autophagosomes) prior to lysosomal degradation of the confined proteins. It seems logical that the two major pathways for removal of abnormal proteins and protein aggregates would share common features or be coordinated in some fashion, and in vitro evidence links the two pathways [28]. In addition, there are reports that lysine 29 and lysine 63 ubiquitin linkages may target substrates for autophagic, rather than proteasomal degradation [29, 30]. In animal models with impaired autophagy, protein inclusions are enriched in ubiquitin, but it is not yet known whether their presence signifies that under normal circumstances, (1) the ubiquitin tag facilitates degradation of the protein aggregates, (2) ubiquitylated proteins are trapped in inclusions in which they are then degraded by autophagy, and/or (3) the ubiquitin tag plays a non-degradative role in autophagy [31]. It is known that ubiquitin has a recruiting function in autophagosome formation and may interact with proteins that recognize cargo molecules or have other roles in autophagy, but whether this function of ubiquitin is sufficient is unclear at present [31]. In stress conditions autophagy can be regarded as a cellular defense mechanism. In addition to its multiple proapoptotic effects, bortezomib has been reported to increase autophagy [32], so treatment with a combination of bortezomib and an inhibitor of autophagy may be beneficial. Clinical studies should answer this question in the near future.

12.2.2.4 Resistance to Proteasome Inhibitors

A principal limitation to the ability of antitumor agents to be generally curative is the development of resistance. Because the complex cellular response to proteasome inhibition involves numerous molecular pathways, resistance could arise through the alteration of a variety of proteins that are critical to these pathways. Resistance is being studied using resistant cultured cell lines as well as gene profiling of patients. In the case of bortezomib, clinical experience shows evidence of primary resistance (refractory disease in naïve patients) as well as secondary resistance (developing during the course of treatment) [6, 13].

Resistance must be considered in the context of the demonstrated cytotoxic effects of bortezomib. Initially, proteins left un-degraded owing to proteasome inhibition accumulate in the ER, where they generate a stress response [2]. The unfolded protein response (UPR) is activated initially to help the cell survive the stress generated by ER unfolded/misfolded protein overload; this complex series of molecular events is coordinated by activated transcription of specific genes, general reduction in the initiation of translation, and altered translation patterns [33]. Expression of chaperone proteins is increased to increase the folding capacity of the ER, and ER-associated protein degradation (ERAD) is activated to relieve proteotoxic stress [34]. While the molecular mechanism has not yet been completely elucidated, it is clear that the initial stress response to treatment with proteasome inhibitors is subverted to an apoptotic response that is responsible for the antitumor effect and various side effects.

Several potential mechanisms of bortezomib resistance have been identified, based on both its inhibition of the catalytic activity of the proteasome and the extensive, multicomponent signal transduction network through which it exerts its cellular, antitumor effects. Since the inhibitor binds the β5 proteasomal subunit, mutations at the binding site of β5 would be expected to impart resistance; this type of mutation has been found in cultured cell lines made resistant to bortezomib [13, 35–37]. Resistance can also originate downstream of the proteasome from a multitude of proteasome-dependent growth inhibitory pathways. Because bortezomib induces apoptosis, modulation of proteins that control the induced apoptotic events (either genetically [38] or epigenetically [39]) can desensitize cells to treatment with the proteasome inhibitor ([40]; reviewed in [2, 35]). Another common mechanism of resistance to anticancer agents of various chemotypes is their binding to transporter proteins for efflux from the cell. Numerous in vitro studies of expression of P-glycoprotein and other transporters in bortezomib-resistant cell lines, cross resistance of these resistant cell lines to known MDR drugs, and binding of bortezomib to multidrug transporters suggest, with the exception of one report [41], that MDR is at best a minor mechanism of resistance to this proteasome inhibitor ([42–45], reviewed in [35]). It is interesting to note, in addition, that a clinical retrospective study of multiple myeloma patient polymorphisms in P-glycoprotein-1 and MRP1 demonstrated that selected drug transporter SNPs were associated with extended progression-free survival in patients given bortezomib plus pegylated liposomal doxorubicin (but not in those given bortezomib alone); the authors speculate that these polymorphisms may be useful for patient selection strategies [46].

Prospective clinical studies with bortezomib and the newer proteasome inhibitors will determine the relative significance of MDR in proteasome inhibitor resistance. In fact, a clear picture of all of the bortezomib (and other proteasome inhibitor) resistance mechanisms actually encountered in the clinical setting is necessary to address resistance successfully.

12.2.3 Next-Generation Proteasome Inhibitors

12.2.3.1 Proteasome Inhibitors in Clinical Trial

The clinical standard of treatment for proteasome inhibitors was established by bortezomib, a *reversible* inhibitor of the *constitutive* proteasome. Several properties of the mechanism of action of bortezomib against proteasome activity have been employed as starting points in the development of second-generation inhibitors (Table 12.1). In addition to carfilzomib [47], which was approved in 2012, several small molecules are currently undergoing clinical evaluation for cancer or are in preclinical development (Table 12.1; Fig 12.3). MLN-9708 [48] and CEP-18770 [49], which are reversible inhibitors like bortezomib, have been developed for the oral route of administration, which may improve patient experience even though they may not be superior to bortezomib in therapeutic index or susceptibility to resistance. Other next-generation proteasome inhibitors currently undergoing clinical evaluation (Table 12.1) may have improved therapeutic indices and/or the potential

Table 12.1 Proteasome inhibitors currently approved by the FDA or in development

Compound	Mechanism	Preferred site	Route	Phase
Bortezomib/VELCADE®/ (PS-341)	Reversible catalytic	Chymotrypsin-like β5 subunit	*iv*	Approved by FDA 2003
Carfilzomib/Kyprolis® (PR-171)	Irreversible catalytic	Chymotrypsin-like β5 subunit	*iv*	Approved by FDA 2012
MLN-9708	Reversible catalytic	Chymotrypsin-like β5 subunit	*iv, po*	Phase I/II
CEP-18770/delanzomib	Reversible catalytic	Chymotrypsin-like β5 subunit	*iv, po*	Phase I/II
NPI0052/marizomib	Irreversible catalytic	Chymotrypsin-like, trypsin-like β5, β2 subunits	*iv*	Phase I
ONX 0912/oprozomib	Irreversible catalytic	Chymotrypsin-like β5 subunit	*po*	Phase I
Clioquinol	Binds metals (Cu)	Unknown; may be several	*po*	Phase I
Inhibitors 4, 5	Irreversible catalytic	Caspase-like (β1, β1i); selective for β1i		Preclinical
NC-002, NC-012, NC-022	Irreversible catalytic	Trypsin-like; equipotent vs. β2, β2i		Preclinical
IPSI-001	Catalytic	Specifically targets immunoproteasome β1i subunit		Preclinical
Chloroquine, 5AHQ	Allosteric; α and β subunits	noncompetitive		Preclinical
b-AP15	Proteasome associated DUBs UCH-L5, USP14	Inhibits 19S regulatory protein DUB activity		Preclinical

to be active in bortezomib-resistant patients. To address these clinical challenges, various strategies have emerged, represented by molecules currently in cancer trials. The first strategy addresses the binding mode. The recently approved epoxyketone carfilzomib binds irreversibly to the chymotrypsin-like β5 site, in contrast to bortezomib, which binds this site reversibly. Carfilzomib is a more potent inhibitor than bortezomib, which may translate to an improved therapeutic index [47, 50]. A second strategy takes advantage of proteasome heterogeneity. In addition to the classical ("constitutive") proteasome, which is present in all cells, some cells contain a second proteasome (the immunoproteasome) that differs from the constitutive proteasome in the β1, β2, and β5 catalytic subunits (denoted as β1i, β2i, and β5i for the immunoproteasome) and contains an 11S regulatory particle [19]. An orally bioavailable truncated version of carfilzomib, ONX 0912/oprozomib, is in Phase I clinical trial and should work similarly to carfilzomib [51]. Another example of the potential capacity to overcome resistance to bortezomib is the irreversible Phase I proteasome inhibitor NPI-0052, which inhibits trypsin-like *as well as* chymotrypsin-like protease activity [40]. Recently, a third strategy for overcoming resistance, the use of mechanisms that are distinct from those involving inhibition of proteasomal protease activity, is represented by a class of inhibitor that may work by binding metals that are essential to the proteasome; clioquinol, which works by this mechanism, advanced to a Phase I clinical trial [52, 53]. Additional properties of bortezomib that could be addressed in developing improved proteasome inhibitors include its inability to cross the blood–brain barrier and its rapid metabolism [54].

12.2.3.2 Experimental (Preclinical) Proteasome Inhibitors

Proteasome inhibitors are currently in preclinical development to improve upon the therapeutic index and tumor efficacy spectrum of bortezomib as well as its susceptibility to resistance. A recently described preclinical immunoproteasome inhibitor, IPSI-001, targets the β1i subunit of the immunoproteasome with a high degree of selectivity and, like carfilzomib, overcomes resistance to bortezomib [55]. As one would expect, novel mechanisms are also being explored in preclinical studies of new proteasome inhibitors. Secondary to an observation in the Goldberg laboratory suggesting that allosteric interactions among the proteasome subunits may afford new therapeutic strategies [56], Kisselev et al. developed inhibitors that selectively bind β1 ([57]) or β2 ([58]) subunits and exert allosteric effects. β2 subunit selective inhibitors have been shown to sensitize myeloma cells to β5 subunit site inhibitors such as bortezomib; in combination with β1 subunit inhibitors, they inhibit cell growth in the absence of β5 subunit inhibitors [58]. Chloroquine weakly inhibits proteasome activity by a novel allosteric mechanism and more potent substituted chloroquines such as 5AHQ may offer clinical potential (Table 12.1 [19, 59]). Allosteric proteasome inhibitors similar to these will likely enter clinical trials within the next few years. Another novel proteasome inhibitor target, deubiquitylating activity contained in the 19S regulatory cap of the proteasome, has recently been identified using the small-molecule b-AP15, found in a functional screen [60]. b-AP15 inhibits the deubiquitylating activity of the 19S-associated deubiquitylating enzymes (DUBs) UCH-L5 and USP14, blocking proteasome activity.

These studies with new classes of proteasome inhibitor show that the global effect of proteasome inhibition, found clinically to be tolerated in patients and to be therapeutic, can be replicated via novel targets in hopes of improving upon the profile of bortezomib and other first-generation inhibitors.

12.3 E3 Ligase Inhibitors

While a considerable compendium of clinical data on response, resistance, and other factors permits an assessment of the effectiveness of proteasome inhibitors in patients with multiple myeloma and other cancers, E3 ligase inhibitors, with the possible exception of the immunomodulatory drugs (IMiDs) such as lenalidomide, cannot be evaluated in this fashion (and, in fact, the IMiDs were not developed as ligase inhibitors). In this sense, proteasome inhibitors and ligase inhibitors cannot be compared side by side. Instead, in this section, the preclinical profiles of inhibitors of various E3 ligases associated with cancer will be examined for indications of how they might perform in the clinic.

12.3.1 E3 Ligases Are Complicated Drug Targets

E3 ligase enzymes comprise a superfamily which can be divided by mechanistic criteria into enzymes which (1) bind the ubiquitylation substrate and facilitate transfer of ubiquitin from the E2 to the substrate (RING ligases) or (2) receive ubiquitin from E2 and transfer it to the substrate (HECT ligases) (Fig. 12.1 [61]). Therapeutically interesting E3 ligases contain binding domains that interact with E2 enzymes and substrate proteins as well as ubiquitin; they catalyze ubiquitylation of limited subsets of target proteins that can include the ligases themselves (autoubiquitylation) [62, 63]. Despite the availability of crystal structures, however, details of the relevant molecular mechanisms of E3 enzymes are incompletely understood. Some progress has been made in the search for E3 ligase inhibitors with anticancer potential (summarized below), but the traditional approaches for identifying inhibitors of ubiquitylation mediated by E3s relevant to cancer have not yet been successful. Because each of the several hundred E3 ligases determines which limited subset of proteins are ubiquitylated in concert with E1 and E2 (Fig. 12.1), selective inhibition of a given E3 ligase should result in a selective pharmacological action with relatively few side effects (Fig. 12.2).

12.3.2 New Paradigms for Discovering and Developing E3 Ligase Inhibitors

Results of early attempts by various pharmaceutical companies to identify novel, selective E3 inhibitors were disappointing; it was noted in 2005 that the early history of E3 ligase-based drug discovery had not been a chronicle of unparalleled success, and possible reasons for this failure were elaborated [64]. One of these, a pleiotropic effect argument—i.e., that treatment with a ligase inhibitor which can in theory affect several targets (albeit a limited number) would lead to undesired cellular consequences compromising therapeutic utility—is perhaps less compelling today than at that time, given the demonstrated success of multi-specific kinase inhibitors and the increased ability, with the use of in vivo biomarkers, to determine the actual physiological effect, out of numerous hypothetical ones, of a small-molecule effector [65, 66]. Perhaps more relevant than complex cellular effects is the notion that it is not clear how to target the E3 enzyme, which is linked with E2, a substrate, and ancillary or scaffold proteins in the physiological setting.

Before reviewing the E3 ligase-acting compounds that have finally been put into clinical development for cancer treatment, it is perhaps useful to consider alternative approaches to "drugging" the E3 ligase target, which have led, or promise to lead to clinically viable therapeutic molecules. Two such approaches, one at early stages and the other somewhat more mature, will be discussed. The first approach entails the use of biophysical assays that identify, in a high-throughput fashion, compounds which bind to E3 ligases (or fragments thereof) [67, 68]. The second approach, which has generated actual clinical candidates in the past several years, is the identification of molecules that inhibit binding of E3 ligases to their protein substrates (protein–protein interactions) [69].

12.3.2.1 Assessment of Ligand-Protein Binding in Biophysical Assays

The endpoint of the catalytic reaction assay, ubiquitylation, reflects the complex transfer of ubiquitin from E1 to E2 to a substrate selected by E3, and obliteration of this endpoint by a small molecule may or may not be due to its effect on E3. Alternative approaches to a biochemical endpoint (ubiquitylation) assay model include biophysical assays (Fig. 12.4). As one example, thermal shift (thermofluor)

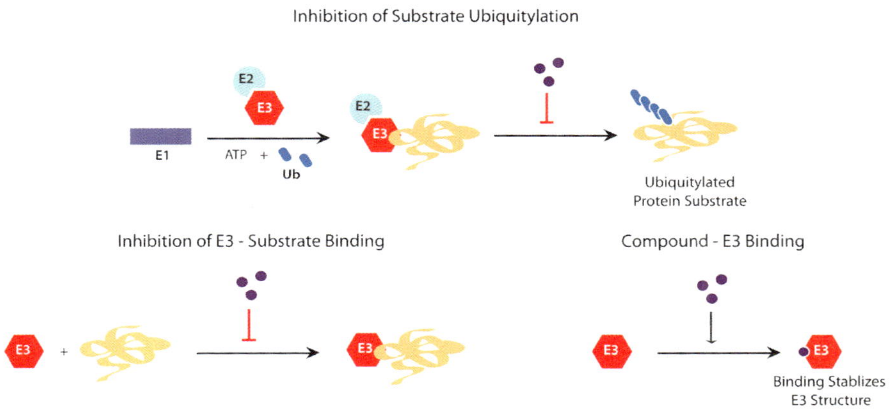

Fig. 12.4 Alternative strategies for developing compounds that act on ubiquitin E3 ligases. *Top*: Traditional strategy for discovering inhibitors of the catalytic activity of E3 ligase complexes. Purified components of the ligase reaction—E1, E2, E3, substrate, and, in the case of multisubunit E3 ligases, scaffold proteins, in addition to ubiquitin and ATP—are incubated together, and the endpoint, polyubiquitination of the substrate (or, in some cases, autoubiquitination of E3), is assayed by various means. *Bottom*: Alternative assay types that do not utilize ubiquitination as the endpoint. *Left*: Binding of E3 to an important reaction component, in this case, the substrate (e.g., MDM2 to p53 (see text)), compounds being tested for their ability to disrupt this binding. This type of assay has resulted in several compounds now in Phase I trials (Table 12.2). *Right*: Thermal shift assay measures binding of test compounds to purified E3 (or a fragment thereof). Binding generally stabilizes the structure of the E3 enzyme, shifting the melting temperature to a higher value than that of the unbound E3. High-throughput configurations of this assay have been used in primary screening and hit compound validation

technology [68] is used to monitor the change in protein conformational stabilization of an E3 ligase or ligase fragment upon binding a high affinity ligand. Compounds identified in such an assay have intrinsic functional relevance to E3, and isolated domains of the E3 molecule can be tested such that highly conserved, nonselective "catalytic site" binders will not be identified. The method employs differential scanning fluorometry to examine how a small molecule that binds to a given protein affects that protein's melting curve. Thermal shift methodology is amenable to reasonably high-throughput screening with proteins or protein fragments that can be produced in high quality and yield, having been used to screen >100,000 compounds in primary screens [70]. It has been used successfully for early drug discovery in the pharmaceutical industry [68], including efforts to find antagonists of the ubiquitin ligase HDM2 [71]. More recently, thermal shift screening has identified compounds that bind to the E3 ligase Idol, which is responsible for degradation of the LDL receptor [72]. These compounds demonstrate reduced ubiquitylation of the LDLR, increased presence of the receptor at the cell surface, and increased LDL (cholesterol) association with the cells [73].

An additional biophysical method that has been employed to identify E3 ligase binders is Surface Plasmon Resonance (SPR) [67]. SPR can be utilized to monitor protein–ligand interactions by the change in refractive index of a solvent at a sensor surface, identifying protein binders [74]. This method is not typically amenable to primary high-throughput screening, although recent advances in instrumentation are changing this picture. SPR technology, at present, can accommodate moderate throughput operations, e.g., fragment-based screening approaches (~5,000 fragments). The technique was used to identify compounds that bind the E3 ligase parkin; new scaffolds and leads were identified that differed from compounds discovered in enzyme inhibitor screening and abandoned because chemical optimization failed to improve potency [67]. Thus, data emerging from the use of thermal shift and SPR screening suggest that high-quality, drug-like small molecules acting on E3 ligases can be discovered [67, 73]. High-throughput biophysical screening methods such as thermal shift and SPR, having achieved cellular proof of concept, likely will find increasing utility in the search for novel, physiologically relevant E3 ligase inhibitors.

12.3.2.2 Protein–Protein Interactions

The mode of action of classical receptor agonists and antagonists and of active site inhibitors of enzymatic activity entails interaction of pharmacophores of small molecules with limited numbers of amino acids that comprise 3-dimensional binding pockets of the active site (or an important regulatory site) on the target molecule. Because the active site/module of HECT or RING E3 ligases is highly conserved [62, 75, 76], even though it may be possible to discover or design tight binding inhibitors, the potential for developing them as selective ligase inhibitors may be small. Nonenzymatic interactions between proteins have important biological roles, and small-molecule disruptors of such interactions have been sought for various therapeutic uses. Efforts to find inhibitors of protein–protein interactions have been relatively unsuccessful until structural biology methods were employed to develop E3 ligase-acting experimental anticancer drugs such as the nutlins and other small molecules that disrupt the binding of the tumor suppressor p53 to its corresponding E3 ligase HDM2/MDM2 (see below) [77–79].

12.3.3 E3 Ligase-Acting Anticancer Compounds

12.3.3.1 E1, E2, and E3 Enzymes Are Anticancer Targets

It should be noted that all three enzymes involved in the ubiquitylation reaction—E1, E2, and E3 (Fig. 12.1)—are active targets in anticancer drug discovery [80]. There are eight known human E1s, the enzyme which activates ubiquitin or ubiquitin-like proteins in an ATP-dependent step [80, 81], in addition to approximately 40 human E2s and ~600 E3s. An inhibitor of E1, E2, or E3 could presumably have the same general impact on cell physiology (allowing for differences in selectivity), and part of the complexity of screening for E3 ligase inhibitors employing ubiquitylation assays is the need to eliminate E1 and E2 as the actual target. Before considering E3 ligase-acting anticancer compounds, therefore, it is useful to review E1 and E2 inhibitors under development for cancer treatment. An adenosine sulfamate analogue, MLN4924, inhibits the E1 enzyme responsible for NEDDylation, the covalent addition of an ubiquitin-like protein, NEDD8, to activate specific target proteins including SCF^{Skp2}, a pro-growth E3 ligase linked to cell cycle regulation [82]. MLN4924 is currently in Phase II clinical trial for hematologic cancers [83]. The experimental E1 inhibitor PYR-41, an irreversible ubiquitin E1 active site binder, is able to enter cells and, while possibly too reactive to be a clinical candidate, is being used as a translational tool compound [84]. Recently, a selective allosteric site inhibitor of the human E2 enzyme hCdc34 (CC0651) was described [85]. One target of this E2 (complexed with the appropriate E3) is p27, which blocks tumor cell cycle progression. Thus, compounds such as CC0651 are in preclinical development for cancer treatment.

12.3.3.2 The "Classical" E3 Ligase Anticancer Targets: MDM2/HDM2 and IAP Ligases

Among the more successful ligase-based drug discovery strategies undertaken have been the development of antagonists of the binding of E3 ligases to their substrates (protein–protein interactions). The E3 ligase MDM2/HDM2 (HDM2 is the human orthologue, and these names are used interchangeably in the cancer literature) was one of the pioneer anticancer targets among non-proteasomal ubiquitin pathway proteins [86, 87]; it is responsible for ubiquitylating the tumor suppressor proapoptotic protein p53. The nearly 50 % of tumors that have a functional p53 represented a huge patient population that would benefit from therapy directed against MDM2. Targeted disruption of MDM2 has been one of many molecular oncology strategies employed in the last 10–15 years to maximize p53 presence and activity in tumors (reviewed in [88]); the seven E3 ligase antagonists currently in Phase I clinical trial for cancer all are directed at MDM2 to regulate its substrate p53 [89–92] (Table 12.2; one completed a lone Phase I trial in 2010 with no additional trials reported and six have only recently been entered).

Nutlin-3 (RO5045337) is a structurally designed small-molecule inhibitor of the MDM2/p53 interaction; it was engineered to bind to the N-terminal hydrophobic pocket domain of MDM2 [69]. Inhibition of the ligase by nutlin-3 afforded non-genotoxic p53 stabilization, activation of cell cycle arrest and apoptosis pathways, and preclinical antitumor efficacy and proof of concept [79]. RO5045337 is being evaluated in Phase I clinical trial as an oral formulation against a spectrum of cancers including refractory solid malignancies and hematologic cancers [93]. Two recent observations on nutlin-3 provide a strong indication of the likely utility of E3 ligase inhibitors, if any, in cancer treatment in the near term. First, the experimental selection and analysis of a broad spectrum of mutant HDM2s resistant to inhibition by nutlin-3 suggests that mutation of the target enzyme will be a factor in clinical resistance and, moreover, that any clinical utility of the nutlins (or, in fact, of E3 ligase inhibitors as a class) will likely reside in combination therapy [94]. Secondly, this prediction finds support in a recent report that nutlin-3 enhances the efficacy of the multi-specific kinase inhibitor sorafenib in the highly refractory disease renal cell carcinoma [95].

Several other small molecules that block HDM2/p53 interaction are currently in Phase I clinical trial (Table 12.2). JNJ-26854165 (serdemetan) is a novel tryptamine derivative which inhibits the interaction of MDM2-p53 complex with the proteasome and increases p53 levels by binding to the RING domain of MDM2 [89] (Fig. 12.5). The compound has undergone extensive preclinical [96, 97] evaluation and has completed one Phase I trial (2006–2010) in Europe as an oral formulation (safety, determination of maximally tolerated dose). Grade 3 prolongation of QTc (cardiotoxicity) was the most prominent dose-limiting toxicity; one patient had a partial response and 22 manifested stable disease [98]. No subsequent Phase I trials have been reported. Additional small-molecule inhibitors having strong affinities for MDM2 and suitable absorption distribution, metabolism, excretion (ADME) properties have entered Phase I trials [98]; most of these trials are in the patient recruitment stage (Table 12.2). As in the case of nutlin-3, these HDM2/MDM2 inhibitors are being evaluated as both single agents and components of combination therapy protocols.

Use of the MDM2/nutlin paradigm has spread to other E3 RING proteins. MDMX, like its homologue MDM2, regulates p53 activity; MDM2 and MDMX act individually or in concert to affect transcription in a variety of ways [99]. For this reason and owing to the success of efforts targeting MDM2/HDM2, considerable efforts are underway to design and develop small-molecule inhibitors of the MDMX-p53 interaction, and potent binders of MDMX (affinities in the nanomolar range) have been synthesized [92, 100]. Inhibitors of a second cancer-associated E3

Table 12.2 E3 inhibitors currently approved or in development

Compound	Mechanism	Pharma	Status
Thalidomide/ THALOMID®	Oral binder of E3 ligase component CRBN, exerting pleiotropic immunomodulatory and anti-tumorigenic effects	Celgene	Approved by FDA 2006
Lenalidomide/ REVLIMID®	Oral binder of E3 ligase component CRBN, exerting pleiotropic immunomodulatory and anti-tumorigenic effects	Celgene	Approved by FDA 2006
Pomalidomide/ POMALYST®	Oral binder of E3 ligase component CRBN, exerting pleiotropic immunomodulatory and anti-tumorigenic effects	Celgene	Approved by FDA 2013
RO5045337 (RG7112, Nutlin-3)	Oral antagonist of MDM2-p53 interaction by binding in the MDM2 pocket (protein–protein)	Roche	Phase I
RO5503781	Oral MDM2 inhibitor (protein–protein)	Roche	Phase I
JNJ-26854165 (serdemetan)	Oral E3 inhibitor: binds to RING domain of MDM2, antagonizes regulation of p53 by MDM2	Johnson & Johnson	Phase I
DS-3032b	Oral MDM2 inhibitor (protein–protein)	Daiichi Sankyo	Phase I
CGM097	Oral MDM2 inhibitor (protein–protein)	Novartis	Phase I
MK-8242 (SCH 900242)	Oral MDM2 inhibitor (protein–protein)	Merck	Phase I
SAR405838	Oral MDM2 inhibitor (protein–protein)	Sanofi	Phase I
GDC-0152	iv IAP (Smac mimetic; binds to and inhibits IAP activity)	Genentech	Phase I
LCL161	Oral IAP (Smac mimetic; binds to and inhibits IAP activity)	Novartis	Phase I, II
AT-406/Debio 1143	IAP (Smac mimetic; binds to and inhibits IAP activity)	Ascenta	Phase I
AEG 35156	IAP (antisense)	Aegera	Phase I,II
AEG 40826 (HGS1029)	IAP (Smac mimetic; binds to and inhibits IAP activity)	Aegera/GSK	Phase I
TL 32711/birinapant	IAP (Smac mimetic; binds to and inhibits IAP activity)	Tetralogics	Phase I,II
YM155	IAP (suppresses expression of IAP family member, survivin)	Astellas	Phase I, II

(continued)

Table 12.2 (continued)

Compound	Mechanism	Pharma	Status
RITA (NSC652287)	Binds to MDM2 binding domain of p53	NCI; Karolinska Inst	Preclinical
AM-8553	Binds MDM2, disrupts MDM2-p53 binding	Univ of Michigan; Amgen	Preclinical
Various small molecules related to MI-219	Bind to MDM2, disrupting MDM2-p53 binding	Univ of Mich., Ascenta, Sanofi	Preclinical

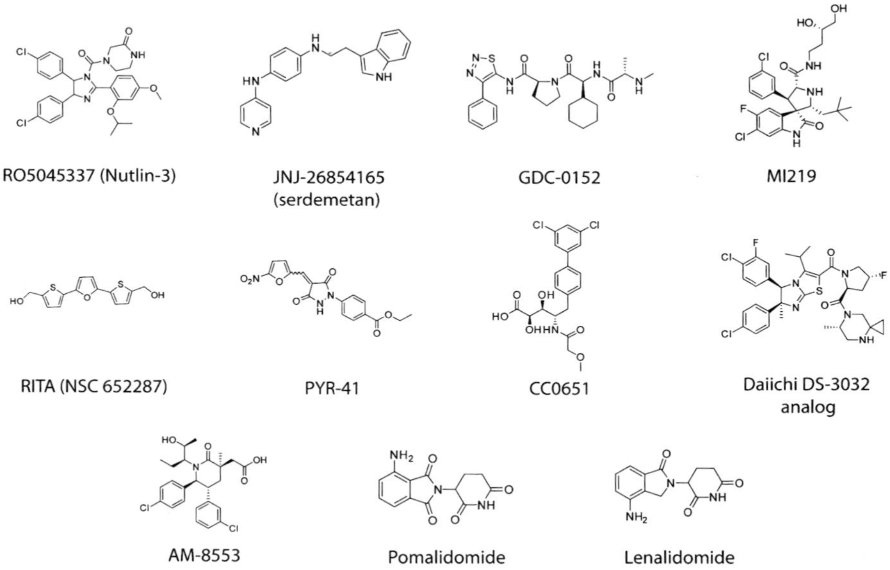

Fig. 12.5 Chemical structures of selected E3 ligase inhibitors (see text)

ligase-substrate pair—the E3 ligase pVHL binding to its substrate Hif-1α—are described in recent reports [78, 101]; such inhibitors, which would favor Hif-1α accumulation, may be useful as tool compounds or as therapeutic agents for hematologic toxicities associated with certain cancer chemotherapies (in a supportive care setting carrying the same secondary cancer risks as erythropoietin replacement therapy).

The ligase binding theme is also utilized in the development and testing of Smac mimetics, compounds designed to bind to members of a family of E3 ligases known as inhibitors of apoptosis (IAPs). Proteins that are essential to apoptosis are the ubiquitylation/degradation targets of IAPs (see Table 12.3); tumor cells, which tend to overexpress IAPs, are equipped to combat apoptosis. Smac (the abbreviation for

Table 12.3 E3 ligases with therapeutic relevance to cancer

E3 ligase	Physiological role(s)
Cbl-b	Simple RING E3 ligase that ubiquitylates ZAP70 and p85 promoting T cell anergy
CRBN	Substrate targeting component of DDB1, Cul4A ligase, a molecular target of the IMiDs
E6-AP	E3 ubiquitin HECT-domain ligase that ubiquitylates the tumor suppressor p53 in oncogenic HPV-infected cells; associated with HPV protein E6, which regulates substrate recognition
Hrd1/synoviolin	Endoplasmic reticulum (ER) resident E3 ligase that is involved in ER-associated protein degradation (ERAD) of a number of substrates including the tumor suppressor p53
cIAP1 and 2	RING E3 ligases that ubiquitylate RIP1 preventing activation of caspase 8
MDM2/HDM2	RING-finger-dependent E3 ligase for tumor suppressor p53
MuRF-1	RING-finger E3 ligase associated with muscle wasting, cachexia
Ring1B	Simple RING E3, epigenetic modifier as a component of polycomb repressive complex 1, monoubiquitinates histone H2A, suppresses $p16^{Ink4a}$
$SCF^{Atrogin\text{-}1/(MFBx1)}$	SCF complex E3 ligase associated with muscle wasting, cachexia
$SCF\beta^{TrCP}$	Multisubunit E3 RING-finger ligase for various targets associated with cellular control mechanisms, including β-catenin and IκBα
SCF^{Skp2}	Multisubunit E3 RING-finger ligase for p27 tumor suppressor (cell-cycle inhibitor)
TRAF6	RING-finger E3 ligase that ubiquitinates and activates IκB kinase (IKK) resulting in activation of NF-κB
pVHL	Tumor suppressor, mutated in various cancers, multisubunit E3 RING-finger complex (pVHL-ElonginC-ElonginB), ubiquitinates and degrades HIF1α
XIAP	E3 RING-finger ligase for various caspases (apoptosis execution phase)

"second mitochondria-derived activator of caspases") is a naturally occurring protein that binds to the IAP and triggers its autoubiquitylation and destruction, thereby favoring apoptosis. In tumors, overexpressed IAPs easily overwhelm the ability of endogenous Smac to defend against their antiapoptotic activity. Small-molecule mimics of Smac are able to supplement the function of endogenous Smac and restore apoptosis, translating to antitumor effect. Several Smac mimetics and an antisense compound targeting IAPs have recently entered clinical trial [102–108]. IAPs comprise a family of E3 ligases, and therapeutic strategies can entail the development of compounds that inhibit one or more IAPs (Table 12.2).

In addition to HDM2/MDM2 and the IAPs, at least ten E3 ligases have been linked to cancer; most of them, like MDM2, act as oncoproteins with antiapoptotic or pro-cycling mechanisms, and one is associated with muscle wasting/cachexia [109]. Inhibitors of these ligase activities would be potential anticancer or supportive care (anti-cachexia) drugs [86, 87, 90, 109–118] (Table 12.3). Although efforts have been made to find inhibitors of the catalytic activity of E3s (ubiquitylation endpoint), the search is complicated by the participation of three enzymes in the conjugation reaction [80], and to date no other E3 inhibitors have entered the clinic, although several such inhibitors have been reported and are useful as tool compounds (for a comprehensive list of potential E3 anticancer targets, see [119]). A recent report describes a selective inhibitor of SCF^{Skp2} ubiquitin ligase, which has long been associated with cancer and was one of the earliest ligase anticancer targets. The compound, discovered by in silico screening [120], demonstrates ligase selectivity and in vivo efficacy, and is being studied as an effector of cancer stem cell progression. It has the potential to be the first acknowledged SCF ligase inhibitor to survive preclinical development.

12.3.3.3 Ex Post Facto E3 Ligase Inhibitors

There is one example of a class of related molecules (thalidomide and its analogues lenalidomide and pomalidomide; collectively known as the IMiDs) approved for anticancer therapy and found, subsequent to their clinical evaluation, to act on an ubiquitin E3 ligase [5]. Pomalidomide (POMALYST®) was approved in 2013 for use in patients with multiple myeloma who received at least two prior therapies including REVLIMID® (lenalidomide) and VELCADE® (bortezomib) and whose disease progressed after the last treatment. All three drugs are currently used against multiple myeloma in triplet combinations, with impressive results [3], and all inhibit the multi-subunit E3 ligase protein substrate targeting component Cereblon (CRBN), the latter observation supported by clinical correlates [5]. CRBN forms a complex with damaged DNA binding protein 1 (DDB1) and Cul4A; the complex is important for limb outgrowth and expression of the fibroblast growth factor Fgf8 in zebrafish and chicks. Thalidomide initiates its teratogenic effects by binding to CRBN and inhibiting the associated ubiquitin ligase activity [121].

Since 2005 or so, views on the potential for turning E3 ligase modulators into anticancer drugs have been moderated. Predictions [64] that (1) the nutlin compounds might not progress to clinical trial owing to poor animal efficacy and (2) E3s in general are perhaps too complex for drug discovery have not been borne out. The fact that today there are seven MDM2-p53 binding inhibitors (including two nutlins) and seven IAP antagonists in Phase I/II clinical trials refutes the notion that E3 ligases are not druggable. The target remains difficult, however, and progress has been made outside the traditional approaches of recapitulating the ubiquitylation reaction and screening for inhibitors of this activity [122, 123]. Protein interaction (with other proteins or with small molecules) has been harnessed in various ways to find new inhibitors of E3 ligases [124, 125]. The approval for marketing of immunomodulatory thalidomide derivatives demonstrates, moreover, that some E3 inhibitors can sustain clinical development and become efficacious therapies.

12.4 Conclusions

Consideration of the current states of proteasome inhibitors and E3 ligase inhibitors in cancer treatment reveals some commonalities, despite the fact that proteasome inhibitors are farther ahead of ligase inhibitors in development and patient use.

Firstly, while details are sometimes sketchy, there is evidence of cancer selectivity in the inhibition of both targets, which is a good starting point for the design or improvement of treatment protocols. Secondly, progress in translational research and assay development has led to proteasome inhibitors that may be even more cancer selective than the original clinical compounds, owing to the type of proteasome or the type of proteasomal protease that they attack, and to ligase inhibitors that disrupt ligase-substrate binding or bind to non-conserved elements of the ligase, thereby inhibiting their target enzymes with vastly improved selectivity. These advances may facilitate ongoing efforts to expand the spectrum of tumor types treatable by both types of anticancer drug. In addition, the development of clinical resistance against proteasome inhibitors and ligase inhibitors suggests that these drugs will perform optimally in combination trials, which is likely to broaden their utility. A final as yet an incompletely answered question concerns the surprising efficacy of proteasome inhibitors, given that they exert numerous effects. Part of the answer may derive from the need to inhibit multiple targets to ensure anti-growth, proapoptotic activity that is minimally impacted by either mechanistic compensation by parallel pathways or development of resistance, both of which are most likely if there is only one target. The first half of the year 2013 witnessed numerous reports of dual or multiple kinase inhibitors with promising antitumor efficacy [126–128], and this model may also be appropriate for therapies derived from the ubiquitin-proteasome pathway.

References

1. Adams J (2002) Development of the proteasome inhibitor PS-341. Oncologist 7(1):9–16
2. McConkey DJ, Zhu K (2008) Mechanisms of proteasome inhibitor action and resistance in cancer. Drug Resist Updat 11(4–5):164–179
3. Anderson KC (2013) Therapeutic advances in relapsed or refractory multiple myeloma. J Natl Compr Canc Netw 11(5 suppl):676–679
4. Adams J (2004) The development of proteasome inhibitors as anticancer drugs. Cancer Cell 5(5):417–421
5. Lopez-Girona A et al (2012) Cereblon is a direct protein target for immunomodulatory and antiproliferative activities of lenalidomide and pomalidomide. Leukemia 26(11):2326–2335
6. Pellom ST Jr, Shanker A (2012) Development of proteasome inhibitors as therapeutic drugs. J Clin Cell Immunol S5:5
7. Hershko A, Ciechanover A (1998) The ubiquitin system. Annu Rev Biochem 67:425–479
8. Ciechanover A (2005) Proteolysis: from the lysosome to ubiquitin and the proteasome. Nat Rev Mol Cell Biol 6(1):79–87
9. Murata S, Yashiroda H, Tanaka K (2009) Molecular mechanisms of proteasome assembly. Nat Rev Mol Cell Biol 10(2):104–115
10. Miller Z et al (2013) Inhibitors of the immunoproteasome: current status and future directions. Curr Pharm Des 19(22):4140–4151
11. Wehenkel M et al (2012) A selective inhibitor of the immunoproteasome subunit LMP2 induces apoptosis in PC-3 cells and suppresses tumour growth in nude mice. Br J Cancer 107(1):53–62
12. Kloetzel PM (2001) Antigen processing by the proteasome. Nat Rev Mol Cell Biol 2(3):179–187

13. Suzuki E et al (2011) Molecular mechanisms of bortezomib resistant adenocarcinoma cells. PLoS One 6(12):e27996
14. Groettrup M, Kirk CJ, Basler M (2010) Proteasomes in immune cells: more than peptide producers? Nat Rev Immunol 10(1):73–78
15. Teicher BA et al (1999) The proteasome inhibitor PS-341 in cancer therapy. Clin Cancer Res 5(9):2638–2645
16. Orlowski RZ et al (2002) Phase I trial of the proteasome inhibitor PS-341 in patients with refractory hematologic malignancies. J Clin Oncol 20(22):4420–4427
17. Orlowski RZ, Kuhn DJ (2008) Proteasome inhibitors in cancer therapy: lessons from the first decade. Clin Cancer Res 14(6):1649–1657
18. Molineaux SM (2012) Molecular pathways: targeting proteasomal protein degradation in cancer. Clin Cancer Res 18(1):15–20
19. Ruschak AM et al (2011) Novel proteasome inhibitors to overcome bortezomib resistance. J Natl Cancer Inst 103(13):1007–1017
20. Frezza M, Schmitt S, Dou QP (2011) Targeting the ubiquitin-proteasome pathway: an emerging concept in cancer therapy. Curr Top Med Chem 11(23):2888–2905
21. Palombella VJ et al (1994) The ubiquitin-proteasome pathway is required for processing the NF-kappa B1 precursor protein and the activation of NF-kappa B. Cell 78(5):773–785
22. Hideshima T et al (2001) The proteasome inhibitor PS-341 inhibits growth, induces apoptosis, and overcomes drug resistance in human multiple myeloma cells. Cancer Res 61(7):3071–3076
23. Shanker A et al (2008) Treating metastatic solid tumors with bortezomib and a tumor necrosis factor-related apoptosis-inducing ligand receptor agonist antibody. J Natl Cancer Inst 100(9):649–662
24. Lesinski GB et al (2008) IFN-alpha and bortezomib overcome Bcl-2 and Mcl-1 overexpression in melanoma cells by stimulating the extrinsic pathway of apoptosis. Cancer Res 68(20):8351–8360
25. Ling YH et al (2002) PS-341, a novel proteasome inhibitor, induces Bcl-2 phosphorylation and cleavage in association with G2-M phase arrest and apoptosis. Mol Cancer Ther 1(10):841–849
26. Landowski TH et al (2005) Mitochondrial-mediated disregulation of Ca2+ is a critical determinant of Velcade (PS-341/bortezomib) cytotoxicity in myeloma cell lines. Cancer Res 65(9):3828–3836
27. Wang F et al (2011) A novel dithiocarbamate analogue with potentially decreased ALDH inhibition has copper-dependent proteasome-inhibitory and apoptosis-inducing activity in human breast cancer cells. Cancer Lett 300(1):87–95
28. Ding WX et al (2007) Linking of autophagy to ubiquitin-proteasome system is important for the regulation of endoplasmic reticulum stress and cell viability. Am J Pathol 171(2):513–524
29. Chastagner P, Israel A, Brou C (2008) AIP4/Itch regulates Notch receptor degradation in the absence of ligand. PLoS One 3(7):e2735
30. Tan JM et al (2008) Lysine 63-linked ubiquitination promotes the formation and autophagic clearance of protein inclusions associated with neurodegenerative diseases. Hum Mol Genet 17(3):431–439
31. Wong E, Cuervo AM (2010) Integration of clearance mechanisms: the proteasome and autophagy. Cold Spring Harb Perspect Biol 2(12):a006734
32. Zhu K, Dunner K Jr, McConkey DJ (2010) Proteasome inhibitors activate autophagy as a cytoprotective response in human prostate cancer cells. Oncogene 29(3):451–462
33. Kaufman RJ (2002) Orchestrating the unfolded protein response in health and disease. J Clin Invest 110(10):1389–1398
34. Travers KJ et al (2000) Functional and genomic analyses reveal an essential coordination between the unfolded protein response and ER-associated degradation. Cell 101(3):249–258
35. Lu S, Wang J (2013) The resistance mechanisms of proteasome inhibitor bortezomib. Biomark Res 1(13):1–9

36. Lu S et al (2008) Point mutation of the proteasome beta5 subunit gene is an important mechanism of bortezomib resistance in bortezomib-selected variants of Jurkat T cell lymphoblastic lymphoma/leukemia line. J Pharmacol Exp Ther 326(2):423–431
37. Oerlemans R et al (2008) Molecular basis of bortezomib resistance: proteasome subunit beta5 (PSMB5) gene mutation and overexpression of PSMB5 protein. Blood 112(6): 2489–2499
38. Letai A et al (2002) Distinct BH3 domains either sensitize or activate mitochondrial apoptosis, serving as prototype cancer therapeutics. Cancer Cell 2(3):183–192
39. Xiao C et al (2008) Lymphoproliferative disease and autoimmunity in mice with increased miR-17-92 expression in lymphocytes. Nat Immunol 9(4):405–414
40. Chauhan D et al (2005) A novel orally active proteasome inhibitor induces apoptosis in multiple myeloma cells with mechanisms distinct from Bortezomib. Cancer Cell 8(5):407–419
41. Wang HH et al (2011) Reversion of multidrug-resistance by proteasome inhibitor bortezomib in K562/DNR cell line. Chin J Cancer Res 23(1):69–73
42. O'Connor R et al (2013) The interaction of bortezomib with multidrug transporters: implications for therapeutic applications in advanced multiple myeloma and other neoplasias. Cancer Chemother Pharmacol 71(5):1357–1368
43. de Wilt LH et al (2012) Proteasome-based mechanisms of intrinsic and acquired bortezomib resistance in non-small cell lung cancer. Biochem Pharmacol 83(2):207–217
44. Shringarpure R et al (2006) Gene expression analysis of B-lymphoma cells resistant and sensitive to bortezomib. Br J Haematol 134(2):145–156
45. Lu S et al (2008) Overexpression of the PSMB5 gene contributes to bortezomib resistance in T-lymphoblastic lymphoma/leukemia cells derived from Jurkat line. Exp Hematol 36(10): 1278–1284
46. Buda G et al (2010) Polymorphisms in the multiple drug resistance protein 1 and in P-glycoprotein 1 are associated with time to event outcomes in patients with advanced multiple myeloma treated with bortezomib and pegylated liposomal doxorubicin. Ann Hematol 89(11):1133–1140
47. Kuhn DJ et al (2007) Potent activity of carfilzomib, a novel, irreversible inhibitor of the ubiquitin-proteasome pathway, against preclinical models of multiple myeloma. Blood 110(9):3281–3290
48. Kupperman E et al (2010) Evaluation of the proteasome inhibitor MLN9708 in preclinical models of human cancer. Cancer Res 70(5):1970–1980
49. Piva R et al (2008) CEP-18770: a novel, orally active proteasome inhibitor with a tumor-selective pharmacologic profile competitive with bortezomib. Blood 111(5):2765–2775
50. Demo SD et al (2007) Antitumor activity of PR-171, a novel irreversible inhibitor of the proteasome. Cancer Res 67(13):6383–6391
51. Chauhan D et al (2010) A novel orally active proteasome inhibitor ONX 0912 triggers in vitro and in vivo cytotoxicity in multiple myeloma. Blood 116(23):4906–4915
52. Daniel KG et al (2005) Clioquinol and pyrrolidine dithiocarbamate complex with copper to form proteasome inhibitors and apoptosis inducers in human breast cancer cells. Breast Cancer Res 7(6):R897–R908
53. Schimmer AD et al (2012) A phase I study of the metal ionophore clioquinol in patients with advanced hematologic malignancies. Clin Lymphoma Myeloma Leuk 12(5):330–336
54. Voorhees PM, Orlowski RZ (2006) The proteasome and proteasome inhibitors in cancer therapy. Annu Rev Pharmacol Toxicol 46:189–213
55. Kuhn DJ et al (2009) Targeted inhibition of the immunoproteasome is a potent strategy against models of multiple myeloma that overcomes resistance to conventional drugs and nonspecific proteasome inhibitors. Blood 113(19):4667–4676
56. Kisselev AF et al (2003) The caspase-like sites of proteasomes, their substrate specificity, new inhibitors and substrates, and allosteric interactions with the trypsin-like sites. J Biol Chem 278(38):35869–35877
57. van Swieten PF et al (2007) A cell-permeable inhibitor and activity-based probe for the caspase-like activity of the proteasome. Bioorg Med Chem Lett 17(12):3402–3405

58. Mirabella AC, Pletnev AA, Downey SL, Florea BI, Shabaneh TB, Britton M, Verdoes M, Filippov DV, Overkleeft HS, Kisselev AF (2011) Specific cell-permeable inhibitor of proteasome trypsin-like sites selectively sensitizes myeloma cells to bortezomib and carfilzomib. Chem Biol 18(5):608–618
59. Sprangers R et al (2008) TROSY-based NMR evidence for a novel class of 20S proteasome inhibitors. Biochemistry 47(26):6727–6734
60. D'Arcy P et al (2011) Inhibition of proteasome deubiquitinating activity as a new cancer therapy. Nat Med 17(12):1636–1640
61. Weissman AM (2001) Themes and variations on ubiquitylation. Nat Rev Mol Cell Biol 2(3):169–178
62. Pickart CM (2001) Mechanisms underlying ubiquitination. Annu Rev Biochem 70:503–533
63. Herman-Bachinsky Y et al (2007) Regulation of the Drosophila ubiquitin ligase DIAP1 is mediated via several distinct ubiquitin system pathways. Cell Death Differ 14(4):861–871
64. Garber K (2005) Missing the target: ubiquitin ligase drugs stall. J Natl Cancer Inst 97(3): 166–167
65. Buchwald M et al (2010) Ubiquitin conjugase UBCH8 targets active FMS-like tyrosine kinase 3 for proteasomal degradation. Leukemia 24(8):1412–1421
66. Rajbhandari P et al (2013) Pin1 modulates ERalpha levels in breast cancer through inhibition of phosphorylation-dependent ubiquitination and degradation. Oncogene 33:1438–1447
67. Regnstrom K et al (2013) Label free fragment screening using surface plasmon resonance as a tool for fragment finding—analyzing parkin, a difficult CNS target. PLoS One 8(7):e66879
68. Salemme FR (2004) High-throughput biochemistry heats up. Nat Biotechnol 22(9): 1100–1101
69. Vassilev LT (2004) Small-molecule antagonists of p53-MDM2 binding: research tools and potential therapeutics. Cell Cycle 3(4):419–421
70. Pantoliano MW et al (2001) High-density miniaturized thermal shift assays as a general strategy for drug discovery. J Biomol Screen 6(6):429–440
71. Grasberger BL et al (2005) Discovery and cocrystal structure of benzodiazepinedione HDM2 antagonists that activate p53 in cells. J Med Chem 48(4):909–912
72. Zelcer N et al (2009) LXR regulates cholesterol uptake through Idol-dependent ubiquitination of the LDL receptor. Science 325(5936):100–104
73. Eddins M (2013) Promising cardiovascular intervention by ubiquitin ligases: LDL-cholesterol regulation by IDOL. In: Ubiquitin drug discovery & diagnostics conference 2013. Conference presentation abstracts, p 29
74. Razinkov VI, Treuheit MJ, Becker GW (2013) Methods of high throughput biophysical characterization in biopharmaceutical development. Curr Drug Discov Technol 10(1):59–70
75. Page RC et al (2012) Structural insights into the conformation and oligomerization of E2~ubiquitin conjugates. Biochemistry 51(20):4175–4187
76. Katoh S et al (2005) Active site residues and amino acid specificity of the ubiquitin carrier protein-binding RING-H2 finger domain. J Biol Chem 280(49):41015–41024
77. Zhao Y et al (2013) Diastereomeric spirooxindoles as highly potent and efficacious MDM2 inhibitors. J Am Chem Soc 135(19):7223–7234
78. Buckley DL et al (2012) Targeting the von Hippel-Lindau E3 ubiquitin ligase using small molecules to disrupt the VHL/HIF-1alpha interaction. J Am Chem Soc 134(10):4465–4468
79. Vassilev LT et al (2004) In vivo activation of the p53 pathway by small-molecule antagonists of MDM2. Science 303(5659):844–848
80. Ciechanover A, Orian A, Schwartz AL (2000) The ubiquitin-mediated proteolytic pathway: mode of action and clinical implications. J Cell Biochem 77(S34):40–51
81. Chen JJ, Tsu CA, Gavin JA, Milhollen MA, Bruzzese FJ, Mallender WD, Sintchak MD, Bump NJ, Yang X, Ma J, Loke H-K, Xu Q, Li P, Bence NF, Brownell JE, Dick LR (2011) Mechanistic studies of substrate-assisted inhibition of ubiquitin-activating enzyme by adenosine sulfamate analogues. J Biol Chem 286(47):40867–40877
82. Chen Q et al (2008) Targeting the p27 E3 ligase SCF(Skp2) results in p27- and Skp2-mediated cell-cycle arrest and activation of autophagy. Blood 111(9):4690–4699

83. Milhollen MA et al (2012) Treatment-emergent mutations in NAEbeta confer resistance to the NEDD8-activating enzyme inhibitor MLN4924. Cancer Cell 21(3):388–401
84. Yang Y, Kitagati J, Dai R-M, Tsai YC, Lorick KL, Ludwig RL, Pierre SA, Jensen JP, Davydov IV, Oberoi P, Li C-CH, Kenten JH, Beutler JA, Vousden KH, Weissman AM (2007) Inhibitors of ubiquitin-activating enzyme (E1), a new class of potential cancer therapeutics. Cancer Res 67(19):9472–9481
85. Ceccarelli DF et al (2011) An allosteric inhibitor of the human Cdc34 ubiquitin-conjugating enzyme. Cell 145(7):1075–1087
86. Boddy MN, Freemont PS, Borden KL (1994) The p53-associated protein MDM2 contains a newly characterized zinc-binding domain called the RING finger. Trends Biochem Sci 19(5):198–199
87. Fakharzadeh SS, Trusko SP, George DL (1991) Tumorigenic potential associated with enhanced expression of a gene that is amplified in a mouse tumor cell line. EMBO J 10(6): 1565–1569
88. Suzuki K, Matsubara H (2011) Recent advances in p53 research and cancer treatment. J Biomed Biotechnol 2011:978312
89. Yuan Y et al (2011) Novel targeted therapeutics: inhibitors of MDM2, ALK and PARP. J Hematol Oncol 4:16
90. Issaeva N et al (2004) Small molecule RITA binds to p53, blocks p53-HDM-2 interaction and activates p53 function in tumors. Nat Med 10(12):1321–1328
91. Patel S, Player MR (2008) Small-molecule inhibitors of the p53-HDM2 interaction for the treatment of cancer. Expert Opin Investig Drugs 17(12):1865–1882
92. Zhao Y, Bernard D, Wang S (2013) Small molecule inhibitors of MDM2-p53 and MDMX-p53 interactions as new cancer therapeutics. Biodiscovery 8(4):1–15
93. Secchiero P et al (2011) Recent advances in the therapeutic perspectives of Nutlin-3. Curr Pharm Des 17(6):569–577
94. Wei SJ et al (2013) In vitro selection of mutant HDM2 resistant to Nutlin inhibition. PLoS One 8(4):e62564
95. Vatsyayan R et al (2013) Nutlin-3 enhances sorafenib efficacy in renal cell carcinoma. Mol Carcinog 52(1):39–48
96. Smith MA et al (2012) Initial testing of JNJ-26854165 (Serdemetan) by the pediatric preclinical testing program. Pediatr Blood Cancer 59(2):329–332
97. Kojima K et al (2010) The novel tryptamine derivative JNJ-26854165 induces wild-type p53- and E2F1-mediated apoptosis in acute myeloid and lymphoid leukemias. Mol Cancer Ther 9(9):2545–2557
98. Tabernero J et al (2011) A phase I first-in-human pharmacokinetic and pharmacodynamic study of serdemetan in patients with advanced solid tumors. Clin Cancer Res 17(19): 6313–6321
99. Biderman L, Manley JL, Prives C (2012) Mdm2 and MdmX as regulators of gene expression. Genes Cancer 3(3–4):264–273
100. Zhao Y et al (2013) A potent small-molecule inhibitor of the MDM2-p53 interaction (MI-888) achieved complete and durable tumor regression in mice. J Med Chem 56:5553–5561
101. Buckley DL et al (2012) Small-molecule inhibitors of the interaction between the E3 ligase VHL and HIF1alpha. Angew Chem Int Ed Engl 51(46):11463–11467
102. Flygare JA et al (2012) Discovery of a potent small-molecule antagonist of inhibitor of apoptosis (IAP) proteins and clinical candidate for the treatment of cancer (GDC-0152). J Med Chem 55(9):4101–4113
103. Cohen P, Tcherpakov M (2010) Will the ubiquitin system furnish as many drug targets as protein kinases? Cell 143:686–693
104. Weisberg E et al (2010) Smac mimetics: implications for enhancement of targeted therapies in leukemia. Leukemia 24(12):2100–2109
105. Cai Q et al (2011) A potent and orally active antagonist (SM-406/AT-406) of multiple inhibitor of apoptosis proteins (IAPs) in clinical development for cancer treatment. J Med Chem 54(8):2714–2726

106. McManus DC et al (2004) Loss of XIAP protein expression by RNAi and antisense approaches sensitizes cancer cells to functionally diverse chemotherapeutics. Oncogene 23(49):8105–8117
107. Allensworth JL et al (2013) Smac mimetic Birinapant induces apoptosis and enhances TRAIL potency in inflammatory breast cancer cells in an IAP-dependent and TNF-alpha-independent mechanism. Breast Cancer Res Treat 137(2):359–371
108. de Almagro MC, Vucic D (2012) The inhibitor of apoptosis (IAP) proteins are critical regulators of signaling pathways and targets for anti-cancer therapy. Exp Oncol 34(3):200–211
109. Bodine SC et al (2001) Identification of ubiquitin ligases required for skeletal muscle atrophy. Science 294(5547):1704–1708
110. Maxwell PH et al (1999) The tumour suppressor protein VHL targets hypoxia-inducible factors for oxygen-dependent proteolysis. Nature 399(6733):271–275
111. Deng L et al (2000) Activation of the IkappaB kinase complex by TRAF6 requires a dimeric ubiquitin-conjugating enzyme complex and a unique polyubiquitin chain. Cell 103(2): 351–361
112. Carrano AC et al (1999) SKP2 is required for ubiquitin-mediated degradation of the CDK inhibitor p27. Nat Cell Biol 1(4):193–199
113. Winston JT et al (1999) The SCFbeta-TRCP-ubiquitin ligase complex associates specifically with phosphorylated destruction motifs in IkappaBalpha and beta-catenin and stimulates IkappaBalpha ubiquitination in vitro. Genes Dev 13(3):270–283
114. Vidal M (2009) Role of polycomb proteins Ring1A and Ring1B in the epigenetic regulation of gene expression. Int J Dev Biol 53(2–3):355–370
115. Paolino M et al (2011) Essential role of E3 ubiquitin ligase activity in Cbl-b-regulated T cell functions. J Immunol 186(4):2138–2147
116. Nakahara T et al (2007) YM155, a novel small-molecule survivin suppressant, induces regression of established human hormone-refractory prostate tumor xenografts. Cancer Res 67(17):8014–8021
117. Yamasaki S et al (2007) Cytoplasmic destruction of p53 by the endoplasmic reticulum-resident ubiquitin ligase 'Synoviolin'. EMBO J 26(1):113–122
118. Scheffner M et al (1993) The HPV-16 E6 and E6-AP complex functions as a ubiquitin-protein ligase in the ubiquitination of p53. Cell 75(3):495–505
119. Shi D, Grossman SR (2010) Ubiquitin becomes ubiquitous in cancer: emerging roles of ubiquitin ligases and deubiquitinases in tumorigenesis and as therapeutic targets. Cancer Biol Ther 10(8):737–747
120. Chan CH et al (2013) Pharmacological inactivation of Skp2 SCF ubiquitin ligase restricts cancer stem cell traits and cancer progression. Cell 154(3):556–568
121. Ito T et al (2010) Identification of a primary target of thalidomide teratogenicity. Science 327(5971):1345–1350
122. Goldenberg SJ et al (2010) Strategies for the identification of ubiquitin ligase inhibitors. Biochem Soc Trans 38(pt 1):132–136
123. Davydov IV et al (2004) Assay for ubiquitin ligase activity: high-throughput screen for inhibitors of HDM2. J Biomol Screen 9(8):695–703
124. Huang KS, Vassilev LT (2005) High-throughput screening for inhibitors of the Cks1-Skp2 interaction. Methods Enzymol 399:717–728
125. Ungermannova D et al (2013) High-throughput screening AlphaScreen assay for identification of small-molecule inhibitors of ubiquitin E3 ligase SCFSkp2-Cks1. J Biomol Screen 18(8):910–920
126. Dy GK et al (2013) Phase Ib trial of the oral angiogenesis inhibitor pazopanib administered concurrently with erlotinib. Invest New Drugs 31(4):891–899
127. Britten CD (2013) PI3K and MEK inhibitor combinations: examining the evidence in selected tumor types. Cancer Chemother Pharmacol 71(6):1395–1409
128. Sheppard KE et al (2013) Synergistic inhibition of ovarian cancer cell growth by combining selective PI3K/mTOR and RAS/ERK pathway inhibitors. Eur J Cancer 49:3936–3944

Chapter 13
Novel Ubiquitin E3 Ligases as Targets for Cancer Therapy: Focus on Breast Cancer-Associated Gene 2 (BCA2)

Yutaka Amemiya, Stephanie Bacopulos, and Arun Seth

Abstract The struggle to find new cancer targets continues unabated. With this in mind, E3 ligases (also called E3 ubiquitin ligases) constitute a large and diverse family of genes that play a role in the ubiquitination of proteins as well as in a myriad of other important activities in cells including, but not limited to, DNA repair and proliferation. Breast cancer-associated protein 2 (BCA2) is an E3 ligase that is expressed in a large number of invasive breast cancers and is involved in several important cellular functions. In this chapter we describe the mechanisms that control the expression and half-life of BCA2 and the association between high expression of BCA2 and breast cancer tumor grade. Furthermore, we explore the role that this E3 ligase may play in cancer progression. Finally, we examine the potential effects of E3 ligases, including BCA2, a novel class of wide-ranging therapeutic cancer targets.

Keywords Breast cancer-associated gene 2 (BCA2) • Ubiquitin-proteasome system (UPS) • E3 ubiquitin ligase • Human homolog of Rad23 variant A (hHR23a) • 14-3-3σ • Breast cancer

---

Y. Amemiya, M.Sc., Ph.D.
Next Generation Sequencing Lab, Sunnybrook Research Institute,
2075 Bayview Avenue, Toronto, ON, Canada M4N 3M5
e-mail: yamemiya@sri.utoronto.ca

S. Bacopulos
Biological Sciences Platform, Sunnybrook Research Institute, Sunnybrook Health Sciences Centre, 2075 Bayview Avenue, Toronto, ON, Canada M4N 3M5
e-mail: stephanie.bacopulos@gmail.com

A. Seth, Ph.D. (✉)
Biological Sciences Platform, Sunnybrook Research Institute, Sunnybrook Health Sciences Centre, 2075 Bayview Avenue, Toronto, ON, Canada M4N 3M5

Department of Laboratory Medicine and Pathobiology, University of Toronto, Toronto, ON, Canada
e-mail: arun.seth@utoronto.ca

Q.P. Dou (ed.), *Resistance to Proteasome Inhibitors in Cancer*, Resistance to Targeted Anti-Cancer Therapeutics, DOI 10.1007/978-3-319-06752-0_13

Abbreviations

ALDH	Aldehyde dehydrogenase
APC	Anaphase-promoting complex
BARD1	BRCA1-associated RING domain 1
BCA2	Breast cancer-associated gene 2
BER	Base excision repair
BZF	BCA2 zinc-finger
C-CBL	Casitas B-lineage lymphoma
Cdc4	Cell division cycle 4
CDK	Cyclin-dependent kinase
CGH	Comparative genomic hybridization
CHX	Cycloheximide
DUBs	Deubiquitinating enzymes
E1	Ubiquitin-activating enzyme
E2s	Ubiquitin-conjugating enzymes
E3s	Ubiquitin ligases
E6-AP	E6-associated protein
EFP	Estrogen-responsive finger protein
EGFR	Epidermal growth factor receptor
ER	Estrogen receptor
FBW7	F-box and WD repeat domain-containing 7
FR	Folate receptor
HER2	Epidermal growth factor receptor 2
hHR23a	Human homolog of Rad23 variant A
HOS	Homolog of Slimb
HPV	Human papillomavirus
HSV-1	Herpes simplex virus-1
K	Lysine
LMP-1	Latent membrane protein 1
MetAP-2	Methionine aminopeptidase-2
NER	Nucleotide excision repair
PDGFRα	Platelet-derived growth factor receptor alpha
PR	Progesterone receptor
Protac	Proteolysis targeting chimeric molecule
RNAi	RNA interference
RTK	Receptor tyrosine kinases
SCF	Skp-Cullin-F-box
TOR	Target of rapamycin
UBL	Ubiquitin-like
UPS	Ubiquitin-proteasome system
VHL	von Hippel-Lindau
XP	Xeroderma pigmentosum
XPC	XP group C protein

13.1 The Ubiquitin-Proteasome System

Ubiquitin is a highly conserved small (8.5 kDa) protein modifier, which is posttranslationally covalently conjugated to target proteins through a number of well-coordinated steps, a process referred to as ubiquitylation (or ubiquitination). The attachment of ubiquitin to substrate proteins can occur as a single moiety or in the form of polymeric chains in which successive ubiquitin molecules are connected through specific isopeptide bonds. The outcomes of this ubiquitination process on target proteins are diverse and depend on the nature of the ubiquitin chain formed, which is reminiscent of a code. The specific linkages of lysine residues within the ubiquitin molecule itself and to subsequent ubiquitin moieties define this "ubiquitin code." The various ubiquitin modifications adopt distinct conformations and lead to different outcomes in cells.

There are seven lysine (K) residues within ubiquitin that can be used to create a chain. Although the ubiquitin code still largely remains a mystery, trends of protein fates following ubiquitination are as follows. K48-linked chains, the most common variation, and K11-linked chains target proteins for degradation via the 26S proteasome [1, 2]. K63-linked chains have been implicated in DNA repair and targeting of proteins to the lysosome [3]. Linear N-terminal-linked ubiquitin chains on target proteins are necessary for NF-κB activation [4, 5]. Chains whose functions are still unknown include K6-, K27-, and K29-linked chains. Moreover, because ubiquitin chains are not always solely composed of one linkage type, branched or forked ubiquitin chains are also generated (reviewed in [6]). These branched chains, as with polyubiquitin chains and monoubiquitination, are signals for various protein functions and fates. Monoubiquitination plays a role in various cellular functions such as internalization of cell surface proteins and receptors and DNA damage responses [6–9]. Furthermore, monoubiquitination is used as a "jumping-off point" for building polyubiquitin chains, as multiple ubiquitin-conjugating enzymes (E2s) and E3 ligases (E3s) can be involved in the modification of a single target [6–9].

Additionally, it has also been recognized that similar to phosphorylation-directed signaling pathways, which can be "turned-off" by phosphatase activity that causes the removal of phosphate groups, ubiquitin signaling is also capable of dynamic regulation of pathways via ubiquitination reversal by deubiquitinating enzymes (DUBs) [6]. These proteases function in the activation of ubiquitin monomers following translation of polyubiquitin precursor proteins, as well as in the selective removal of ubiquitins from growing chains. This provides a mechanism for regulating the processivity of E3s and their substrates [reviewed in [10, 11]. The existence of DUBs adds an important new dimension to the ubiquitin-proteasome system (UPS), by adding another layer of control and specificity to protein degradation and regulation.

There are three specific types of enzymes, involved in the ubiquitin conjugation of target proteins, as shown in Fig. 13.1. (1) Ubiquitin-activating enzyme, or E1, is the first enzyme that activates the ubiquitin moiety through adenylation with ATP, causing a covalent thiol-ester bond to form between ubiquitin and E1 [12]. This step is carried out by only two E1s that function in the ubiquitin pathway, UBA1 and UBA6 [13]; other E1s exist, but they are involved in various ubiquitin-like modifier pathways. (2) The second enzyme is the ubiquitin-conjugating enzyme (E2). Following activation,

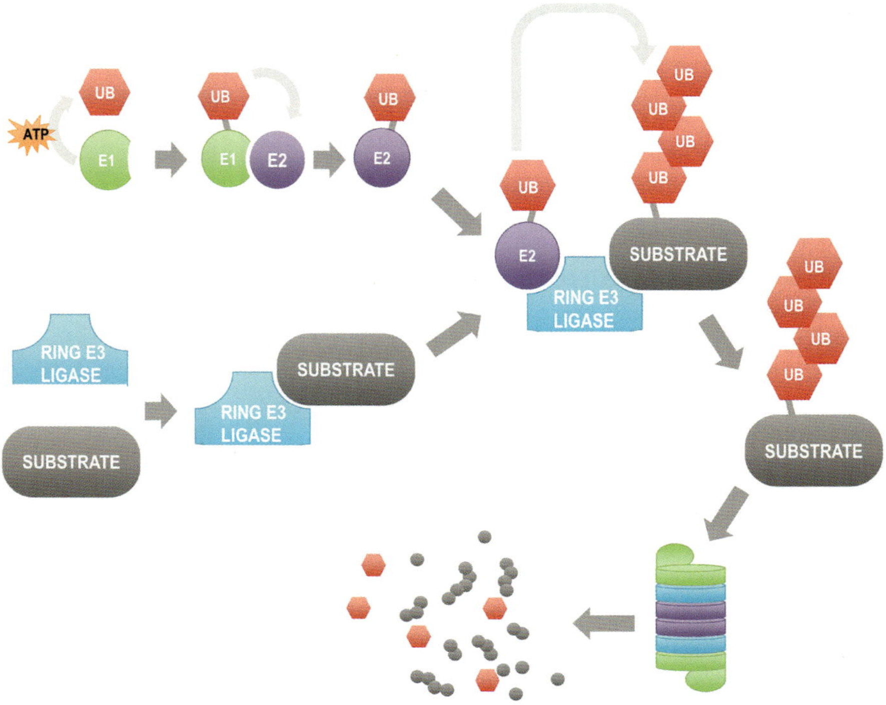

Fig. 13.1 Representation of the ubiquitin-proteasome system (UPS). Ubiquitin (UB) is activated in step 1 by adenylation, which links the UB to the E1 via a thiol-ester bond. UB is then transferred from the E1 to E2, which creates a second thiol-ester bond with the ubiquitin moiety. The RING E3 ligase binds with specificity to the substrate and positions the ubiquitin-loaded E2 in close proximity for transfer of ubiquitin to the substrate. Substrates, on which poly-K-48-linked ubiquitin chains are conjugated, are then typically targeted for degradation by the 26S proteasome

the ubiquitin moiety gets transferred from the donor cysteine residue on E1 to the acceptor cysteine residue on E2 [12]. (3) The third enzyme, the E3 ligase (E3), is involved in linkage, which is a cooperative effort between E3-mediated changes in conformation and proximity, and E2 specificity for a particular linkage type. For example, the E2 UBE2S is specific for the elongation of K11-linked chains, while UBC1, UBC3, and UBC7 E2s elongate and catalyze K48-linked chains, and UBC13 is specific for K63-linked chains. However, not all E2s share this linkage specificity, especially those that associate with HECT-type E3 ligases [13–17].

13.2 The Role of E3 Ligases

E3 (also called an E3 ubiquitin ligase) plays an important role in the UPS. It is a ligase enzyme that associates with a ubiquitin-bound E2, which enables the recognition of the target protein that is to be ubiquitinated and triggers the attachment of ubiquitin to a lysine on the target protein via an isopeptide bond. In this way, E3 can target specific protein substrates for degradation by the proteasome. When proteins are polyubiquitinated by E3, this basically marks the protein for degradation by the proteasome.

In certain circumstances, however, some ubiquitination events are limited to monoubiquitination, whereby only a single ubiquitin is added by E3 to a substrate molecule. These monoubiquitinated proteins are not targeted to the proteasome for degradation, but rather can be altered with respect to their cellular location or function by binding to other proteins that have domains capable of binding ubiquitin.

E3 subclassification is based on the protein structure, which is highly diverse among the subclasses. These include HECT-type, RING-type, U-box, F-box, and PHD domains. E3s function as monomeric units as in the case of CBL, or as a part of a complex, such as the Skp-Cullin-F-box (SCF) protein complex. There are two different approaches used by E3 to transfer ubiquitin to the substrate: (1) Direct transfer of the ubiquitin moiety first to E3 and then, subsequently, from E3 to the substrate. Such an approach is primarily utilized by HECT-type ligases such as E6-AP [18]. (2) Indirect transfer is the preferred route used by other E3 subtypes including RING-type E3s, where E3 acts as a scaffold for both the substrate and E2. The target protein to be ubiquitinated is specified by E3 [12]. The two approaches used by E3 are the most well-characterized methods of substrate ubiquitination; however, it is now becoming more evident that E3s can function in other modes as well. For example, it has been shown that E3s can act cooperatively to perform multi-site ubiquitinations on target proteins, as well as initiate ubiquitin chains to be elongated by a secondary E3. In this case, the second E3 is considered to be functioning in the capacity of an E4 (recently reviewed by Metzger and Weissman [19]).

13.3 Mechanisms of Regulation and Stabilization of E3 Ligases

The mechanisms through which E3 ligases are regulated are virtually unknown. Both proteolytic and non-proteolytic mechanisms are involved in controlling stability, turnover, substrate affinity, and ubiquitination of E3 ligases [20]. Stability can be altered by modifications including phosphorylation, dynamic monoubiquitination, or non-K48-linked multi-ubiquitination and branched multi-ubiquitination, which can also either increase the stability of the E3 ligase or alter its ability to bind substrate, as has been shown to be the case with E3 ligase RING1B and its substrate histone H2A [21, 22]. By and large, the most common method of E3 ligase regulation is through autoubiquitination, resulting in proteasome-mediated degradation. However, it is precisely this ability of E3 ligases to self-degrade that is problematic in terms of investigating ligase functions and consequences. Thus, studies have been conducted in which a novel E3 ligase, BCA2 (breast cancer-associated gene 2, also designated RNF115, ZNF364, and T3A12; see below), has been overexpressed, hence allowing for investigations of both BCA2 and its stability. Additionally, theses studies aim to characterize its interactions with partner protein modifications that result in modifications to BCA2 itself and the effects this has on protein function.

The presence of substrate or other interacting partners has been found to diminish the self-destructive behavior of E3 ligases [23]. This stabilization through binding inhibits the autoubiquitination of the E3 ligases, since the binding of ubiquitin and substrate is a mutually exclusive event. E3 ligases that have been demonstrated to be stabilized through substrate binding, to date, include homolog of Slimb (HOS), whose protein turnover is stabilized by the presence of the substrate IκBα [24]. This is also the case for cell division cycle 4 (Cdc4), which in the absence of substrate binds ubiquitin, thereby promoting its own degradation. Conversely, in the presence of an increasing concentration of substrate, Cdc4 is stabilized [25].

In general, E3 ligases usually interact with other components of the UPS, including proteins that have seemingly antagonistic roles. An example of this is the RING-type E3 ligase, ICP0, which has been shown to stimulate the lytic infection of herpes simplex virus-1 (HSV-1). When ICP0 binds to the deubiquitinase, USP7, it is unable to self-ubiquitinate, and therefore, fails to target itself for degradation. Another mechanism used in the stabilization of E3 ligases is dimerization. This has been seen with E3 ligases such as TRAF3, BRCA1/BARD1, and LMP-1. When TRAF3 heterodimerizes with the Epstein-Barr virus-encoded latent membrane protein 1 (LMP-1), this interaction may have functional consequences as well as results in the stabilization of TRAF3 by preventing its autoubiquitination [26].

13.4 E3 Link to Cancer

Each of the over 600 E3 ligase genes plays a specific role in the UPS, and given their potential link to cancer, this opens the door to prospective novel treatments for breast and other cancers that involve targeting E3 ligases. There are a number of E3 ligases that are potential targets for various therapeutic approaches, which are being developed to either prevent a specific protein from being degraded or promote its degradation (see Sect. 13.10). Given the combination of differential tumor expression and substrate specificity, this family of over 600 genes becomes a potentially rich source of novel and promising cancer targets.

13.5 Discovery and Expression of Breast Cancer-Associated Gene 2

Subtractive hybridization is a powerful technique that has been used successfully to discover novel differentially expressed genes in specific normal or cancerous tissues or cell types [27]. This technique was used to identify changes in expressed genes in the breast carcinoma cell line Hs578Bst (HTB 126) compared with an immortalized control cell line, which were derived from tumor and adjacent normal tissues, respectively. There were a total of 950 cDNAs that were found to be enriched in the breast cancer cell line compared to the control, and 28 of these were

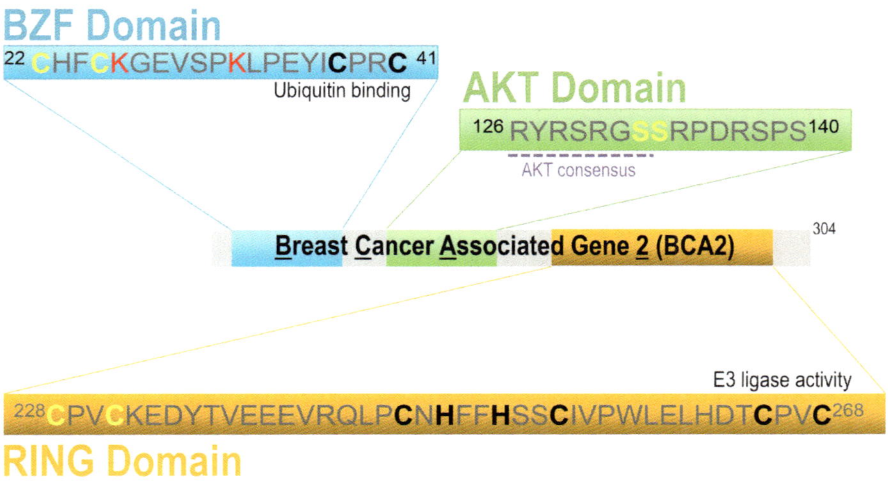

Fig. 13.2 Schematic representing the domains of BCA2. The *bolded black* amino acids represent key residues which are imperative to the structural integrity of the BZF and RING domains. The *bolded yellow* residues indicate amino acids that have been modified to alanine by site-directed mutagenesis. The *blue* domain, BZF, is responsible for non-covalent ubiquitin binding, which is also the site of BCA2 autoubiquitination. Lysine residues to which ubiquitins are conjugated are shown in *red*. The AKT domain, depicted in *green*, is determined to be the most likely site of AKT-mediated phosphorylation of BCA2 and predicted by in silico analysis. Amino acids shown in *yellow* are the serine residues most likely to be phosphorylated and have been mutated to alanine, the BCA2 S132, 133A mutant. The RING domain, depicted in *orange*, is responsible for BCA2-mediated ubiquitination. The *yellow* cysteine residues have been mutated to create a ligase-dead variation, the BCA2 RING mutant

identified as novel genes [28]. One of these cDNA clones encoded a novel 304 amino acid with a RING H2-domain [29] and was named BCA2. The gene for BCA2 is found on chromosome 1q21.1. Interestingly, this region on chromosome 1 has been found to be a "hot spot" for upregulated genes in breast cancer as well as a region of genomic instability and driver genes in other cancers [30].

The BCA2 protein contains three domains, depicted in Fig. 13.2, an amino-terminal BCA2 zinc-finger (BZF) domain, an AKT-phosphorylation domain, and a carboxy-terminal RING H2 domain [31, 32]. The RING domain confers autoubiquitination activity, which is similar to other E3 ubiquitin ligases such as RING proteins MDM2 and SIAH1 [29, 33, 34]. Another E3 ligase, RNF126, recently shown to promote cancer cell proliferation by targeting p21 for ubiquitin-mediated degradation [35], has been shown to be structurally homologous to BCA2 in the similarity of protein domains.

1. *RING-H2 domain*: This domain coordinates two zinc ions using the following consensus sequence, Cys-X2-Cys-X(9-39)-Cys-X(1-3)-His-X(2-3)-Cys-X2-Cys-X(4-48)-Cys-X2-Cys, where X may be any amino acid [36]. This domain is critically involved in ubiquitination of substrates and self, and is the binding site

Table 13.1 Effects of mutations on function and stability of BCA2 protein

Mutation	Ligase positive/negative	Stability
BCA2 (wild type)	Normal	Normal
C22A, C25A (BZF mutant)	Increased ligase activity	Unstable
K26R, K32R	No ligase activity	Very stable
S132A, S133A (AKT mutant)	Normal	Normal
C228A, C231A (RING mutant)	No ligase activity	Very stable
K260R	Very high ligase activity	Very unstable

for ubiquitin transfer enzymes (E2s). Disruption or mutation of these domains results in the inactivation of the ligase. This has been shown to be the case for BCA2, whereby the RING domain is involved in autoubiquitination and this E3 ligase activity is completely eliminated by mutations of C228 and C231 to alanines [31, 29] (Table 13.1).

2. *AKT domain*: This domain was initially identified following in silico analysis of the BCA2 sequence. It is found in the mid-protein region and it was initially proposed that AKT could bind to either of two AKT consensus sequences. Phosphorylation assays in vitro were used to confirm that this consensus sequence was indeed sites for AKT phosphorylation of BCA2, most likely on serine residues 132 and 133 [31, 32]. When BCA2 is mutated to alanine at S132 and S133, ligase activity is unaffected in vitro; however, these mutations indicate that phosphorylation may be important with regard to conformational changes in the protein that concern partner binding [31].
3. *BZF domain*: This last novel domain, which is unique to BCA2 and RNF126, is the principle location involved in autoubiquitination, in particular at lysines 26 and 32 [31]. These residues are both highly ubiquitinated, as shown by time-course in vitro ubiquitination assays [31]. Furthermore, these two lysines play functionally redundant roles in that mutation in one is rescued by the other non-mutated lysine; however, mutations in both positions lead to the elimination of autoubiquitination in vitro [31]. This strongly suggests that these two lysines are an important regulatory feature of BCA2. Of note, non-covalent ubiquitin binding also occurs through the BZF domain, which displays a particular affinity for polyubiquitin chains [31]. The affinity of ubiquitin chains for BCA2 depends on their length; monoubiquitin has less affinity than two ubiquitin moieties, with BCA2 having the highest affinity for ubiquitin chains of six molecules. The BZF domain of BCA2 displays a high affinity for ubiquitin binding that is second only to the A20 domain of Rabex-5 [31].

BCA2 mRNA expression occurred at a moderate level in a number of normal tissues including heart, skeletal muscle, and testis. Basal expression was also detected in normal breast, prostate, lung, and colon. In breast cancer cell lines and tissues, however, BCA2 was overexpressed. For example, BCA2 mRNA was very highly expressed in the estrogen receptor (ER)-positive MCF7 breast cancer cell line as well as in invasive breast carcinomas [29]. This potential link between BCA2, binding partners, and breast cancer is explored later in the chapter.

13.6 BCA2-Binding Partners

Autoubiquitination activity of the wild-type BCA2 protein renders it unstable, which is mediated by its RING domain. This results in substantial protein degradation as has been shown in vivo and in vitro for the wild-type protein; however, of note, ligase-dead BCA2 variants do not show signs of degradation [29, 31]. Interaction with a binding partner can play an important role in stabilizing BCA2.

Various groups, including our own, have investigated binding partners for BCA2 [37–39]. Recently, one of the targets for BCA2-mediated substrate ubiquitination has been identified as the cyclin-dependent kinase (CDK) inhibitor $p21^{Waf/Cip1}$ [40]. To date, several binding partners of BCA2 that have been confirmed include ubiquitin, Rab7, tetherin, and UBC9 [31, 37, 38, 41]. A yeast-II-hybrid screen with murine cell lines was used to identify Rab7, which was further confirmed using a GST pull-down assay on a human homolog of Rab7 [38, 41].

We have recently identified 16 new BCA2 interacting proteins (Table 13.2), two of which were human homolog of Rad23 variant A (hHR23a) and 14-3-3σ. HHR23a is a known chaperone in the UPS [42] and 14-3-3σ is a multifunctional adaptor protein that has been found to play a role in various cancers including breast. [43] The effects of hHR23a and 14-3-3σ on the stability and autoubiquitination activity of BCA2, as well as co-expression with BCA2 in breast cancer, are discussed in turn below.

13.6.1 HHR23a: A Multifunctional Ubiquitin Receptor

It was shown that HHR23a is a component of the DNA nucleotide excision repair (NER) pathway and to a lesser extent the base excision repair (BER) pathway, where, like its homolog hHR23b, it was found to regulate and stabilize the XP group C protein (XPC) [44, 45]. Mutations in hHR23a, resulting in protein deletion or malfunction, contribute to known rare genetic disorders, including xeroderma pigmentosum (XP), Cockayne syndrome, and trichothiodystrophy [45]. In the case of XP patients, they are unable to properly correct DNA damage resulting from the formation of UV-induced dimers; thus, they display an increased sensitivity to sunlight and therefore, have a greatly increased risk for developing skin cancer [45].

In addition to the role hHR23a plays in NER/BER pathways, it also functions as a ubiquitin receptor, which has widespread and far-reaching roles throughout the cell. This relatively recent classification of hHR23a as a member of the ubiquitin receptor family is due to its affinity for binding ubiquitin moieties. In particular, hHR23a regulates the longevity of its binding partners. This is accomplished in one of two ways: (1) through proteasomal shuttling, where hHR23a simultaneously binds to the target protein and the 26S proteasomal subunit, or (2) by stabilizing the target protein through sequestration of ubiquitin moieties in the emerging polyubiquitin chain, thereby preventing chain elongation and deubiquitinase activity [46]. Two domains of hHR23a, the N-terminal ubiquitin-like domain (UBL) and two C-terminal ubiquitin-associating domains, are largely responsible for the dichotomous and dual nature of this protein [46].

Table 13.2 Putative binding partners of BCA2 identified through two hybrid screening

Gene	Official symbol	Accession number	Function
14-3-3σ	*SFN*	*NP_006133.1*	*Proliferation, signal transduction and apoptosis*
Atrophin-1	ATN1	NP_001007027.1	Transcription factor
CDC2-related protein kinase 10	CDK10	NP_001092003.2	Cell proliferation
Cystatin C	CST3	NP_000090.1	Inhibitor of cysteine proteases
Microfibril-associated glycoprotein 4	MFAP4	NP_001185624.1	Cell adhesion and cell-cell interactions
Immunoglobulin heavy constant alpha 1 (SNC73)	IGHA1	AF067420	Colorectal cancer marker
Human homolog of Rad23 variant A	*RAD23A*	*NP_005044.1*	*DNA repair, chaperone*
DOCK4 dedicator of cytokinesis 4	DOCK4	NP_055520.3	Regulates cell-cell adhesion
Folate receptor 3	FOLR3	NP_000795.2	Internalization of folic acid
UBE2I ubiquitin-conjugating enzyme E2I (UBC9)	UBE2I	NP_003336.1	SUMO E2-conjugating enzyme
RAB7A, member RAS oncogene family	RAB7A	NP_004628.4	Vesicle traffic in endosomes
Ubiquitin C	UBC	NP_066289	Precursor of ubiquitin
Ubiquitin A-52 residue ribosomal protein fusion product 1	UBA52	NP_001029102.1	Precursor of ubiquitin
Ribosomal protein L18a	RPL18A	NP_000971.1	Component of the 60S ribosome subunit
Bone marrow stromal cell antigen 2, tetherin	BST2	NP_004326.1	Bone marrow stromal cell antigen
Cyclin-dependent kinase inhibitor 1A	CDKN1A	NP_000380.1	Cyclin-dependent kinase inhibitor

One of the known critical functions of hHR23a acting as a ubiquitin receptor is in the regulation of p53 protein levels through its interaction with p53. Binding of hHR23a to p53 inhibits the ability of MDM2 to polyubiquitinate p53, targeting it for degradation [44]. With its dual role in mutation repair at the DNA level and in modulation of proteins involved in mutation checkpoints, hHR23A may play a bigger role in cancer formation/progression.

13.6.2 Implications of the BCA2 and hHR23a Interaction

Binding experiments with GST-tagged BCA2 proteins were used to validate the interaction between BCA2 and hHR23a [36]. Through recombinant expression studies in HEK293T cells, the binding affinity of wild-type and the S132, 133A

BCA2 mutant with hHR23a appeared to be much greater than with BCA2 BZF and RING mutants, implying that the RING and BZF domains may both be necessary for interaction between hHR23a and BCA2. Interestingly, because the S132, 133A mutant, which is AKT-phosphorylation deficient, interacts with hHR23a with a high binding affinity, this suggests that hHR23a may interact with BCA2 when BCA2 is in a dephosphorylated state. Furthermore, BCA2 has been shown to interact non-covalently with polyubiquitin chains [31], a trait shared with hHR23a; specifically hHR23a preferentially interacts with tetra-ubiquitin chains [46, 47]. This further suggests that this shared affinity for polyubiquitin chains is what forms the basis for the interaction between BCA2 and hHR23a.

While hHR23a interacts with BCA2, it is not a substrate for BCA2-mediated degradation. When increasing amounts of BCA2 were co-transfected with stable amounts of hHR23a, there was no decrease in the concentration of hHR23a; on the contrary, the interaction with BCA2 appeared to increase the level of hHR23a expression [37].

In yeast, Rad23, the ortholog of hHR23a, may be monoubiquitinated and/or multi-ubiquitinated in vivo [48]; however this does not lead to its degradation. It has recently come to light that degradation of Rad23 does not occur due to the lack of an effective initiation region at which the proteasome can engage the protein and unfold it [49]. Furthermore, the authors showed that the unstructured loops found in Rad23 were too short to support degradation, which is not specific to Rad23 but rather appears to be a common property of the UPS. An ancestral relative of BCA2 exists as Znf364 in yeast, which may be involved in the ubiquitination of Rad23; however, since it cannot be degraded by the proteasome, ubiquitin signaling fate may determine protein localization. Similarly, BCA2 may be involved in the ubiquitination of hHR23a in mammalian cells, which may play a role in the intracellular localization of hHR23a.

Co-expression of BCA2 and hHR23a was first validated in breast cancer cell lines and co-expression of BCA2 and hHR23a, using immunofluorescence, revealed that co-localization of BCA2 and hHR23a occurred over large areas in both the nucleus and cytoplasm [50]. The characteristic punctate staining observed for BCA2 likely indicates localization at the endosome given its association with Rab7, an important regulator of vesicular transport. [41, 38, 39] Co-localization of BCA2 and hHR23a was also found to occur in breast cancer cases with intense staining seen in both the cytoplasm and nucleus (see below).

What is most critical concerning the interaction between BCA2 and hHR23a may not be the effect that BCA2 exerts on hHR23a, but rather the impact that hHR23a has on the stability of BCA2. Degradation of BCA2 occurs via autoubiquitination through its interaction with E2s of the UbcH5 family, but not by other degradation-specific E2 ubiquitin-conjugating enzymes, such as UBC3 [41]. Furthermore, it has been clearly demonstrated that these E2 enzymes are responsible for the rapid and complete degradation of wild-type BCA2 protein in vitro and in vivo [31, 29].

Expression of increasing amounts of hHR23a protein correlated with an increase in the amount of BCA2 protein in a recombinant expression system [50]. Stabilization of BCA2 is thought to occur through interaction with hHR23a, which prevents the autoubiquitination of BCA2 from taking place. This is consistent with hHR23a acting as a ubiquitin receptor, which binds to polyubiquitin chains [46, 51]. In the recombinant system, when BCA2 is expressed alone or with E2, intense ubiquitin laddering is observed, indicative of highly degraded BCA2. In sharp contrast, ubiquitin smears are absent from cells co-expressing hHR23a, as hHR23a binding sequesters the growing ubiquitin chains [50].

Previous experiments in our lab regarding protein turnover of BCA2 have clearly shown that the wild-type BCA2 is rapidly degraded in cells but not the RING mutant, which does not undergo autoubiquitination [29]. Furthermore, when half-life determinations were conducted in the presence of the protein synthesis inhibitor cycloheximide (CHX), BCA2 was found to be present substantially longer when co-expressed with hHR23a. Thus, by stabilizing BCA2, hHR23a also contributes to lengthening its half-life in cells [50], which may be quite important regarding function given its relatively short half-life in the absence of any stabilization.

13.6.3 Interaction of BCA2 with 14-3-3σ

14-3-3σ is a member of the ubiquitously expressed 14-3-3 family of seven highly conserved adaptor proteins, which are integral to a number of important cellular activities and have far-reaching implications in cancer [52]. They characteristically bind as either homo- or heterodimers to specific phosphopeptide consensus sequences [52]. One of the main roles for 14-3-3σ is as a prominent regulator of cell cycle checkpoints, while also being involved in multiple and diverse cellular pathways through its interaction with numerous known ligands [43, 53–55]. In addition, 14-3-3σ is the only member of its family that is induced by DNA damage [53].

Because of its important role in mediating cell cycle progression, it is not unexpected that 14-3-3σ regulation is also associated with carcinogenesis pathways; in particular, it has been found to be downregulated in breast cancer [56]. Expression of 14-3-3σ is often regulated by epigenetic silencing through hypermethylation of CpG islands in the promoter region [57].

14-3-3σ was isolated from a bacteria-II-hybrid partner-screening assay with wild-type BCA2. The association between BCA2 and 14-3-3σ was established using recombinant pull-down assays [50] for both the wild-type protein and the RING mutant, but not for the BZF or S132, 133A BCA2 mutants, signifying that the interaction may rely on sequences in these domains. Importantly, surrounding S132 and S133 are two 14-3-3σ binding motifs. The principal site is likely to correspond to the motif R(S/X)XpSXP (as reviewed by Manning and Cantley [58],), which is highly similar to the BCA2 sequence 130-RG<u>SS</u>RP-135.

Evidence for an interaction between BCA2 and 14-3-3σ was obtained from expression analysis of these two proteins in breast cancer cell lines, which were found to co-localize in the cytoplasm of the breast cancer cell line MCF7 using immunofluorescent staining of endogenous proteins [50] (see below). Phosphorylation was also found to be an essential component in the binding of

14-3-3σ to BCA2, because samples exposed to the AKT inhibitor, LY294002, were less apt to co-immunoprecipitate [50].

It was also noted that although the BCA2 S132, 133A mutant was less efficient at binding 14-3-3σ, it was not entirely eliminated, suggesting the likelihood of a second functional AKT-phosphorylation site and 14-3-3σ binding site, predicted to be located in the adjacent sequence 133-SRPDRSPS-140 [50].

Interestingly, tandem 14-3-3σ sites (see above) have been detected in other proteins, such as Cbl and c-Raf-1. These tandem 14-3-3σ sites present in BCA2 can have one of two potential consequences. Firstly, it may impart a tight bidentate binding with a single 14-3-3σ dimer, which may result in sequestering of the bound protein [59]. Secondly, both sites may be necessary to promote binding with 14-3-3σ, as has been shown to be the case with Cbl [59]. In addition, results of experiments conducted with the BCA2 S132, 133A mutant highlight the potential importance of AKT phosphorylation of BCA2 in mediating binding with partner proteins and substrate interactions.

Interaction of BCA2 with 14-3-3σ has an apparent impact on the degradation of 14-3-3σ as shown by the dose-dependent effect that increased expression of BCA2 had on 14-3-3σ protein levels [50]. Conversely, 14-3-3σ appears to stabilize BCA2 through substrate interactions. Co-expression of 14-3-3σ and BCA2 in HEK cells in the presence of the proteasomal inhibitor MG-132 resulted in greater stabilization of BCA2 than when BCA2 was expressed alone [50]. 14-3-3σ presumably stabilizes BCA2 by sterically or conformationally precluding access of the RING finger domain to the target lysines (K26 and K32) in the BZF domain [31].

Degradation of BCA2 still occurred in the presence of a proteasome inhibitor alone, which gives credence to the argument that the UPS is not solely involved in the degradation of BCA2. Rab7, a binding partner of BCA2, plays an important role in the trafficking of proteins between late endosomes and lysosomes and subsequent degradation [60]. In a comparable manner, BCA2 may be subjected to lysosomal degradation as a potential transferred cargo [61, 20]. This is similar to the E3 ligase Cbl-b, which has been shown to be involved in the coordinated degradation of the EGFR signaling complex in the lysosome [62].

13.7 Mechanisms of BCA2 Stabilization: The Role of AKT

The role of the highly dynamic process of phosphorylation is to regulate proteins through modification, including changes to conformation and thus substrate affinity and specificity for many enzyme types, including E3 ligases [63, 64]. Phosphorylation of E3 ligases can also result in protein activation and turnover. The RING-type E3 ligase, c-Cbl, is activated by phosphorylation to its ubiquitination-ready state, where it is responsible for the internalization and degradation of EGFR [65]. Once c-Cbl is activated by phosphorylation, however, it also becomes targeted for degradation by other ligases. Through the involvement of CD28, Cbl-b is phosphorylated by PKC-θ, which targets it for degradation by the NEDD4 E3 ligase [66].

With respect to BCA2, in addition to stabilization by hHR23a, AKT phosphorylation can also enhance the stability of BCA2. Phosphorylation of BCA2 has been shown to occur in the presence of AKT [32]. When wild-type BCA2 is co-expressed with constitutively active AKT, it is more stable, but not when co-expressed with inactive AKT mutants [50]. Conversely, the BCA2 mutant variant, S132, S133A, which does not contain the predicted AKT-phosphorylation site, displayed no noticeable change in stability, strongly supporting the role of these serine residues as the primary site of AKT-mediated BCA2 phosphorylation.

13.8 The Role of BCA2 in Cell Internalization Pathways

To date, all evidence points to BCA2 functioning in the trafficking and internalization of membrane-bound proteins/complexes, either directly or indirectly. As we have seen, UPS is not the only pathway responsible for BCA2 degradation, but BCA2 may also be degraded in the lysosome. Rabring7, the mouse homolog of BCA2, was shown to be a Rab7 target protein that was recruited to the late endosome/lysosome by the GTP-bound form of Rab7 [38] and that Rabring7 ubiquitinates itself but not Rab7 [39]. BCA2 also binds Rab7 and similarly, is not involved in its degradation [41]. Rabring7 through its interaction with Rab7 has also been shown to play a role in EGFR internalization and degradation [38, 39].

Rab7 is principally involved in lysosomal biogenesis and receptor degradation [60]. According to the one study, Rabring7 in conjunction with c-Cbl was found to accelerate EGFR degradation [39]. C-Cbl has emerged as a key regulator of EGFR downregulation by playing an important role in receptor ubiquitination [67], which is required for trafficking of the receptor towards the lysosome for degradation. In a recent report, RNF126 and Rabring7 were found to associate with EGFR through a ubiquitin-binding zinc-finger domain and both murine E3 ubiquitin ligases stimulated ubiquitination of EGFR. In the absence of c-Cbl, the binding of RNF126 and Rabring7 to EGFR decreased, suggesting that the two E3 ligases function downstream of c-Cbl [68]. They also showed that in HeLa cells, depletion of either RNF126 or Rabring7 resulted in EGFR being retained in a late endocytic compartment where it was inefficiently degraded. Furthermore, depletion of Rabring7 or RNF126 could also attenuate the degradation of other receptors including MET and CXCR4. Therefore, the authors suggested that these two ligases may play a role in ubiquitin-dependent sorting and downregulation of membrane receptors [68].

Additionally, BCA2 has been found to be associated with the host response to nascent virus particles in HIV-1-infected individuals. Newly formed virus particles that have not been released from the cell bind to tetherin, a cell-membrane protein. Internalization and degradation of both tetherin and tetherin-bound bodies is then mediated by BCA2 [37]. Taken together, these studies implicate BCA2/Rabring7 as playing an important role in the internalization of cell surface proteins and lysosomal degradation pathways.

13.9 The BCA2 Cancer Connection

13.9.1 Co-expression of BCA2 and Binding Partners in Breast Cancer Cell Lines

Previous studies have implicated BCA2 as playing a role in breast cancer progression and metastasis. Overexpression of BCA2 in breast cancer cell lines, such as MCF7, has been shown to correlate with an increase in the proliferative capacity and motility of cells [29]. These effects were decreased in breast cancer cells in which RNA interference (RNAi) was used to knock down endogenous BCA2 [29]. Additionally, exogenous expression of wild-type BCA2 in MCF7 cells rendered them more susceptible to wound closure than cells transfected with BCA2 with impaired ligase activity [31]. In the same study, cells transfected with the BZF mutant of BCA2, which is defective in ubiquitin binding, were slightly more motile than cells expressing the wild-type protein; however, what is underlying this observation has yet to be explored [31]. BCA2 functions in breast cancer cells are depicted in Fig. 13.3.

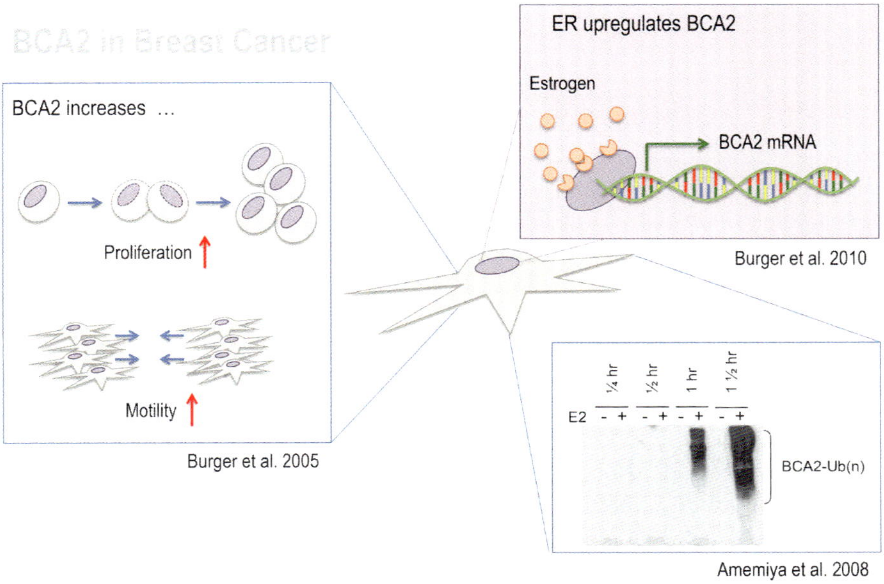

Fig. 13.3 Functions of BCA2 and how they relate to cellular behavior in breast cancer. BCA2 has been shown to be estrogen responsive; transcription of BCA2 is upregulated in the presence of estrogen [69]. BCA2 is unstable in vivo and in vitro in the presence of E2 enzyme as show in Amemiya et al. [31]. Increased BCA2 expression is correlated with increased proliferation and increased cellular motility [29, 31]

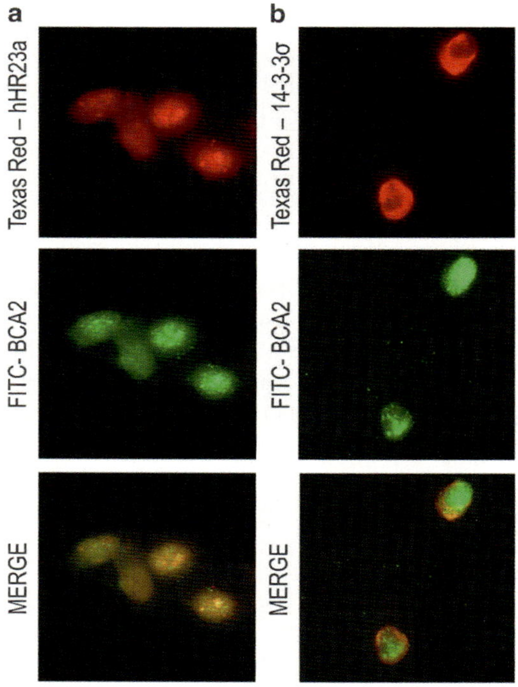

Fig. 13.4 Co-localization of BCA2 with hHR23 and 14-3-3σ in MCF7 cells. (**a**) Endogenous BCA2 and hHR23a tagged with either a secondary antibody conjugated to FITC dye or Texas Red in MCF7 cells. The *bottom panel* shows the co-localization of the proteins. (**b**) Endogenous BCA2 and 14-3-3σ tagged with either a secondary antibody conjugated to FITC dye or Texas Red in MCF7 cells. The *bottom panel* shows the co-localization of the proteins

BCA2, as well as its binding partners hHR23a and 14-3-3σ, were assessed in a number of breast cancer cell lines using Western blotting and TMAs. Transcriptional upregulation of BCA2 was previously shown to occur in ER-positive mammary epithelial cell lines [29, 69]. Similarly, BCA2 protein expression, determined using whole cell extracts on Western blots, was greater in ER-positive cell lines, BT474 and MCF7, compared with ER-negative cell lines, MDA MB 231, MDA MB 435, MDA MB 436, and MDA MB 45 [41]. HHR23a protein was shown to co-localize with BCA2 in MCF7 cells (Fig. 13.4a), and hHR23a levels correlated positively with BCA2 levels in the various other breast cancer cell lines, both ER-positive and ER-negative.

On the other hand, while 14-3-3σ protein expression was only found in cell lines that expressed BCA2, there was an inverse relationship in expression levels. This was also seen in breast cancer tissues such that cells with high BCA2 tended to express low amounts of 14-3-3σ, implying that BCA2 may be negatively regulating 14-3-3σ, although this inverse correlation was not shown to be statistically significant [50]. Co-localization of BCA2 and 14-3-3σ occurred in the cytoplasm in MCF7 cells (Fig. 13.4b) as well as in breast cancer tissues using immunofluorescence [50].

Cellular localization of BCA2 and hHR23a in MCF7 was shown to occur in both the cytoplasm and nucleus using immunofluorescent staining, albeit with more intense staining in the nucleus. The nuclear staining pattern was different between the two proteins in that BCA2 showed a more punctate pattern while staining of hHR23a was more diffuse [50]. In contrast to BCA2, which was found throughout MCF7 cells, 14-3-3σ was found exclusively in the cytoplasm. Thus, BCA2 is co-expressed and co-localized with hHR23a and 14-3-3σ in MCF7 cells [50].

13.9.2 BCA2 and Partner Proteins Are Co-expressed in Breast Cancer

Evaluation of co-expression of BCA2, hHR23a, and 14-3-3σ proteins in both the cytoplasmic and nuclear compartments was conducted in multiple breast cancer cases using TMAs and was analyzed in the context of potential diagnostic and prognostic value. BCA2 staining in the cytoplasm was found in nearly all 105 tumors (97 %), and although nuclear staining was detected in a lower percentage of cases, it was still detected in the majority of them (60 %). A similar picture emerged for hHR23a with 93 % of the tumors showing positive staining in the cytoplasm and 54 % in the nucleus. On the other hand, 14-3-3σ staining was only detected in the cytoplasm of tumor cells, albeit in the majority of cases (62 %). The staining pattern in tumor cells was consistent with that found in MCF7 cells [50].

A statistically significant positive correlation ($p=0.0113$) was observed for the cytoplasmic expression of BCA2 with hHR23a. This was also seen for nuclear co-expression, where there was an even greater statistical significance for the positive correlation between BCA2 and hHR23a in the nucleus ($p \leq 0.0001$). In contrast, while there was a nonsignificant statistical trend ($p=0.0804$) related to the negative correlation between low levels of 14-3-3σ expression in the face of high BCA2 expression, this was only found in 42 % of the 105 tumor samples [50].

There was also a correlation between hHR23a expression, ER-positive status, and negative nodal status, although the latter did not reach statistical significance, possibly due to the small sample size. Increased expression of BCA2, especially in the nucleus, may be regulated through interaction with hHR23a and possibly 14-3-3σ. Furthermore, given that BCA2 levels in the nucleus correlated with tumor grade, ER-positive status, negative nodal status, and increased >5-year survival, suggested that BCA2 may play a role, albeit an indirect one, in the physiology of breast carcinogenesis, growth, and metastasis, as well as in the predictability of tumor response to treatment [29].

13.9.3 BCA2 Is Associated with ER-Positive Breast Cancer

Historically, classification of breast tumors and treatment strategies have relied on immunohistochemical techniques in order to characterize biomarkers such as the estrogen receptor (ER), progesterone receptor (PR), and epidermal growth factor receptor 2 (HER2). However, these markers have been found to be somewhat lacking in fully predicting a patient's response to a given breast cancer treatment such as endocrine therapy. A thorough understanding of the key molecular drivers and the appropriate molecular signals should then provide a comprehensive list of therapeutic targets and predictive biomarkers.

Given the potential role that BCA2 plays in breast cancer and towards investigating its potential as a biomarker in breast cancer, positive staining of BCA2 has been detected in both the nucleus and cytoplasm in 56 % of tumor samples on a TMA [29]. When the TMA was analyzed with respect to hormone status, there was a significant co-localization and co-expression of BCA2 with ER, with 634 (67.1 %) and 526 (83 %) of the 945 samples staining positively for ER and BCA2 overexpression, respectively [29].

Co-expression of ER and BCA2 suggested a potential involvement of estrogen in the hormone-induced transcriptional regulation of BCA2 in ER-positive cells. This was supported by evidence obtained with the ER/PR/HER2-negative cell line MDA MB 231. When exogenous ER was overexpressed in this cell line, addition of estrogen caused an increase in the expression of BCA2 mRNA compared with mock transfected cells [69].

BCA2 expression was also associated with more positive prognostic factors and ER status. A RING E3 ligase, MDM2, has been shown to be prognostic of both poor and favorable outcomes in various cancers. Overexpression of MDM2 was a marker of poor outcome in sarcomas, gliomas, and acute lymphocytic leukemia; however, it was a marker of favorable prognosis in melanoma, non-small cell lung cancers, and ER-positive breast cancers [70–73].

The chromosomal location of BCA2, 1q21.1, is intriguing in that the chromosomal region, 1q21-31, has been shown to have a high frequency of allelic loss in breast carcinomas [74]. Conversely, a common finding in breast tumors using comparative genomic hybridization (CGH) was an increased 1q copy number, which in one study, was shown to occur in 55 % of primary invasive breast cancers [74, 75]. This chromosomal aberration has been shown to correlate with positive ER and PR status and higher survival rates compared with patients with other aberrations [75]. Given that BCA2 expression has been detected to occur in a majority of invasive breast tumors that are ER-positive [29], this chromosomal amplification may play a role in this.

In summary, BCA2 expression was shown to correlate with positive estrogen receptor status, negative lymph node status, and an increase in disease-free survival for regional recurrence [29]. Further studies will be required to understand the nature of the link between BCA2 and ER, whether BCA2 and ER expressions are co-regulated and whether a causal connection between ER status and BCA2 expression can be established. For breast cancer patients with hormone-refractory tumors, targeting BCA2 may provide an alternative treatment strategy to pursue.

13.9.4 BCA2 Expression in Other Cancers

BCA2 is not solely a characteristic of invasive breast cancers, but has also been implicated in other pathologies, including lymphoma and HIV host mechanisms. [37, 30] Furthermore, BCA2 is being investigated as a potential biomarker in renal cancer.

In a recent pilot study using TMAs, BCA2 was found to be highly expressed in oncocytoma, a typically benign tumor that is thought to arise from the intercalated epithelial cells of collecting ducts of the kidney, but was not detectable in any of the 114 cases of renal cell carcinoma examined that included cases of the rare chromophobe renal cell carcinoma [76]. This study highlights the potential of using BCA2 as a marker in the differential diagnosis of kidney tumors distinguishing between renal oncocytoma from both chromophobe and renal cell carcinoma.

13.10 Implications for E3 Ligases in Cancer Therapeutics

There are many new targeted therapies that are currently being evaluated in clinical trials. With respect to UPS-related therapies, initial efforts have been aimed at non-specific targeting of components of the proteasome. One of the most promising is bortezomib (Velcade), a reversible proteasome inhibitor that blocks the chymotryptic activity of the proteasome [77, 78]. Bortezomib has been approved for the treatment of relapsed multiple myeloma and mantle cell lymphoma and has shown limited toxicity [18].

In terms of specifically targeting components of the UPS, E3 ligases make for a large and diverse family of interesting proteins to study. There are over 600 E3 ligases [79], an astounding number of proteins not including the 70 deubiquitinating enzymes and hundreds of ubiquitin-like proteins. It will be a huge and daunting, but also a potentially very rewarding, process to sort out their individual functions and further our knowledge of diseases in general and cancer in particular.

Thus, targeting E3 ligases will open up new potential avenues of treatment in breast and other cancers. A summary of E3 ligases of different types, their substrates, links to cancer, and the potential therapies currently being developed to either prevent substrate degradation or promote substrate degradation is shown in Table 13.3. E3 ligases that have already emerged as tempting anticancer targets include:

1. E6-AP (E6-associated protein), a HECT-type E3 ligase that binds to the human papillomavirus (HPV) type 16 oncoprotein E6 and is involved in E6-mediated cellular transformation. This binding can be interfered with using zinc-ejecting compounds such as 4,4′-dithiodimorpholine that can potentially be used to inhibit the pathology of HPV and therefore, in the treatment of cervical cancer [80].
2. Mdm2, a RING-type ubiquitin ligase that is involved in the degradation of p53, a major tumor suppressor. Inhibiting Mdm2 should elevate p53 levels, driving damaged cancer cells into apoptosis. For example, there are a number of tactics that are being attempted to block the activity of the E3 ligase, Mdm2. These include the Nutlins [81], cis-imidazoline analogs that inhibit the interaction between Mdm2 and p53 resulting in the stabilization of p53, which leads to senescence of cancer cells [82]. Additional strategies being investigated include MDM2 gene silencing using antisense and p53-GAr domain chimeras (gene therapy) [83, 81, 84]; both are designed to prevent p53 degradation mediated by Mdm2.
3. C-CBL (casitas B-lineage lymphoma), a RING-type E3 [85], behaved as a bone tumor suppressor when overexpressed in osteosarcoma cells mainly through the

Table 13.3 Ubiquitin ligase as potential targets for specific cancer therapies

Ligase	Substrate(s)	Contribution to cancer	Therapies	References
E6-AP (H)	p53	Degradation of p53	Zinc ejectors (C16), Nutlins	[80]
Mdm2 (R)	p53	Degradation of p53	Mdm2 antisense (silencing), p53-GAr domain chimeras (gene therapy)	[81–84]
c-CBL (R)	EGFR	Mutation in c-CBL leads to upregulation of EGFR		[85]
BCA2 (R)	14-3-3, p21	Degradation of cell cycle checkpoint 14-3-3	Disulfiram	[86]
		Degradation of CDK inhibitor p21		
EFP (R)	14-3-3	Degradation of cell cycle checkpoint 14-3-3	Antisense therapy	[71]
TRAF6 (R)	IKK	Upregulation of NF-κB pathway	Benzoxadiazole derivatives	[87]
BRCA1/ BCAD1 (C)	p53	Degradation of p53		[89]
VHL (C)	HIF	Increased HIF levels—tumor vascularization	Gene therapy	[90]
SCF^{SKP2} (F)	p27	Degradation of p27		[92]
$SCF\beta^{-TRCP}$ (F)	IkB	Upregulation of NF-κB pathway	Protac-1, methionine aminopeptidase-2 chimera with ovalicin	[93–95]
FBW7 (F)	MYC	Inhibition leads to upregulation of oncoproteins	Small-molecule inhibitors	[96]
SCF^{Met30} (F)	Met4	Cell cycle progression	Small-molecule inhibitors	[97, 98]
CHIP (U)	Abnormal proteins		Geldanamycins	[99, 100]

Note: E3 ligase types are bracketed beside E3 name, where (H), HECT-type; (R), RING-type; (C), E3 ligase complex; (F), F-box; and (U), U-box

increased degradation of the epidermal growth factor receptor (EGFR) and platelet-derived growth factor receptor alpha (PDGFRα). Elevating c-CBL levels in tumors may be an approach for targeting tumors in which receptor tyrosine kinases play an important role in tumorigenesis.

4. Given the potential role that BCA2 plays in breast cancer progression, targeting BCA2 in the treatment of breast cancer may be an interesting approach. A zinc-ejecting aldehyde dehydrogenase (ALDH) inhibitor, disulfiram, inhibits BCA2 and displays potent antitumor activity. A new series of BCA2-selective dithio(peroxo)thioate compounds were synthesized and found to display potent antiproliferative activity (0.1–0.3 μM IC_{50}) against breast cancer cell lines that

express endogenous BCA2 (MCF-7 and T47D), but not those that do not (MDA-MB-231 or MCF10A) [86]. These are interesting candidates to explore further, given their potency and selectivity.

5. EFP (estrogen-responsive finger protein), a RING-type E3, is an ER target gene that was cloned using a genomic binding site approach [71]. The resistance to endocrine therapy that occurs frequently in breast cancer patients may be overcome by targeting estrogen-responsive genes that regulate tumor proliferation. EFP was shown to be involved in proliferation using MCF7 cells in a xenograft model of breast cancer. Inhibiting EFP using antisense targeting reduced tumor growth, while EFP overexpression resulted in tumor formation even in an estrogen-deprived environment. Furthermore, EFP interacted with and caused the ubiquitin-dependent degradation of 14-3-3σ, which is involved in cell cycle arrest in G2 [71]. Therefore, inhibiting EFP may be an interesting protein to target in estrogen-resistant breast cancer.
6. The development of drugs such as benzoxadiazole derivatives inhibits the E3 RING-type ligase TRAF6, which prevents upregulation of the NF-κB pathway [87]. New evidence regarding copy number variations indicated that TRAF6 acted as an oncogene in lung cancer. Overexpression of TRAF6 resulted in tumor formation and malignant transformation of fibroblasts, and RNAi-mediated knockdown of TRAF6 decreased adenocarcinoma in two lung cell lines that had TRAF6 amplification [88]. Inhibition of TRAF6 in human lung cancer cell lines suppressed NF-κB activation, anchorage-independent growth, and tumor formation. In these two lung cell lines, RAS required TRAF6 for its oncogenic activities. This finding provides an explanation for the constitutive NF-κB activation observed in RAS-driven lung cancers.
7. BRCA1-BARD1 (BRCA1-associated RING domain 1) are part of an E3 ligase complex. Within the nucleus of cells, BARD1 interacts with BRCA1 and together these two proteins act as tumor suppressors. The BRCA1-BARD1 heterodimer is essential for BRCA1 stability and specifically mediates the formation of Lys-6-linked polyubiquitin chains and coordinates the activities of a diverse range of cellular pathways such as DNA damage repair, ubiquitination, and transcriptional regulation to maintain genomic stability. It also interacts with p53 [89] as well as a number of other proteins. Activation of BRCA1-BARD1 could potentially be used therapeutically to suppress tumor formation.
8. VHL (von Hippel-Lindau) is also part of an E3 ligase complex, and is another tumor suppressor implicated in cancer [90]. Mutations in the VHL gene result in von Hippel-Lindau disease, in which individuals develop a variety of tumors as the result of an attenuation of the ubiquitination and degradation of HIF-1α, leading to the accumulation and overexpression of HIF-1α and its target genes. Inhibitors that target USP20 (VDU2) and/or USP33 (VDU1) could enhance the polyubiquitination of HIF-1α and, therefore, may be used as novel cancer agents. Recently, small-molecule inhibitors of the VHL/HIF-1α protein–protein interaction have been developed and can be used to probe the hypoxic response and the role of HIF-1α in cancer [91].

9. Skp2 (SCF^{SKP2}) is an F-box ubiquitin ligase, which has been implicated in the degradation of the key tumor suppressor gene p27kip1. It is expected that Skp2 inhibitors would have antitumor effects. A compound that has been identified can prevent the incorporation of Skp2 into the SCFskp2 complex, resulting in cell death (i.e., autophagy) by stabilizing p27kip1 and inducing G1/S cell cycle arrest. The compound was also shown to synergize with bortezomib and could also overcome resistance to bortezomib in models of multiple myeloma. Furthermore, the compound was shown to be active against aggressive leukemia blasts as well as plasma cells derived from patients [92].
10. $SCF^{ß\text{-}TrCP1}$ (Skp1-Cullin-F-box), an F-box or Cullin RING E3 ligase, can trigger the degradation of IκBα, the inhibitory component of the proinflammatory transcription factor NF-κB. Therefore, drugs that target $SCF^{ß\text{-}TrCP1}$ may have potential as anti-inflammatory and anticancer agents. To this end, Nakajima et al. have identified an inhibitor of $SCF^{ß\text{-}TrCP1}$, which prevents the polyubiquitination and degradation of IκBα [93]. Using a very different approach, Sakamoto et al. employed the SCF ubiquitin ligase complex and artificially targeted a normally stable protein, methionine aminopeptidase-2 (MetAP-2), to this complex for ubiquitination and degradation through a chimeric bridging molecule or Protac (proteolysis targeting chimeric molecule) [94]. They then went on to show that an estradiol-based Protac could cause the ubiquitination and degradation of ERα in vitro, and a dihydroxytestosterone-based Protac introduced into cells could promote the rapid disappearance of the androgen receptor in a proteasome-dependent manner [95]. This very interesting technology could potentially be used to target cancer as well as many other diseases.
11. FBW7 (F-box and WD repeat domain-containing 7) is a mammalian F-box or Cullin RING E3 ligase and Cdc4 is the yeast ortholog for which one of the first small-molecule allosteric inhibitors of an E3 ligase has been identified [96].
12. More recently, a small-molecule inhibitor of the SCF^{Met30} ligase was identified in a screen for small-molecule enhancers of the drug rapamycin, which inhibits the target of rapamycin (TOR) [97]. TOR has been found to play a predominant role in mammalian cell growth and has been implicated in many different cancers [98].
13. It has also been shown that CHIP, a U-box E3 involved in the degradation of mutated proteins in tumor cells as well as in the degradation of overexpressed receptor tyrosine kinases (RTK) such as HER2, can be interfered with the benzoquinone ansamycin antibiotic geldanamycin [99, 100]. Two of the above, Skp2 and Mdm2, have also been shown to be overexpressed in various tumors.

Additional E3 ligase targets include the anaphase-promoting complex (APC), an E3 that causes the degradation of key cell cycle proteins and is responsible for completing the final steps of mitosis. Blocking APC, in theory, could halt cell division. Therefore, drugs that target individual ligases should be more effective than those that target the proteasome, and given the specificity of substrates for E3 ligases, drugs that target these proteins are ripe for personalized therapy.

The path forward, however, is fraught with obstacles. While there is more specificity by targeting specific E3 ligases, each ligase degrades multiple proteins, so inhibition may have unexpected off-target effects. For example, Skp2 degrades p27 but can also degrade the Myc oncogene; therefore, selective inhibition of Skp2 may cause tumors to become more aggressive, not less. Developing drugs that target E3 ligases will be difficult given the uncertainty that such perturbations will have on the host, but it may also lead to very effective cancer therapies.

13.11 Conclusion and Future Directions for BCA2 in Cancer

The role of E3 ligases in cancer is far from clear. They can play the role of both a tumor suppressor and oncogene, depending on their substrates in the context of cancer therapeutics. Investigations that lead to uncovering the mechanisms in which this family of proteins are deregulated and/or stabilized are paramount to understanding their functions. Given our current knowledge of how E3 ligases are stabilized, the following models have been put forth to account for what is known regarding the likely behavior of BCA2 and its interaction with hHR23a and 14-3-3σ, as depicted in Figs. 13.5 and 13.6, respectively. BCA2, in the absence of any binding partner or substrate, catalyzes its own ubiquitination, whereby the addition and elongation of a ubiquitin chain to the known accepting lysines in the BZF domain [31] is facilitated

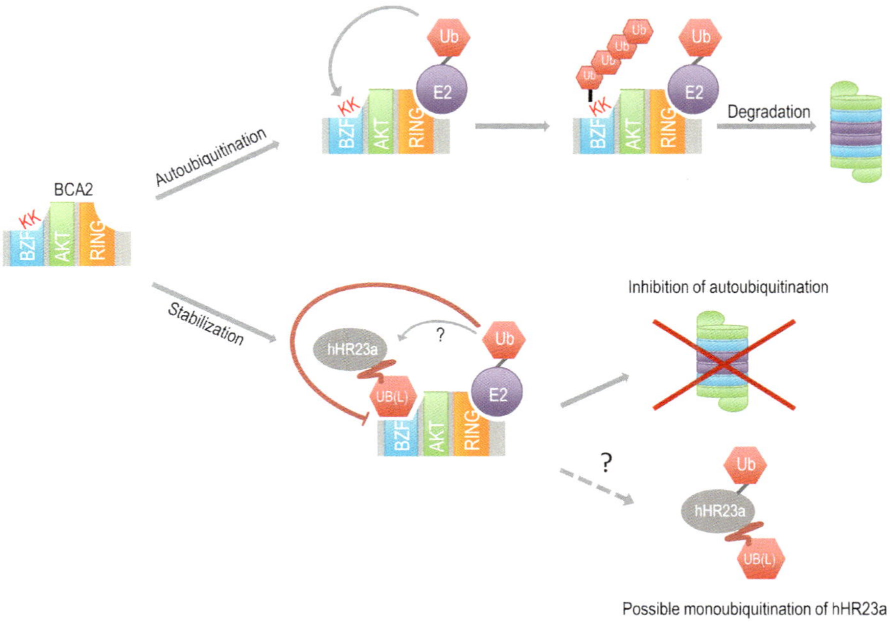

Fig. 13.5 Model for BCA2 interaction with hHR23a. When BCA2 is alone (*top*), it is ubiquitinated upon binding of E2 and targeted for proteasomal degradation. When hHR23a is present (*bottom*), hHR23a binds BCA2 preventing Ub-chain elongation, which stabilizes BCA2. Furthermore, hHR23a is possibly mono-/multi-ubiquitinated by BCA2, which does not lead to degradation

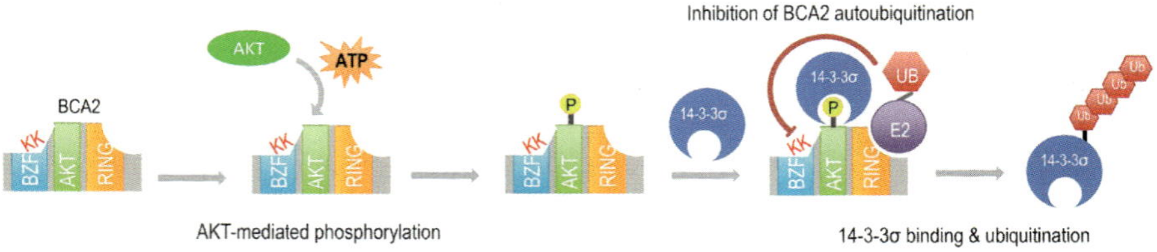

Fig. 13.6 Model for BCA2 interaction with 14-3-3σ. BCA2 is phosphorylated in the AKT domain by AKT kinase (*top*). Following modification, it is then able to bind 14-3-3σ, which sterically prevents autoubiquitination of BCA2 and also likely targets 14-3-3σ for degradation through conjugation of polyubiquitin chains

by the RING domain. Target or interacting proteins such as hHR23a or 14-3-3σ can bind to the BZF domain resulting in the inhibition of autoubiquitination activity. This in turn can stabilize BCA2. Through this interaction, the half-life of BCA2 is prolonged, allowing it to more readily take part in the ubiquitination of a substrate or incorporation into a complex. The BZF domain of BCA2 has a high affinity for ubiquitin and also for UBA52 [31], a ubiquitin fusion protein; therefore, the substrate for BCA2 may be previously monoubiquitinated or contain a ubiquitin-like domain. When BCA2 is phosphorylated, the interaction with 14-3-3σ prevents self-ubiquitin conjugation by BCA2, which is then followed by the catalysis of polyubiquitin chain formation and elongation on 14-3-3σ, and subsequent degradation.

The folate receptor (FR) was also identified as a possible BCA2 partner protein through yeast screening. Expression of FR has been linked to several cancers including breast and renal cancers among others, where overexpression of FR is correlated with poor prognosis [101, 102]. BCA2 may play an important role in FR internalization and regulation, which is worthy of further investigation. The role of other putative BCA2 interactants (Table 13.3) remains to be elucidated.

The precise role that BCA2 plays in breast cancer in particular and cancer in general is fertile ground for future research. Many questions still remain regarding protein modifications, substrates, and binding partners. It will be important to determine the impact that differential regulation and stability have on BCA2 in the context of breast cancer and other tumor types. With the recent interest of the pharmaceutical industry in developing drugs that target E3 ligases, BCA2 may evolve into a promising target to pursue in the clinic in the area of tumor biology; only time will tell.

References

1. Thrower JS, Hoffman L, Rechsteiner M, Pickart CM (2000) Recognition of the polyubiquitin proteolytic signal. EMBO J 19(1):94–102. doi:10.1093/emboj/19.1.94
2. Xu P, Duong DM, Seyfried NT, Cheng D, Xie Y, Robert J, Rush J, Hochstrasser M, Finley D, Peng J (2009) Quantitative proteomics reveals the function of unconventional ubiquitin chains in proteasomal degradation. Cell 137(1):133–145. doi:10.1016/j.cell.2009.01.041

3. Duncan LM, Piper S, Dodd RB, Saville MK, Sanderson CM, Luzio JP, Lehner PJ (2006) Lysine-63-linked ubiquitination is required for endolysosomal degradation of class I molecules. EMBO J 25(8):1635–1645. doi:10.1038/sj.emboj.7601056
4. Iwai K, Tokunaga F (2009) Linear polyubiquitination: a new regulator of NF-kappaB activation. EMBO Rep 10(7):706–713. doi:10.1038/embor.2009.144
5. Tokunaga F (2013) Linear ubiquitination-mediated NF-kappaB regulation and its related disorders. J Biochem 154(4):313–323. doi:10.1093/jb/mvt079
6. Komander D (2009) The emerging complexity of protein ubiquitination. Biochem Soc Trans 37(Pt 5):937–953. doi:10.1042/BST0370937
7. Alpi AF, Pace PE, Babu MM, Patel KJ (2008) Mechanistic insight into site-restricted monoubiquitination of FANCD2 by Ube2t, FANCL, and FANCI. Mol Cell 32(6):767–777. doi:10.1016/j.molcel.2008.12.003
8. Haglund K, Sigismund S, Polo S, Szymkiewicz I, Di Fiore PP, Dikic I (2003) Multiple monoubiquitination of RTKs is sufficient for their endocytosis and degradation. Nat Cell Biol 5(5):461–466. doi:10.1038/ncb983
9. Sigismund S, Polo S, Di Fiore PP (2004) Signaling through monoubiquitination. Curr Top Microbiol Immunol 286:149–185
10. Komander D, Clague MJ, Urbe S (2009) Breaking the chains: structure and function of the deubiquitinases. Nat Rev Mol Cell Biol 10(8):550–563. doi:10.1038/nrm2731
11. Reyes-Turcu FE, Ventii KH, Wilkinson KD (2009) Regulation and cellular roles of ubiquitin-specific deubiquitinating enzymes. Annu Rev Biochem 78:363–397. doi:10.1146/annurev.biochem.78.082307.091526
12. Pickart CM, Eddins MJ (2004) Ubiquitin: structures, functions, mechanisms. Biochim Biophys Acta 1695(1–3):55–72. doi:10.1016/j.bbamcr.2004.09.019
13. Chen Z, Pickart CM (1990) A 25-kilodalton ubiquitin carrier protein (E2) catalyzes multi-ubiquitin chain synthesis via lysine 48 of ubiquitin. J Biol Chem 265(35): 21835–21842
14. Haas AL, Reback PB, Chau V (1991) Ubiquitin conjugation by the yeast RAD6 and CDC34 gene products. Comparison to their putative rabbit homologs, E2(20K) AND E2(32K). J Biol Chem 266(8):5104–5112
15. Hofmann RM, Pickart CM (1999) Noncanonical MMS2-encoded ubiquitin-conjugating enzyme functions in assembly of novel polyubiquitin chains for DNA repair. Cell 96(5):645–653
16. Van Nocker S, Vierstra RD (1991) Cloning and characterization of a 20-kDa ubiquitin carrier protein from wheat that catalyzes multiubiquitin chain formation in vitro. Proc Natl Acad Sci U S A 88(22):10297–10301
17. Wang M, Cheng D, Peng J, Pickart CM (2006) Molecular determinants of polyubiquitin linkage selection by an HECT ubiquitin ligase. EMBO J 25(8):1710–1719. doi:10.1038/sj.emboj.7601061
18. Burger AM, Seth AK (2004) The ubiquitin-mediated protein degradation pathway in cancer: therapeutic implications. Eur J Cancer 40(15):2217–2229. doi:10.1016/j.ejca.2004.07.006
19. Metzger MB, Weissman AM (2010) Working on a chain: E3s ganging up for ubiquitylation. Nat Cell Biol 12(12):1124–1126. doi:10.1038/ncb1210-1124
20. de Bie P, Ciechanover A (2011) Ubiquitination of E3 ligases: self-regulation of the ubiquitin system via proteolytic and non-proteolytic mechanisms. Cell Death Differ 18(9):1393–1402. doi:10.1038/cdd.2011.16
21. Ben-Saadon R, Zaaroor D, Ziv T, Ciechanover A (2006) The polycomb protein Ring1B generates self atypical mixed ubiquitin chains required for its in vitro histone H2A ligase activity. Mol Cell 24(5):701–711. doi:10.1016/j.molcel.2006.10.022
22. Cao R, Tsukada Y, Zhang Y (2005) Role of Bmi-1 and Ring1A in H2A ubiquitylation and Hox gene silencing. Mol Cell 20(6):845–854. doi:10.1016/j.molcel.2005.12.002
23. Canning M, Boutell C, Parkinson J, Everett RD (2004) A RING finger ubiquitin ligase is protected from autocatalyzed ubiquitination and degradation by binding to ubiquitin-specific protease USP7. J Biol Chem 279(37):38160–38168. doi:10.1074/jbc.M402885200

24. Li Y, Gazdoiu S, Pan ZQ, Fuchs SY (2004) Stability of homologue of Slimb F-box protein is regulated by availability of its substrate. J Biol Chem 279(12):11074–11080. doi:10.1074/jbc.M312301200
25. Pashkova N, Gakhar L, Winistorfer SC, Yu L, Ramaswamy S, Piper RC (2010) WD40 repeat propellers define a ubiquitin-binding domain that regulates turnover of F box proteins. Mol Cell 40(3):433–443. doi:10.1016/j.molcel.2010.10.018
26. Rothenberger S, Burns K, Rousseaux M, Tschopp J, Bron C (2003) Ubiquitination of the Epstein-Barr virus-encoded latent membrane protein 1 depends on the integrity of the TRAF binding site. Oncogene 22(36):5614–5618. doi:10.1038/sj.onc.1206497
27. Wu M, Tu T, Huang Y, Cao Y (2013) Suppression subtractive hybridization identified differentially expressed genes in lung adenocarcinoma: ERGIC3 as a novel lung cancer-related gene. BMC Cancer 13:44. doi:10.1186/1471-2407-13-44
28. Burger AM, Zhang X, Li H, Ostrowski JL, Beatty B, Venanzoni M, Papas T, Seth A (1998) Down-regulation of T1A12/mac25, a novel insulin-like growth factor binding protein related gene, is associated with disease progression in breast carcinomas. Oncogene 16(19):2459–2467. doi:10.1038/sj.onc.1201772
29. Burger AM, Gao Y, Amemiya Y, Kahn HJ, Kitching R, Yang Y, Sun P, Narod SA, Hanna WM, Seth AK (2005) A novel RING-type ubiquitin ligase breast cancer-associated gene 2 correlates with outcome in invasive breast cancer. Cancer Res 65(22):10401–10412. doi:10.1158/0008-5472.CAN-05-2103
30. Toujani S, Dessen P, Ithzar N, Danglot G, Richon C, Vassetzky Y, Robert T, Lazar V, Bosq J, Da Costa L, Perot C, Ribrag V, Patte C, Wiels J, Bernheim A (2009) High resolution genome-wide analysis of chromosomal alterations in Burkitt's lymphoma. PLoS One 4(9):e7089. doi:10.1371/journal.pone.0007089
31. Amemiya Y, Azmi P, Seth A (2008) Autoubiquitination of BCA2 RING E3 ligase regulates its own stability and affects cell migration. Mol Cancer Res 6(9):1385–1396. doi:10.1158/1541-7786.MCR-08-0094
32. Connor MK, Azmi PB, Subramaniam V, Li H, Seth A (2005) Molecular characterization of ring finger protein 11. Mol Cancer Res 3(8):453–461. doi:10.1158/1541-7786.MCR-04-0166
33. Fang S, Jensen JP, Ludwig RL, Vousden KH, Weissman AM (2000) Mdm2 is a RING finger-dependent ubiquitin protein ligase for itself and p53. J Biol Chem 275(12):8945–8951
34. Hu G, Fearon ER (1999) Siah-1 N-terminal RING domain is required for proteolysis function, and C-terminal sequences regulate oligomerization and binding to target proteins. Mol Cell Biol 19(1):724–732
35. Zhi X, Zhao D, Wang Z, Zhou Z, Wang C, Chen W, Liu R, Chen C (2013) E3 ubiquitin ligase RNF126 promotes cancer cell proliferation by targeting the tumor suppressor p21 for ubiquitin-mediated degradation. Cancer Res 73(1):385–394. doi:10.1158/0008-5472.CAN-12-0562
36. Deshaies RJ, Joazeiro CA (2009) RING domain E3 ubiquitin ligases. Annu Rev Biochem 78:399–434. doi:10.1146/annurev.biochem.78.101807.093809
37. Miyakawa K, Ryo A, Murakami T, Ohba K, Yamaoka S, Fukuda M, Guatelli J, Yamamoto N (2009) BCA2/Rabring7 promotes tetherin-dependent HIV-1 restriction. PLoS Pathog 5(12):e1000700. doi:10.1371/journal.ppat.1000700
38. Mizuno K, Kitamura A, Sasaki T (2003) Rabring7, a novel Rab7 target protein with a RING finger motif. Mol Biol Cell 14(9):3741–3752. doi:10.1091/mbc.E02-08-0495
39. Sakane A, Hatakeyama S, Sasaki T (2007) Involvement of Rabring7 in EGF receptor degradation as an E3 ligase. Biochem Biophys Res Commun 357(4):1058–1064. doi:10.1016/j.bbrc.2007.04.052
40. Wang Z, Nie Z, Chen W, Zhou Z, Kong Q, Seth AK, Liu R, Chen C (2013) RNF115/BCA2 E3 ubiquitin ligase promotes breast cancer cell proliferation through targeting p21Waf1/Cip1 for ubiquitin-mediated degradation. Neoplasia 15(9):1028–1035
41. Burger A, Amemiya Y, Kitching R, Seth AK (2006) Novel RING E3 ubiquitin ligases in breast cancer. Neoplasia 8(8):689–695. doi:10.1593/neo.06469

42. Dantuma NP, Heinen C, Hoogstraten D (2009) The ubiquitin receptor Rad23: at the crossroads of nucleotide excision repair and proteasomal degradation. DNA Repair 8(4):449–460. doi:10.1016/j.dnarep.2009.01.005
43. Benzinger A, Muster N, Koch HB, Yates JR III, Hermeking H (2005) Targeted proteomic analysis of 14-3-3 sigma, a p53 effector commonly silenced in cancer. Mol Cell Proteomics 4(6):785–795. doi:10.1074/mcp.M500021-MCP200
44. Hsieh HC, Hsieh YH, Huang YH, Shen FC, Tsai HN, Tsai JH, Lai YT, Wang YT, Chuang WJ, Huang W (2005) HHR23A, a human homolog of Saccharomyces cerevisiae Rad23, regulates xeroderma pigmentosum C protein and is required for nucleotide excision repair. Biochem Biophys Res Commun 335(1):181–187. doi:10.1016/j.bbrc.2005.07.067
45. Li L, Lu X, Peterson C, Legerski R (1997) XPC interacts with both HHR23B and HHR23A in vivo. Mutat Res 383(3):197–203
46. Kang Y, Chen X, Lary JW, Cole JL, Walters KJ (2007) Defining how ubiquitin receptors hHR23a and S5a bind polyubiquitin. J Mol Biol 369(1):168–176. doi:10.1016/j.jmb.2007.03.008
47. Kang Y, Vossler RA, Diaz-Martinez LA, Winter NS, Clarke DJ, Walters KJ (2006) UBL/UBA ubiquitin receptor proteins bind a common tetraubiquitin chain. J Mol Biol 356(4):1027–1035. doi:10.1016/j.jmb.2005.12.001
48. Watkins JF, Sung P, Prakash L, Prakash S (1993) The Saccharomyces cerevisiae DNA repair gene RAD23 encodes a nuclear protein containing a ubiquitin-like domain required for biological function. Mol Cell Biol 13(12):7757–7765
49. Fishbain S, Prakash S, Herrig A, Elsasser S, Matouschek A (2011) Rad23 escapes degradation because it lacks a proteasome initiation region. Nat Commun 2:192. doi:10.1038/ncomms1194
50. Bacopulos S, Amemiya Y, Yang W, Zubovits J, Burger A, Yaffe M, Seth AK (2012) Effects of partner proteins on BCA2 RING ligase activity. BMC Cancer 12:63. doi:10.1186/1471-2407-12-63
51. Raasi S, Orlov I, Fleming KG, Pickart CM (2004) Binding of polyubiquitin chains to ubiquitin-associated (UBA) domains of HHR23A. J Mol Biol 341(5):1367–1379. doi:10.1016/j.jmb.2004.06.057
52. Lodygin D, Hermeking H (2005) The role of epigenetic inactivation of 14-3-3sigma in human cancer. Cell Res 15(4):237–246. doi:10.1038/sj.cr.7290292
53. Hermeking H, Lengauer C, Polyak K, He TC, Zhang L, Thiagalingam S, Kinzler KW, Vogelstein B (1997) 14-3-3 sigma is a p53-regulated inhibitor of G2/M progression. Mol Cell 1(1):3–11
54. Laronga C, Yang HY, Neal C, Lee MH (2000) Association of the cyclin-dependent kinases and 14-3-3 sigma negatively regulates cell cycle progression. J Biol Chem 275(30):23106–23112. doi:10.1074/jbc.M905616199
55. Wilker EW, Grant RA, Artim SC, Yaffe MB (2005) A structural basis for 14-3-3sigma functional specificity. J Biol Chem 280(19):18891–18898. doi:10.1074/jbc.M500982200
56. Nacht M, Ferguson AT, Zhang W, Petroziello JM, Cook BP, Gao YH, Maguire S, Riley D, Coppola G, Landes GM, Madden SL, Sukumar S (1999) Combining serial analysis of gene expression and array technologies to identify genes differentially expressed in breast cancer. Cancer Res 59(21):5464–5470
57. Ferguson AT, Evron E, Umbricht CB, Pandita TK, Chan TA, Hermeking H, Marks JR, Lambers AR, Futreal PA, Stampfer MR, Sukumar S (2000) High frequency of hypermethylation at the 14-3-3 sigma locus leads to gene silencing in breast cancer. Proc Natl Acad Sci U S A 97(11):6049–6054. doi:10.1073/pnas.100566997
58. Manning BD, Cantley LC (2007) AKT/PKB signaling: navigating downstream. Cell 129(7):1261–1274. doi:10.1016/j.cell.2007.06.009
59. Yaffe MB, Rittinger K, Volinia S, Caron PR, Aitken A, Leffers H, Gamblin SJ, Smerdon SJ, Cantley LC (1997) The structural basis for 14-3-3:phosphopeptide binding specificity. Cell 91(7):961–971

60. Vanlandingham PA, Ceresa BP (2009) Rab7 regulates late endocytic trafficking downstream of multivesicular body biogenesis and cargo sequestration. J Biol Chem 284(18):12110–12124. doi:10.1074/jbc.M809277200
61. Alwan HA, van Zoelen EJ, van Leeuwen JE (2003) Ligand-induced lysosomal epidermal growth factor receptor (EGFR) degradation is preceded by proteasome-dependent EGFR de-ubiquitination. J Biol Chem 278(37):35781–35790. doi:10.1074/jbc.M301326200
62. Ettenberg SA, Magnifico A, Cuello M, Nau MM, Rubinstein YR, Yarden Y, Weissman AM, Lipkowitz S (2001) Cbl-b-dependent coordinated degradation of the epidermal growth factor receptor signaling complex. J Biol Chem 276(29):27677–27684. doi:10.1074/jbc.M102641200
63. Cheng PL, Lu H, Shelly M, Gao H, Poo MM (2011) Phosphorylation of E3 ligase Smurf1 switches its substrate preference in support of axon development. Neuron 69(2):231–243. doi:10.1016/j.neuron.2010.12.021
64. Nacerddine K, Beaudry JB, Ginjala V, Westerman B, Mattiroli F, Song JY, van der Poel H, Ponz OB, Pritchard C, Cornelissen-Steijger P, Zevenhoven J, Tanger E, Sixma TK, Ganesan S, van Lohuizen M (2012) Akt-mediated phosphorylation of Bmi1 modulates its oncogenic potential, E3 ligase activity, and DNA damage repair activity in mouse prostate cancer. J Clin Invest 122(5):1920–1932. doi:10.1172/JCI57477
65. Levkowitz G, Waterman H, Ettenberg SA, Katz M, Tsygankov AY, Alroy I, Lavi S, Iwai K, Reiss Y, Ciechanover A, Lipkowitz S, Yarden Y (1999) Ubiquitin ligase activity and tyrosine phosphorylation underlie suppression of growth factor signaling by c-Cbl/Sli-1. Mol Cell 4(6):1029–1040
66. Gruber T, Hermann-Kleiter N, Hinterleitner R, Fresser F, Schneider R, Gastl G, Penninger JM, Baier G (2009) PKC-theta modulates the strength of T cell responses by targeting Cbl-b for ubiquitination and degradation. Sci Signal 2(76):ra30. doi:10.1126/scisignal.2000046
67. Umebayashi K, Stenmark H, Yoshimori T (2008) Ubc4/5 and c-Cbl continue to ubiquitinate EGF receptor after internalization to facilitate polyubiquitination and degradation. Mol Biol Cell 19(8):3454–3462. doi:10.1091/mbc.E07-10-0988
68. Smith CJ, Berry DM, McGlade CJ (2013) The E3 ubiquitin ligases RNF126 and Rabring7 regulate endosomal sorting of the epidermal growth factor receptor. J Cell Sci 126(Pt 6):1366–1380. doi:10.1242/jcs.116129
69. Burger AM, Kona F, Amemiya Y, Gao Y, Bacopulos S, Seth AK (2010) Role of the BCA2 ubiquitin E3 ligase in hormone responsive breast cancer. Open Cancer J 3(1):116–123
70. Higashiyama M, Doi O, Kodama K, Yokouchi H, Kasugai T, Ishiguro S, Takami K, Nakayama T, Nishisho I (1997) MDM2 gene amplification and expression in non-small-cell lung cancer: immunohistochemical expression of its protein is a favourable prognostic marker in patients without p53 protein accumulation. Br J Cancer 75(9):1302–1308
71. Horie K, Urano T, Ikeda K, Inoue S (2003) Estrogen-responsive RING finger protein controls breast cancer growth. J Steroid Biochem Mol Biol 85(2–5):101–104
72. Onel K, Cordon-Cardo C (2004) MDM2 and prognosis. Mol Cancer Res 2(1):1–8
73. Polsky D, Melzer K, Hazan C, Panageas KS, Busam K, Drobnjak M, Kamino H, Spira JG, Kopf AW, Houghton A, Cordon-Cardo C, Osman I (2002) HDM2 protein overexpression and prognosis in primary malignant melanoma. J Natl Cancer Inst 94(23):1803–1806
74. Bieche I, Champeme MH, Lidereau R (1995) Loss and gain of distinct regions of chromosome 1q in primary breast cancer. Clin Cancer Res 1(1):123–127
75. Rennstam K, Ahlstedt-Soini M, Baldetorp B, Bendahl PO, Borg A, Karhu R, Tanner M, Tirkkonen M, Isola J (2003) Patterns of chromosomal imbalances defines subgroups of breast cancer with distinct clinical features and prognosis. A study of 305 tumors by comparative genomic hybridization. Cancer Res 63(24):8861–8868
76. Ehsani L, Seth R, Bacopulos S, Seth A, Osunkoya AO (2013) BCA2 is differentially expressed in renal oncocytoma: an analysis of 158 renal neoplasms. Tumour Biol 34(2):787–791. doi:10.1007/s13277-012-0608-8
77. Bortezomib (Velcade) for Multiple Myeloma (2003) The Medical Letter on Drugs and Therapeutics 45(1161):57–58

78. Mitchell BS (2003) The proteasome—an emerging therapeutic target in cancer. N Engl J Med 348(26):2597–2598. doi:10.1056/NEJMp030092
79. Cohen P, Tcherpakov M (2010) Will the ubiquitin system furnish as many drug targets as protein kinases? Cell 143(5):686–693. doi:10.1016/j.cell.2010.11.016
80. Beerheide W, Bernard HU, Tan YJ, Ganesan A, Rice WG, Ting AE (1999) Potential drugs against cervical cancer: zinc-ejecting inhibitors of the human papillomavirus type 16 E6 oncoprotein. J Natl Cancer Inst 91(14):1211–1220
81. Vassilev LT, Vu BT, Graves B, Carvajal D, Podlaski F, Filipovic Z, Kong N, Kammlott U, Lukacs C, Klein C, Fotouhi N, Liu EA (2004) In vivo activation of the p53 pathway by small-molecule antagonists of MDM2. Science 303(5659):844–848. doi:10.1126/science.1092472
82. Shangary S, Wang S (2009) Small-molecule inhibitors of the MDM2-p53 protein-protein interaction to reactivate p53 function: a novel approach for cancer therapy. Annu Rev Pharmacol Toxicol 49:223–241. doi:10.1146/annurev.pharmtox.48.113006.094723
83. Lai Z, Yang T, Kim YB, Sielecki TM, Diamond MA, Strack P, Rolfe M, Caligiuri M, Benfield PA, Auger KR, Copeland RA (2002) Differentiation of Hdm2-mediated p53 ubiquitination and Hdm2 autoubiquitination activity by small molecular weight inhibitors. Proc Natl Acad Sci U S A 99(23):14734–14739. doi:10.1073/pnas.212428599
84. Wang H, Zeng X, Oliver P, Le LP, Chen J, Chen L, Zhou W, Agrawal S, Zhang R (1999) MDM2 oncogene as a target for cancer therapy: an antisense approach. Int J Oncol 15(4):653–660
85. Severe N, Dieudonne FX, Marty C, Modrowski D, Patino-Garcia A, Lecanda F, Fromigue O, Marie PJ (2012) Targeting the E3 ubiquitin casitas B-lineage lymphoma decreases osteosarcoma cell growth and survival and reduces tumorigenesis. J Bone Miner Res 27(10):2108–2117. doi:10.1002/jbmr.1667
86. Brahemi G, Kona FR, Fiasella A, Buac D, Soukupova J, Brancale A, Burger AM, Westwell AD (2010) Exploring the structural requirements for inhibition of the ubiquitin E3 ligase breast cancer associated protein 2 (BCA2) as a treatment for breast cancer. J Med Chem 53(7):2757–2765. doi:10.1021/jm901757t
87. Ande SR, Chen J, Maddika S (2009) The ubiquitin pathway: an emerging drug target in cancer therapy. Eur J Pharmacol 625(1–3):199–205. doi:10.1016/j.ejphar.2009.08.042
88. Starczynowski DT, Lockwood WW, Delehouzee S, Chari R, Wegrzyn J, Fuller M, Tsao MS, Lam S, Gazdar AF, Lam WL, Karsan A (2011) TRAF6 is an amplified oncogene bridging the RAS and NF-kappaB pathways in human lung cancer. J Clin Invest 121(10):4095–4105. doi:10.1172/JCI58818
89. Dong Y, Hakimi MA, Chen X, Kumaraswamy E, Cooch NS, Godwin AK, Shiekhattar R (2003) Regulation of BRCC, a holoenzyme complex containing BRCA1 and BRCA2, by a signalosome-like subunit and its role in DNA repair. Mol Cell 12(5):1087–1099
90. Hoeller D, Dikic I (2009) Targeting the ubiquitin system in cancer therapy. Nature 458(7237):438–444. doi:10.1038/nature07960
91. Buckley DL, Van Molle I, Gareiss PC, Tae HS, Michel J, Noblin DJ, Jorgensen WL, Ciulli A, Crews CM (2012) Targeting the von Hippel-Lindau E3 ubiquitin ligase using small molecules to disrupt the VHL/HIF-1alpha interaction. J Am Chem Soc 134(10):4465–4468. doi:10.1021/ja209924v
92. Chen Q, Xie W, Kuhn DJ, Voorhees PM, Lopez-Girona A, Mendy D, Corral LG, Krenitsky VP, Xu W, Moutouh-de Parseval L, Webb DR, Mercurio F, Nakayama KI, Nakayama K, Orlowski RZ (2008) Targeting the p27 E3 ligase SCF(Skp2) results in p27- and Skp2-mediated cell-cycle arrest and activation of autophagy. Blood 111(9):4690–4699. doi:10.1182/blood-2007-09-112904
93. Nakajima H, Fujiwara H, Furuichi Y, Tanaka K, Shimbara N (2008) A novel small-molecule inhibitor of NF-kappaB signaling. Biochem Biophys Res Commun 368(4):1007–1013. doi:10.1016/j.bbrc.2008.01.166
94. Sakamoto KM, Kim KB, Kumagai A, Mercurio F, Crews CM, Deshaies RJ (2001) Protacs: chimeric molecules that target proteins to the Skp1-Cullin-F box complex for ubiquitination and degradation. Proc Natl Acad Sci U S A 98(15):8554–8559. doi:10.1073/pnas.141230798

95. Sakamoto KM, Kim KB, Verma R, Ransick A, Stein B, Crews CM, Deshaies RJ (2003) Development of Protacs to target cancer-promoting proteins for ubiquitination and degradation. Mol Cell Proteomics 2(12):1350–1358. doi:10.1074/mcp.T300009-MCP200
96. Orlicky S, Tang X, Neduva V, Elowe N, Brown ED, Sicheri F, Tyers M (2010) An allosteric inhibitor of substrate recognition by the SCF(Cdc4) ubiquitin ligase. Nat Biotechnol 28(7):733–737. doi:10.1038/nbt.1646
97. Aghajan M, Jonai N, Flick K, Fu F, Luo M, Cai X, Ouni I, Pierce N, Tang X, Lomenick B, Damoiseaux R, Hao R, Del Moral PM, Verma R, Li Y, Li C, Houk KN, Jung ME, Zheng N, Huang L, Deshaies RJ, Kaiser P, Huang J (2010) Chemical genetics screen for enhancers of rapamycin identifies a specific inhibitor of an SCF family E3 ubiquitin ligase. Nat Biotechnol 28(7):738–742. doi:10.1038/nbt.1645
98. Wullschleger S, Loewith R, Hall MN (2006) TOR signaling in growth and metabolism. Cell 124(3):471–484. doi:10.1016/j.cell.2006.01.016
99. Xu W, Marcu M, Yuan X, Mimnaugh E, Patterson C, Neckers L (2002) Chaperone-dependent E3 ubiquitin ligase CHIP mediates a degradative pathway for c-ErbB2/Neu. Proc Natl Acad Sci U S A 99(20):12847–12852. doi:10.1073/pnas.202365899
100. Zhou P, Fernandes N, Dodge IL, Reddi AL, Rao N, Safran H, DiPetrillo TA, Wazer DE, Band V, Band H (2003) ErbB2 degradation mediated by the co-chaperone protein CHIP. J Biol Chem 278(16):13829–13837. doi:10.1074/jbc.M209640200
101. Hartmann LC, Keeney GL, Lingle WL, Christianson TJ, Varghese B, Hillman D, Oberg AL, Low PS (2007) Folate receptor overexpression is associated with poor outcome in breast cancer. Int J Cancer 121(5):938–942. doi:10.1002/ijc.22811
102. Yuan Y, Nymoen DA, Dong HP, Bjorang O, Shih Ie M, Low PS, Trope CG, Davidson B (2009) Expression of the folate receptor genes FOLR1 and FOLR3 differentiates ovarian carcinoma from breast carcinoma and malignant mesothelioma in serous effusions. Hum Pathol 40(10):1453–1460. doi:10.1016/j.humpath.2009.02.013

Chapter 14
The 26S Proteasomal ATPases: Structure, Function, Regulation, and Potential for Cancer Therapies

Young-Chan Kim and David M. Smith

Abstract The 26S proteasome is the only protein degradation machine in the cell that selectively degrades proteins, and as such it regulates the vast majority of cellular processes (e.g., cell proliferation, differentiation, transcription, and signal transduction), and it is essential for cell survival. The multistep process of protein degradation by the 26S proteasome begins with the recognition of substrates by the 19S regulatory particle and ends with their degradation inside the 20S core particle. Inhibitors of the 20S proteolytic sites (e.g., by bortezomib and carfilzomib) have proven useful for the treatment of hematological cancers, especially multiple myeloma, where bortezomib is used as a first-line treatment. However, relapse typically occurs in these patients and drug resistance is observed. Alternative therapeutic targets within the 26S proteasome—especially in 19S regulatory complex—are highly attractive due to the proven requirement for ubiquitin-dependent protein degradation in multiple myeloma. Because the 19S regulatory particle must catalyze a complex multiple step processes to stimulate the degradation of proteins, there are many attractive sites that could be targeted for new cancer therapies. We summarize recent developments in our understanding of the structure, function, and regulation of the 19S ATPases complex and the potential for pharmacological manipulation of the 19S and its ATPases to develop new classes of compounds that inhibit proteasomal regulation rather than global protein degradation, which we expect will have therapeutic advantages.

Keywords 26S proteasome • 19S proteasomal ATPases • Rpt • Substrate binding • Deubiquitylation • ATP binding and hydrolysis • Gating • Unfolding and Translocation • Proteasome • ATPases • Allosteric • Proteasome inhibitor • Protein degradation • AAA • Ubiquitin

Y.-C. Kim • D.M. Smith (✉)
Department of Biochemistry, West Virginia University School of Medicine,
1 Medical Center Drive, Morgantown, WV 26506, USA
e-mail: dmsmith@hsc.wvu.edu

Q.P. Dou (ed.), *Resistance to Proteasome Inhibitors in Cancer*, Resistance to Targeted Anti-Cancer Therapeutics, DOI 10.1007/978-3-319-06752-0_14

Abbreviations

AAA+ATPases	ATPases associated with diverse cellular activities
CaMKII	Ca2+/calmodulin-dependent kinase II
CC	Coiled coil
CP	Core particle
DUB	Deubiquitinating enzyme
EM	Electron microscopy
HbYX	Hydrophobic (Hb), tyrosine (Y), and any residue (X)
OB	Oligonucleotide/oligosaccharide binding
OGT	O-GlcNAc transferase
PA28	Proteasome activator 28 kDa
PAN	Proteasome-activating nucleotidase
PI31	Proteasome inhibitor 31 kDa
PKA	Protein kinase A
PTMs	Posttranslational modifications
RP	Regulatory particle
RPN	Regulatory particle non-ATPase
RPT	Regulatory particle ATPase
UBA-UBL domain	Ubiquitin-associated-ubiquitin-like domain

14.1 Introduction

The 26S proteasome catalyzes the degradation of misfolded, damaged, and short-lived regulatory proteins in the cell, and as such it is a key player in maintaining protein homeostasis. It does so by selectively degrading proteins that have been "tagged" for degradation by the conjugation of a ubiquitin chain to the substrate. This is the first step of selectivity in protein degradation. The 26S is a multisubunit proteolytic machine and it requires ATP to drive a multistep process that processively degrades its protein substrates. This 2.5 MDa complex is made up of ~33 different types of subunits and consists of two subcomplexes: a core protease (20S proteasome or CP) and a regulatory particle (19S, RP, or PA700) that caps one or both ends of the 20S. Two subcomplexes make up the 19S, the lid and the base. The lid contains mostly scaffolding subunits and also some ubiquitin processing subunits, while the base contains a ring of ATPases and other ancillary subunits discussed below. This 19S binds to and regulates the 20S core particle. The 20S is a barrel-shaped compartmentalized protease that is composed of four stacked rings. The outer α-rings are heteroheptameric and their subunits are labeled α1–α7. The two inner β-rings are also heteroheptameric and are labeled β1–β7. The proteolytic sites are located on the central pore area of the beta subunits. To form the functional 26S proteasome complex, the base of the 19S associates with the α-ring of the 20S, but this interaction requires the binding of ATP to the 19S ATPases [1, 2].

Most of the steps in the multistep process of substrate degradation are regulated by the 19S. The 19S must: (1) recognize polyubiquitylated substrates, (2) open a gate

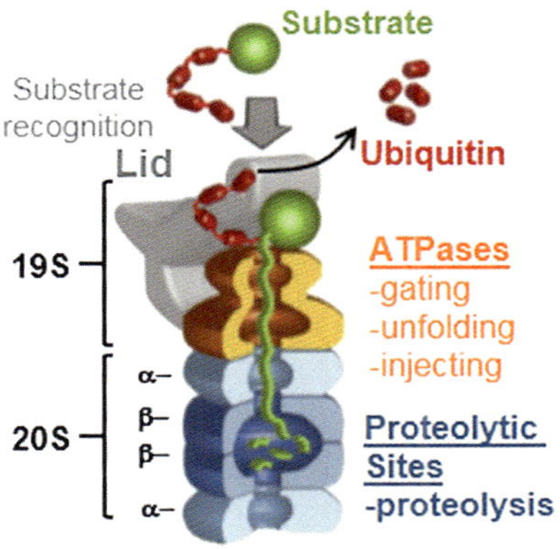

Fig. 14.1 The ATP-dependent multistep process of protein degradation by the 26S proteasome. Ubiquitination of a protein allows it to be recognized by the 19S regulatory particle. The hexameric complex of ATPases opens a gate in the 20S proteasome and translocates the protein through its central pore causing unfolding of upstream regions. Deubiquitinating enzymes (DUBs) on the 19S remove the ubiquitin chain, and the ATPases complete the injection of the substrate into the 20S where it is degraded to small peptides. The 19S can bind to one or both ends of the 20S to form the 26S proteasome. This cartoon was altered and adapted from Maupuin-Furlow 2012

that occludes the 20S central chamber, (3) unfold the proteins so they can pass through the narrow channel leading to the degradation chamber, (4) remove any conjugated ubiquitin chains, and (5) inject the unfolded and deubiquitylated polypeptide into the 20S catalytic chamber where it can be degraded to small peptides (Fig. 14.1) [3]. The ATPase ring in the 19S can be thought of as the control center of the 26S proteasome, regulating and catalyzing all of these critical steps. The field has sought for many years to understand this multistep process, but difficulties in obtaining high-resolution structures of this highly dynamic 26S complex have slowed progress. Recently, however, several subnanometer cryo-EM structures of eukaryotic 26S proteasome were elucidated and the subunit arrangement of the 19S was finally solved. These recent structural advancements have provided significant insights into the mechanisms and function of the 26S proteasome [4–7]. The following sections summarize the current knowledge of structure, function, and regulation of the 19S ATPases complex and the therapeutic potential for cancer treatment by targeting this complex.

14.2 Structural Organization of 19S Proteasomal ATPases Complex

14.2.1 Overall Architecture and Function

The 19S is an ATP-dependent activator of the 20S proteasome and is composed of 19 stoichiometric subunits each belonging to either the base or lid subcomplex. The base is a central and pivotal part of RP that consists of six different but homologous AAA+ATPase, called Rpt1–6 as well as three non-ATPase subunits: Rpn1, Rpn2,

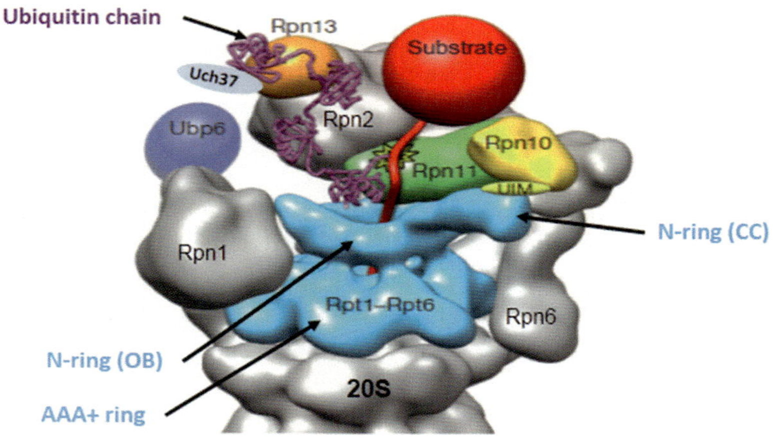

Fig. 14.2 Schematic structural organization of the 19S regulatory particle. The subunit organizations of the 19S subunits are shown and only the subunits (and key domains) that are discussed are labeled. The substrate (*red*) and the conjugated ubiquitin chain (*purple*) are also depicted. The N-ring contains two domains, the OB domain and the CC domain; see the text for more details. This cartoon was adapted with permission from [4]

and Rpn13. The lid is composed of the non-ATPase subunits (Rpn3, Rpn5–9, Rpn11, Rpn12, and Rpn15). Rpn10 was previously proposed to connect the base and lid and stabilize them because deletion of this subunit caused dissociation of base and lid. This traditional structural organization of the 19S complex has been revised in many aspects due to the recent generation of cryo-EM reconstruction studies which revealed complete subunit architectures of the 19S particle (Fig. 14.2) [4–11]. In addition, these studies revealed several new structural features of the 26S, which we discuss in brief here: (1) the ubiquitin receptors Rpn10 and Rpn13 are flexibly attached to the periphery of the RP well above the ATPase ring and the distance between these two Ub receptors approximately matches the length of tetra-ubiquitin chains. It was a surprise to find that Rpn10 primarily binds to lid subunits Rpn11 and Rpn9; however, in some conformational states it also binds to the ATPase subunits Rpt4 and Rpt5, which may explain Rpn10's presumed role in joining the base and the lid subcomplexes. (2) The deubiquitinating enzyme (or DUB), Rpn11, is located above but in close proximity to the substrate entrance pore of the ATPase ring. Further, Rpn11 shows significant conformational changes upon lid integration into holoenzyme, and again after substrate engagement which is driven by conformational changes in the ATPase ring [4, 11]. These conformational changes help explain how allosteric changes in Rpn11's position link deubiquitination to the degradation of proteins degradation. (3) Several lid subunits, Rpn5 and Rpn6, are shown to interact with the 20S subunits, α1 and α2, respectively, and appear to act as important regulatory points for the 19S–20S interaction. (4) Surprisingly, the base subunits Rpn2 and Rpn13 are found distant from the 20S at the top of the 19S complex above the lid (Fig. 14.2), and thus, the traditional "base" and "lid" terminology could benefit from revision. (5) The DUB Ubp6 (Usp14) is associated with Rpn1 at the periphery of the 19S complex and Uch37 (UchL5) is shown to bind to Rpn13 via indirect linkage to Rpn2. (6) A big surprise was that the pore loops of the large AAA+domains of the six Rpts show a helical staircase or lockwasher-like conformation, except for one subunit (Rpt6) that is intermediate in height and bridges the highest (Rpt3) and lowest (Rpt2) subunits in the presence of saturating amount of ATP. Oddly, in the structure with ATP present, the pore of the ATPase ring is not in alignment with the pore of the 20S and that the ATPase pore was found to be in a fairly closed state [4, 6]. (7) However, the ATPases undergo conformational switching in the presence of ubiquitinated substrate: the ATPase ring is shown to rearrange so that the interface between each of the ATPase subunits becomes more uniform and its central pore widens. In addition, the ATPase pore now aligns with the 20S substrate translocation pore. This suggests that a rapid progression of ATP hydrolysis is induced upon substrate engagement that generates this conformation, which appears to be translocation-competent. Interestingly, the pore loops of the Rpt ring are also rearranged but they still exhibit a spiral staircase although with a lower pitch. In addition, the lockwasher-like conformation appears to have rotated through the ring after substrate binding, so that the highest subunit now becomes Rpt1, the lowest Rpt4, and the bridging one Rpt5 [11]. Similar translocation-competent topology and subunits rearrangement are also observed upon binding of the non-hydrolyzable analog ATPγS, even without substrate present [10]. (8) These large conformational changes in the ATPase ring also cause a large rotation of the 19S around the long axis of the 26S. One obvious function of this rotation is to bring Rpn11 into proximity directly above the ATPase pore, where it is positioned to remove ubiquitin chains before they enter the ATPase ring. This is important since ubiquitin chains could slow or even halt the translocation of proteins into the 20S. Therefore, multiple EM reconstruction studies clearly show that both ATP binding (ATPγS) and substrate binding induce large, and similar conformational changes, which affect all of the 19S subunits to some extent.

14.2.2 The Ring of ATPases

The eukaryotic heterohexameric 26S ATPases (Rpts) are thought to have evolved from a simpler AAA+proteasomal ATPase in archaea. This archaeal proteasomal ATPase is called PAN (proteasome-activating nucleotidase), which forms a homohexameric ring complex and shows remarkable similarities to the 26S ATPases in many aspects of structure and function. Both the eukaryotic and archaeal proteasomal ATPases consist of four structural domains and a key C-terminal tail motif: (1) N-terminal coiled-coil (CC) domain, (2) OB (oligonucleotide/oligosaccharide binding) domain, (3) AAA+ATPase domain, (4) C-terminal helical domain, and (5) the C-terminal HbYX motif. Crystal structures of PAN and related bacterial ARC show that the ATPases complex forms a hexameric ring structure, the N-ring (CC-OB hexamer), which makes a small ring that sits on top of the larger AAA+ring [12–15].

14.2.3 The CC Domain

The CC domain is shown to form a trimer of α-helical dimers. At the base of the CC domain adjacent to the OB domain, there is a highly conserved proline residue which is in a *cis* conformation in one subunit and a *trans* conformation in its neighbor, which alternates around the ring. The *cis*-proline containing subunits allow the CC domain to bend back toward its neighbor, allowing for coiled coiling to occur. This *cis–trans* subunit pairing is also conserved in the eukaryotic Rpt ring, where the *cis*-proline-containing subunits are Rpt2, Rpt3, and Rpt5 and the expected *trans* subunits are Rpt1, Rpt6, and Rpt4, respectively, demonstrating a conserved structural asymmetry in N-terminal ring. In agreement with this assumption, previous studies have also demonstrated that the N-terminal domains of proteasomal ATPases have a chaperone activity and are capable of preventing the aggregation of misfolded proteins [14–17]. One hypothesis for this chaperone activity is that as substrates are translocated, they become unfolded at the mouth of the ATPase ring, and to prevent aggregation of the unfolded domains with other cytosolic proteins, the CC domains bind to and chaperone these newly unfolded domains.

14.2.4 The OB Domain

The OB domain is a five-stranded β sandwich fold with surface loops. Based on conservation with other OB fold proteins, it's suggested that these loops may bind substrates. In addition, based on the contact surface area of neighboring OB domains, it has been suggested that conformational changes in one domain would be recapitulated to others in the ring in an allosteric fashion [14]. Interestingly, many point mutations made in these domains drastically affect the activity of the ATPase domains, which are somewhat distant and connected by a flexible linker, which is also sensitive to point mutations [14]. This suggests these domains may be critical regulatory points. Therefore, the OB domain together with the CC domain is thought to play an important role in initial substrate binding, substrate handling, and threading through the central pore.

14.2.5 The C-Terminal HbYX Motif and 20S Gating

The crystal structure of the 20S CP complex shows that the entrance route for substrates into the proteolytic chamber is closed-off by interactions between the N-termini of certain α-subunits [18, 19]. These N-termini thus form a gate, which prevents unwanted protein degradation. How is this gate opened to allow substrate entry? The C-termini of 19S ATPases, as well as PAN, have the autonomous ability to induce opening of this 20S gate. Studies of PAN's ability to activate degradation by the 20S proteasome first identified a three-residue motif, the HbYX motif that had the ability to induce gate opening (HbYX—Hb, hydrophobic; Y, Tyrosine; X, variable but ultimate residue). Biochemical, cryo-EM, and crystal structural studies have shown in detail how the HbYX motif opens the archaeal 20S gate and defines the associated conformational changes in the α-ring. Because the HbYX motif is autonomous in its ability to induce gate opening, peptides that correspond to the C-terminus of PAN (or Rpt2, Rpt3, or Rpt5) can bind to the 20S by themselves and stimulate gate opening. However, ATP binding to PAN (or the 19S) is essential to cause a conformational change in its C-termini to allow for the HbYX to bind to the 20S proteasome and to induce gate opening (Fig. 14.3) [20], though these

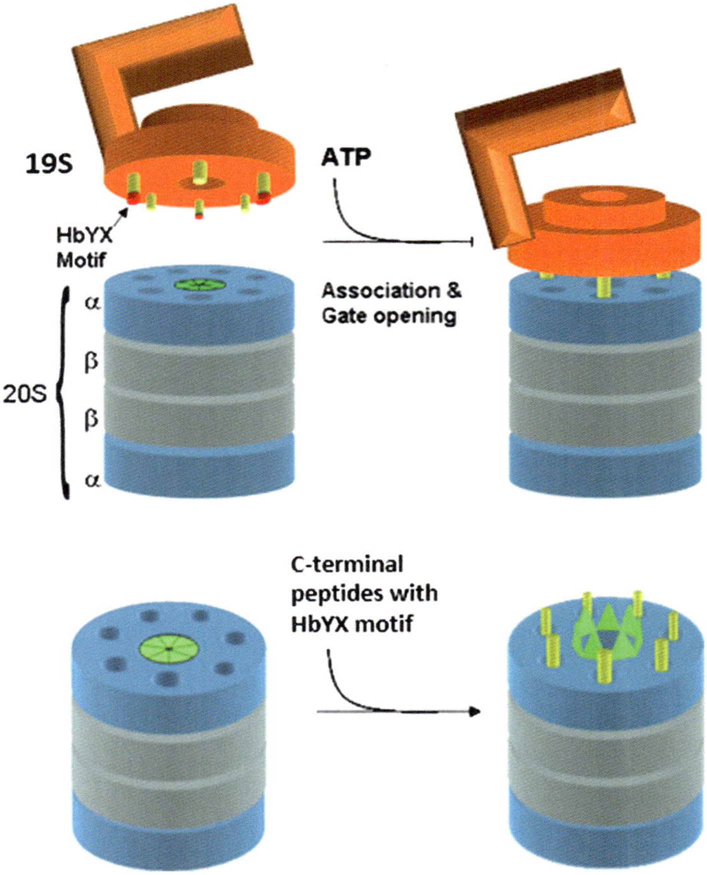

Fig. 14.3 Model depicting the association of 19S with the α-ring of the 20S proteasome. The C-termini (*yellow*) of 19S (*orange*) dock into the intersubunit pockets on the top of the 20S upon the binding of ATP. Schematic model showing that peptides that contain the HbYX motif from the 19S proteasomal ATPase C-termini (e.g., Rpt2, Rpt3, and Rpt5) can be functional by themselves to induce gate opening. To do this, they bind to the intersubunit pockets of the 20S and induce rotation of the α-subunits to cause stabilization of the open-gate conformation

conformational changes are not yet understood. The HbYX motif binds to pockets located between the α-subunits in the 20S and this binding induces a rotation in the α-subunits, which displaces a reverse-turn loop destabilizing the closed-gated conformation and stabilizing the open-gate conformation [21]. These closed- and open-gate conformations involving the reverse-turn loop were previously described by Hill and colleagues in their studies of how PA26 activates gate opening [22, 23], which apparently works by a different mechanism that does not utilize α-subunit rotations. The archaeal 20S gate is also shown to be highly dynamic by an NMR study, which shows that the N-terminal tails of the α-subunit interchanges between open and closed states on the second time scale [24]. This may suggest why the 20S always shows a basal level of peptide hydrolysis activity that is accelerated upon stabilization of the open-gate structure by proteasome activators. The HbYX motif is also highly conserved in the ATPases of the eukaryotic 26S complex, where it plays the same role in triggering gate opening in the 20S [20, 25]. However, only three of the six different ATPase subunits have a conserved HbYX motif, and recent EM structural studies show that the C-terminal HbYX tails of Rpt2, Rpt3, and Rpt5 are shown to be docked into their specific 20S α-subunit binding pockets at the interfaces of the α3 and α4, α1 and α2, and α5 and α6, respectively, whereas densities for the non-HbYX tails of Rpt1, Rpt4, and Rpt6 were not observed [4]. Besides their role in gate opening, the HbYX tails of Rpt3 and Rpt5 are also shown to be essential for the 26S proteasome assembly [26]. Furthermore, the Rpt6 C-terminal tail is demonstrated to play an important role in maintaining 26S stability and base-20S complex formation and subsequent reconfiguration of the 26S complex [26, 27], which is not yet fully understood. Sufficient to say, the 19S–20S assembly process appears to be dynamic and complicated and further work is necessary to understand it, but what is known is that the C-termini of the ATPases play an essential and critical role in the 26S assembly.

14.3 Function

14.3.1 ATP Binding Regulates 26S Assembly and Gate Opening

While the role of the C-terminal HbYX motif in the Rpt subunits is certainly critical, an important regulatory factor is the binding of ATP to the ATPase subunits. ATP binding is essential to allow the ATPase C-termini to bind to the 20S and stimulate gate opening. It's assumed that binding of ATP induces some conformational change in the ATPase subunits that allows the HbYX motif to become available for binding to the 20S proteasome (Fig. 14.3). Interestingly, the non-hydrolyzable analog of ATP (ATPγS) induces complex formation and 20S gate opening in vitro better than ATP does [12, 28], presumably because ATP is cleaved to ADP, which cannot support ATPase-20S association and gate opening. Mutational analyses of the Walker A motif (required for ATP binding) in various Rpt subunits revealed that ATP binding to Rpt1, Rpt2, Rpt3, and Rpt4 is indispensable in forming the 26S, but presumed ATP binding defects in Rpt5 and Rpt6 are tolerable, suggesting ATP binding to some of the Rpt subunits is more critical for the 26S assembly than other subunits [29]. This also suggests that different α-subunit pockets are utilized for 19S–20S association to different extents.

14.3.2 *Substrate Binding, Unfolding, and Translocation*

The AAA+ATPases are involved in protein degradation and protein remodeling in archaea, bacteria, and eukaryotic cells. To catalyze ATP-dependent protein substrate remodeling, all of these AAA+ATPases utilize six key functional motifs (i.e., Walker A, Walker B, Sensor 1, arginine finger, Sensor 2, and pore loop) [30–32]. The proteasomal ATPases and other bacterial AAA+unfoldases, ClpX, ClpA, FtsH, ClpB, and HslU, belong to the AAA+protein superfamily. Because the 26S proteasome is an ATP-dependent molecular machine, it's obvious that understanding how ATP binding and hydrolysis are coordinated to drive function will be important for targeting the regulatory aspects of the proteasome. ATP binding and hydrolysis are known to be required for several of the proteasome's functions including: (1) substrate binding, (2) gate opening, (3) 26S assembly (or ATPase-20S association), (4) initial substrate threading (engagement) [29, 33, 34], and (5) substrate unfolding [35]. Moreover, the binding of ubiquitinated conjugates to the 19S complex is known to stimulate ATPase activity and gate opening in the 26S proteasome, which presumably aids their own degradation [29, 36–39]. Therefore, based on these observations and known functions, a complex network of interactions and allosteric pathways, mediated by the ATPase ring, must exist in the 26S proteasome, which is essential for its ability to degrade proteins.

Unfolding of structured substrates requires ATP hydrolysis by the proteasomal ATPases, although the exact ATP costs and time for processing substrates vary depending on the stability of the tertiary structure of the substrates [28, 35, 40, 41]. Substrate translocation by the proteasome per se is known not to require ATP hydrolysis, given that unfolded proteins are rapidly degraded in the ATPγS state or by the open-gated 20S [12, 28]. However, it is widely accepted that unfolding and translocation are a coupled process (translocation through a narrow pore is what causes unfolding). Nevertheless, this mechanism has not been directly shown for the 26S or PAN-20S complex [2], though several studies corroborate it [42].

14.3.3 *ATP Binding Pattern, Stoichiometry, and ATPase Cycle*

The cycle of ATP hydrolysis lays the basis for all the ATP-dependent functions of the proteasome as this event drives the conformational changes in the ATPase ring that do work. This ATP binding and hydrolysis mechanism has been directly examined using the PAN-20S and eukaryotic 26S complex. Surprisingly, it was found that though the proteasomal ATPase is a hexamer, it could only bind to two ATPs and two ADPs at a time [34]. These studies suggested a cooperative and coordinated cyclic ATP binding and hydrolysis model. This "paired" ATP binding model explains the presence of three different types of nucleotide binding sites on the hexameric ATPase ring, two high-affinity (ATP), two low-affinity (ADP), and two non-binding (empty) subunits per hexamer. Further evidence, using Walker A mutants, suggests a sequential progression of these different subunit conformations around the ring driven by ATP hydrolysis [29, 41]. Given that the two ATP-bound state maximally regulates 20S binding and gating, this model also explains that the symmetric fixed-order arrangement of alternating HbYX and non-HbYX Rpt subunits (-Rpt1-*Rpt2*-Rpt6-*Rpt3*-Rpt4-*Rpt5*-) ensures simultaneous interactions of at least one HbYX- and one non-HbYX-containing Rpt subunits with the 20S proteasome at all times during ATP-dependent hydrolysis of substrates. Since the two-ATP-bound state is the active one, the elucidation of the allosteric pathways that control these ATP binding effects will be important to understanding how to target these critical functions.

14.4 Regulation

Selective degradation of proteins by the proteasome is crucial for proper proteostasis (protein homeostasis) and cell physiology. Above we discussed several layers of regulation in the 26S proteasome that maintain proper proteasome function and protein degradation capacity. Below we discuss mechanisms by which the 26S proteasome can be regulated by ancillary factors.

14.4.1 Proteasome-Interacting Proteins (PIPs)

Several proteasome-interacting proteins (PIPs) are known to regulate proteasome activity. In addition to intrinsic Ub receptors (Rpn10 and Rpn13), the shuttling factors (UBA-UBL proteins which can bind to both ubiquitin and ubiquitin receptors)—Rad23 (hHR23b), Dsk1 (PLIC2), Ddi1, and p62 (SQSTM1)—have been known to bind ubiquitinated proteins and transport them to the proteasome (Rpn1 or Rpn10/Rpn13) [2]. This substrate targeting to the proteasome is the first regulatory point in controlling proteasome activity. Some Rpt interacting proteins (called base assembly chaperones) have been shown to influence ATPase ring assembly. Overexpression of the base assembly chaperones (p27, PAAF1, and S5b) and in vitro binding characterizations showed negative effect on proteasome assembly and activity by these Rpt assembly chaperones [43–46]. PI31, which is also sometimes considered a PIP, has been shown to modulate proteasome activity by inhibiting 20S activity and stimulating 26S activity [47–49]. Interestingly, recent findings demonstrated that ADP-ribosylation of drosophila-dPI31 promotes 26S assembly by sequestering dp27 and dS5b. Inhibition of the PI31 ADP-ribosylation process shows reduction of 26S assembly, resulting in partial inhibition of cancer cell growth [50].

14.4.2 Deubiquitinating Enzymes (DUBs)

While ubiquitination of substrates is important for their recognition by the 26S proteasome, the regulated and timely removal of ubiquitin from substrates by proteasome-associated DUBs is also important for proper substrate processing. Three DUBs have been known to be associated with the 26S proteasome. Rpn11 is a proteasomal lid subunit and it cleaves the entire ubiquitin chain from the substrate (en bloc) near the mouth of ATPase ring. Moreover, it is known to require ATP hydrolysis to promote substrate degradation, suggesting the coupling of Rpn11 activity and translocation of the substrate through the ATPase ring [28, 51–53]. In addition, two DUBs, Ubp6 (Usp14) and Uch37 (UchL5), trim the polyubiquitin chains from the distal side of the chain, in essence shortening it. Ubp6's chain trimming activity has been known to inhibit the efficiency of the proteasome's ability to degrade proteins, presumably because the ubiquitin chain shortening decreases the substrates affinity for the proteasome, which may act as a timing mechanism [54]. Moreover, an inhibitor of Ubp6/Usp14 has been shown to activate degradation of certain ubiquitinated substrates [55]. In addition, Usp14 is overexpressed in colorectal cancer and appears to play a role in Wnt signaling [56]. Uch37's chain editing activity is also known to suppress the breakdown of lightly ubiquitinated proteins in vitro [57]. RNAi depletion study of Uch37 or Usp14 in HeLa cells showed stimulation of model substrate (i.e., Ub-R-GFP) degradation [58], further supporting the notion that these DUBs play a negative role in regulating substrate degradation. Though their physiological functions are not fully understood, it appears that proteasome-bound DUBs are an important control point in regulating proteasome activity.

14.4.3 Posttranslational Modifications (PTMs) of the Proteasome Subunits

Like other regulatory proteins, several proteasome subunits are also regulated by various posttranslational modifications (PTMs). These PTMs have a wide range of effects including: modulation of biochemical activity, intracellular localization, stability, and protein–protein interactions. Several different types of PTMs have been observed, usually by mass-spectrometry-based proteomic approaches (and some biochemical studies) including: phosphorylation, dephosphorylation, acetylation, glycosylation (O-GlcNAc), ADP-ribosylation, monoubiquitination, proteolytic processing, oxidation, nitration, and myristoylation [59, 60]. A few examples include phosphorylation of Rpt6 by PKA, and CaMKII was known to activate proteasome activity, most probably by facilitating the 26S assembly [61, 62]. In contrast, phosphorylation of Rpt5 by ASK1 was shown to inhibit Rpt5 ATPase activity and resulting in 26S proteasome activity [63]. Additionally, O-GlcNAcylation of Rpt2 by O-GlcNAc transferase (OGT) was known to inhibit the proteasome's ATPase activity and resulting in protein degradation activity [64]. As expected, these various PTMs of the proteasome and their downstream effects on controlling function, assembly, and localization are important for maintaining overall protein degradation capacity. These above discussed structures, functions, and PTMs highlight inherent points of regulation in the proteasome that provide mechanisms for fine-tuning the proteasome function for specific cellular needs and indicate potential targets for pharmacological modulation.

14.5 Potential for Cancer Therapies

As described above, the 26S proteasome has a complex structural organization, whose function is driven primarily by ATP-dependent allosteric networks with many layers of regulatory elements. While the core functions of the 19S are essential for most ubiquitin-dependent protein degradation, the additional layers of ancillary regulatory points are presumed to be necessary for regulating the degradation of different types of substrates depending on the different cellular states or types. Since the 26S proteasome regulates the degradation of the majority of proteins in the cell, a detailed understanding of its many regulatory points will be highly useful for drug development of agents that can selectively modulate these proteasome regulatory features. While current proteasome inhibitors in the clinic are useful to treat hematological cancers, these inhibitors target protein degradation globally since they target the function of the 20S protease sites. Presumably, the inhibition of proteasome regulatory factors, which are discussed above, that may be specific to certain cell types (e.g., cancer) could prove to be more useful to treat other cancers (e.g., solid tumors) and would, at a minimum, be expected to be less toxic, since only subsets of the proteasome substrates would be affected.

14.5.1 26S Assembly Modulator

Although the 26S assembly process is complex involving multiple 20S and 19S assembly chaperones [1], it has critical regulatory points involving specific interactions (e.g., HbYX motif and 20S pocket), and ATP binding to certain subunits controls this assembly process. Therefore, these crucial protein–protein interactions and the allosteric pathways that mediate selective ATP binding effects are expected to be important therapeutic targets. The HTS and follow-up characterizations of 26S assembly modulator candidates are under way, which promises to identify new 26S assembly inhibitors and which could affect a variety of mechanisms discussed above.

Such agents would be expected to block ubiquitin-dependent protein degradation while leaving the assembled 20S intact and free to degrade proteins by itself or with other proteasome-activating complexes.

14.5.2 Gating Modulators

The substrate gate in the isolated 20S proteasomes typically remains in a closed state and is said to be latent. But several proteasome activators can bind the proteasome and stimulate gate opening. One example we discussed above is the 19S regulatory particle, whose HbYX motif binds to specific pockets in the 20S α-subunits. However, several other regulators also bind to a set of these seven different 20S intersubunit pockets, including PA200, PA28αβ, PA28γ, and potentially PI31. Presumably these different regulators regulate the degradation of different subsets of proteins in the cell. Because the intersubunit pockets are well defined, it's likely that competitive agents could be found that bind to these seven different pockets on top of the 20S. In addition, it is expected that such agents could differentially affect the binding of these different proteasome activators, in which case each agent could have different physiological effects. Essentially, such agents would be expected to inhibit degradation of proteins that require the specific proteasome activator for their degradation. If any one of the HbYX binding sites could be targeted, it would be expected that such agents would block 19S-dependent gate opening, and thus, ubiquitin-dependent protein degradation should be perturbed due to inhibition of gate opening. In addition, since the HbYX motif induces gate opening in these sites, it could also be expected that some compounds could bind and stabilize the closed state of the gate, perhaps even in the latent 20S, which still has a capacity to degrade unstructured proteins due to gate fluctuations. Agents that block the HbYX mechanism without affecting the degradation of unstructured proteins by the 20S proteasome alone would add a new layer of specificity. Similarly, such agents would not be expected to inhibit gate opening due to PA28αβ or PA28γ, since these activators do not use an HbYX-dependent mechanism for gate opening. Such gating modulators could be a new generation of proteasome inhibitors and would be expected to have anticancer activities due to their ability to specifically inhibit ubiquitin-dependent protein degradation. Such agents are expected to have remarkably different physiological effects compared to traditional proteasome inhibitors.

14.5.3 Modulating PTM Enzymes

Developing agents that modulate PTMs that occur on the 19S proteasomal Rpt subunits (i.e., Rpt6 phosphorylation) or the PTMs of proteasome regulators (i.e., PI31 ADP-ribosylation) by pharmacological methods also have merit. In addition, such approaches could be more readily developed, since the target (the posttranslational modifying enzyme) will be a simpler enzyme, which has advantages in drug development, unlike with the proteasome complex. Validation of target choice would be easier experimentally, as siRNA approaches could be used to downregulate the proteasome modifying enzyme. Similar approaches (i.e., using siRNA) for the 26S subunits are less attractive, since knockdown of their constitutive subunits halt proteasome assembly, which causes a different type of functional defect than pharmacological inhibition of regulatory subunits that are part of a functionally assembled proteasome.

14.5.4 DUB Modulator

Proteasomal DUBs have already been identified and targeted as novel targets for therapeutic intervention. To date, the compound named b-AP-15 has been identified as a dual inhibitor of Usp14 and Uch37 (UchL5). The treatment of cancer cells by b-AP-15 elicits biological effects which are similar to those of the 20S inhibitors including accumulation of polyubiquitylated proteins, induction of apoptosis, and inhibition of tumor cell proliferation [65]. As mentioned above, Rpn11 (Poh1) has shown an ATP-dependent stimulatory role in substrate degradation [51, 52] and has been shown to be important for proteasome activity and cell proliferation [58]. Thus, targeting Rpn11 looks promising and screening is under way to find new Rpn11 modulators, which hold promise as new cancer therapeutic reagents.

14.5.5 Inhibiting the Unfolding and Translocation Process

Targeting the proteasomal ATPases has been attempted previously without resounding success thus far. Only one known peptoid inhibitor (RIP-1) which was shown to bind to the Rpt4 subunit has demonstrated some efficacy for inhibiting the 19Ss unfoldase activity in vitro and possibly also substrate degradation (p53) in cells [38, 66, 67]. However, off-target effects of this compound have not been rigorously tested in cells, and further validation as a specific 19S ATPase inhibitor is needed. Although the development of ATP mimics is challenging, especially considering the issue of selectivity in AAA+ATPases, specific agents for the ATP hydrolysis sites could make for very interesting proteasomal modulators. Compounds that mimic the ATP-bound state but inhibit ATP hydrolysis could theoretically allow for the degradation of unfolded substrates, perhaps even in a ubiquitin-dependent manner, since translocation of unfolded substrates into the open-gated proteasome does not require ATP hydrolysis [12]. However, the degradation of folded substrates should be inhibited since they do require ATP hydrolysis. While it's difficult to predict the physiological outcome of using such inhibitors, such agents would allow for the inhibition of a unique subset of cellular proteasome substrates. ADP mimics that specifically bind the proteasomal ATPases would be expected to block substrate binding, gating, unfolding, and translocation, which would also have differential effects on the cells' physiology. Targeting the proteasomal ATPases is still an opportunity and remains as an important drug target; we expect that such agents will be identified in the future.

14.6 Conclusion

The proteasome is an interesting target for the development of drugs that can regulate the levels of different subsets of proteins in the cell. Due to the importance of the proteasome to cellular physiology, its function is strictly and highly regulated, not only in the context of ubiquitin-dependent protein degradation by the 26S, but also by other types of proteasome regulatory complexes and proteins, which are discussed here. That being said, our above discussion of possible therapeutic targets in the proteasome is in no way exhaustive, and many other interesting sites for regulation are also available that are not discussed here. This extensive regulatory system for controlling the degradation of individual proteins provides a rich ground for drug development, especially in diseases where general proteasome inhibitors have already proven useful to treat disease, such as hematological cancers. We imagine the new generation of proteasome modulators may also prove to be useful in solid tumors as well and perhaps even other diseases not specifically related to cancer.

References

1. Tomko RJ Jr, Hochstrasser M (2013) Molecular architecture and assembly of the eukaryotic proteasome. Annu Rev Biochem 82:415–445
2. Finley D (2009) Recognition and processing of ubiquitin-protein conjugates by the proteasome. Annu Rev Biochem 78:477–513
3. Bar-Nun S, Glickman MH (2012) Proteasomal AAA-ATPases: structure and function. Biochim Biophys Acta 1823:67–82
4. Lander GC, Estrin E, Matyskiela ME, Bashore C, Nogales E, Martin A (2012) Complete subunit architecture of the proteasome regulatory particle. Nature 482:186–191
5. Lasker K, Forster F, Bohn S, Walzthoeni T, Villa E, Unverdorben P, Beck F, Aebersold R, Sali A, Baumeister W (2012) Molecular architecture of the 26S proteasome holocomplex determined by an integrative approach. Proc Natl Acad Sci U S A 109:1380–1387
6. Beck F, Unverdorben P, Bohn S, Schweitzer A, Pfeifer G, Sakata E, Nickell S, Plitzko JM, Villa E, Baumeister W, Forster F (2012) Near-atomic resolution structural model of the yeast 26S proteasome. Proc Natl Acad Sci U S A 109:14870–14875
7. da Fonseca PC, He J, Morris EP (2012) Molecular model of the human 26S proteasome. Mol Cell 46:54–66
8. Bohn S, Beck F, Sakata E, Walzthoeni T, Beck M, Aebersold R, Forster F, Baumeister W, Nickell S (2010) Structure of the 26S proteasome from Schizosaccharomyces pombe at subnanometer resolution. Proc Natl Acad Sci U S A 107:20992–20997
9. Sakata E, Bohn S, Mihalache O, Kiss P, Beck F, Nagy I, Nickell S, Tanaka K, Saeki Y, Forster F, Baumeister W (2012) Localization of the proteasomal ubiquitin receptors Rpn10 and Rpn13 by electron cryomicroscopy. Proc Natl Acad Sci U S A 109:1479–1484

10. Sledz P, Unverdorben P, Beck F, Pfeifer G, Schweitzer A, Forster F, Baumeister W (2013) Structure of the 26S proteasome with ATP-gammaS bound provides insights into the mechanism of nucleotide-dependent substrate translocation. Proc Natl Acad Sci U S A 110:7264–7269
11. Matyskiela ME, Lander GC, Martin A (2013) Conformational switching of the 26S proteasome enables substrate degradation. Nat Struct Mol Biol 20:781–788
12. Smith DM, Kafri G, Cheng Y, Ng D, Walz T, Goldberg AL (2005) ATP binding to PAN or the 26S ATPases causes association with the 20S proteasome, gate opening, and translocation of unfolded proteins. Mol Cell 20:687–698
13. Zhang F, Hu M, Tian G, Zhang P, Finley D, Jeffrey PD, Shi Y (2009) Structural insights into the regulatory particle of the proteasome from Methanocaldococcus jannaschii. Mol Cell 34:473–484
14. Zhang F, Wu Z, Zhang P, Tian G, Finley D, Shi Y (2009) Mechanism of substrate unfolding and translocation by the regulatory particle of the proteasome from Methanocaldococcus jannaschii. Mol Cell 34:485–496
15. Djuranovic S, Hartmann MD, Habeck M, Ursinus A, Zwickl P, Martin J, Lupas AN, Zeth K (2009) Structure and activity of the N-terminal substrate recognition domains in proteasomal ATPases. Mol Cell 34:580–590
16. Braun BC, Glickman M, Kraft R, Dahlmann B, Kloetzel PM, Finley D, Schmidt M (1999) The base of the proteasome regulatory particle exhibits chaperone-like activity. Nat Cell Biol 1:221–226
17. Benaroudj N, Goldberg AL (2000) PAN, the proteasome-activating nucleotidase from archaebacteria, is a protein-unfolding molecular chaperone. Nat Cell Biol 2:833–839
18. Groll M, Ditzel L, Lowe J, Stock D, Bochtler M, Bartunik HD, Huber R (1997) Structure of 20S proteasome from yeast at 2.4 A resolution. Nature 386:463–471
19. Groll M, Bajorek M, Kohler A, Moroder L, Rubin DM, Huber R, Glickman MH, Finley D (2000) A gated channel into the proteasome core particle. Nat Struct Biol 7:1062–1067
20. Smith DM, Chang SC, Park S, Finley D, Cheng Y, Goldberg AL (2007) Docking of the proteasomal ATPases' carboxyl termini in the 20S proteasome's alpha ring opens the gate for substrate entry. Mol Cell 27:731–744
21. Rabl J, Smith DM, Yu Y, Chang SC, Goldberg AL, Cheng Y (2008) Mechanism of gate opening in the 20S proteasome by the proteasomal ATPases. Mol Cell 30:360–368
22. Whitby FG, Masters EI, Kramer L, Knowlton JR, Yao Y, Wang CC, Hill CP (2000) Structural basis for the activation of 20S proteasomes by 11S regulators. Nature 408:115–120
23. Forster A, Masters EI, Whitby FG, Robinson H, Hill CP (2005) The 1.9 A structure of a proteasome-11S activator complex and implications for proteasome-PAN/PA700 interactions. Mol Cell 18:589–599
24. Religa TL, Sprangers R, Kay LE (2010) Dynamic regulation of archaeal proteasome gate opening as studied by TROSY NMR. Science 328:98–102
25. Gillette TG, Kumar B, Thompson D, Slaughter CA, DeMartino GN (2008) Differential roles of the COOH termini of AAA subunits of PA700 (19 S regulator) in asymmetric assembly and activation of the 26 S proteasome. J Biol Chem 283:31813–31822
26. Kim YC, Demartino GN (2011) C termini of proteasomal ATPases play nonequivalent roles in cellular assembly of mammalian 26 S proteasome. J Biol Chem 286:26652–26666
27. Park S, Li X, Kim HM, Singh CR, Tian G, Hoyt MA, Lovell S, Battaile KP, Zolkiewski M, Coffino P, Roelofs J, Cheng Y, Finley D (2013) Reconfiguration of the proteasome during chaperone-mediated assembly. Nature 497:512–516
28. Liu CW, Li X, Thompson D, Wooding K, Chang TL, Tang Z, Yu H, Thomas PJ, DeMartino GN (2006) ATP binding and ATP hydrolysis play distinct roles in the function of 26S proteasome. Mol Cell 24:39–50
29. Kim YC, Li X, Thompson D, DeMartino GN (2013) ATP binding by proteasomal ATPases regulates cellular assembly and substrate-induced functions of the 26 S proteasome. J Biol Chem 288:3334–3345
30. Sauer RT, Baker TA (2011) AAA+proteases: ATP-fueled machines of protein destruction. Annu Rev Biochem 80:587–612

31. Hanson PI, Whiteheart SW (2005) AAA+proteins: have engine, will work. Nat Rev Mol Cell Biol 6:519–529
32. Erzberger JP, Berger JM (2006) Evolutionary relationships and structural mechanisms of AAA+proteins. Annu Rev Biophys Biomol Struct 35:93–114
33. Peth A, Uchiki T, Goldberg AL (2010) ATP-dependent steps in the binding of ubiquitin conjugates to the 26S proteasome that commit to degradation. Mol Cell 40:671–681
34. Smith DM, Fraga H, Reis C, Kafri G, Goldberg AL (2011) ATP binds to proteasomal ATPases in pairs with distinct functional effects, implying an ordered reaction cycle. Cell 144:526–538
35. Benaroudj N, Zwickl P, Seemuller E, Baumeister W, Goldberg AL (2003) ATP hydrolysis by the proteasome regulatory complex PAN serves multiple functions in protein degradation. Mol Cell 11:69–78
36. Bech-Otschir D, Helfrich A, Enenkel C, Consiglieri G, Seeger M, Holzhutter HG, Dahlmann B, Kloetzel PM (2009) Polyubiquitin substrates allosterically activate their own degradation by the 26S proteasome. Nat Struct Mol Biol 16:219–225
37. Peth A, Besche HC, Goldberg AL (2009) Ubiquitinated proteins activate the proteasome by binding to Usp14/Ubp6, which causes 20S gate opening. Mol Cell 36:794–804
38. Li X, Demartino GN (2009) Variably modulated gating of the 26S proteasome by ATP and polyubiquitin. Biochem J 421:397–404
39. Peth A, Kukushkin N, Bosse M, Goldberg AL (2013) Ubiquitinated proteins activate the proteasomal ATPases by binding to Usp14 or Uch37 homologs. J Biol Chem 288:7781–7790
40. Henderson A, Erales J, Hoyt MA, Coffino P (2011) Dependence of proteasome processing rate on substrate unfolding. J Biol Chem 286:17495–17502
41. Peth A, Nathan JA, Goldberg AL (2013) The ATP costs and time required to degrade ubiquitinated proteins by the 26S proteasome. J Biol Chem 288(40):29215–29222
42. Lee C, Schwartz MP, Prakash S, Iwakura M, Matouschek A (2001) ATP-dependent proteases degrade their substrates by processively unraveling them from the degradation signal. Mol Cell 7:627–637
43. Kaneko T, Hamazaki J, Iemura S, Sasaki K, Furuyama K, Natsume T, Tanaka K, Murata S (2009) Assembly pathway of the mammalian proteasome base subcomplex is mediated by multiple specific chaperones. Cell 137:914–925
44. Lassot I, Latreille D, Rousset E, Sourisseau M, Linares LK, Chable-Bessia C, Coux O, Benkirane M, Kiernan RE (2007) The proteasome regulates HIV-1 transcription by both proteolytic and nonproteolytic mechanisms. Mol Cell 25:369–383
45. Park Y, Hwang YP, Lee JS, Seo SH, Yoon SK, Yoon JB (2005) Proteasomal ATPase-associated factor 1 negatively regulates proteasome activity by interacting with proteasomal ATPases. Mol Cell Biol 25:3842–3853
46. Shim SM, Lee WJ, Kim Y, Chang JW, Song S, Jung YK (2012) Role of S5b/PSMD5 in proteasome inhibition caused by TNF-alpha/NFkappaB in higher eukaryotes. Cell Rep 2:603–615
47. McCutchen-Maloney SL, Matsuda K, Shimbara N, Binns DD, Tanaka K, Slaughter CA, DeMartino GN (2000) cDNA cloning, expression, and functional characterization of PI31, a proline-rich inhibitor of the proteasome. J Biol Chem 275:18557–18565
48. Zaiss DM, Standera S, Holzhutter H, Kloetzel P, Sijts AJ (1999) The proteasome inhibitor PI31 competes with PA28 for binding to 20S proteasomes. FEBS Lett 457:333–338
49. Bader M, Benjamin S, Wapinski OL, Smith DM, Goldberg AL, Steller H (2011) A conserved f box regulatory complex controls proteasome activity in Drosophila. Cell 145:371–382
50. Cho-Park P, Steller H (2013) Proteasome regulation by ADP-ribosylation. Cell 153:614–627
51. Verma R, Aravind L, Oania R, McDonald WH, Yates JR 3rd, Koonin EV, Deshaies RJ (2002) Role of Rpn11 metalloprotease in deubiquitination and degradation by the 26S proteasome. Science 298:611–615
52. Yao T, Cohen RE (2002) A cryptic protease couples deubiquitination and degradation by the proteasome. Nature 419:403–407
53. Lee MJ, Lee BH, Hanna J, King RW, Finley D (2011) Trimming of ubiquitin chains by proteasome-associated deubiquitinating enzymes. Mol Cell Proteomics 10(5):R110.003871

54. Hanna J, Hathaway NA, Tone Y, Crosas B, Elsasser S, Kirkpatrick DS, Leggett DS, Gygi SP, King RW, Finley D (2006) Deubiquitinating enzyme Ubp6 functions noncatalytically to delay proteasomal degradation. Cell 127:99–111
55. Lee BH, Lee MJ, Park S, Oh DC, Elsasser S, Chen PC, Gartner C, Dimova N, Hanna J, Gygi SP, Wilson SM, King RW, Finley D (2010) Enhancement of proteasome activity by a small-molecule inhibitor of USP14. Nature 467:179–184
56. Jung H, Kim BG, Han W, Lee J, Cho JY, Park W, Maurice M, Han JK, Lee M, Finley D, Jho EH (2013) Deubiquitination of Dishevelled by Usp14 is required for Wnt signaling. Oncogenesis 2:e64
57. Lam YA, Xu W, DeMartino GN, Cohen RE (1997) Editing of ubiquitin conjugates by an isopeptidase in the 26S proteasome. Nature 385:737–740
58. Koulich E, Li X, DeMartino GN (2008) Relative structural and functional roles of multiple deubiquitylating proteins associated with mammalian 26S proteasome. Mol Biol Cell 19:1072–1082
59. Aiken CT, Kaake RM, Wang X, Huang L (2011) Oxidative stress-mediated regulation of proteasome complexes. Mol Cell Proteomics 10:R110.006924
60. Schmidt M, Finley D (2014) Regulation of proteasome activity in health and disease. Biochim Biophys Acta 1843(1):13–25
61. Zhang F, Hu Y, Huang P, Toleman CA, Paterson AJ, Kudlow JE (2007) Proteasome function is regulated by cyclic AMP-dependent protein kinase through phosphorylation of Rpt6. J Biol Chem 282:22460–22471
62. Djakovic SN, Schwarz LA, Barylko B, DeMartino GN, Patrick GN (2009) Regulation of the proteasome by neuronal activity and calcium/calmodulin-dependent protein kinase II. J Biol Chem 284:26655–26665
63. Um JW, Im E, Park J, Oh Y, Min B, Lee HJ, Yoon JB, Chung KC (2010) ASK1 negatively regulates the 26 S proteasome. J Biol Chem 285:36434–36446
64. Zhang F, Su K, Yang X, Bowe DB, Paterson AJ, Kudlow JE (2003) O-GlcNAc modification is an endogenous inhibitor of the proteasome. Cell 115:715–725
65. D'Arcy P, Brnjic S, Olofsson MH, Fryknas M, Lindsten K, De Cesare M, Perego P, Sadeghi B, Hassan M, Larsson R, Linder S (2011) Inhibition of proteasome deubiquitinating activity as a new cancer therapy. Nat Med 17(12):1636–1640
66. Lim HS, Archer CT, Kodadek T (2007) Identification of a peptoid inhibitor of the proteasome 19S regulatory particle. J Am Chem Soc 129:7750–7751
67. Lim HS, Cai D, Archer CT, Kodadek T (2007) Periodate-triggered cross-linking reveals Sug2/Rpt4 as the molecular target of a peptoid inhibitor of the 19S proteasome regulatory particle. J Am Chem Soc 129:12936–12937

Chapter 15
Deubiquitinating Enzymes as Novel Targets for Cancer Therapies

Kwang-Hyun Baek, Key-Hwan Lim, and Jang-Joon Park

Abstract Most ubiquitinated proteins can be recognized and degraded by the 26S proteasome. In the meantime, protein deubiquitination by various deubiquitinating enzymes (DUBs) regulates protein stability within cells, and it can counterbalance intracellular homeostasis mediated by ubiquitination. Numerous reports have demonstrated that an aberrant process of the ubiquitin-proteasome pathway (UPP) regulated by the ubiquitination and deubiquitination systems results in failure of balancing between protein stability and degradation, and this failure can lead to tumorigenesis in various organs and tissues of mammals. The identification of molecular properties for various DUBs is very critical to understand cancer development and tumorigenesis. Therefore, knowledge of DUBs and their association with cancer and diseases is indispensible for developing effective inhibitors for DUBs. This chapter describes various features and functions of cancer-related DUBs. In addition, we summarize several inhibitors that specifically target certain DUBs in cancer and suggest that DUBs may be one of the most ideal and attractive therapeutic targets.

Keywords Anticancer drug • Bortezomib • Deubiquitination • Oncogene • Proteasome • Tumor suppressor • Ubiquitin-specific protease • Ubiquitination

Abbreviations

CLL	Chronic lymphoid leukemia
CML	Chronic myeloid leukemia
DUB	Deubiquitinating enzyme
HR	Homologous recombination
ICL	Interstrand cross-link
JAMM	JAB1/MPN/MOV34 metalloenzyme
MCL	Mantle cell lymphoma

K.-H. Baek (✉) • K.-H. Lim • J.-J. Park
Department of Biomedical Science, CHA University, Bundang CHA General Hospital, 502 Yatap-Dong, Bundang-Gu, Seongnam-Si, Gyeonggi-Do 463-840, Republic of Korea
e-mail: baek@cha.ac.kr; limkhwan@gmail.com; wkdwnsp@gmail.com

Q.P. Dou (ed.), *Resistance to Proteasome Inhibitors in Cancer*, Resistance to Targeted Anti-Cancer Therapeutics, DOI 10.1007/978-3-319-06752-0_15

MFT	Multiple familiar trichoepithelioma
MJD	Machado-Joseph disease
MM	Multiple myeloma
OTU	Ovarian-tumor protease
PDA	Pancreatic ductal adenocarcinoma
TLS	Translesion DNA synthesis
UCH	Ubiquitin carboxy-terminal hydrolase
UPP	Ubiquitin-proteasome pathway
USP	Ubiquitin-specific protease

15.1 Introduction

As a reverse process against ubiquitination, deubiquitination accomplished by deubiquitinating enzymes (DUBs) acts as counterbalancing regulation for the fate of proteins. The requirement of catalytic activity for DUBs in cellular processes has been shown in numerous studies. In terms of cellular homeostasis, controlled expression levels of proteins are essential, and abnormal expression of certain proteins can be directly linked to cancer and other diseases causing breakdown of the coordinated cellular system. A number of unregulated proteins are mediated by ubiquitination and deubiquitination. Therefore, it is necessary to understand and investigate in detail the cellular and molecular mechanisms underlining deubiquitinating activity. In addition, the targeting of DUBs as anticancer therapies is becoming an important field in cancer therapeutics. Knowledge of DUBs, their association with cancer and diseases, and use of DUB inhibitors in clinical and preclinical studies will be presented in this chapter.

15.2 Overview of DUBs

15.2.1 Classification of Proteases in Mammals

Proteases are essential enzymes that catalyze protein-peptide bonds in all species, and they have various cellular functions such as in food digestion, ovulation, fertilization, and inflammatory responses. Many studies have analyzed and revealed the roles of proteases, and the research results have been applied to the medical treatment of cancer and diverse diseases. Recent studies have suggested that the human genome encodes a total of 600 proteases [1]. Human proteases can be divided into five classes according to their catalytic characteristics: serine proteases, threonine proteases, cysteine proteases, aspartate proteases, and metalloproteases. The glutamic proteases are limited to fungal species. Of the 600 proteases, 176 are serine proteases (32 %), 74 are threonine proteases (4 %), 143 are cysteine proteases (26 %), 21 are aspartate proteases (4 %), and 186 are metalloproteases (34 %)

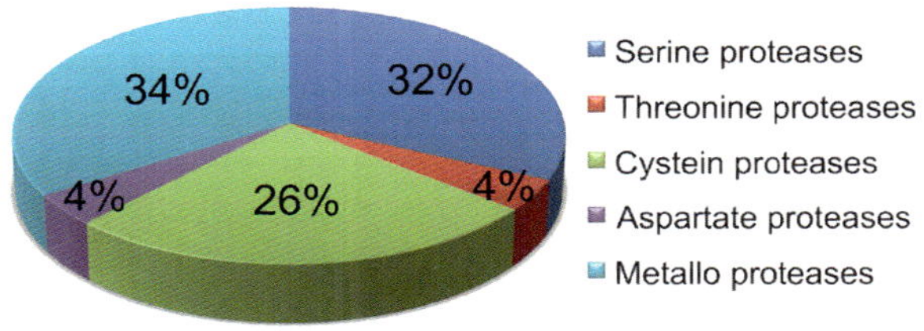

Fig. 15.1 Pie chart of mammalian protease classification. A pie chart representing the percentage of mammalian proteases classified by the expression pattern based on a genome encoding database

according to genomics and bioinformatics research on proteasomes (Fig. 15.1). To the cysteine proteases family, this chapter will focus on cysteine proteases to understand the biological functions of DUBs.

15.2.2 DUB and Its Family

DUBs are a subfamily of cysteine proteases and have reversible abilities against E3 ligases, in which they detach ubiquitin molecules from ubiquitinated substrates via their enzymatic activities (Fig. 15.2). This DUB-mediated process, which is the opposite of ubiquitination, is called deubiquitination. Like ubiquitination, deubiquitination can give signals to functional proteins to modulate their activities. Therefore, DUBs are involved in numerous cellular functions including cell cycle regulation, signal transduction, membrane trafficking, DNA damage response, immune response, and apoptosis or programmed cell death. The major known signal of ubiquitination guides ubiquitinated proteins heading to the 26S proteasome for protein degradation (the ubiquitin-proteasome pathway, UPP), while DUB-mediated deubiquitination can prevent the proteasomal degradation of the substrates. Thus, the orchestration of reversible posttranslational regulations by ubiquitination and deubiquitination affects cellular homeostasis and cell viability, based on not only protein levels, but also on protein functions. It is critical to systemically maintain expression levels and functions of cellular proteins for the healthy cells, tissues, organs, and individuals. Indeed, as we will discuss later in this chapter, the breakdown of coordinated regulation of functional proteins caused by altered activities or abnormal expression level of DUBs can induce severe diseases including cancer.

To date, almost 100 human genes encoding DUB enzymes have been identified; these can be grouped into the following five classes according to their properties: ubiquitin-specific proteases (USPs), ubiquitin carboxy-terminal hydrolases (UCHs), ovarian-tumor proteases (OTUs), Machado-Joseph diseases (MJDs), and JAB1/MPN/MOV34 metalloenzymes (JAMMs). This classification can be expanded to six categories, in order to include the recently identified monocyte chemotactic protein-induced protein (MCPIP) [2]. The DUBs which have been identified so far are listed in Table 15.1. Except for JAMMs, which are zinc metalloproteases, all DUBs have conserved domains including Cys, Asp/Asn, and His domains, which are associated with their catalytic activity [3].

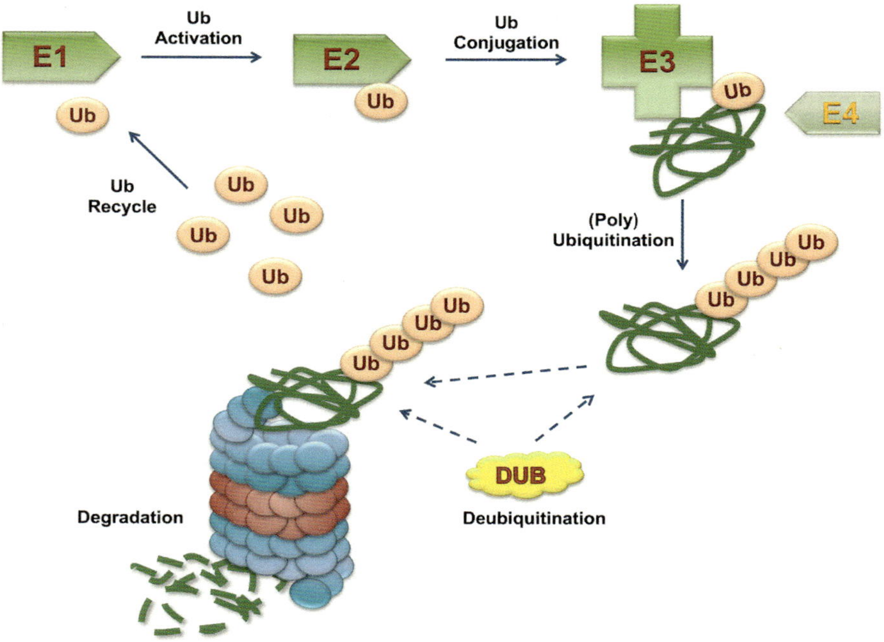

Fig. 15.2 Ubiquitination and deubiquitination. The proteasomal degradation of ubiquitinated proteins occurs via the ubiquitin-proteasome pathway (UPP). The coordinated ubiquitination and deubiquitination of target proteins are mediated by specific enzymes. For ubiquitination, successive action of several enzymes is required. For the first step, ubiquitin (Ub), which consists of 76 amino acids, is activated by a ubiquitin-activating enzyme (E1) in an ATP-dependent manner. This is followed by interaction with the ubiquitin-conjugating enzyme (E2). Lastly, the E2-bound ubiquitin is transferred to the E3 ubiquitin ligase. In some cases, E4 enzymes are needed for efficient ubiquitination. In addition to mono-ubiquitination, additional ubiquitins can be conjugated to the attached ubiquitin to form polyubiquitin chains. In a reversible process, deubiquitinating enzymes (DUBs) detach ubiquitin molecules from ubiquitinated substrates via their enzymatic activities. In this process, ubiquitin chains from proteasome-targeted proteins should be removed, thereby promoting protein degradation and recycling free ubiquitins. Deconjugating ubiquitin in proteasomal processing is mediated by certain DUBs including UCHL5, USP14, and POH1. Through these processes, DUBs generate free ubiquitin molecules, prevent proteasomal degradation of target proteins, and stabilize target proteins

15.2.3 Structure of DUBs

Structural analysis has been performed for diverse DUBs [4]. This is the most reliable way of gaining information about target protein activity, functions, and interaction motifs. The generalization of several 3D structures has emerged from diverse studies in which the molecular key features of DUBs as ubiquitin moieties have been established [4]. Each DUB subfamily shares similar sequences and structures.

Table 15.1 Subfamily types of deubiquitinating enzymes classified into six categories

Subfamily types	DUB names
USP family	USP1, USP2, USP3, USP4, USP5, USP6, USP7, USP8, USP9X, USP9Y, USP10, USP11, USP12, USP13, USP14, USP15, USP16, DUB3, USP18, USP19, USP20, USP21, USP22, USP24, USP25, USP26, USP27X, USP28, USP29, USP30, USP31, USP31, USP32, USP33, USP34, USP35, USP36, USP37, USP38, USP39, USP40, USP41, USP42, USP43, USP44, USP45, USP46, USP47, USP48, USP49, USP50, USP51, USP52, USP53, USP54, CYLD, USPL1
UCH family	UCH-L1, UCH-L3, UCH-L5, BAP1
JAMM family	BRCC36, CSN5, POH1, AMSH, AMSH-LP, MPND, MYSM1, PRPF8, EIF3
OTU family	OTUB1, OTUB2, OTUD1, OTUD3, OTUD4, OTUD5, OTUD6A, OTUD6B, OTU1, HIN1L, A20, Cezanne, Cezanne2, VCPIP, TRABID
MJD family	ATXN3, ATXN3L, JOSD1, JOSD2
MCPIP family[a]	MCPIP1, MCPIP2, MCPIP3, MCPIP4, MCPIP5, MCPIP6, MCPIP7

[a]MCPIP family, which is newly discovered, can be grouped as a subfamily of DUBs

In general, most USP family members have six homologue-conserved USP domains and consist of three domains organizing as a palm, a thumb, and fingers [4]. Among them, the finger domains interact with ubiquitin. In addition, a number of diverse motifs exist through USPs, and these specific domains and structures give unique functions to USPs. USP3, USP5, USP39, USP44, USP45, USP49, and USP51 have the zinc-finger USP domain, while the domain present in USP (DUSP) is located in USP4, USP11, USP15, USP20, USP33, and USP48. Moreover, other functional domains are present through different USPs [5]. It is known that UCHs are small in size and target only small peptides because of their structures, which include a confined loop [5]. The OTU family can be subdivided into three classes depending on their characteristics—otubains (OTUB1 and OTUB2), A20-like OTUs (A20/TNFα-induced protein 3 {TNFAIP3}; Cezanne, Cezanne2, TRABID, and VCPIP1), and OTUDs (OTUD1, OTUD2/YOD1, OTUD3, OTUD4, OTUD5, OTUD6A, OTUD6B, and ALG13). The Josephin family of DUBs also consists of four different subfamilies, including ataxin-3 (ATXN3), ATXN3L, JOSD1, and JOSD2. Unlike other DUBs, the JAMMs have zinc metalloprotease activity and contain an AMSH-LP structure and two conserved motifs that are related to the capacity for cleaving K63-linked polyubiquitin chains [5].

15.3 Various Roles of DUBs in Cancer

Most vertebrates have a balance that maintains cell birth and cell death through intracellular signaling from various stimuli. Cells disproportionated by abnormal protein expression or oncogene transcription from several stimuli can be transformed into cancer cells. For example, treatment of normal cells with viruses, carcinogenic compounds, UV, or IR can transform cell characterization, leading to a cancerous state by deregulating gene or protein expression. DUBs widely participate in biological functions such as DNA repair, chromatin remodeling, transcription, the signal transduction cascade, protein localization, cell cycle progression, and apoptosis in cancer cells [6].

15.3.1 Oncogenic Functions of DUBs

The functions of USP2a (also known as USP2-69) were first found in prostate cancer. It exhibits oncogenic behavior and depletion of USP2a induces cancer cell apoptosis [7, 8]. USP2a mainly regulates and stabilizes the fatty acid synthase (FAS) which is frequently overexpressed in malignant tumors [7]. The deubiquitinating activity of USP2a in FAS regulation may lead to tumorigenesis. In addition, USP2a is associated with Mdm2 and MdmX [9]. Both Mdm2 and MdmX, known as oncogenic proteins, are negative regulators of p53. Depletion of USP2a enhances both Mdm2 and MdmX protein degradation [8, 9]. USP2a overexpression increases the c-MYC level and is able to inactivate p53 in prostate cancer cells [10]. With these findings, one might expect that USP2a would be strongly associated with tumorigenesis through the regulation of Mdm2 and MdmX and collaboration with c-Myc. A recent study has added the function of USP2a expression to cell death by targeting RIP and tumor necrosis factor receptor-associated factor 2 (TRAF2) degradation during tumor necrosis factor (TNF) response, and USP2a consequently promotes the activation of NF-κB [11].

Although USP4/UNP is associated with the TNF response and activates NF-κB as shown with USP2a, it has a different role, wherein USP4 regulates TAK-1 stability upon TNF response. Interestingly, USP4 deubiquitinates not only TRAF2 but also TRAF6 and leads to the regulation of cell migration [12]. Further, a genome-wide gain-of-function study revealed that AKT acts as a kinase for USP4 phosphorylation and phosphorylated USP4 moves into the cytoplasm from the nucleus. Molecular mechanism studies have shown that USP4 is strongly associated with the transforming growth factor-β (TGF-β) type I receptor (TβRI) and deubiquitinates and stabilizes TβRI at the plasma membrane. In addition, USP4 depletion inhibits breast cancer cell migration, which is induced by AKT [13]. ARF-BP1 is a p53-specific E3 ligase that binds to USP4. Through USP4 overexpression, stabilized ARF-BP1 reduces the stability of p53. The in vivo molecular mechanism study by which depleted USP4 in MEF cells showed resistance to tumorigenic transformation [14].

USP6 (also known as Tre17, Tre-2) was isolated as an oncogene in Ewing's sarcoma, and a further study revealed that the *Usp6* gene encodes a deubiquitinating enzyme and regulates mammalian cell growth [15, 16]. Moreover, the domain studies showed that *Usp6* is homologous to *Bub2* and *cdc16*, mitosis-regulating genes [17]. Aneurysmal bone cyst (ABC) can generate malignant bone tumor, and *Usp6* transcription is deregulated in ABCs [18]. The intracellular function of USP6 has been identified in the regulation of Arf6 as a GTPase. USP6 interacts with Arf6 through its N-terminus Tre2/Bub2/Csc16 (TBC) domain, and depletion of USP6 decreases Arf6 activity [19].

USP7 (known as herpesvirus-associated ubiquitin-specific protease, HAUSP) is the most studied deubiquitinating enzyme in the USP family. Herpes simplex virus (HSV) protein ICP0 was initially identified as a USP7/HAUSP-associated protein, and interaction between these two proteins facilitates viral replication [20]. In addition, as a herpes virus regulatory protein, Vmw110 is also bound to and stabilized by USP7/HAUSP, and their interaction leads to the regulation of ND10 as a PML nuclear body [21]. Further, USP7/HAUSP interacts with EBNA1 as an Epstein-Barr virus (EBV) protein and regulates EBNA1 replication [22]. EBV infection is closely associated with nasopharyngeal carcinoma (NPC), and the EBNA1 protein disrupts ND10 [23]. Study of the mechanisms of cellular EBNA1 function showed that EBNA1 is required for binding of USP7/HAUSP to disrupt ND10 [23]. The tumor suppressor phosphatase and tensin homologue (PTEN) has been studied with cancer progression, and a recent study showed that USP7/HAUSP and PTEN interaction leads to the regulation of PTEN localization [24]. PTEN ubiquitinated by E3 ligase is translocated and accumulated in the nucleus. However, PTEN is deubiquitinated by USP7/HAUSP and released to the cytoplasm on the PML-RARα signaling network [24]. The tumor suppressor p53 has been identified as a USP7/HAUSP binding substrate in the nuclear extract of human lung carcinoma H1299 cells (known as p53 null cells) [25]. The expression of USP7/HAUSP prevents p53 ubiquitination from Mdm2 as a p53-specific E3 ligase and increases the p53 protein stability [25]. The overexpression of USP7/HAUSP induces cancer cell apoptosis, and this phenotype depends on p53 existence in the cells [25]. Further, USP7/HAUSP can make a complex with p53-Mdm2 and regulates the balancing of p53 expression between normal and stressed cell states [26]. USP7/HAUSP can elongate p53; however, depletion of USP7/HAUSP also induces upregulation of p53 protein expression [27]. USP7/HAUSP stability is regulated by phosphorylation and dephosphorylation via the ataxia-telangiectasia-mutated (ATM)-dependent pathway, and dephosphorylated USP7/HAUSP undergoes the proteasomal degradation [28]. For example, USP7/HAUSP is phosphorylated by CK2 as a serine/threonine kinase and leads to stabilization of USP7/HAUSP in a normal state [28]. The stabilized USP7/HAUSP can enhance Mdm2 and decrease p53 protein expression. In the DNA-damaged state, however, USP7/HAUSP is dephosphorylated by PPM1G as a phosphatase and then degraded, and it decreases the Mdm2 protein and accumulates the p53 protein [28]. In addition, approximately 60–80 % of phosphorylated USP7/HAUSP exists in human cells [28]. Thus, USP7/HAUSP expression is reduced to 45 % in adenocarcinoma [27]. Recently, one study identified a novel gene that is associated with oncogenesis in the breast, called *TSPYL5* [29]. TSPYL5 is frequently overexpressed in breast cancer, and the study showed that an increasing level of TSPYL5 decreased USP7/HAUSP expression and led to the accumulation of p53 ubiquitination [29].

USP9X/FAM is known as an X-linked deubiquitinating enzyme and the homologue of the *Drosophila fat facets* gene [30]. An oncogenic function of USP9X was found in human lymphomas [31]. MCL1 is a substrate of USP9X that is abundantly expressed in mantle cell lymphoma (MCL), chronic myeloid leukemia (CML), and multiple myeloma (MM) [31]. The overexpression of USP9X stabilizes the MCL1 protein in human lymphomas, and the depletion of USP9X increases MCL1 ubiquitination, which leads to MM cell apoptosis [31]. A feature of this USP9X in cancer was confirmed by a further study on pancreatic ductal adenocarcinoma (PDA) [32]. More than 50 % of tumors exhibit inactive USP9X protein, and the deletion of *Usp9x* increases pancreatic tumorigenesis in mice [32].

Usp15 has sequence similarity with *Usp4/Unp* as a proto-oncogene [33]. The COP9 signalosome (CSN), as a conserved protein complex, is involved in the transformation of eukaryotic cells and is associated with the UPP [34]. USP15 is bound to the CSN complex, and a recent study showed that the Cullin-RING ubiquitin ligase (CRL), as a CSN-binding partner, is associated with USP15 [34, 35]. Under NF-κB degradation by CRL, USP15 is involved in Iκ-Bα as an NF-κB-inhibiting protein in the process of deubiquitination [35]. However, USP15 does not have deubiquitinating activity for other CSN-binding proteins, such as the microtubule end-binding protein 1 (EB1) [36]. This indicates that the enzyme activity of USP15 may work differently and selectively in CSN-mediated protein regulation.

Previously, the cancer cell marker was not fully defined, and several studies suggested that *Polycomb* genes could be markers for the identification of cancer stem cells [37]. An initial study of USP22 showed that USP22 is overexpressed in malignant tumors linked to the Polycomb group [38]. Furthermore, USP22 acts as an enzymatic component of the SAGA transcriptional cofactor complex and is activated by Myc as an oncogene [38]. Thus, it is considered that USP22 itself can be a positive marker of cancer stem cells [38, 39]. Further, several studies have shown that the level of USP22 in colorectal cancer tissues is highly expressed compared with that in noncancerous mucosa tissues, and colorectal cancer growth is significantly decreased by depletion of USP22 [40–42]. In addition, recent studies have demonstrated that USP22 is also increased in several cancer tissues such as breast cancer and oral squamous cell carcinoma [43, 44].

The function of USP44 was found in the duration of the mitotic spindle checkpoint. Anaphase-promoting complex (APC) as an E3 ubiquitin ligase is activated by Cdc20 to promote the progression of anaphase, and these two proteins' interaction regulates sister chromatin separation [45]. Several studies have indicated that the overexpression of Cdc20 and dysfunction of APC lead to genomic instability in various cancers [46]. USP44 does not affect the spindle checkpoint, but it exhibits deubiquitinating activity for Cdc20 regulation [46]. A further study has supported this result, in which non-transformed murine embryonic fibroblasts showed aneuploidy with the overexpression of USP44 [47]. In addition, the level of USP44 was increased in T-cell leukemia [47]. However, a recent study showed that USP44 expression is decreased in lung cancer [48].

Several studies have also shown the involvement of oncogenic functions of DUBs in various tumors. For instance, USP33 contributes to Slit-mediated breast cancer cell migration [49]. Tumor biopsy results have indicated that USP17 was overexpressed in the lung, colon, esophagus, and cervix, and USP36 was overexpressed in ovarian cancer [50, 51].

15.3.2 DUBs Involved in Tumor Suppression

The tumor-suppressive functions of DUBs are mainly derived from their association with p53. Since p53, as a transcription factor, is a final gatekeeper between DNA damage repair and cell death in the case of untouchable DNA damage, stabilization and activation of p53 are essential requirements in tumor suppression. Therefore, the failure in defending p53 can be linked to cell survival signaling, and partially, to cancer development. Several DUBs are identified as p53 regulating and stabilizing DUBs including USP10, USP29, USP42, and Ub aldehyde-binding protein (Otub1, Otubain 1) [52]. In normal conditions (unstressed conditions), p53 is located in the cytosol and regulated by Mdm2 E3 ligase for its proteasomal degradation and nuclear export. However, under stress conditions, p53 is stabilized and translocated to the nucleus. USP10 is involved in the stress response of p53. USP10, upon ATM-dependent phosphorylation at threonine 42 and serine 337 residues, is stabilized and translocated to the nucleus to activate p53 through deubiquitinating activity, inducing tumor cell suppression [53]. USP29 is expressed by JTV1 and FBP transcriptional factors. Because these factors are activated by stressed condition or physiological signaling, USP29 can also be mediated through external stress signals. USP29, in turn, protects and upregulates p53 by directly deubiquitinating it [54]. USP42 has also been found to have deubiquitinating activity for p53. During the early phase of response to a stress signal, USP42 preferentially makes up a complex with and deubiquitinates p53, leading to the rapid activation of p53 for cell cycle arrest and p53-dependent transcription [55]. Otub1 has a somewhat different capacity from other DUBs toward p53. Unlike the catalytic activities of DUBs, the deubiquitinating activity of Otub1 for p53 rescue is weak. Instead, Otub1 has the ability to block the ubiquitin-conjugating activity of Mdm2. The Asp88 residue of Otub1 turns out to be essential for Mdm2 inhibition. Thus, Otub1-mediated stabilization and activation of p53 result from downregulated Mdm2 functions inducing p53-mediated apoptosis and inhibition of cell proliferation [56].

Another important pathway related to DUB-associated tumor suppression is NF-κB signaling. NF-κB is a transcription factor that induces several downstream genes for cell survival and inflammation. However, several oncogenic mutations lead to the abnormal activation of NF-κB in cases of many solid tumors as well as lymphoid malignancies [57]. In many cases, these affected factors are regulated by ubiquitination. Thus, as opposite processes, deubiquitination of NF-κB signaling factors has been considered as a vital mechanism for balancing systemic regulation and potential therapeutic targets. Many works to identify DUBs and substrates for these DUBs, involved in NF-κB signaling, have shown the relevance of several DUBs in NF-κB-associated tumor progression (described in a previous section) or suppression. A classic example of tumor-suppressive DUB is cylindromatosis

(CYLD). After the first identification of CYLD as a tumor suppressor, mutations in certain types of cancers, including familial cylindromatosis (FC) and multiple familiar trichoepithelioma (MFT), were found, and a number of studies underlining the molecular mechanisms of CYLD-mediated tumor-suppressive function have delineated the importance and pivotal roles of CYLD in the regulation of the NF-κB signaling pathway [58]. In addition, various studies using yeast two-hybrid, co-immunoprecipitation, and RNAi-based screening were performed to identify CYLD-regulated substrates of NF-κB signaling components. As a result, it was confirmed that the deubiquitinating activity of CYLD can regulate several factors of the NF-κB signaling pathway such as TRAF2, TRAF6, and NF-κB essential modulator (NEMO), resulting in negative regulation of NF-κB signaling and tumor-suppressive function [59, 60]. In contrast, deficiency in CYLD leads to increased ubiquitination of target proteins. Further studies using CYLD knockout mice have also supported critical functions of CYLD in tumor suppression, by showing enhanced susceptibility to tumor development [61, 62]. Indeed, recent studies involving clinical patients have revealed that the downregulation of CYLD is correlated with human colon and hepatocellular carcinoma and chronic lymphoid leukemia (CLL) [63, 64].

In addition to CYLD, A20 is another DUB that negatively regulates NF-κB signaling. Diverse components of the NF-κB signaling pathway are regulated by the deubiquitinating capacity of A20 [65]. RNAi and knockout model-based validation of A20-mediated deubiquitination has uncovered that receptor-interacting serine/threonine protein kinase 1 (RIPK1), RIPK2, TRAF2, TRAF6, and NEMO are substrates for A20 [66–71]. Overall, CYLD and A20 negatively regulate NF-κB pathway-mediated tumor progression by deubiquitinating and modulating upstream signal mediators.

USP46 is known to have a tumor-suppressive characteristic due to its activity for PH domain leucine-rich repeat protein phosphatase (PHLPP). PHLPP is a serine/threonine protein phosphatase and has a role in the negative regulation of AKT, a mediator of cell survival signaling. Li et al. showed that PHLPP is downregulated by UPP, and USP46 can protect PHLPP through deubiquitination and stabilization of PHLPP. Indeed, reduced expression of USP46 and PHLPP is often found in colon cancer patients. Thus, USP46 is possibly an important regulator that has antiproliferative roles via the stabilization of PHLLP and inhibition of Akt in colon cancer [72].

15.4 DUB Inhibitors for Cancer Therapy: Clinical and Preclinical Studies

In the previous section, we categorized DUBs as oncogenic or tumor suppressors depending on their major involvement in cellular functions such as cell proliferation or apoptosis. In accordance with the relevance of DUBs to cancer, it has been proposed that selective inhibition of the catalytic activity of DUBs can be efficient as anticancer therapeutics. Although there are many inhibitors of cysteine proteases, the efficacy of these inhibitors is poor due to the difficulty of targeting these enzymes. The hardship of generating inhibitors specific for enzymes is derived from limited specificity and metabolic instability. Further, in the case of the USP family, only small numbers of inhibitors are reported. To date, however, there have been much effort in overcoming these difficulties, and several biological assays using high-throughput screening technology and fluorescence polarization assays have led to the development of small inhibitors for specific DUBs. Numerous endeavors have provided the possibility of using DUBs as therapeutic targets. It is considered as one of the leading therapeutic approaches to deal with such severe diseases including cancer [73, 74]. Here, we will describe specific DUB inhibitors, which have been generated and/or tested as effective drugs for cancer and neural disorders.

15.4.1 Targeting the 26S Proteasome

Bortezomib (Velcade®) is well known and is the most successful anticancer drug, which inhibits the 26S proteasome. After FDA approval, the use of bortezomib for the treatment of multiple myeloma and MCL patients showed remarkable therapeutic efficacy. The consequences of proteasome blockade are increased apoptosis and reduced cancer cell survival. Toward the goal of developing proteasome-targeting anticancer drugs and applying to subsequent preclinical and clinical studies,

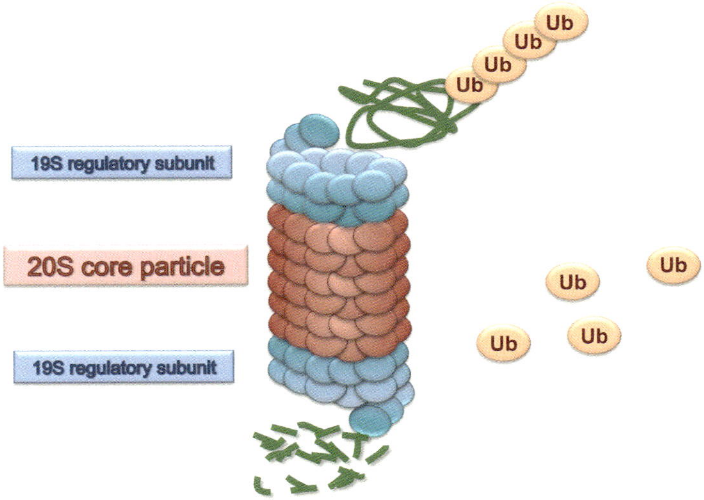

Fig. 15.3 The 26S proteasome. The 26S proteasome is a huge complex of 20,000 kDa in mass. This structure consists of two different large subunits. In the center of the 26S structure, there is a hollow with the 20S core particle, and each end of the core subunit is covered with the 19S regulatory subunits existing "cap"-like shape. The 19S regulatory subunit has ubiquitin-binding sites and ATPase active sites that allow entry of substrates into the catalytic core. The 20S core particle provides a chamber for protein degradation

numerous biochemical studies have been performed and newly developed proteasome inhibitors have been tested [75]. The 26S proteasome is composed of a 20S catalytic "core" particle forming pore inside and two 19S regulatory "cap" subunits located at each end of the core particle (Fig. 15.3). The 19S subunit recognizes ubiquitinated target proteins destined for proteasomal degradation through its ATPase active sites and ubiquitin-binding sites. For the next step, deubiquitinated targets are transferred to the catalytic core particle for degradation [76]. Besides direct blockade of proteasome function, there are also further efforts to target components of the 26S proteasome thereby preventing the transfer or degradation process. One example of this effort is b-AP15. This small molecule selectively blocks UCH-L5 and USP14 [77]. Both UCH-L5 and USP14 are DUBs, components of the 19S subunit of the 26S proteasome; they detach ubiquitin molecules from ubiquitinated proteins targeted to the 26S proteasome. Currently, b-AP15 is being used in preclinical trials; its effective inhibition of proteasomal activity gives a hope that it will be a strong proteasome inhibitory anticancer drug. IU1 is a newly developed USP14 inhibitor. Lee and his colleagues showed that IU1 specifically inhibits USP14 activity of the proteasome and thereby enhances proteasomal degradation of the substrates [78]. Another DUB associated with the 26S proteasome is POH1 (Rpn11). POH1 is localized in the "lid" region of the 19S regulatory subunit. Several studies have revealed that POH1 is pivotal for cell survival in certain cancers [76, 79, 80]. In addition, it affects drug resistance to the anticancer drugs in clinical use. There are some debates over whether b-AP15 can block not only UCH-L5 and USP14 but also inhibit POH1. Although the effect of b-AP15 on POH1 is uncertain, inhibitors targeting POH1 are also expected to be suitable anticancer drugs in certain types of cancers.

15.4.2 *Specific DUB Inhibitors*

One of the important proteins during cancer development is the p53 tumor suppressor; thus, p53 is often called a "guardian gene." More than 50 % of cancers are derived from p53 mutation or alteration in its function. In addition to the modulation of p53 function, the expression level of p53 also affects cellular viability and cancer progression. The p53 protein level is regulated by the ubiquitination system mediated by diverse enzymes, including E3 ligases and DUBs [52]. Mdm2 is an E3 ligase targeting p53. In its normal state, Mdm2 ubiquitinates p53 and leads to the proteasomal degradation. However, upon DNA damage, Mdm2 undergoes proteasomal degradation and, subsequently, p53 can be prevented from Mdm2-mediated degradation. The key regulating protein between p53 and Mdm2 is USP7/HAUSP [25]. USP7/HAUSP can deubiquitinate and stabilize both Mdm2 and p53 depending on cellular stress. Accordingly, targeting p53-regulating proteins including Mdm2 and USP7/HAUSP is attractive for cancer therapy.

In addition to the development of numerous inhibitors for Mdm2-p53 interaction [81], leading studies for the development of inhibitors targeting USP7/HAUSP have recently been conducted. HBX 19,818, P005091 and analogues such as P045204 and P022077, HBX 41,108, and others are found to be USP7/HAUSP inhibitors showing effective anticancer effects. HBX 19,818 has the ability to covalently bind with USP7/HAUSP, and thereby blocks USP7/HAUSP activity, leading to the possible activation of p53-mediated apoptosis in cancer cells [82]. P005091 has a great effect on reducing multiple myeloma growth and overcoming bortezomib resistance when combined with other drugs such as dexamethasone, lenalidomide, and/or suberoylanilide hydroxamic acid (SAHA). However, these treatments are currently under preclinical stage, and clinical trials are required to confirm their efficacy for cancer patients [83].

UCH-L1 is a well-known DUB due to its association with Parkinson's disease. The E3 ligase enzyme activity of UCH-L1 is linked to occurring of Parkinson's disease. UCH-L1 can be dimerized, and the UCH-L1 dimer has the ability to ligate ubiquitin molecules. In addition, UCH-L1 has shown different expression patterns in certain cancers including lung cancer. Based on a recent study on whether several lung cancers and lung cancer cell lines express more UCH-L1 than normal lung tissue, continual efforts to develop UCH-L1-specific inhibitors using high-throughput screening have been made. Isatin O-acyl oximes efficiently inhibit UCH-L1 and tumor growth in lung cancer cells. The importance of the enzymatic activity of UCH-L1 regarding association with diseases has also brought about the development of other specific inhibitors for UCH-L1. For instance, 3-amino-2-keto-7*H*-thieno[2,3-*b*]pyridin-6-one derivatives and other compounds discovered through in silico drug screening have been tested for inhibitory effects against UCH-L1 [84, 85]. UCH-L1 inhibitors showed a potential therapeutic activity for targeting neural disorders and cancers. HBX 90,397, another DUB-specific inhibitor, blocks USP8 activity. Small-molecule inhibitors targeting USP8 can prevent cell growth in several cancer cell lines including HCT116, colon cancer cells, and PC3, prostate cancer cells. USP1 is one of the well-characterized DUBs, and it plays an important role in the DNA repair processes [86]. USP1 combined with USP1-associated factor 1 (UAF1) deubiquitinates PCNA or FANCD2 during DNA repair process such as interstrand cross-link (ICL) repair, homologous recombination (HR) repair, and translesion DNA synthesis (TLS) [87]. Importantly, USP1 expression is deregulated in certain types of cancers, suggesting that USP1 may be an attractive target for cancer therapy. Indeed, treatment with pimozide, a USP1-specific inhibitor, showed synergistic effect in non-small cell lung cancer (NSCLC) when treated with the anticancer drug cisplatin [88].

15.4.3 DUB Inhibitors Targeting Multiple DUBs

The most important and unique feature of DUBs, as mentioned above, is its catalytic activity, whereby it can specifically recognize and target ubiquitinated substrates. Therefore, in many cases, DUBs share similar domains for their ability. This has brought about two advancements in developing inhibitors for DUBs. In general, it is thought to be difficult to generate inhibitors targeting the "hot spot" of a specific DUB, whereas it usefully generates inhibitors that block multiple DUBs at the same time. Indeed, in addition to the specific DUB inhibitors described in Sect. 4.2, there are several inhibitors that could target two or more DUBs. Examples of such inhibitors will be introduced in this section.

WP1130 (degrasyn) was originally used to inhibit Janus-activated kinase2 (JAK2), thereby blocking the JAK-STAT pathway. This small molecule is also known to have an inhibitory effect toward the Bcr-Abl fusion protein, which is a major cause of several types of leukemias. However, many recent studies have demonstrated that the WP1130 treatment induces polyubiquitinated proteins, followed by the inhibition of several DUBs including USP5, USP9x, USP14, and UCH-L5. The effects of WP1130 have been further investigated, and it has been demonstrated that WP1130 can induce apoptosis by affecting anti- and proapoptotic factors, including MCL-1 and p53 [89, 90]. In addition, the effectiveness of WP1130 as a therapeutic drug is supported by the study of Bartholomeusz et al., which showed that WP1130 treatment combined with bortezomib had a synergistic effect as anticancer therapy concomitant with the inhibition of tumor cell growth, modulation of apoptosis, and prolonged survival period of animals [90].

PR619 is a well-known small molecule that inhibits a broad range of DUBs and other cysteine proteases. Activity-based chemical proteomics revealed that treatment with PR619 results in the accumulation of ubiquitinated proteins, suggesting it as an anticancer chemotherapeutic agent [91]. Chalcone-based derivatives such as AM114 and RA-1 were originally known to have an inhibitory effect on the 26S proteasome. However, further investigation of chalcone derivatives showed that AM146, RA-9, and RA-14 act as inhibitors for DUBs. These molecules induce a remarkable accumulation of polyubiquitinated proteins leading to an altered expression level of cell cycle regulating proteins, cell cycle arrest, and tumor cell death via apoptosis. In particular, they are able to block UCH-L1, UCH-L3, USP2, USP5, and USP8, which are known to have important functions in cell survival and proliferation [92]. These experimental results provide the rationale for and support the possibility of chalcone derivatives as anticancer drugs.

HBX 41,108 was originally identified as an USP7/HAUSP-specific inhibitor. Colland et al. showed that HBX 41,108 has a great effect in blocking USP7/HAUSP enzyme activity. The inactivity of USP7/HAUSP causes stabilization of p53 and an increase in p53-mediated apoptosis in cancer cells [93]. However, it was recently found that HBX 41,108 has an inhibitory effect on not only USP7/HAUSP but also other DUBs.

Cyclopentenone prostaglandins (cyPGs) are a type of prostaglandin (PG); they are biological metabolites found in animal bodies, and certain cyPGs are thought to increase apoptosis and ubiquitinated proteins. For example, PGD_2, a D series PG, can be modified to take a biologically active form, specifically as cyPGs of the J_2 series such as PGJ_2, Δ^{12}-PGJ_2, and 15-deoxy- $\Delta^{12,14}$-PGJ_2 (15d-PGJ_2). 15d-PGJ_2 has the ability to covalently modify and subsequently inhibit the hydrolase activity of UCH-L1 [94]. Treatment with Δ^{12}-PGJ_2 in cells also inhibited UCH-L1 and UCH-L3 without alteration of proteasomal activity, indicating that prostaglandins can be suitable for neural disorder therapy [95].

15.5 Therapeutic Prediction of DUB Inhibitors

Although there are only a few DUBs inhibitors, all the results discussed here raise the line of evidence for their possibility and importance as potential anticancer agents. Indeed, blocking DUBs, which are involved in abnormal regulation and cause cancer development, is one emerging anticancer therapeutic strategy. Moreover, the inhibition of DUBs is not limited to treating cancer, as shown in the case of targeting UCH-L1 and UCH-L3. There are also other classes of DUB inhibitors. Papain-like protease (PLpro) of coronavirus is a viral deubiquitinating enzyme that has a pivotal role in evading the immune system of human host cells inducing severe acute respiratory syndrome (SARS-CoV); it also has the ability to cleave viral polyprotein into functional derivatives. Thus, targeting PLpro can be considered as a primary target for antiviral drugs. Ratia et al. investigated efficient inhibitors specific for PLpro by screening around 50,000 library compounds. Among them, GRL0617 showed the most effective inhibition of PLpro and replication of the virus without cytotoxicity. More importantly, they uncovered a 3D binding structure between GRL0617 and PLpro. GRL0617 can dock with the catalytic active site of PLpro [96]. Their study suggests that GRL0617 can be developed as a promising antiviral drug with specificity that targets viral DUB but not host DUBs.

The functions and turnover of proteins are some of the most pivotal regulating mechanisms in a cellular process. These are followed by posttranslational modification by protein phosphorylation, methylation, or ubiquitination. In particular, for cellular homeostasis, proteins need to be degraded and newly synthesized. Proteins undergo two different degradation pathways through either the lysosome or the 26S proteasome. Over 80 % of cellular proteins are tagged with ubiquitin, followed by proteasomal degradation. For the well-organized UPP, several hundreds of E3 ligases help proteins to be conjugated with ubiquitin, whereas far fewer numbers of DUBs are responsible for reversely removing ubiquitin from ubiquitinated proteins. In this regard, each DUB has numerous substrates, and deregulation of a certain DUB can alter cellular processes via substrate-related functions, indicating that DUB is an important regulator in cells. Here, we have described the relevance of DUBs with cancer caused by deregulation of DUB expression, altered enzymatic activity, and complex effect on substrates' functions. In many cases, DUB inhibitors have shown anticancer effect mainly in preclinical levels. Their applications as anticancer drugs should be validated in clinical settings. Bortezomib is now used as an anticancer drug, but there are some problems associated with its use, including bortezomib resistance, severe toxicities, or a lower therapeutic effect in some individuals with solid tumors. Thus, treatments involving a combination of agents are recommended in current cancer therapy. As a result, we need more effective drugs to target not only cancer, but also other diseases. Through numerous studies and hypotheses that have been validated so far, DUBs may be one of the most ideal and attractive targets.

References

1. Puente XS, Sanchez LM, Overall CM, Lopez-Otin C (2003) Human and mouse proteases: a comparative genomic approach. Nat Rev Genet 4(7):544–558. doi:10.1038/nrg1111
2. Fraile JM, Quesada V, Rodriguez D, Freije JM, Lopez-Otin C (2012) Deubiquitinases in cancer: new functions and therapeutic options. Oncogene 31(19):2373–2388. doi:10.1038/onc.2011.443
3. Lim KH, Ramakrishna S, Baek KH (2013) Molecular mechanisms and functions of cytokine-inducible deubiquitinating enzymes. Cytokine Growth Factor Rev 24:427–431. doi:10.1016/j.cytogfr.2013.05.007
4. Lim KH, Baek KH (2013) Deubiquitinating enzymes as therapeutic targets in cancer. Curr Pharm Des 19(22):4039–4052
5. Komander D, Clague MJ, Urbe S (2009) Breaking the chains: structure and function of the deubiquitinases. Nat Rev Mol Cell Biol 10(8):550–563. doi:10.1038/nrm2731
6. Hussain S, Zhang Y, Galardy PJ (2009) DUBs and cancer: the role of deubiquitinating enzymes as oncogenes, non-oncogenes and tumor suppressors. Cell Cycle 8(11):1688–1697
7. Graner E, Tang D, Rossi S, Baron A, Migita T, Weinstein LJ, Lechpammer M, Huesken D, Zimmermann J, Signoretti S, Loda M (2004) The isopeptidase USP2a regulates the stability of fatty acid synthase in prostate cancer. Cancer Cell 5(3):253–261
8. Mahul-Mellier AL, Datler C, Pazarentzos E, Lin B, Chaisaklert W, Abuali G, Grimm S (2012) De-ubiquitinating proteases USP2a and USP2c cause apoptosis by stabilising RIP1. Biochim Biophys Acta 1823(8):1353–1365. doi:10.1016/j.bbamcr.2012.05.022
9. Allende-Vega N, Sparks A, Lane DP, Saville MK (2010) MdmX is a substrate for the deubiquitinating enzyme USP2a. Oncogene 29(3):432–441. doi:10.1038/onc.2009.330
10. Benassi B, Flavin R, Marchionni L, Zanata S, Pan Y, Chowdhury D, Marani M, Strano S, Muti P, Blandino G, Loda M (2012) MYC is activated by USP2a-mediated modulation of microRNAs in prostate cancer. Cancer Discov 2(3):236–247. doi:10.1158/2159-8290.CD-11-0219
11. Mahul-Mellier AL, Pazarentzos E, Datler C, Iwasawa R, AbuAli G, Lin B, Grimm S (2012) De-ubiquitinating protease USP2a targets RIP1 and TRAF2 to mediate cell death by TNF. Cell Death Differ 19(5):891–899. doi:10.1038/cdd.2011.185
12. Xiao N, Li H, Luo J, Wang R, Chen H, Chen J, Wang P (2012) Ubiquitin-specific protease 4 (USP4) targets TRAF2 and TRAF6 for deubiquitination and inhibits TNFalpha-induced cancer cell migration. Biochem J 441(3):979–986. doi:10.1042/BJ20111358
13. Zhang L, Zhou F, Drabsch Y, Gao R, Snaar-Jagalska BE, Mickanin C, Huang H, Sheppard KA, Porter JA, Lu CX, ten Dijke P (2012) USP4 is regulated by AKT phosphorylation and directly deubiquitylates TGF-beta type I receptor. Nat Cell Biol 14(7):717–726. doi:10.1038/ncb2522
14. Zhang X, Berger FG, Yang J, Lu X (2011) USP4 inhibits p53 through deubiquitinating and stabilizing ARF-BP1. EMBO J 30(11):2177–2189. doi:10.1038/emboj.2011.125
15. Onno M, Nakamura T, Mariage-Samson R, Hillova J, Hill M (1993) Human TRE17 oncogene is generated from a family of homologous polymorphic sequences by single-base changes. DNA Cell Biol 12(2):107–118
16. Papa FR, Hochstrasser M (1993) The yeast DOA4 gene encodes a deubiquitinating enzyme related to a product of the human tre-2 oncogene. Nature 366(6453):313–319. doi:10.1038/366313a0
17. Richardson PM, Zon LI (1995) Molecular cloning of a cDNA with a novel domain present in the tre-2 oncogene and the yeast cell cycle regulators BUB2 and cdc16. Oncogene 11(6):1139–1148
18. Oliveira AM, Perez-Atayde AR, Dal Cin P, Gebhardt MC, Chen CJ, Neff JR, Demetri GD, Rosenberg AE, Bridge JA, Fletcher JA (2005) Aneurysmal bone cyst variant translocations upregulate USP6 transcription by promoter swapping with the ZNF9, COL1A1, TRAP150, and OMD genes. Oncogene 24(21):3419–3426. doi:10.1038/sj.onc.1208506
19. Martinu L, Masuda-Robens JM, Robertson SE, Santy LC, Casanova JE, Chou MM (2004) The TBC (Tre-2/Bub2/Cdc16) domain protein TRE17 regulates plasma membrane-endosomal

trafficking through activation of Arf6. Mol Cell Biol 24(22):9752–9762. doi:10.1128/MCB.24.22.9752-9762.2004
20. Everett RD, Meredith M, Orr A, Cross A, Kathoria M, Parkinson J (1997) A novel ubiquitin-specific protease is dynamically associated with the PML nuclear domain and binds to a herpesvirus regulatory protein. EMBO J 16(7):1519–1530. doi:10.1093/emboj/16.7.1519
21. Everett RD, Freemont P, Saitoh H, Dasso M, Orr A, Kathoria M, Parkinson J (1998) The disruption of ND10 during herpes simplex virus infection correlates with the Vmw110- and proteasome-dependent loss of several PML isoforms. J Virol 72(8):6581–6591
22. Holowaty MN, Zeghouf M, Wu H, Tellam J, Athanasopoulos V, Greenblatt J, Frappier L (2003) Protein profiling with Epstein-Barr nuclear antigen-1 reveals an interaction with the herpesvirus-associated ubiquitin-specific protease HAUSP/USP7. J Biol Chem 278(32):29987–29994. doi:10.1074/jbc.M303977200
23. Sivachandran N, Sarkari F, Frappier L (2008) Epstein-Barr nuclear antigen 1 contributes to nasopharyngeal carcinoma through disruption of PML nuclear bodies. PLoS Pathog 4(10):e1000170. doi:10.1371/journal.ppat.1000170
24. Song MS, Salmena L, Carracedo A, Egia A, Lo-Coco F, Teruya-Feldstein J, Pandolfi PP (2008) The deubiquitinylation and localization of PTEN are regulated by a HAUSP-PML network. Nature 455(7214):813–817. doi:10.1038/nature07290
25. Li M, Chen D, Shiloh A, Luo J, Nikolaev AY, Qin J, Gu W (2002) Deubiquitination of p53 by HAUSP is an important pathway for p53 stabilization. Nature 416(6881):648–653. doi:10.1038/nature737
26. Li M, Brooks CL, Kon N, Gu W (2004) A dynamic role of HAUSP in the p53-Mdm2 pathway. Mol Cell 13(6):879–886
27. Becker K, Marchenko ND, Palacios G, Moll UM (2008) A role of HAUSP in tumor suppression in a human colon carcinoma xenograft model. Cell Cycle 7(9):1205–1213
28. Khoronenkova SV, Dianova II, Ternette N, Kessler BM, Parsons JL, Dianov GL (2012) ATM-dependent downregulation of USP7/HAUSP by PPM1G activates p53 response to DNA damage. Mol Cell 45(6):801–813. doi:10.1016/j.molcel.2012.01.021
29. Epping MT, Meijer LA, Krijgsman O, Bos JL, Pandolfi PP, Bernards R (2011) TSPYL5 suppresses p53 levels and function by physical interaction with USP7. Nat Cell Biol 13(1):102–108. doi:10.1038/ncb2142
30. Wood SA, Pascoe WS, Ru K, Yamada T, Hirchenhain J, Kemler R, Mattick JS (1997) Cloning and expression analysis of a novel mouse gene with sequence similarity to the Drosophila fat facets gene. Mech Dev 63(1):29–38
31. Schwickart M, Huang X, Lill JR, Liu J, Ferrando R, French DM, Maecker H, O'Rourke K, Bazan F, Eastham-Anderson J, Yue P, Dornan D, Huang DC, Dixit VM (2010) Deubiquitinase USP9X stabilizes MCL1 and promotes tumour cell survival. Nature 463(7277):103–107. doi:10.1038/nature08646
32. Perez-Mancera PA, Rust AG, van der Weyden L, Kristiansen G, Li A, Sarver AL, Silverstein KA, Grutzmann R, Aust D, Rummele P, Knosel T, Herd C, Stemple DL, Kettleborough R, Brosnan JA, Li A, Morgan R, Knight S, Yu J, Stegeman S, Collier LS, ten Hoeve JJ, de Ridder J, Klein AP, Goggins M, Hruban RH, Chang DK, Biankin AV, Grimmond SM, Wessels LF, Wood SA, Iacobuzio-Donahue CA, Pilarsky C, Largaespada DA, Adams DJ, Tuveson DA (2012) The deubiquitinase USP9X suppresses pancreatic ductal adenocarcinoma. Nature 486(7402):266–270. doi:10.1038/nature11114
33. Baker RT, Wang XW, Woollatt E, White JA, Sutherland GR (1999) Identification, functional characterization, and chromosomal localization of USP15, a novel human ubiquitin-specific protease related to the UNP oncoprotein, and a systematic nomenclature for human ubiquitin-specific proteases. Genomics 59(3):264–274. doi:10.1006/geno.1999.5879
34. Hetfeld BK, Helfrich A, Kapelari B, Scheel H, Hofmann K, Guterman A, Glickman M, Schade R, Kloetzel PM, Dubiel W (2005) The zinc finger of the CSN-associated deubiquitinating enzyme USP15 is essential to rescue the E3 ligase Rbx1. Curr Biol 15(13):1217–1221. doi:10.1016/j.cub.2005.05.059

35. Schweitzer K, Bozko PM, Dubiel W, Naumann M (2007) CSN controls NF-kappaB by deubiquitinylation of IkappaBalpha. EMBO J 26(6):1532–1541. doi:10.1038/sj.emboj.7601600
36. Peth A, Boettcher JP, Dubiel W (2007) Ubiquitin-dependent proteolysis of the microtubule end-binding protein 1, EB1, is controlled by the COP9 signalosome: possible consequences for microtubule filament stability. J Mol Biol 368(2):550–563. doi:10.1016/j.jmb.2007.02.052
37. Valk-Lingbeek ME, Bruggeman SW, van Lohuizen M (2004) Stem cells and cancer; the polycomb connection. Cell 118(4):409–418. doi:10.1016/j.cell.2004.08.005
38. Zhang XY, Varthi M, Sykes SM, Phillips C, Warzecha C, Zhu W, Wyce A, Thorne AW, Berger SL, McMahon SB (2008) The putative cancer stem cell marker USP22 is a subunit of the human SAGA complex required for activated transcription and cell-cycle progression. Mol Cell 29(1):102–111. doi:10.1016/j.molcel.2007.12.015
39. Goodliffe JM, Wieschaus E, Cole MD (2005) Polycomb mediates Myc autorepression and its transcriptional control of many loci in Drosophila. Genes Dev 19(24):2941–2946. doi:10.1101/gad.1352305
40. Liu YL, Yang YM, Xu H, Dong XS (2010) Increased expression of ubiquitin-specific protease 22 can promote cancer progression and predict therapy failure in human colorectal cancer. J Gastroenterol Hepatol 25(11):1800–1805. doi:10.1111/j.1440-1746.2010.06352.x
41. Liu Y, Yang Y, Xu H, Dong X (2010) Implication of USP22 in the regulation of BMI-1, c-Myc, p16INK4a, p14ARF, and cyclin D2 expression in primary colorectal carcinomas. Diagn Mol Pathol 19(4):194–200. doi:10.1097/PDM.0b013e3181e202f2
42. Xu H, Liu YL, Yang YM, Dong XS (2012) Knock-down of ubiquitin-specific protease 22 by micro-RNA interference inhibits colorectal cancer growth. Int J Colorectal Dis 27(1):21–30. doi:10.1007/s00384-011-1275-8
43. Zhang Y, Yao L, Zhang X, Ji H, Wang L, Sun S, Pang D (2011) Elevated expression of USP22 in correlation with poor prognosis in patients with invasive breast cancer. J Cancer Res Clin Oncol 137(8):1245–1253. doi:10.1007/s00432-011-0998-9
44. Piao S, Liu Y, Hu J, Guo F, Ma J, Sun Y, Zhang B (2012) USP22 is useful as a novel molecular marker for predicting disease progression and patient prognosis of oral squamous cell carcinoma. PLoS One 7(8):e42540. doi:10.1371/journal.pone.0042540
45. Wang Z, Wan L, Zhong J, Inuzuka H, Liu P, Sarkar FH, Wei W (2013) Cdc20: a potential novel therapeutic target for cancer treatment. Curr Pharm Des 19(18):3210–3214
46. Wasch R, Engelbert D (2005) Anaphase-promoting complex-dependent proteolysis of cell cycle regulators and genomic instability of cancer cells. Oncogene 24(1):1–10. doi:10.1038/sj.onc.1208017
47. Zhang Y, van Deursen J, Galardy PJ (2011) Overexpression of ubiquitin specific protease 44 (USP44) induces chromosomal instability and is frequently observed in human T-cell leukemia. PLoS One 6(8):e23389. doi:10.1371/journal.pone.0023389
48. Zhang Y, Foreman O, Wigle DA, Kosari F, Vasmatzis G, Salisbury JL, van Deursen J, Galardy PJ (2012) USP44 regulates centrosome positioning to prevent aneuploidy and suppress tumorigenesis. J Clin Invest 122(12):4362–4374. doi:10.1172/JCI63084
49. Yuasa-Kawada J, Kinoshita-Kawada M, Rao Y, Wu JY (2009) Deubiquitinating enzyme USP33/VDU1 is required for Slit signaling in inhibiting breast cancer cell migration. Proc Natl Acad Sci U S A 106(34):14530–14535. doi:10.1073/pnas.0801262106
50. Li J, Olson LM, Zhang Z, Li L, Bidder M, Nguyen L, Pfeifer J, Rader JS (2008) Differential display identifies overexpression of the USP36 gene, encoding a deubiquitinating enzyme, in ovarian cancer. Int J Med Sci 5(3):133–142
51. McFarlane C, Kelvin AA, de la Vega M, Govender U, Scott CJ, Burrows JF, Johnston JA (2010) The deubiquitinating enzyme USP17 is highly expressed in tumor biopsies, is cell cycle regulated, and is required for G1-S progression. Cancer Res 70(8):3329–3339. doi:10.1158/0008-5472.CAN-09-4152
52. Hock AK, Vousden KH (2014) The role of ubiquitin modification in the regulation of p53. Biochim Biophys Acta 1843:137–149. doi:10.1016/j.bbamcr.2013.05.022
53. Yuan J, Luo K, Zhang L, Cheville JC, Lou Z (2010) USP10 regulates p53 localization and stability by deubiquitinating p53. Cell 140(3):384–396. doi:10.1016/j.cell.2009.12.032

54. Liu J, Chung HJ, Vogt M, Jin Y, Malide D, He L, Dundr M, Levens D (2011) JTV1 co-activates FBP to induce USP29 transcription and stabilize p53 in response to oxidative stress. EMBO J 30(5):846–858. doi:10.1038/emboj.2011.11
55. Hock AK, Vigneron AM, Carter S, Ludwig RL, Vousden KH (2011) Regulation of p53 stability and function by the deubiquitinating enzyme USP42. EMBO J 30(24):4921–4930. doi:10.1038/emboj.2011.419
56. Sun XX, Challagundla KB, Dai MS (2012) Positive regulation of p53 stability and activity by the deubiquitinating enzyme Otubain 1. EMBO J 31(3):576–592. doi:10.1038/emboj.2011.434
57. Karin M (2009) NF-kappaB as a critical link between inflammation and cancer. Cold Spring Harb Perspect Biol 1(5):a000141. doi:10.1101/cshperspect.a000141
58. Sun SC (2010) CYLD: a tumor suppressor deubiquitinase regulating NF-kappaB activation and diverse biological processes. Cell Death Differ 17(1):25–34. doi:10.1038/cdd.2009.43
59. Kovalenko A, Chable-Bessia C, Cantarella G, Israel A, Wallach D, Courtois G (2003) The tumour suppressor CYLD negatively regulates NF-kappaB signalling by deubiquitination. Nature 424(6950):801–805. doi:10.1038/nature01802
60. Brummelkamp TR, Nijman SM, Dirac AM, Bernards R (2003) Loss of the cylindromatosis tumour suppressor inhibits apoptosis by activating NF-kappaB. Nature 424(6950):797–801. doi:10.1038/nature01811
61. Massoumi R, Chmielarska K, Hennecke K, Pfeifer A, Fassler R (2006) Cyld inhibits tumor cell proliferation by blocking Bcl-3-dependent NF-kappaB signaling. Cell 125(4):665–677. doi:10.1016/j.cell.2006.03.041
62. Zhang J, Stirling B, Temmerman ST, Ma CA, Fuss IJ, Derry JM, Jain A (2006) Impaired regulation of NF-kappaB and increased susceptibility to colitis-associated tumorigenesis in CYLD-deficient mice. J Clin Invest 116(11):3042–3049. doi:10.1172/JCI28746
63. Wu W, Zhu H, Fu Y, Shen W, Xu J, Miao K, Hong M, Xu W, Liu P, Li J (2014) Clinical significance of down-regulated cylindromatosis gene in chronic lymphocytic leukemia. Leuk Lymphoma 55:588–594. doi:10.3109/10428194.2013.809077
64. Hellerbrand C, Bumes E, Bataille F, Dietmaier W, Massoumi R, Bosserhoff AK (2007) Reduced expression of CYLD in human colon and hepatocellular carcinomas. Carcinogenesis 28(1):21–27. doi:10.1093/carcin/bgl081
65. Hymowitz SG, Wertz IE (2010) A20: from ubiquitin editing to tumour suppression. Nat Rev Cancer 10(5):332–341. doi:10.1038/nrc2775
66. Lee EG, Boone DL, Chai S, Libby SL, Chien M, Lodolce JP, Ma A (2000) Failure to regulate TNF-induced NF-kappaB and cell death responses in A20-deficient mice. Science 289(5488):2350–2354
67. Wertz IE, O'Rourke KM, Zhou H, Eby M, Aravind L, Seshagiri S, Wu P, Wiesmann C, Baker R, Boone DL, Ma A, Koonin EV, Dixit VM (2004) De-ubiquitination and ubiquitin ligase domains of A20 downregulate NF-kappaB signalling. Nature 430(7000):694–699. doi:10.1038/nature02794
68. Hitotsumatsu O, Ahmad RC, Tavares R, Wang M, Philpott D, Turer EE, Lee BL, Shiffin N, Advincula R, Malynn BA, Werts C, Ma A (2008) The ubiquitin-editing enzyme A20 restricts nucleotide-binding oligomerization domain containing 2-triggered signals. Immunity 28(3):381–390. doi:10.1016/j.immuni.2008.02.002
69. Turer EE, Tavares RM, Mortier E, Hitotsumatsu O, Advincula R, Lee B, Shifrin N, Malynn BA, Ma A (2008) Homeostatic MyD88-dependent signals cause lethal inflamMation in the absence of A20. J Exp Med 205(2):451–464. doi:10.1084/jem.20071108
70. Boone DL, Turer EE, Lee EG, Ahmad RC, Wheeler MT, Tsui C, Hurley P, Chien M, Chai S, Hitotsumatsu O, McNally E, Pickart C, Ma A (2004) The ubiquitin-modifying enzyme A20 is required for termination of Toll-like receptor responses. Nat Immunol 5(10):1052–1060. doi:10.1038/ni1110
71. Mauro C, Pacifico F, Lavorgna A, Mellone S, Iannetti A, Acquaviva R, Formisano S, Vito P, Leonardi A (2006) ABIN-1 binds to NEMO/IKKgamma and co-operates with A20 in inhibiting NF-kappaB. J Biol Chem 281(27):18482–18488. doi:10.1074/jbc.M601502200

72. Li X, Stevens PD, Yang H, Gulhati P, Wang W, Evers BM, Gao T (2013) The deubiquitination enzyme USP46 functions as a tumor suppressor by controlling PHLPP-dependent attenuation of Akt signaling in colon cancer. Oncogene 32(4):471–478. doi:10.1038/onc.2012.66
73. Eldridge AG, O'Brien T (2010) Therapeutic strategies within the ubiquitin proteasome system. Cell Death Differ 17(1):4–13. doi:10.1038/cdd.2009.82
74. Ernst A, Avvakumov G, Tong J, Fan Y, Zhao Y, Alberts P, Persaud A, Walker JR, Neculai AM, Neculai D, Vorobyov A, Garg P, Beatty L, Chan PK, Juang YC, Landry MC, Yeh C, Zeqiraj E, Karamboulas K, Allali-Hassani A, Vedadi M, Tyers M, Moffat J, Sicheri F, Pelletier L, Durocher D, Raught B, Rotin D, Yang J, Moran MF, Dhe-Paganon S, Sidhu SS (2013) A strategy for modulation of enzymes in the ubiquitin system. Science 339(6119):590–595. doi:10.1126/science.1230161
75. Mattern MR, Wu J, Nicholson B (2012) Ubiquitin-based anticancer therapy: carpet bombing with proteasome inhibitors vs surgical strikes with E1, E2, E3, or DUB inhibitors. Biochim Biophys Acta 1823(11):2014–2021. doi:10.1016/j.bbamcr.2012.05.005
76. D'Arcy P, Linder S (2012) Proteasome deubiquitinases as novel targets for cancer therapy. Int J Biochem Cell Biol 44(11):1729–1738. doi:10.1016/j.biocel.2012.07.011
77. D'Arcy P, Brnjic S, Olofsson MH, Fryknas M, Lindsten K, De Cesare M, Perego P, Sadeghi B, Hassan M, Larsson R, Linder S (2011) Inhibition of proteasome deubiquitinating activity as a new cancer therapy. Nat Med 17(12):1636–1640. doi:10.1038/nm.2536
78. Lee BH, Lee MJ, Park S, Oh DC, Elsasser S, Chen PC, Gartner C, Dimova N, Hanna J, Gygi SP, Wilson SM, King RW, Finley D (2010) Enhancement of proteasome activity by a small-molecule inhibitor of USP14. Nature 467(7312):179–184. doi:10.1038/nature09299
79. Gallery M, Blank JL, Lin Y, Gutierrez JA, Pulido JC, Rappoli D, Badola S, Rolfe M, Macbeth KJ (2007) The JAMM motif of human deubiquitinase Poh1 is essential for cell viability. Mol Cancer Ther 6(1):262–268. doi:10.1158/1535-7163.MCT-06-0542
80. Liu H, Buus R, Clague MJ, Urbe S (2009) Regulation of ErbB2 receptor status by the proteasomal DUB POH1. PLoS One 4(5):e5544. doi:10.1371/journal.pone.0005544
81. Guedat P, Colland F (2007) Patented small molecule inhibitors in the ubiquitin proteasome system. BMC Biochem 8(Suppl 1):S14. doi:10.1186/1471-2091-8-S1-S14
82. Reverdy C, Conrath S, Lopez R, Planquette C, Atmanene C, Collura V, Harpon J, Battaglia V, Vivat V, Sippl W, Colland F (2012) Discovery of specific inhibitors of human USP7/HAUSP deubiquitinating enzyme. Chem Biol 19(4):467–477. doi:10.1016/j.chembiol.2012.02.007
83. Nicholson B, Suresh Kumar KG (2011) The multifaceted roles of USP7: new therapeutic opportunities. Cell Biochem Biophys 60(1–2):61–68. doi:10.1007/s12013-011-9185-5
84. Mitsui T, Hirayama K, Aoki S, Nishikawa K, Uchida K, Matsumoto T, Kabuta T, Wada K (2010) Identification of a novel chemical potentiator and inhibitors of UCH-L1 by in silico drug screening. Neurochem Int 56(5):679–686. doi:10.1016/j.neuint.2010.01.016
85. Mermerian AH, Case A, Stein RL, Cuny GD (2007) Structure-activity relationship, kinetic mechanism, and selectivity for a new class of ubiquitin C-terminal hydrolase-L1 (UCH-L1) inhibitors. Bioorg Med Chem Lett 17(13):3729–3732. doi:10.1016/j.bmcl.2007.04.027
86. Colland F (2010) The therapeutic potential of deubiquitinating enzyme inhibitors. Biochem Soc Trans 38(Pt 1):137–143. doi:10.1042/BST0380137
87. Murai J, Yang K, Dejsuphong D, Hirota K, Takeda S, D'Andrea AD (2011) The USP1/UAF1 complex promotes double-strand break repair through homologous recombination. Mol Cell Biol 31(12):2462–2469. doi:10.1128/MCB.05058-11
88. Garcia-Santisteban I, Peters GJ, Giovannetti E, Rodriguez JA (2013) USP1 deubiquitinase: cellular functions, regulatory mechanisms and emerging potential as target in cancer therapy. Mol Cancer 12:91. doi:10.1186/1476-4598-12-91
89. Kapuria V, Peterson LF, Fang D, Bornmann WG, Talpaz M, Donato NJ (2010) Deubiquitinase inhibition by small-molecule WP1130 triggers aggresome formation and tumor cell apoptosis. Cancer Res 70(22):9265–9276. doi:10.1158/0008-5472.CAN-10-1530
90. Bartholomeusz GA, Talpaz M, Kapuria V, Kong LY, Wang S, Estrov Z, Priebe W, Wu J, Donato NJ (2007) Activation of a novel Bcr/Abl destruction pathway by WP1130 induces apoptosis of chronic myelogenous leukemia cells. Blood 109(8):3470–3478. doi:10.1182/blood-2006-02-005579

91. Altun M, Kramer HB, Willems LI, McDermott JL, Leach CA, Goldenberg SJ, Kumar KG, Konietzny R, Fischer R, Kogan E, Mackeen MM, McGouran J, Khoronenkova SV, Parsons JL, Dianov GL, Nicholson B, Kessler BM (2011) Activity-based chemical proteomics accelerates inhibitor development for deubiquitylating enzymes. Chem Biol 18(11):1401–1412. doi:10.1016/j.chembiol.2011.08.018
92. Issaenko OA, Amerik AY (2012) Chalcone-based small-molecule inhibitors attenuate malignant phenotype via targeting deubiquitinating enzymes. Cell Cycle 11(9):1804–1817. doi:10.4161/cc.20174
93. Colland F, Formstecher E, Jacq X, Reverdy C, Planquette C, Conrath S, Trouplin V, Bianchi J, Aushev VN, Camonis J, Calabrese A, Borg-Capra C, Sippl W, Collura V, Boissy G, Rain JC, Guedat P, Delansorne R, Daviet L (2009) Small-molecule inhibitor of USP7/HAUSP ubiquitin protease stabilizes and activates p53 in cells. Mol Cancer Ther 8(8):2286–2295. doi:10.1158/1535-7163.MCT-09-0097
94. Liu H, Li W, Ahmad M, Miller TM, Rose ME, Poloyac SM, Uechi G, Balasubramani M, Hickey RW, Graham SH (2011) Modification of ubiquitin-C-terminal hydrolase-L1 by cyclopentenone prostaglandins exacerbates hypoxic injury. Neurobiol Dis 41(2):318–328. doi:10.1016/j.nbd.2010.09.020
95. Li Z, Melandri F, Berdo I, Jansen M, Hunter L, Wright S, Valbrun D, Figueiredo-Pereira ME (2004) Delta12-Prostaglandin J2 inhibits the ubiquitin hydrolase UCH-L1 and elicits ubiquitin-protein aggregation without proteasome inhibition. Biochem Biophys Res Commun 319(4):1171–1180. doi:10.1016/j.bbrc.2004.05.098
96. Ratia K, Pegan S, Takayama J, Sleeman K, Coughlin M, Baliji S, Chaudhuri R, Fu W, Prabhakar BS, Johnson ME, Baker SC, Ghosh AK, Mesecar AD (2008) A noncovalent class of papain-like protease/deubiquitinase inhibitors blocks SARS virus replication. Proc Natl Acad Sci U S A 105(42):16119–16124. doi:10.1073/pnas.0805240105

Index

Q.P. Dou (ed.), *Resistance to Proteasome Inhibitors in Cancer*, Resistance to Targeted Anti-Cancer Therapeutics, DOI 10.1007/978-3-319-06752-0

Printed by Printforce, the Netherlands